DIETETICS

DIETETICS

NINTH
Multi Colour
EDITION

B Srilakshmi
M.Sc., M.Ed., M.Phil.

NEW AGE
TECHNO
PRESS

An Imprint of

NEW AGE INTERNATIONAL (P) LIMITED, PUBLISHERS
LONDON • NEW DELHI
Bangalore • Chennai • Cochin • Guwahati • Hyderabad • Kolkata • Mumbai
Visit us at **www.newagepublishers.com**

Published by New Age International (P) Ltd., Publishers
First Edition: 1993
Ninth Multi Colour Edition: 2024
Reprint: 2026

GLOBAL OFFICES

- **New Delhi** — **NEW AGE INTERNATIONAL (P) LIMITED, PUBLISHERS**
  7/30 A, Daryaganj, New Delhi-110002, (INDIA), **Tel.:** (011) 23253472, 23253771, **Mob.:** 9315905300
  E-mail: contactus@newagepublishers.com • Visit us at www.newagepublishers.com

- **London** — **NEW AGE INTERNATIONAL (UK) LTD.**
  27 Old Gloucester Street, London, WC1N 3AX, UK
  E-mail: info@newacademicscience.co.uk • Visit us at www.newacademicscience.co.uk

BRANCHES

- **Bangalore** — 37/10, 8th Cross (Near Hanuman Temple), Azad Nagar, Chamarajpet, Bangalore- 560 018
  Tel.: (080) 26756823, **Mob.:** 9315905288, **E-mail: bangalore@newagepublishers.com**

- **Chennai** — 26, Damodaran Street, T. Nagar, Chennai-600 017, **Tel.:** (044) 24353401, **Mob.:** 9315905309
  E-mail: chennai@newagepublishers.com

- **Cochin** — CC-39/1016, Carrier Station Road, Ernakulam South, Cochin-682 016
  Tel.: (0484) 4051304, **Mob.:** 9315905289, **E-mail: cochin@newagepublishers.com**

- **Guwahati** — Hemsen Complex, Mohd. Shah Road, Paltan Bazar, Near Starline Hotel
  Guwahati-781 008, **Tel.:** (0361) 2513881, **Mob.:** 9315905296
  E-mail: guwahati@newagepublishers.com

- **Hyderabad** — 105, 1st Floor, Madhiray Kaveri Tower, 3-2-19, Azam Jahi Road, Near Kumar Theater
  Nimboliadda Kachiguda, Hyderabad-500 027, **Tel.:** (040) 24652456, **Mob.:** 9315905326
  E-mail: hyderabad@newagepublishers.com

- **Kolkata** — RDB Chambers (Formerly Lotus Cinema) 106A, 1st Floor, S N Banerjee Road
  Kolkata-700 014, **Tel.:** (033) 22273773, **Mob.:** 9315905319, **E-mail: kolkata@newagepublishers.com**

- **Mumbai** — 142C, Victor House, Ground Floor, N.M. Joshi Marg, Lower Parel, Mumbai-400 013
  Tel.: (022) 24927869, 24915415, **Mob.:** 9315905282, **E-mail: mumbai@newagepublishers.com**

- **New Delhi** — 22, Golden House, Daryaganj, New Delhi-110 002, **Tel.:** (011) 23262368, 23262370
  Mob.: 9315905300, **E-mail: sales@newagepublishers.com**

C-25-07-14973

Printed in India at Ajit Printers, Delhi.
Typeset at In-house, Delhi.

NEW AGE INTERNATIONAL (P) LIMITED, PUBLISHERS
7/30 A, Daryaganj, New Delhi - 110002
Visit us at **www.newagepublishers.com**
(CIN: U74899DL1966PTC004618)

Dedicated

To
'Amma'

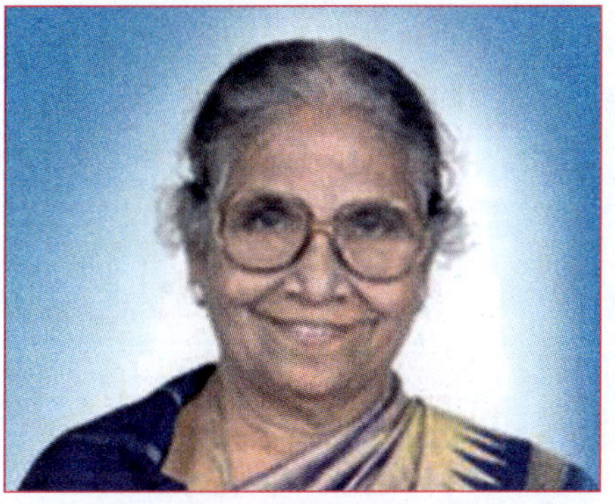

(Late) Dr. Rajammal P. Devadas
Chancellor, Avinashilingam
Deemed University, Coimbatore

"who is a source of inspiration"

Foreword

Food and nutrition are important for human beings during health and disease. Nutrition and dietetics are basic to all developmental programmes. A knowledge of diet is essential for teachers, health professionals, administrators and students of health science. Written by Mrs. B. Srilakshmi, Lecturer, Anna Adarsh College for Women, Chennai, this book explains the dietetic care needed during the different periods and stages of life and the specific diet therapy for several disease conditions. With a variety of diets, illustrations and tables in appropriate chapters, the book has been written well. The book also displays a knowledge of physiology, biochemistry, pathology and clinical medicine as related to nutrition.

'Dietetics' will be a valuable guide and reference for physicians, other medical professionals, teachers, students nurses, practicing dietitians and health workers.

This book fills a timely need.

LATE RAJAMMAL P. DEVADAS

Preface to the Ninth Edition

Diet and health are two sides of the same coin. They are inseparable. Dietetics is like all disciplines an ever expanding and consequently evolving field. Textbooks on Nutrition focus mainly on the theoretical aspects of clinical nutrition and there is a growing need for comprehensive source of up to date and essentially practical information. "**Dietetics**" aims precisely to do that.

This edition gives normal nutrition with the revised Recommended Dietary Allowances - 2020 suggested by ICMR. This edition also emphasises new developments in the field of therapeutic nutrition.

The new frontiers of research include functional foods, glycemic index, importance of vegan diets and diet in mental illness. All these are given due importance in this edition. As more and more people are working in shifts, dietary modifications are also suggested for them.

To understand therapeutic diets the student need to know certain aspects in detail like dietary supplements, diet in inflammation and prebiotics and probiotics, gut microbiome which are all discussed in detail.

This book is intended to be a textbook for undergraduates and postgraduates specialising in Nutrition and Dietetics. This book is valuable as a reference book for medical and paramedical students. Practicing dietitians would find this book a ready reckoner. For the common man this book can be a source of authentic information.

Globalisation has affected society and changed the food habits and lifestyle of people. Media is constantly pouring information on food and diet. In this context there is a need for the dietetian to equip with scientific information. This book satisfies this need.

I strongly believe that knowledge is seamless and a textbook cannot provide all the details. The students are expected make an effort to learn 'beyond' the textbook.

B. Srilakshmi

Acknowledgements

In compiling this book, I have extensively referred and presented information from a vast number of standard books, journals, proceedings of seminars and conferences and workshop manuals. Various ICMR and American Dietetic Association publications have been used in this edition. I tried to present source of information at the appropriate location.

I express my deep sense of indebtedness to all these scientists and publishers.

Students, past and present, have contributed to a great extent in the conception, formation and development of this book. The discussions with dietitians of different hospitals have helped me to understand the present scenario and to structure this book. I am thankful to all these dietitians. No doubt, encouragement of students constantly has inspired me to bring new editions.

I am thankful to my daughter, Dr. Swathi, for sending books and scientific journals related to Diet from the USA. She is also helpful in clarifying my doubts related to clinical nutrition. I am also thankful to my daughter, Ms. Kranthi and to my sons-in-law for their constant encouragement in this endeavour.

I am indebted to Mr. Saumya Gupta for bringing out the ninth edition of this book. I am also grateful to the production department of 'New Age International (P) Ltd' for their cooperation.

Above all, I am grateful to God Almighty for blessing me with good physical and mental health while carrying out this task.

B. Srilakshmi

Contents

1

Menu Planning

Diet has a powerful yet complex effect on health. Dietetics is a science that deals with the adequacy of diets during normal life cycle and modifications required during diseased conditions. According to American Dietetic Association 'Dietetics is the integration and application of principles derived from the science of nutrition, biochemistry, physiology, food management and behavioral and social sciences to achieve and maintain people's health'.

Menu planning is the process of planning and scheduling intake of meals for general or specific individual requirements.

The following terms and concepts are widely used and a clear understanding of these terms makes menu planning efficient.

EXPLANATION OF TERMS

Health is defined by the World Health Organisation as the "state of complete physical, mental and social well-being and not merely the absence of disease and infirmity."

The essential requisites (or dimensions) of "health" would include the following:

- Achievement of optimal growth and development, reflecting the full expression of one's genetic potential.
- Maintenance of the structural integrity and functional efficiency of body tissues necessary for an active and productive life.
- Mental well-being.
- Ability to withstand the inevitable process of ageing with minimal disability and functional impairment, and
- Ability to combat disease, such as
  - (*a*) resistance to infections (immunocompetence)
  - (*b*) preventing the onset and retarding the progress of degenerative diseases such as cancer and
  - (*c*) resistance to effect of environmental toxins and pollutants.

Nutrient requirement can be defined as the minimum amount of the absorbed nutrient that is necessary for maintaining the normal physiological functions of the body.

Dietary standards: Recommended Dietary Allowances, Recommended Nutrient Intakes, Recommended Daily Amounts of Nutrients, or Safe Intakes of Nutrients—are the average daily amounts of essential nutrients estimated, on the basis of available scientific knowledge, to be sufficiently high to meet the physiological needs of practically all healthy persons in a group with specified characteristics.

Dietary Reference Intake (DRI) values are replacing the traditional Recommended Dietary Allowances. This nutrient reference provides four sources of information:

- ***Recommended Dietary Allowance (RDA):*** The average daily dietary nutrient intake level sufficient to meet the nutrient requirement of nearly all (97 to 98 per cent) healthy individuals in a particular life stage and gender group.
- ***Adequate Intake:*** A recommended average daily intake level based on observed or experimentally determined approximations or estimates of nutrient intake by a group (or groups) of apparently healthy people, that are assumed to be adequate—used when an RDA cannot be determined. In the Indian context, this is referred to as acceptable intake.
- ***Tolerable Upper Intake Level (UL):*** The highest average daily nutrient intake level that is likely to pose no risk of adverse health effects for almost all individuals in the general population. As intake increases above the UL, the potential risk of adverse effects increases.
- ***Estimated Average Requirement (EAR):*** The average daily nutrient intake level estimated to meet the requirement of half of the healthy individuals in a particular life stage and gender group. It is primarily used to evaluate population groups.

Phytochemicals: These are of plant origin like terpenes, phytosterols, flavonoids, theols and allylic sulphides which are antimutagenic, anticarcinogenic or have antioxidant properties.

Nutraceuticals: They combine 'nutrition' and 'pharmaceuticals' to mean that food or parts of food or food extracts can be used as preventive drugs or food supplements.

Dietary/food supplements: These are concentrated sources of nutrients or other substances with a nutritional or physiological effect whose purpose is to supplement the normal diet.

Nutritional Genomics: Nutritional genomics encompasses both nutrigenetics, the influence of genetic variation on nutrient utilisation/metabolism, food tolerances and nutrient requirements; and nutrigenomics, the modulatory role of nutrients and genome evolution, mutation rate, in-utero programming and expression. Nutritional genomics offers insight into ways to tailor the diets of individuals and populations more closely to genetic abilities, to gain the health benefits inherent in this approach. This discipline holds significance for the dietetics profession.

Index of Nutritional Quality: It is a method of quantitative and qualitative analysis of single foods, meals and diets which as special significance in assessing clinical nutritional problems.

The INQ is a ratio of the nutrient to calorie content of foods which may be calculated by computer and printed as bar graphs and tabular data. The number of nutrients and the nutrient standards used for analysis are flexible parameters which may be varied for each clinical situation for example INQ analysis of simple foods, an institutional house diet, the diabetic exchange list and the diagnostic evaluation of the dietary intake of a hospitalised patient.

Orthorexia nervosa: It is characterized by obsessive thoughts about food, self-punishment with fasts or over exercise, restrictive eating behaviours and a belief that one's self esteem is based on dietary choices.

Healthy Eating Index: It is a measure to assess how well a diet conforms to the recommendations of the dietary guidelines.

Diet quality: It aims to describe overall diet and its effect on human health rather than focussing on associations with specific nutrients. This multidimensional concept includes adequate amounts and diversity of healthy foods, limited intakes of unhealthy foods and over all balance of macro and micro nutrients.

Allostatic load: The concept of cumulative biological risk from chronic stressful exposure, may provide a framework with which to examine the links between diet, physiological stress and disease.

DETERMINANTS OF FOOD CHOICE

Food choice is affected by many factors like biological, economic, physical, social, psychological and attitudes, beliefs in addition to stage of life.

Biological Determinants

Hunger and Satiety: The central nervous system is involved in controlling the balance between hunger, appetite stimulation and food intake. The macro nutrients, carbohydrates, proteins and fats generate satiety signals of varying strength. An important satiety signal may be the volume of food or portion size consumed.

Palatability: There is an increase in food intake as palatability increases. Increasing food variety can also increase food and energy intake. Food is not solely regarded as a source of nourishment but is often consumed for the pleasure value it imparts.

Economic and Physical Determinants

Cost and accessibility: Cost of food is a primary determinant of food choice. Low income groups have a greater tendency to consume foods from few food groups and have low intake of fruit and vegetables. Accessibility to shops is another important physical factor influencing food choice. Tribals who live in remote areas have poor access to shops – even ration shops and food choice is limited.

Education and knowledge: Studies indicate that the level of education can influence dietary behaviour during adulthood. Nutrition knowledge is gained by public through various media, reading food package and of course through health professionals.

Social Determinants of Food Choice

Cultural influences: Cultural influences lead to differences in the habitual consumption of certain foods and in traditions of preparations. It can lead to restrictions such as exclusion of meat or milk or some vegetables from the diet.

Social context: Social influences on food intake refer to the impact that one or more persons have on the eating behaviour of others. Social support can have a beneficial effect on food choice and healthful dietary change. Shaping of food choices takes place in the home. Family and friends influence food choice. There are clear differences in social classes with regard to food and nutrient intakes.

Societal trends, the media and peer pressure also influence on food intake.

It is often considered rude, to refuse food or drink being shared by a group or offered by a host. Often one becomes accepted as a member of a social gathering only if one accepts the food served.

Values: People's values, environmental ethics, religious beliefs, and political views also influence their food choices. By choosing to eat some foods or avoid others, people make statements about themselves that reflect their values. For example, people may select only foods that come in containers that can be reused or recycled. People are also influenced by the advice of religious heads in making food choice.

Social setting: Although the majority of food is eaten in the home, people also eat outside home like in schools, colleges, at work and in restaurants. The availability of health food at home and 'away from home' increases the consumption of such foods.

Meal patterns: People follow different meal patterns. Some have three meals and some have five meals. Some snack more frequently. Some have early meals and some have late meals.

Psychological Factors

Stress: The influence of stress on food choice is complex. The mechanisms for stress induced changes in eating and food choice are motivation differences (reduced concern about weight control) and physiological (reduced appetite) associated with stress. If work stress is prolonged or frequent, then adverse dietary changes could result.

Mood: Food influences mood and mood has a strong influence over choice of food. Attempts to restrict intake of certain foods can increase the desire for these particular foods. Depressed mood appears to influence the cravings.

Image: The fashion and movie industries, not the medical community, have defined what people believe to be the ideal body—sometimes an excessively thin body for women, or an excessively muscular body for men. Both men and women seek "beautiful bodies," and in doing so, they select or avoid foods that they believe will improve or impair their physical appearance. Such intentions are rational when based on sound nutrition and fitness knowledge, but when based on faddism or carried to extremes, they undermine good health.

Eating disorders: Food choice is affected if an individual suffers from eating disorders like anorexia nervosa or bulimia. The aetiology of eating disorders is usually a combination of factors including biological, psychological, familial and socio-cultural.

Consumer Attitudes, Beliefs, Knowledge and Optimistic Bias

Consumer attitudes and beliefs: Attitudes and beliefs can change food choice. Attitude to dietary fat has changed in the last 50 years with a corresponding decrease in the absolute amount of fat eaten.

Optimistic bias: If people believe that their diets are already healthy, they are not inclined to alter their diets. Thus a perceived need to undertake change is a fundamental requirement for initiating dietary change.

Dietary change is not easy because it requires alterations in habits that have been built up over a life time. Athlete's strong desire to exceed in sports can act as a strong motivational factor and the food choices can be appropriate. A pregnant mother changes her food habits for better as she is strongly motivated to get healthy baby.

Medical Conditions

Sometimes medical conditions and the medications used to treat the conditions limit which foods a person can select. Ageing and exposure to medications and chronic diseases can modify the oral sensation and food acceptance.

Food choices are personal and not always sensible and to a great extent they resist change.

Before undertaking diet planning, the planner must understand the dynamics of food choices, because people will alter their eating habits only if their preferences are honoured.

FUNCTIONAL FOODS

Functional food can be regarded as functional if it is satisfactorily demonstrated to affect beneficially one or more target functions of the body, beyond adequate nutritional effects. Functional foods must remain as foods and they must demonstrate their effects in amounts that can normally be expected to be consumed in the diet. They are not pills or capsules but part of a normal food pattern.

Functional food has a positive effect on a person's health, physical performance or state of mind. Food also acts like an antioxidant, detoxifying agent, blocking or suppressing agent. Food rich in fibre helps in excreting harmful substances. Probiotics help in maintaining intestinal bacterial balance. Food, not the nutrient, plays an important role in the prevention of disease and in promoting health.

Functional foods should be included in balanced diets of all age groups.

Antioxidant Effect

The normal functioning of cells is dependent on a proper balance of prooxidants and antioxidants. The former promote the release of oxygen to provide the energy needed for cell functioning. In this process, different biochemical reactions take place, which continuously produce various free radicals. Antioxidants help to neutralise and counteract the deleterious free radicals but the natural mechanisms may prove to be inadequate, especially in poor environments. In addition to free radicals generated as part of the natural metabolic process, the body also has to deal with free radical species derived from environmental contaminants such as smoke, carcinogenic chemicals derived from food additives and industrial effluent and radiation.

Free radicals promote lipid peroxidation of membrane lipids, impairing cell function, they could damage cellular proteins and DNA. They could cause peroxidation of circulating lipoprotein lipids thus converting them into more deleterious form. Cumulative tissue injury thus caused by free radicals is now known to underlie the pathogenesis of such diverse conditions as cancer, atherosclerosis and heart diseases, radiation damage and accelerated ageing.

The natural antioxidants are easily absorbable in human system.

Dietary components identified as antioxidants are β-carotene, vitamins C and E, niacin, riboflavin, sulphur containing amino acids. They provide the reducing thiol groups for proteins and glutathione, GSH, and have positive antioxidant properties. Phytochemicals with antioxidant properties are mostly phenolic acids and flavonoids occurring in living cells as glycosides. Examples include flavones, isoflavones, flavanones, chalcone, coumarins and cinnamic acid. Naturally occurring isoflavones are found mainly in the leguminosae family.

Dietary antioxidants can be nutrients or non-nutrients as shown in Table 1.1.

Table 1.1 Dietary antioxidants

Nutrients	*Non-nutrients*
β-carotene-Provitamin A	Carotenoids (Lycopene, Xanthophylls)
Ascorbic acid-Vitamin C	Lutein, α- and γ-carotenes
Tocopherols	(cryptoxanthine, zeaxanthine)
Tocotrienols	Flavonoids (quercetin, myricetin,
Riboflavin	quercetagatin, gossypetin)
Sulphur containing amino acids : Cysteine	Isoflavones
and methionine	Anthocyanins
Selenium	Phenolic compounds (catechin) indoles

Some of the foods which are considered as rich sources of antioxidant phytochemicals are garlic, onion, ginger, oats, sweet potato, soybean, tea, oilseeds, herbs and spices. Black pepper, clove, oregano, rosemary, thyme and turmeric have been shown to possess antioxidant activity.

Table 1.2 Sources of nutrient antioxidants

Nutrient	*Sources*
β-Carotene	Green leafy vegetables, ripe yellow fruits and vegetables like papaya, musk melon, mango, pumpkin, carrots.
Vitamin C	Citrus fruits like orange, lemon, sweet lime; guava, goose berry, sprouted pulses.
Vitamin E	Cereals, cereal products, oil seeds, nuts.
Selenium, Zinc	Meat, sea foods and cereals.
Copper	Oysters, liver, mushroom, nuts, chocolate.
Iron	Meat, liver, green leafy vegetables, cereals, millets, pulses.

Cereals: Whole grains contain phenolic compounds such as ferulic, caffeic acid and phytic acid. Phenolic content contributes to antioxidant activity. Ragi and wheat semolina contain more amount of phenolic content compared to other cereals (NIN). According to studies conducted at NIN domestic processing of wheat like boiling, deep frying, sprouting and malting significantly increase phenolic content.

Selenium a trace element, plays an important role in cellular function as it forms the integral part of an important antioxidant enzyme, glutathione peroxidase (Se – GSH – Px) which protects the body against the oxidative tissue damage. Among cereals, selenium content is more in jowar and bajra. Rice is not rich in selenium compared to other cereals. Polishing rice reduces γ-oryzanol and polyphenol content. Oats contain phenols which have antioxidant property.

It was found that the process of baking bread produces a novel type of antioxidant, called pronyl-lysine that is eight times more abundant in the crust than in the crumb. Pronyl-lysine is formed by the reaction of protein bound amino acid L-lysine and starch as well as reducing sugars in the presence of heat. Maillard reaction produces flavour compounds and also antioxidants.

Pulses: Soya protein contains isoflavones like daidzein and genistein. Total isoflavone content increases in the sprouts of chick-pea seeds. These are compounds that act as antioxidants and protective agents against cancer and heart disease. Phytoestrogen found in soybean is a polyphenolic compound and has anticarcinogenic effect on the breast tissue and positive effects on the lipoprotein profile and bone density.

Rajmah, black gram dal and green gram contain good quantities of phenolic content. By boiling and pressure cooking total phenolic content increases in whole grams like green gram, black gram and bengal gram. Soaking and sprouting increases total phenolic content in green gram.

Table 1.3 Antioxidant activity of cereals, millets and pulses

Cereal/millets	*DPPH* Trolox equivalents mg/100 g*
Rice (milled)	123
Rice parboiled (milled)	75
Wheat flour (whole)	24
Jowar	127
Rice puffed	49
Bajra	126
Finger millet (Ragi)	173
Semolina	27
Maize	139
Red gram dal	61
Green gram dal	30
Black gram dal	27
Bengal gram dal	49
Lentil	44
Green gram whole	86
Bengal gram dal roasted	26
Bengal gram whole	53
Peas green	88
Soybean	97
Rajmah	107

*2,2′-Diphenyl-1-picryl hydrazyl (DPPH) radical scavenging activity.

Source: Annual report, 2006-07, National Institute of Nutrition, Hyderabad.

Pulses like red gram (203 ng/g) and bengal gram (180 ng/g) are rich source of selenium. Green gram contains 98 ng/g of selenium.

Vegetables and fruits: Plants produce vitamins like vitamin C, β-carotene and tocopherols. These chemicals are known as high value, low volume chemicals. The secondary plant metabolites other than vitamins are referred to as nutraceuticals. Most of these compounds are flavonoids of polyphenols which are also known to inhibit free radicals generated in the cellular system when they are obtained through the diet.

Green leafy vegetables are exceptionally rich source of β-carotene, the nature's most potent antioxidant that can inhibit atherosclerosis and prevent heart disease. Studies conducted at NIN 2013-2014, showed that curry leaves which are rich in polyphenolic content have potential benefit for the prevention and treatment of breast cancer.

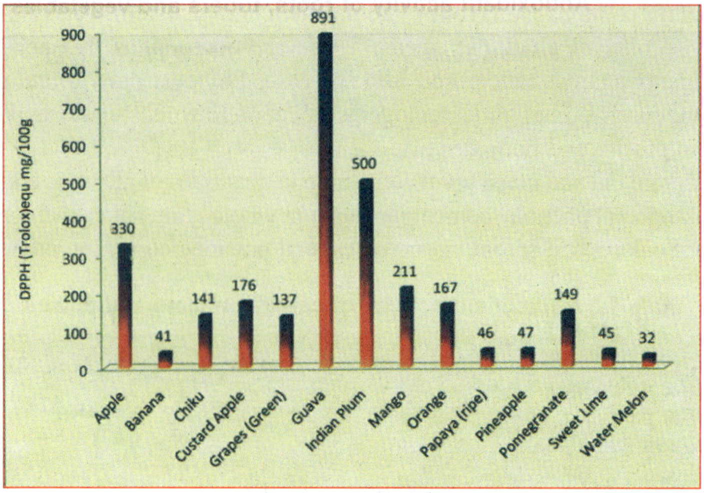

Fig. 1.1 Antioxidant activity of fruits

Source: Sreeramulu, D., *et al.*, Antioxidant activity and phenolic content of fruits, roots, tubers, nuts and vegetables commonly consumed in India, Nutrition News. NIN 2010, 31.

Polyphenolic content of spinach is significantly increased during pressure cooking (NIN, 2005). Lutein carotenoid is found in green leafy vegetables. Evidence suggests that eating foods high in lutein may prevent/slow macular degeneration, a leading cause of blindness in the elderly. As an antioxidant, it may also prevent formation of cataracts, reduce the risk of heart disease and protect against breast cancer.

Guava and amla, are rich in antioxidants due to their vitamin C content. Red grapes and pomegranates contribute to antioxidants due to the presence of anthocyanins. Strawberries, raspberries and black berries contain polyphenols. An apple a day (110 g/day) prevents heart attack by providing flavonoids. Apples contain polyphenols. Banana is poor in antioxidants.

Flavonoids are found in a wide variety of fruits and vegetables. They act as antioxidants. Resveratrol, anthocyanins, quercetin, hesperidin, tangerin, myricetin, kaempferol and apigenin are some flavonoids. They act as anticarcinogen, antiallergen, antiinflammatory and reduce the risk of heart diseases, cancer and urinary tract infection. They are found in apples, pears, cherries, grapes, citrus fruits, onion, broccoli and lettuce.

Terpenes are found in citrus fruits, carrots, parsley, broccoli, cabbage, cucumber and mint.

Dry fruits, oil seeds and nuts: The antioxidant present in walnuts is melatonin which is readily absorbed. Walnuts have the highest antioxidant activity followed by brown raisins. The phytochemicals in nuts include ellagic acid, flavonoid phenolic compounds, luteolin (a major antioxidant) and tocopherols. Dry fruits are rich in antioxidant activity. Phenolic compounds appear to be significant contributors to their antioxidant activity. Consumption of dry fruits may therefore augment the antioxidant status and protect against chronic diseases.

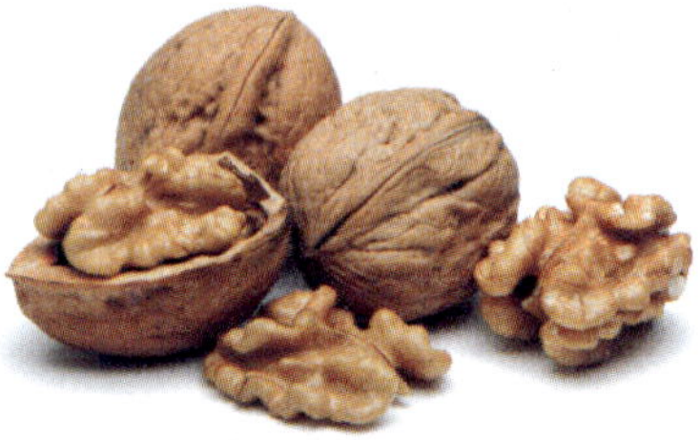

Fig. 1.2 Consumption of seven whole walnuts per day can give health benefits.

Table 1.4 **Antioxidant activity of roots, tubers and vegetables**

Common Name	*DPPH (Trolox equ) mg/100 g*
Roots and Tubers	
Beetroot	125
Carrot	11
Colacasia	71
Onions big	23
Spring onions	12
Potato	16
Radish	29
Sweet potato	25
Tapioca	51
Yam	74
Vegetables	
Beans	83
Bitter gourd	18
Bottle gourd	36
Broad beans	333
Brinjal	150
Cabbage (green)	78
Cabbage (red)	405
Capsicum	96
Cauliflower	66
Cluster beans	102
Cucumber	63
Drumstick	52
Kovai	78
Lady's finger	466
Mango raw (green)	276
Plantain green	34
Pumpkin	38
Ridge gourd	12
Snake gourd	38

Source: Sreeramulu, D, *et al.*, Antioxidant activity and phenolic content of fruits, roots, tubers, nuts and vegetables commonly consumed in India, Nutrition News, NIN 2010, 31.

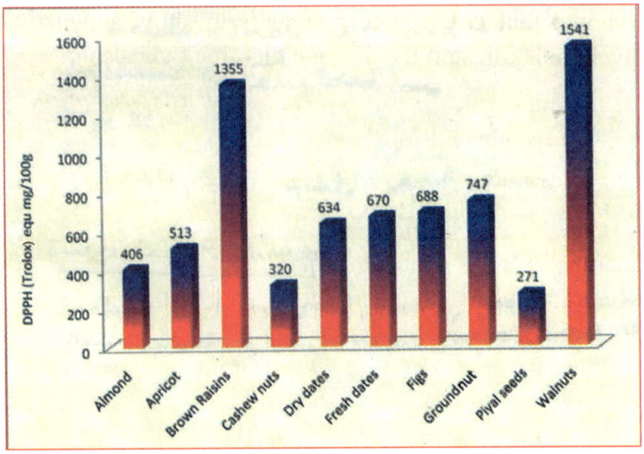

Fig. 1.3 **Antioxidant activity of dry fruits and nuts (Dry weight basis)**

Source: Sreeramulu, D, *et al.*, 2010, Antioxidant activity and phenolic content of fruits, roots, tubers, nuts and vegetables commonly consumed in India, Nutrition News, NIN, 31.

Spices: Saffron and annoto contain carotenoids which are effective antioxidants. Observations in animal studies show that ginger has the ability to stimulate protective enzymes involved in xenobiotic metabolism. Stimulation of quinone reductase activity suggests that ginger can counteract the oxidative damage in tissues of liver and lungs.

Curcumin, a diferuloyl methane, present in turmeric, reduces the mutagenicity in a smoker and promotes mechanisms for detoxification and production of GSH. It is also antiinflammatory. The antioxidant properties of curcumin are attributed to its ability to inhibit lipid peroxidation and scavenging capacity of superoxide anion and hydroxyl radicals. Turmeric provides a viable food base as well as a pharmacological approach in the treatment of diabetic complications like cataract (NIN). The amount of turmeric required appears to be well within cultural norms and safety limits.

Eugenol, 4-allyl-2-methoxyphenol, active principle of clove oil has antioxidant properties.

The selenium content of coriander seeds (136 ng/g) and mustard (128 ng/g) contributes to their antioxidant activity.

The components of garam masala like cloves, cinnamon, bay leaves, star anise have high antioxidant property. Poppy seeds have lowest amount of antioxidant activity.

Population surveys indicate that consumption of spices in general ranges between 10 and 30 g. This amount is enough to protect the body profoundly against cancer and other diseases.

Tea and Coffee: Tea has been shown to contain several polyphenolic compounds and their derivatives which are reported to possess antioxidant activity. Polyphenols like chlorogenic acid present in coffee beans and tea leaves are antioxidants. Flavonoids like catachins and quercetin are found to have antioxidant properties. Tea derived from the plant *camellia sinensis* contains polyphenols in the form of flavonoids and its sub group flavonols, which gives tea its antioxidant properties.

NIN studies indicated that flavonoids in green and black tea have stronger antioxidant activity than standard antioxidant vitamins.

A cup of tea supplies around 200 mg of flavonoids. The antioxidant potency in a cup of tea is 400 per cent greater than a cup of orange juice. Black tea contains other polyphenols such as thearubigins and theaflavins which are very powerful.

Studies have shown that colon cancer appears to show a negative association with tea consumption. Polyphenols can stop the damage that free radicals do to cells, neutralise enzymes essential for tumour growth and deactivate cancer promoters. Catechin in tea play an important role in limiting oxidation of LDL through the radical scavenging activity. Higher the flavonoid intake lower is the risk of death from coronary heart disease. Men who drink more than four cups of tea a day (about 500 ml) are benefited most.

Seeds and Oils: Oilseeds like mustard and rapeseed contain phenolic compounds. Canola and mustard flour as such or their extracts possess strong antioxidant activity. The oil from sesame seeds has a superior oxidative stability when compared with other vegetable oils. Rice bran oil contains a high amount of unsaponifiable components such as tocotrienols and oryzanol. These possess antioxidant activity. Palm oil is a rich source of tocopherols and tocotrienols. The remarkable stability of sesame oil is attributed to its inherent lignans (sesamol, sesamin and sesamolin) present in its non-glyceride fraction. Sesame lignans have antioxidant properties. Blends of sesame oil with other oils may increase the antioxidant potential of oils. Sesame seeds in snacks or pickles help in fortification of foods.

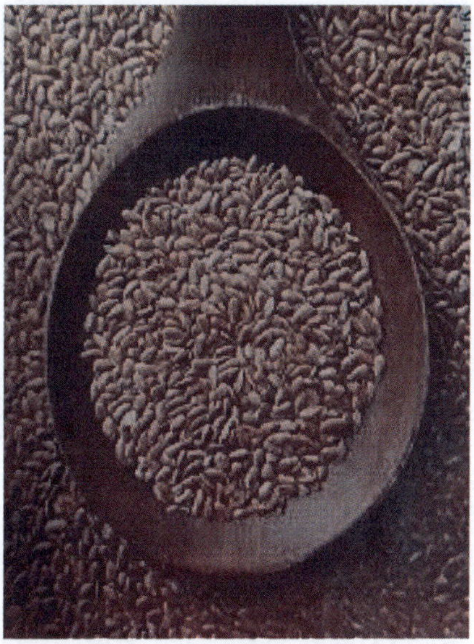

Fig. 1.4 Flax seeds are effective in powder form. It should be consumed two table spoons per day to get the health value

Flax seeds contain ω-3 fatty acids that benefit cardiovascular and immune system. Antioxidants and phytoestrogens such as lignans, phenolic acids, phytic acids and flavonoids present in flax seeds have protective roles in preventing cancer, diabetes and heart disease. Flax seeds contain both soluble and insoluble fibre and benefit both gastro intestinal and cardiovascular systems.

Whey Proteins: Whey proteins have been shown to stimulate cell mediated and humoral immunity in stressed individuals. Whey proteins have an antioxidant role by increasing tissue glutathione and inhibiting the growth of several types of tumours. Water soluble antioxidant components are present in a low molecular weight ultrafiltration permeate obtained from milk or whey.

Red wine: Crushing the grapes and allowing the skins, seeds and stems to ferment together with the pulp and juice creates a mixture rich in antioxidant compounds. Grape seeds in particular contain large amounts of flavonoid substances known as proanthocyanidins. In red wine, flavonols form part of a wider group of antioxidant chemicals called polyphenols. Resveratrol present in red wine may delay the ageing process. Grape seeds and grape skins used in wineries showed a significant decrease in total cholesterol and LDL in subjects having high cholesterol.

Jaggery: Jaggery is a good antioxidant due to the high content of phenol. (NIN-2009-10)

The natural antioxidants are easily absorbable in human system and protect from oxidative stress and associated diseases of humans and therefore, play an important role in health care. Plant foods are the primary source of natural antioxidants. Fruits, vegetables, roots and tubers are important dietary sources of antioxidant polyphenols to humans.

Detoxifying Effect

Detoxification is achieved in the body through two phase mechanism. In the phase-I the reactions are mediated through the Microsomal Mixed Function Oxidase System (MFO). In the phase-II, set of key enzymes render toxins more readily excretable. Limonene present in citrus fruit peel protects against cancer by inducing the glutathione transferase group of phase II enzymes which conjugate various carcinogens and xenobiotics prior to excretion.

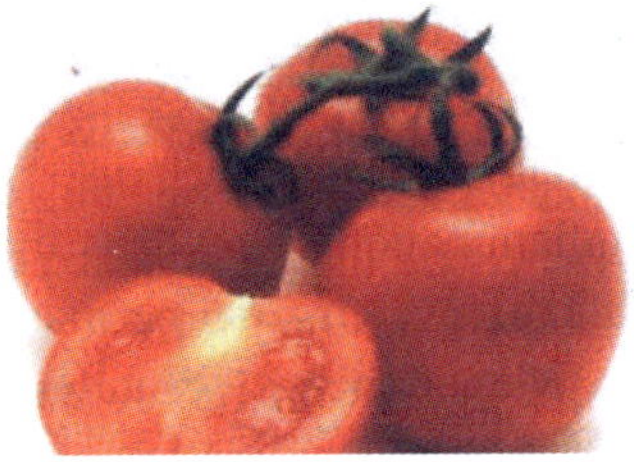

Fig. 1.5 Tomatoes have detoxifying effect.

Foods which contain such detoxifying chemicals are cabbage, tomatoes, strawberries, pineapples, green peppers and green and black tea.

Theols are a major sulphur containing class of phytonutrients. The food sources having theolic nutraceutical properties include garlic, onions, mustard and other cruciferous vegetables like cabbage and turnip. Important subclasses under theols are glucosinolates, allelic sulphides, indoles, isoprenoids and tocopherols. Cruciferous vegetables form rich sources of glucosinolates. They activate liver detoxification enzymes and can reduce the incidence of tumours.

Blocking/Suppressing Effect

There are other chemicals in foods which act by sequestering and preventing potential toxic agents and carcinogens from reaching the target tissues or by suppressing their action. Garlic for example, is known to contain allelic sulphides which not only induce phase-II enzymes, but also inactivate carcinogens.

Allelic sulphides are potent antimutagenic and anticarcinogenic agents. They protect against tumours and give cardiovascular protection. They can block the activity of toxins produced by bacteria and viruses, thereby building immunity against diseases.

Phytosterols form major class of phytonutrients, which are present in all plants. However, the rich sources having nutraceutical functions include yellow vegetables, seeds of pumpkins and yams. This phytochemical competes with dietary cholesterol for uptake in the intestine thereby blocking cholesterol absorption into the body. It facilitates the excretion of cholesterol from the body. It can also prevent the development of tumour in breast and prostate glands.

Flavonoids are phytochemicals that enhance the effectiveness of vitamin C. They can also act against allergies, ulcers, tumours and platelet aggregation. They are effective in controlling high blood pressure and can reduce the risk of oestrogen induced cancer.

Isoflavones can prevent tumour growth. Beans and other legumes are rich sources with nutraceutical properties. Important isoflavones, genistein and daidzein found in soybeans have nutraceutical properties against tumour growth. People who consume soya food rarely experience breast, uterus and prostate cancer.

Anti-inflammatory Effect

ω-3 fatty acid rich foods like fatty fish increase the cell membrane content of both eicosapentaenoic acid, EPA and docosahexaenoic acid, DHA, which increase the production of anti-inflammatory group, eicosanoid. ω-3 fatty acids decrease the production of interleukin-1 and tumour necrosis factor, TNF, by down regulating inflammatory response. Fish oil supplementation in patients with inflammatory diseases such as rheumatoid arthritis and inflammatory bowel disorders result in significant improvements. ω-3 fatty acids reduce inflammation of mucous membrane of the uterus and reduce abdominal pain before, during and after menstrual periods.

Monoterpenes, sesquiterpenes and gingerols present in ginger have anti-inflammatory action by exerting modulation of eicosanoid synthesis. Thus ginger has ameliorate symptoms of pain and swelling in musculo skeletal disorders. Cinnamon has anti-inflammatory activity.

Hypocholesteraemic Effect

Soya protein reduces the plasma cholesterol concentration due to the presence of isoflavones, genistein and daidzein. Garlic also reduces plasma LDL cholesterol and triglyceride concentration. Yogurt and milk reduce cholesterol synthesis. High fibre diet also reduces cholesterol by enhancing the excretion of faecal steroids.

Presence of soluble dietary fibre increases the viscosity of the intestinal contents, decreases the peristaltic movements of the gut. Large molecular complexes from fatty acids, bile salts and cholesterol–miscelles cannot easily go through the molecular sieve formed by soluble non-starch polysaccharides thus slowing down the process of fat absorption. For example, pectin of apples and guavas and β-glucan of oats have hypocholesteraemic effect.

Hypoglycaemic Effect

The soluble dietary fibre fraction of fenugreek seeds is known for its hypoglycaemic effects in humans. Viscous fibres impair mixing of intestinal contents, and impair digestion due to limited access of the food to the enzymes. Hence, the hypoglycaemic effect of dietary fibre could be due to the delaying of starch hydrolysis and glucose absorption and also improvement in glucose utilisation and insulin sensitivity in target tissues.

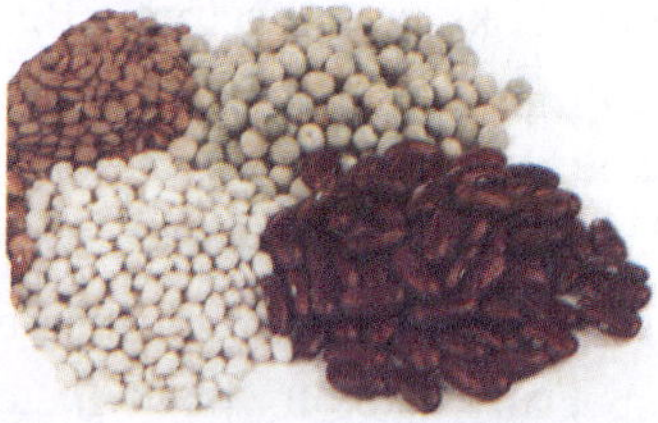

Fig. 1.6 Beans and whole grams have hypoglycaemic effect

Several dietary intervention studies have shown that increasing dietary intake of legumes, including beans, and whole grams affect positively blood glucose management and insulin sensitivity.

Antibacterial Effect

Probiotics, live microbial food supplements that beneficially affect the host by improving its intestinal microbial balance. Probiotics act on prebiotics which are nondigestible carbohydrates. Probiotics modify gut pH and antagonise the pathogens. The pathogens are suppressed by the production of antimicrobial compounds. Probiotics compete for pathogen binding and receptor sites as well as for available nutrients and growth factors. There is some preliminary evidence that probiotic bacteria may inhibit gastric colonisation and activity of *Helicobacter pylori.*

The antibacterial factors are found in the essential oils of spices. Two of the most germicidal spices are cinnamon and cloves. Cinnamon contains cinnamic aldehyde and cloves contain eugenol. Garlic has antibacterial properties against gram positive and gram negative bacteria.

Digestive and Related Effect

Spices in general stimulate salivation, acid secretion and digestive enzymes. Spices are used to reduce flatulence. Omum or ajwain is a household remedy for indigestion. Ajwain is valued for its antispasmodic and carminative effects. Aniseed or fennel seed and ginger are used to counteract flatulence. It is used in colic pain. Asafoetida has similar effect.

Chillies contain a substance called capsaicin which increases the gastric secretion. Capsaicin stimulates digestive system. Cloves have antiflatulent and antihelminthic properties. Fenugreek is used with butter milk in the treatment of dysentery.

Immunopotentiating Effect

Probiotics can enhance both specific and nonspecific immune response. These effects are believed to be mediated through activating macrophages, increasing levels of cytokines, natural killer cell activity and levels of immunoglobulins. The immune response may be further enhanced when one or more probiotics are consumed together and work synergistically, for example *lactobacillus* and *bifidobacteria*. Garlic exerts immunopotentiating effect by stimulating natural killer cell activity. Beet juice boosts man's immune building function.

Thus food has many functions other than providing nutrients.

Modified Functional Foods

Modified foods like fortified or enriched are functional foods *e.g.*, iodised salt. Medical foods specially made for phenylketonuria and foods made for infants are also functional foods.

FOOD GROUP SYSTEM

Food group system helps in planning balanced diets and to achieve nutrient intake specific to the individual.

Five Food Group System

The five food group system suggested by ICMR is given in Table 1.5.

Table 1.5 The five food groups and their major nutrients

Food group	*Main nutrients*
1. **Cereal grains and its products:** Rice, Wheat, Ragi, Bajra, Maize, Jowar, Barley, Rice flakes, wheat flour.	Energy, Protein, Invisible fat, Vitamin-B_1, Vitamin-B_2, Folic acid, Iron, Fibre.
2. **Pulses and Legumes:** Bengal gram, Black gram, Green gram, Red gram, Lentil (whole as well as dhals), Cowpea, Peas, Rajma, Soybean, Beans.	Energy Protein, Invisible fat, Vitamin-B_1, Vitamin-B_2, Folic acid, Calcium, Iron, Fibre.
3. **Milk and Meat Products:** Milk, Curd, Skimmed Milk, Cheese, Chicken, Liver, Fish, Egg, Meat.	Protein, Fat, Vitamin-B_2, Calcium.
4. **Fruits and Vegetables:** Fruits: Mango, Guava, Tomato, Papaya, Orange, Sweet lime, Water melon.	Carotenoids, Vitamin-C, Fibre, Invisible fat, Vitamin-B_2, Folic acid, Iron.
Vegetables (green leafy): Amaranth, Spinach, Gogu, Drumstick leaves, Coriander leaves, Fenugreek leaves.	Carotenoids, Vitamin-B_2, Folic acid, Calcium, Iron, Fibre.
Other Vegetables: Carrots, Brinjal, Lady's finger, Beans, Capsicum, Onion, Drumstick, Cauliflower.	Carotenoids, Folic acid, Calcium, Fibre.
5. **Fats and Sugar:** Fats: Butter, Ghee, Hydrogenated fat, Cooking oils like groundnut, Mustard, Coconut.	Energy, Fat, Essential fatty acids.
Sugar: Jaggery and sugar	Energy

Four Food Group System

The four food groups suggested by ICMR in 2011 are given in Table 1.6.

Table 1.6 Food groups suggested by ICMR (2011)

Food group	*Main nutrients*
1. **Cereals, Millets and Pulses:**	
Rice, Wheat, Ragi, Bajra, Maize, Jowar, Barley, Rice flakes, Wheat flour, Breakfast cereals.	Energy, Protein, Invisible fat, Vitamin-B_1, Vitamin-B_2 Folic acid, Iron, Fibre.
Pulses and Legumes: Bengal gram, Black gram, Green gram, Red gram, Lentil (whole as well as dhal), Cowpea, Peas, Rajmah, Soybean, Beans.	Energy, Protein, Invisible fat, Vitamin-B_1, Vitamin-B_2, Folic acid, Calcium, Iron, Fibre.
2. **Milk and Animal Products:**	
Milk, Curd, Skimmed Milk, Cheese, Chicken, Liver, Fish, Egg, Meat.	Protein, Fat, Vitamin-B_1, Vitamin-B_2, Calcium, Iron.
3. **Vegetables and Fruits:**	
Fruits: Mango, Guava, Tomato, Papaya, Orange, Sweet lime, Watermelon.	Carotenoids, Vitamin-C, Fibre, Invisible fat, Vitamin-B_2, Folic acid, Iron.
Green leafy vegetables: Amaranth, Spinach, Gogu, Drumstick leaves, Coriander leaves, Fenugreek leaves.	Carotenoids, Vitamin-B_2, Folic acid, Calcium, Iron, Fibre.
Other vegetables: Carrots, Brinjal, Lady's finger, Beans, Capsicum, Onion, Drumstick, Cauliflower.	Carotenoids, Folic acid, Calcium, Fibre.
4. **Oils, Fats and Nuts:**	
Fats: Butter, Ghee, Hydrogenated fat, Cooking oils like groundnut, mustard, sunflower.	Energy, Fat, Essential fatty acids.
Sugar: Jaggery and Cane sugar.	Energy
Almonds, walnuts and gingelly seeds.	Protein, ω-3 fatty acids.

The food group system can be used by health professionals for the following purposes:

- *Tool for nutritional assessment and screenings*: A brief dietary history system can disclose inadequacies of nutrient from any of the groups. The information can be the first clue that the subject may be at the risk of developing nutritional deficiency.
- *Tool for nutritional counselling*: The dietary history based on the four food group system allows a health team to counsel or teach a patient about nutrition.
- *Explaining therapeutic diets to the patient*: Therapeutic diets are scientifically based on nutrient composition and groups which can be used in menu planning.
- *Food labelling and surveillance system*: Food groups can be used for food labelling and for nutrition surveillance system.

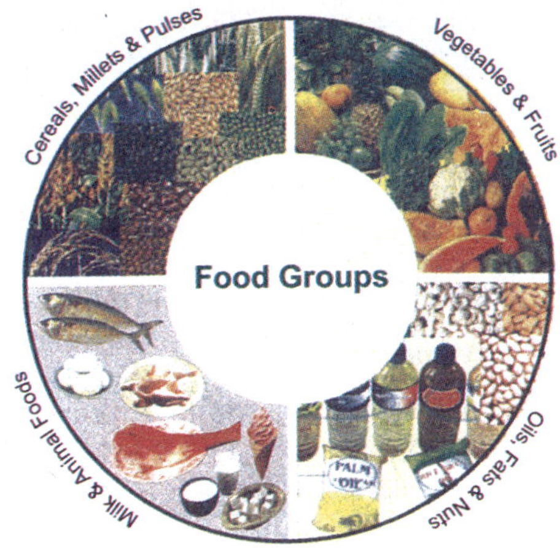

Fig. 1.7 **Food Groups suggested by ICMR (2011)**

Source: Dietary guidelines for Indians—A manual, 2011, NIN, Hyderabad.

THE FOOD GUIDE

Food Pyramid

Food Pyramid is suggested by ICMR. This is made based on the principles of balanced diet. This pyramid also suggests that one needs to do exercise regularly and abstain from drinking alcohol and taking tobacco.

General Dietary Guidelines suggested by ICMR

- Eat variety of foods to ensure a balanced diet.
- Ensure provision of extra food and healthcare to pregnant and lactating women.
- Promote exclusive breastfeeding for six months and encourage breast-feeding till two years or as long as one can.
- Feed home based semi solid foods to the infant after six months.
- Ensure adequate and appropriate diets for children and adolescents, both in health and sickness.

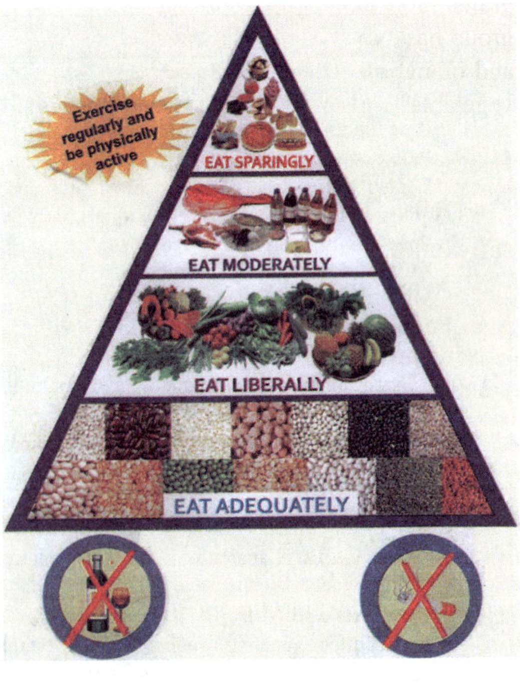

Fig. 1.8 **Food Pyramid**

- Eat plenty of vegetables and fruits.
- Ensure moderate use of edible oils and animal foods and very less use of *ghee/butter/ vanaspati*.
- Avoid overeating to prevent overweight and obesity.
- Exercise regularly and be physically active to maintain ideal body weight.
- Restrict salt intake to minimum.
- Ensure the use of safe and clean foods.
- Adopt right pre-cooking processes and appropriate cooking methods.
- Drink plenty of water and take beverages in moderation.
- Minimize the use of processed foods rich in salt, sugar and fats.
- Include micronutrient-rich foods in the diets of elderly people to enable them to be fit and active.

MyPlate

In 2011, the USDA with an assistance from first lady Michelle Obama, launched a new visual guide called MyPlate, which replaced Food Pyramid.

MyPlate is USDA's primary food group symbol, a food icon that serves as a powerful reminder to make healthy food choices and to build a healthy plate at mealtimes. It is a visual cue that identifies the five basic food groups from which consumers can choose healthy foods to build a healthy plate.

The plate is divided into four groups that is, fruits (20%), vegetables (30%), protein group (20%) and grains (30%) and a bowl of dairy product. Vegetable group has sub groups like dark green vegetables, red and orange vegetables fresh beans and peas, starchy vegetables and other vegetables.

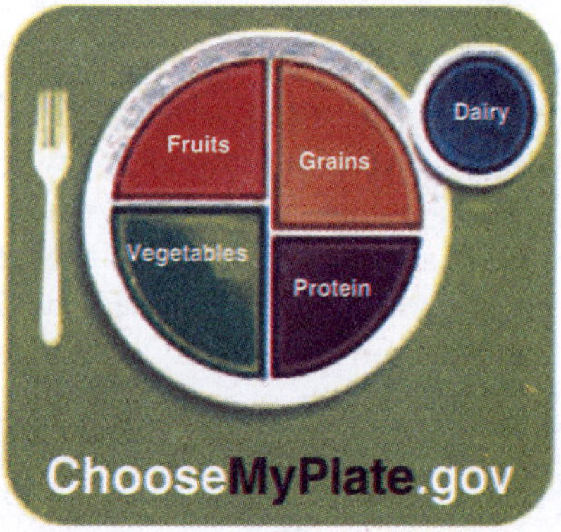

Fig. 1.9 The Food Guide—MyPlate
Source: USDA

Dietary Guidelines of MyPlate

- Balance calories
- Enjoy your food but eat less.
- Avoid over sized portions.
- Foods to eat more often are vegetables, fruits, whole grains and fat free or 1% milk and dairy products.
- Compare sodium in foods.
- Make half your grains whole grains.
- Foods to eat less often are solid fats, added sugars and salt.
- Drink water instead of sugary drinks.

Every family has unique needs and MyPlate helps to discover a personalized healthy eating style that works within their lifestyle.

My Healthy Plate

Figure 1.10 shows Indian Healthy Plate. It is designed in accordance with RDA by National Institute of Nutrition. It is meant for use by the general healthy population and is a guide for the amount and types of food to be included in the daily diet.

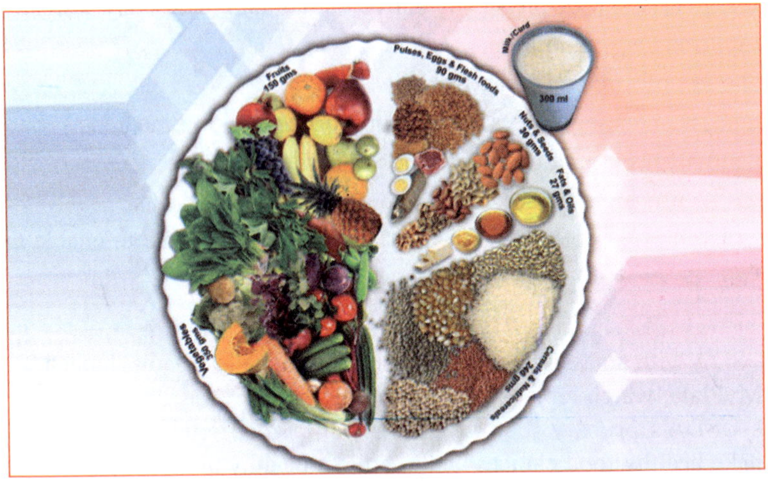

Fig. 1.10 My Healthy Plate-2020 is suggested for Indians by National Institute of Nutrition, Hyderabad

Mediterranean Diet

Mediterranean diet contains high amounts of fruits, vegetables, beans and grains; low in red meat; and modest amounts of fish, eggs, poultry and diary. Red wine is another component of the diet. Olive oil is the primary source of added fat. Research shows that Mediterranean diet lowers total cholesterol, low-density lipoprotein cholesterol and triglycerides and raises high-density lipoprotein cholesterol. Antioxidants present in the diet prevent LDL cholesterol from being oxidized. Studies have shown that Mediterranean diet is inversely associated with blood pressure levels. Studies have shown an inverse relationship between adherence to the Mediterranean dietary pattern and weight gain and diabetes.

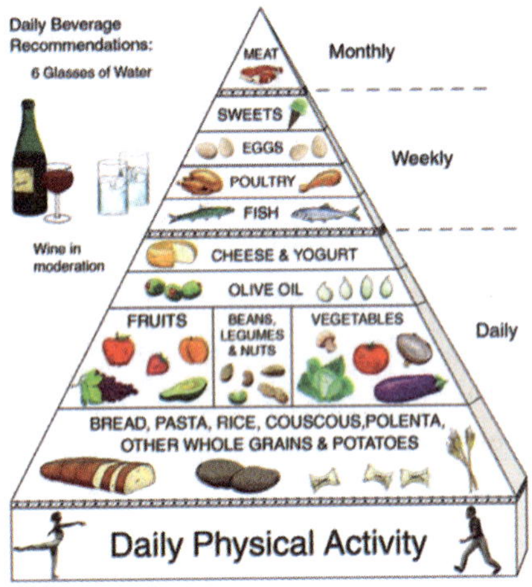

Fig. 1.11 The Traditional Healthy Mediterranean Diet Pyramid

A typical meal includes a nut laden salad tossed with olive oil, red wine, lightly cooked fish, cereals, vegetables, garlic and fresh fruit. Herbs and spices are also used. This diet is cardio protective.

PLANNING BALANCED DIET

Balanced Diet

Balanced diet is one which contains different types of foods in such quantities and proportions so that the need for calories, proteins, minerals, vitamins and other nutrients is adequately met and a small provision is made for extra nutrients to withstand short duration of leanness and it covers energy expenditure and for tissue maintenance, repair and growth. In addition, a balanced diet should provide bioactive photochemicals such as dietary fibre, antioxidants and other nutraceuticals which have positive health benefits. Low glycaemic index foods are preferred.

A balanced diet should provide around 60–70 per cent of total calories from carbohydrate, 10–12 per cent from protein and 20–25 per cent of total calories from fat. It should have good carbohydrate, good protein and good fats. Balanced diet

- meets nutritional requirement
- provides phytochemicals
- prevents degenerative diseases
- improves longevity
- prolongs productive life
- improves immunity
- increases endurance level
- develops optimum cognitive ability
- helps in coping up stress
- ability to withstand short duration of leanness.
- covers energy expenditure and for tissue maintenance, repair and growth.

Food Exchange Lists

Food Exchange Lists are the basis of meal planning. Food exchange lists are groups of measured foods of the same calorific value and similar protein, fat and carbohydrate. All foods of exchange lists make a specific contribution to a good diet. None of the exchange groups can itself supply all the nutrients needed for a well balanced diet. Exchange lists are based on principles of good nutrition that apply to everyone though extremely helpful for diabetics. Food exchange lists help in manipulation of carbohydrate, protein, calories and micro nutrients.

Food Composition Tables

In 2017 National Institute of Nutrition has published Indian Food Composition Tables. These tables are data repository for the content of nutritionally relevant chemical constituents and energy values of foods. These tables in addition to nutritive value of Indian foods, also give data on organic acids, polyphenols, oligosaccharides, phytosterols, saponins and phytates. The data compiled in the Food Composition Tables normally comprises of analytical, achival, calculated and/or derived values weighted towards the most representative of the true content in a given food.

Compositional values of foods are useful in manifold ways; in nutritional surveillance, consumer nutrition appraisal, nutrition labeling, etiology of disease prevalence, setting institutional (school) menu standards – meal planning and issue of dietary guidelines or recommendations.

Principles of Planning Diets

- ***Meeting nutritional requirements:*** A good menu is one which will not only provide adequate calories, fat and proteins but also minerals, vitamins essential for the well being of each member of family. In 2020 ICMR suggested cereal-legume milk composition of the diet should be 3:1:2.5. The diet should contain 'Basic food groups'. The diet should contain healthy fats and carbohydrate.

- ***Meal pattern must fulfil family needs:*** Meal pattern varies with age, occupation and life stage of the family members. A family meal should cater to the needs of the different members. A growing adolescent boy may need variety of foods to satisfy appetite, whereas a young child may require soft and bland diet. Pregnant women require more greens in the diet. A heavy worker requires more calories and B vitamins than other members of the family. The family meal must offer children enough fat and flexibility in caloric density so that their energy needs are met.
- ***Meal planning should save time and energy:*** Planning of meals should be done in such a way, that the recipes should be simple and nutritious. Labour and time saving devices can be used.
- ***Meal planning should consider economic constraints:*** Meals planned that are not within budget, cannot be put into practice. The cost of meals can be reduced by bulk purchasing and using seasonal fruits and vegetables.
- ***Meal plan should give maximum nutrients:*** Losses of nutrients during processing and cooking should be minimised. Sprouted grams, malted cereals and fermented foods enhance the nutritive value. Good quality protein should be distributed in all meals. Pressure cooker can be used to conserve the nutrients.
- ***Meal planning considers individual likes and dislikes:*** The meal plan should not only meet RDA but also individual preferences, like vegetarian or non-vegetarian preferences. If a person does not like particular greens, it can be tried in a different form or substituted by some other equally nourishing food. Food habits and dietary pattern should also be considered. Religion, traditions and customs of the individual should be considered in planning the menu.
- ***Meals planned should provide variety:*** If meals are monotonous they are not relished. Variety can be introduced in colour, texture and taste, by using different kinds of foods and cooking methods. Variety also helps in meeting the nutritional requirement.

  This helps the child to appreciate different flavours and to accept many foods in his later life.
- ***Meals should give satiety:*** Each meal should have some amount of protein, fat and fibre to give satiety. While planning menu, the interval between meals is also considered.
- ***Menus should include locally available foods:*** One can plan balanced diet with locally available millets, green leafy vegetables, fruits, meat and milk products. They are fresh, nutritious and less processed. They are less expensive. If the food travels distance, it should have been processed.
- ***Meals should include health foods:*** Ideal diets should provide besides nutrients those bioactive chemicals which can help to prevent and retard disease processes. Foods should be rich in antioxidants. Meals cooked at home contain more fruits and vegetables unlike outside foods.

Following the International Conference of Nutrition in 1992 the WHO and FAO recommended that all regions of the world provide advice to the public through qualitative and/or quantitative dietary guidelines relevant for different age groups and lifestyles appropriate for the population. Food based dietary guidelines published as a technical bulletin by the WHO expresses the principles of nutrition education in terms of foods and reinforces the link between dietary pattern and reduced risk of certain diseases.

Table 1.7 Summary of Recommended Dietary Allowances for Indians suggested by ICMR-NIN—2020

Age Group	Category of work	Body Wt	Protein	Dietary Fiber*	Cal-cium	Magne-sium	Iron	Zinc	Iodine	Thia-mine	Ribo-flavin	Niacin	Vit B6	Folate	Vit B12	Vit C	Vit A	Vit D
		(kg)	(g/d)	(g/d)	(mg/d)	(mg/d)	(mg/d)	(mg/d)	(mg/day)	(mg/d)	(mg/d)	(mg/d)	(mg/d)	(µg/d)	(µg/d)	(mg/d)	(µg/d)	(IU/d)
Men	Sedentary			30						1.4	2.0	14	1.9					
	Moderate	65	54.0	40	1000	440	19	17	140	1.8	2.5	18	2.4	300	2.2	80	1000	600
	Heavy			50						2.3	3.2	23	3.1					
Woman	Sedentary			25						1.4	1.9	11	1.9					
	Moderate	55	46.0	30	1000	370	29	13.2	140	1.7	2.4	14	1.9	220	2.2	65	840	600
	Heavy			40						2.2	3.1	18	2.4					
	Pregnant woman	55 + 10	+9.5 (2nd trimester) +22.0 3rd trimester)	–	1000	440	27	14.5	220	2.0	2.7	+2	2.3	570	+0.25	+15	900	600
	Lactation 0-6 m		+17.0	–	1200	400	23	14.1	280	2.1	3.0	+5	+0.26	330	+1.0	+50	950	600
	7-12m		+13.0								2.9		+0.17					
Infants	0-6 m*	5.8	8.0	–	300	30	–	–	100	0.2	0.4	2	0.1	25	1.2	20	350	400
	6-12 m	8.5	10.5	–	300	75	3	2.5	130	0.4	0.6	5	0.6	85	1.2	30	350	400
Children	1-3 y	12.9	12.5	15	500	90	8	3.3	90	0.7	1.1	7	0.9	120	1.2	30	390	600
	4-6 y	18.3	16.0	20	550	125	11	4.5	90	0.9	1.3	9	1.2	135	2.2	35	510	
	7-9 y	25.3	23.0	26	650	175	15	5.9	90	1.1	1.6	11	1.5	170	2.2	45	630	
Boys	10-12 y	34.9	32.0	33	850	240	16	8.5	100	1.5	2.1	15	2.0	220	2.2	55	770	600
Girls	10-12 y	36.4	33.0	30	850	250	28	8.5	100	1.4	1.9	14	1.9	225	2.2	50	790	600
Boys	13-15 y	50.5	45.0	43	1000	345	22	14.3	140	1.9	2.7	19	2.6	285	2.2	70	930	600
Girls	13-15 y	49.6	43.0	36	1000	340	30	12.8	140	1.6	2.2	16	2.2	245	2.2	65	890	600
Boys	16-18 y	64.4	55.0	50	1050	440	26	17.6	140	2.2	3.1	22	3.0	340	2.2	85	1000	600
Girls	16-18 y	55.7	46.0	38	1050	380	32	14.2	140	1.7	2.3	17	2.3	270	2.2	70	860	600

* Adequate Intake (AI)

Note : For adequate intake of Biotin and Pantothenic acid, refer a report of the expert group, Nutrient requirements of Indians, ICMR 2020.

Table 1.8 Summary of Estimated Average Requirements for Indians-ICMR-NIN, 2020

Age Group	Category of work	Body Wt	Energy (**)	Protein	Cal-cium	Magne-sium	Iron	Zinc	Iodine	Thia-mine	Ribo-flavin	Niacin	Vit B6	Folate	Vit B12	Vit C	Vit A	Vit D
		(kg)	(Kcal/d)	(g/d)	(mg/d)	(mg/d)	(mg/d)	(mg/d)	(mg/day)	(mg/d)	(mg/d)	(mg/d)	(mg/d)	(µg/d)	(µg/d)	(mg/d)	(µg/d)	(IU/d)
Men	Sedentary	65	2110	43.0	800	370	11	14.1	95	1.2	1.6	12	1.6	250	2	65	460	400
	Moderate		2710							1.5	2.1	15	2.1					
	Heavy		3470							1.9	2.7	19	2.6					
Woman	Sedentary	55	1660	36.0	800	310	15	11.0	95	1.1	1.6	9	1.6	180	2	55	390	400
	Moderate		2130							1.4	2.0	12	1.6					
	Heavy		2720							1.8	2.6	15	2.1					
	Pregnant woman	55 + 10	+ 350	+7.6 (2nd trimester) +17.6 3rd trimester)	800	370	21	12.0	160	1.6	2.3	+2	1.9	480	+0.2	+10	406	400
	Lactation 0-6 m	–	+600	+13.6	1000	335	16	11.8	200	1.7	2.5	+4	+0.22	280	+0.8	+40	720	400
	7-12m		+520	+10.6							2.4		+0.16					
Infants	0-6 m*	5.8	530	7.0	–	–	–	–	–	–	–	–	–	–	–	–	–	–
	6-12 m	8.5	680	9.0	–	–	2	2.1	–	–	–	–	0.5	71	1	–	170	–
Children	1-3 y	12.9	1110	10.0	400	73	6	2.8	65	0.6	0.8	6	0.8	97	1	24	180	400
	4-6 y	18.3	1360	13.0	450	104	8	3.7	65	0.8	1.1	8	1.0	111	2	27	240	
	7-9 y	25.3	1700	19.0	500	144	10	4.9	65	1.0	1.3	10	1.3	142	2	36	290	
Boys	10-12 y	34.9	2220	27.0	650	199	12	7.0	70	1.3	1.7	12	1.7	180	2	45	360	400
Girls	10-12 y	36.4	2060	27.0	650	207	16	7.1	70	1.2	1.6	12	1.6	186	2	44	370	400
Boys	13-15 y	50.5	2860	36.0	800	287	15	11.9	100	1.6	2.2	16	2.2	238	2	60	430	400
Girls	13-15 y	49.6	2400	35.0	800	282	17	10.7	100	1.3	1.9	13	1.8	204	2	55	420	400
Boys	16-18 y	64.4	3320	45.0	850	367	18	14.7	100	1.9	2.5	19	2.5	286	2	70	480	400
Girls	16-18 y	55.7	2500	37.0	850	317	18	11.8	100	1.4	1.9	14	1.9	223	2	57	400	400

* Adequate Intake (AI)

** There is no RDA for energy, the EAR for energy is equivalent to the Estimated Energy Requirement (EER)

Note: For adequate intake of Biotin and Pantothenic acid, refer a report of the expert group, 'Nutrient requirements for Indians', ICMR-2020.

STEPS INVOLVED IN PLANNING A DIET

There are three steps involved in planning a menu.

Step I: Recommended dietary allowances

To calculate balanced diet, as a first step there is a need to know the Recommended Dietary Allowances for different age groups prescribed by Nutrition Expert Committee of ICMR. Table 1.8 shows Recommended Dietary Allowances for Indians 2020 and Estimated Average requirements are given in Table 1.9.

Step II: Food list

Food list can be prepared either by using ICMR Tables or Exchange lists.

A. Using ICMR Tables

As a second step while planning the daily diet the foods are chosen from all food groups. To make menu planning more convenient ICMR has suggested the portion size and balanced diets for adults and for different age groups (Tables 1.9, 1.10 and 1.11).

The balanced diets for adults and different age groups are given as multiples of these portion sizes. The portion sizes are given in terms of raw food.

Table 1.9 Portion size for menu plan

Food groups	*Portion g*	*Energy kcal*	*Protein g*	*Carbohydrate g*	*Fat g*
Cereals and millets	30	100	3.0	20	0.8
Pulses	30	100	6.0	15	0.7
Egg	50	85	7.0	–	7.0
Meat, Chicken or Fish	50	100	9	–	7.0
Milk and milk products	100	70	3.0	5	3.0
Roots and tubers	100	80	1.3	19	–
Green leafy vegetables	100	45	3.6	–	0.4
Other vegetables	100	30	1.7	–	0.2
Fruits	100	40	–	10	–
Sugar	5	20	–	5	–
Fats & Oils	5	45	–	–	5

Source: Dietary Guidelines for Indians—A manual, 2011, National Institute of Nutrition, ICMR, Hyderabad.

Table 1.10 Balanced diet for infants, children and adolescents (number of portions)

Food groups	*Portion g*	*Infants 6–12 months*	*1–3*	*4–6*	*7–9*	*Years 10–12 Girls*	*10–12 Boys*	*13–15 Girls*	*13–15 Boys*	*16–18 Girls*	*16–18 Boys*
Cereals and millets	30	0.5	2	4	6	8	10	11	14	11	15
Pulses	30	0.25	1	1.0	2	2	2	2	2	2.5	3
Milk and milk products	100	4*	5	5	5	5	5	5	5	5	5

Roots and tubers	100	0.5	0.5	1	1	1	1	1	1.5	2	2
Green leafy vegetables	100	0.25	0.5	0.5	1	1	1	1	1	1	1
Other vegetables	100	0.25	0.5	1	1	2	2	2	2	2	2
Fruits	100	1	1	1	1	1	1	1	1	1	1
Sugar	5	2	3	4	4	6	6	5	4	5	6
Fats/Oils (visible)	5	4	5	5	6	7	7	8	9	7	10

*Quantity indicates top milk. For breast-fed infants, 200 ml top milk is required.
One portion of pulse may be exchanged with one portion (50 g) of egg/meat/chicken/fish.
For infants, egg/meat/chicken/fish can be introduced around 9 months.

Table 1.11 Balanced diet for adults—sedentary/moderate/heavy activity (number of portions)

Food groups	*Portion g*	*Type of work*					
		Sedentary		*Moderate*		*Heavy*	
		Man	*Woman*	*Man*	*Woman*	*Man*	*Woman*
Cereals and millets	30	12.5	9	15	11	20	16
Pulses	30	2.5	2	3	2.5	4	3
Milk and milk products	100	3	3	3	3	3	3
Roots and tubers	100	2	2	2	2	2	2
Green leafy vegetables	100	1	1	1	1	1	1
Other vegetables	100	2	2	2	2	2	2
Fruits	100	1	1	1	1	1	1
Sugar	5	4	4	6	6	11	9
Fats and Oils (visible)	5	5	4	6	5	8	6

B. Using Cooked Food Exchange Lists

The diet can also be prescribed in terms of cooked exchange lists. Each exchange provides 100 kcals.

There is no fat exchange as the calorie value of the recipes include fat that is used. If additional fat or sugar is used, calorie value can be calculated by multiplying with 9 and 4 per gram respectively.

All the food portions in the given list provide approximately the same amount of kilocalories. Portion sizes are strictly defined so that every item on a given list provides roughly the same amount of energy. Any food on a list can be exchanged for any other food on that same list without affecting balance or total calories.

Recipes from exchange lists are selected from all groups and energy and protein values are calculated and compared with the RDA. If energy and protein RDA are met, most of the time all the other nutrients would be met in the diet provided principles of balanced diet are followed.

Table 1.12 Exchange list of 100 kcal

Capacity of one standard katori (k) is 150 ml.

Cereal exchange – 1.5–3.5 g protein	
Idli (big)	1
(medium)	1½
Dosa (big)	½
(small)	1
Phulka	2
Chapathi	1
Puri	1½
Rava idli	1
Veg. sandwich	3/4
Bread toast (medium)	1½
Plain rice	3/4 k
Upma	1/2 k
Veg. noodles	1 k
Coconut rice	1/2 k
Pongal	1/2 k
Boiled wheat rava	1 k
Sweet pongal	2 tsp
Paniyaram	1¼ pieces
Verrmicelli payasam	2 tsp
Kesari	1½ tsp
Rice flakes upma	1/2 k
Naan	2/3
Cheese Sandwich	1/3
Ragi puttu	3/4 k
Ragi adai	3/4
Pulao	1/2 k
Bise bela bath	1/2 k
Tamarind rice	1/2 k
Curd rice	1/2 k
Idiappam	1
Pulse exchange – 3–5 g protein	
Sambar	1½ k
Rasam	2½ k
Thick dal	1/2 k
Thin dal	1 k
Channa masala	1/2 k
Dry peas sundal	3/4 k
Roasted bengal gram chutney (without coconut)	1/2 k
Sprouted moong salad	1 heaped katori
Pesarattu	3/4

Baked masala Vada (with negligible amount of fat)	2 nos
Adai	1
Vada	1
Keerai vada	3/4
Bajji	2
Bonda	1
Meat exchange – 5 g protein	
Egg omelette	1
Scrambled egg	1/2 k
Fish Kolambu	3/4 k
Fish fry small piece	1
Egg gravy	3/4 k
Meat curry	1 k
Egg custard	1/2 k
Milk exchange – 4.5 g protein	
Milk	1 k
Curd	1 k
Cheese	1 cube
Paneer	40 g
Butter milk	1 glass–(350 ml)
Badam milk shake	1/4 glass
Banana milk shake	1/3 glass
Milk kheer	1/2 k
Carrot kheer	3/4 k
Vegetable A exchange	
Curry without coconut and gravy (with simple seasoning)	1 heaped katori
Plain tomato soup without fat and crotous	2 k (1 soup bowl)
Soup with white sauce	1 k (1/2 soup bowl)
Mint chutney	1/2 k
Onion chutney	1/2 k
Vegetable B exchange	
Roots and tubers curry	1/2 k
Cutlet	1/2
Fruit exchange	
Apple	1 medium
Banana	1 small
Custard apple	1
Pine apple	3 slices
Orange	2½
Sapota	2 (small)
Guava	1 (Big)
Fruit salad (no sugar or dressing)	3/4 k

*Work out details are given in appendix.

Step III: Making menu

The foods that are listed in step II are converted into recipes if taken as portions from ICMR tables and distributed in different meals like breakfast, lunch, evening tea and dinner. Recipes in cooked exchange lists are distributed in different meals.

People's eating habits vary enormously and dietitians must respect dietary freedom and diversity when making recommendations. Dietary diversity is one of our culture's strengths and sources of pleasure. There are many ways to eat to be healthy. The best way to achieve balanced diet is to plan meals in relation to other food for the whole day. It is advisable to eat small regular meals rather than one huge meal.

Apart from diet, factors like no smoking, alcohol in moderation, regular physical activity, adequate rest and medical attention when needed all contribute to a healthy life. Establishing these healthy habits early in life seems to be the most important step one can take to reduce the risks of diseases, in later life.

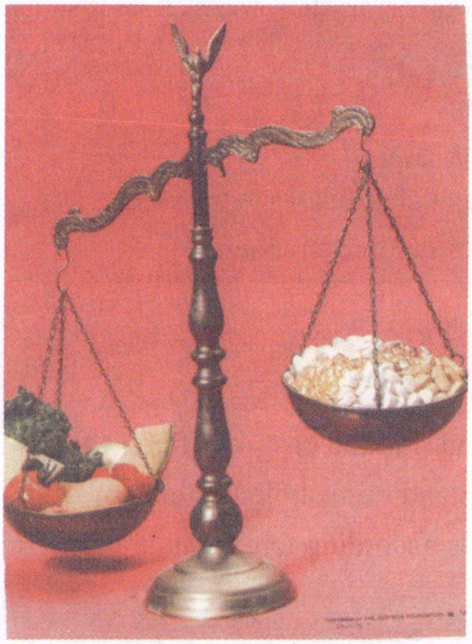

Fig. 1.12 Balanced diets are farm based but not pharmacy based.
Source: **The Arthritis Foundation, USA.**

January 7th is World Dietetics Day

April 7th is World Health Day

SUGGESTED READINGS

- Dietary Guidelines for Indians – A Manual 2011, National Institute of Nutrition, Hyderabad.
- Longvah T., R. Ananthan, K. Bhaskarachary and K. Venkaiah 2017, Indian Food Composition Tables, National Institute of Nutrition, Hyderabad.
- Nutrient Requirements for Indians. A Report of the Expert Group 2020 National Institute of Nutrition ICMR, Hyderabad.
- USDA Food Guide. www.mypyramid.gov, www.choosemyplate.gov.
- American Dietetic Association. www.eatright.org.

Questions

1. Define and explain balanced diet.
2. Write short notes on food composition tables bringing out the limitations.
3. Give the four food group system suggested by ICMR and explain the importance of it.
4. Explain the principles of planning a diet.
5. Discuss in detail the steps involved in planning a menu.
6. Give the importance of planning a menu.
7. What are food exchange lists? How are they used in planning diets?
8. Explain determinants of food choice.
9. Define RDA, nutraceuticals and nutritional genomics.
10. Define functional food. Mention any five and explain their functional value.
11. Explain 'My Healthy Plate'.
12. Write short notes on

    (*a*) Flax seeds (*b*) Walnuts
13. Bring out the importance of antioxidants in the diet.
14. Explain the characteristics of Mediterranean diet.

TOPICS FOR ACTIVITY

- Do market survey and find the cost of different foods.
- Make a list of edible and non edible portions of fruits and vegetables.
- Group different foods according to exchange lists.

2

Adjuncts to Diet Therapy

All issues of health are addressed holistically with the modification of lifestyle. The adjuncts of diet therapy like regular physical activity and coping with stress and overall modification of lifestyle are to be followed by all age groups to prevent and cure diseases.

PHYSICAL ACTIVITY

Physical activity is defined as "any body movement produced by skeletal muscles that requires energy expenditure." Physical activity describes the actions or movements that one makes whereas physical fitness describes the limits on the actions that one is capable of making.

The second largest component of energy expenditure after BMR/REE is physical activity. It is one of the lifestyle factors that can be controlled. Increased physical activity leads to improved physical fitness and to other physiologic changes. Physical activity leads to better health and fitness for all age groups. It is a need from birth to death.

Protein supplementation increases muscle mass when accompanied by physical activity.

Impact of Physical Activity on different Systems of the Body

Table 2.1 highlights the impact of physical activity.

Table 2.1 **The Comprehensive impact of physical activity**

Increase	*Decrease*
Cardiorespiratory	
Circulation	Heart disease risk
Aerobic capacity	Resting HR
VO_2 maximum	Blood pressure
Stroke volume	Bad cholesterol (LDL)
Cardiac output	
Oxygen transport	
Blood distribution	
Lung capacity	
Good cholesterol (HDL)	

Musculoskeletal	
Bone density	Risk of injuries
Lean muscle tissue	Postural problems
Functional strength	Risk of osteoporosis
Functional endurance	Inflexibility
Joint stability	Muscle/joint soreness
Functional abilities of ligaments	Body fat percentage
Functional abilities of tendons	
Resting length of muscles	
Range of motion	
Joint Integrity	
Neuromuscular	
Reaction speed	
Sensory awareness	
Coordination and balance	
Metabolic/Neuroendocrine	
Basal metabolic rate	Body fat
Balanced blood glucose levels	Need for insulin
Number of mitochondria in cells	
Psychoemotional	
Self-esteem	Premature ageing
Self-confidence	Mood swings
Mental alertness	Anxiety
Enhances sleep	PMS symptoms
Sexual health	Effect of chronic stress
Relaxation	
Stress management	
Immunological	
Resistance to illness and disease	Risk of cancer

Source: De Mond, E. Troy, 1997, Improving health and fitness through aerobic fitness, cited from Fitness Theory and Practice Aerobic and Fitness Association of America, California.

Effect of Physical Activity on Appetite

Physical activity regulates appetite. Physical activity significantly affects the hormones acylated ghrelin and leptin. Ghrelin produced by stomach cells increases appetite. Leptin is secreted by adipose tissue and higher concentration of leptin reduces appetite. Physical activity helps in regulating these hormones and in turn appetite. A single workout consisting of three 20 minute tread mill runs causes a decrease in appetite that last upto six hours.

Benefits of Physical Activity

Regular physical activity can reduce the risk of heart disease. It can improve cardiovascular fitness, decrease blood pressure and in losing and maintaining weight and alter blood lipid and lipoprotein levels. Brisk walking for atleast 40 minutes several times a week significantly reduces the heart failure.

Regular physical activity decreases the risk of colon cancer, stroke and hypertension. It can also delay the onset of or help treat type 2 diabetes mellitus, depression, osteoporosis and obesity. Physical activity burns kilocalories, increases the proportion of lean to fat body tissue and raises the BMR.

Daily physical activity improves health, fitness and quality of life. It can help relieve stress and can provide an overall feeling of well being. Being physically active is a key element in living a longer, healthier and happier life.

Physical activity not only helps physically but also mentally and socially. According to WHO, physical activity provides young people opportunities for self expression building self-confidence, social interaction and integration. Physically active young people more reaily adopt other healthy behaviours, for example, avoidance of tobacco, alcohol and drug use.

Other Benefits

- Improves self-esteem and feelings of well being.
- Helps build and maintain bones, muscles and joints.
- Builds endurance and muscle strength.
- Enhances flexibility and posture.
- Helps in maintaining weight
- Reduces feelings of depression and anxiety.
- Improves sleep quality.

EXERCISE

Exercise is a physical activity that is planned, structured and repetitive for the purpose of conditioning any part of the body. Exercise is used to improve health, maintain fitness and is importance as a means of physical rehabilitation. Range of motion is one aspect of exercise importance for increasing or maintaining joint function. Strengthening exercise provides appropriate resistance to the muscles to increase endurance and strength. Exercise in combination with a reduced-calorie diet is the safest and most effective method of weight loss.

Types of Exercise

Exercise and physical activity fall into four basic categories – endurance, strength, balance and flexibility. Some activities fit into more than one category.

Endurance or aerobic activities increase breathing and heart rate and over all fitness. Building endurance makes it easier to carry out many every day activities. Brisk walking, jogging, gardening and dancing improve endurance.

Strength exercise makes muscles stronger. Even small increase in strength can make a big difference in the ability to stay independent. Lifting weights and using a resistance band are examples of strength exercise.

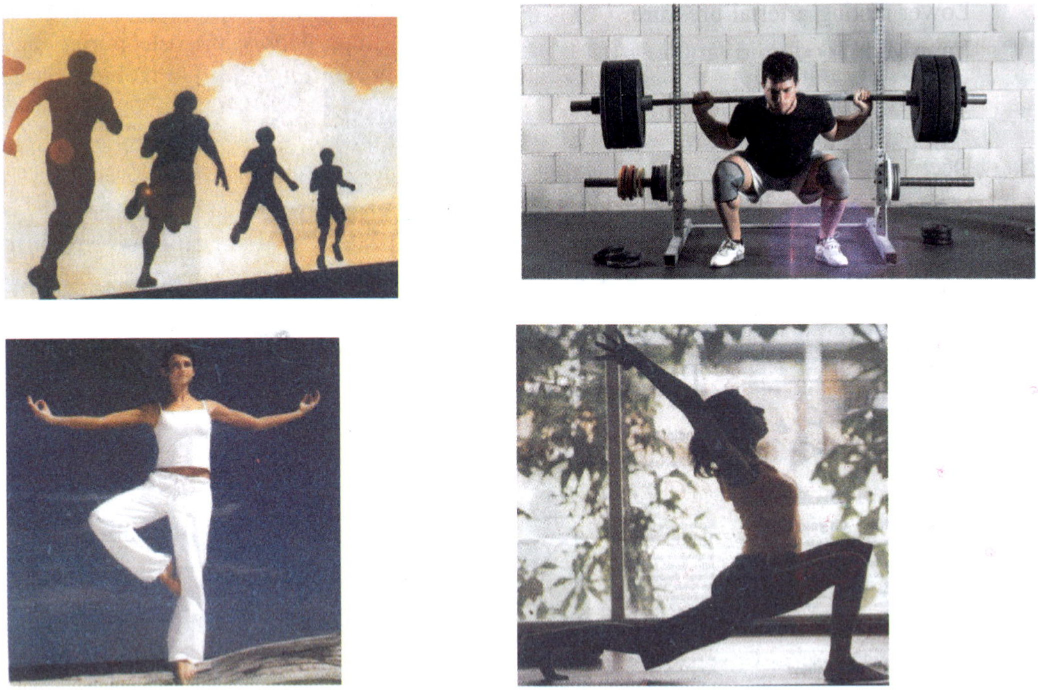

Fig. 2.1 **Exercise of medicine Types of exercise**

Balance exercises help prevent falls, a common problem in older adults. Many lower body strength exercises also improve balance. Standing on one foot and Taichi improve balance.

Flexibility exercise stretches muscles and can help body being flexible. Flexibility gives more freedom of movement for other exercises. Shoulder and upper arm stretch, calf stretch and yoga help flexibility.

Aerobic Exercise

Aerobic exercise also known as cardiovascular exercise, strengthens the muscles and provides the cardiovascular endurance (by targeting a specific heart rate). As the name suggests, aerobic exercise aims at improving the oxygen intake by the blood cells. It involves movement of the muscle groups from a moderate to intense level exercise, for an extended period (at least 20 minutes). There are many aerobic exercise types such as running, jogging, cycling, swimming, dancing and playing sports. It is the most effective form of exercise for losing weight. In an aerobic exercise session, a moderate intensity exercise should be preceded by a warm-up period and by a cooling down period.

The selected health benefits of aerobic exercise are:

- Increased life expectancy.
- Reduced risk of premature heart attack and stroke.

- Lower resting arterial pressure.
- Improved blood lipid profile
  - Decreased total serum cholesterol
  - Increased HDL cholesterol
- Decreased body weight and body fat.
- Modest improvement in bone density.
- Improved control of blood glucose.
- Improved psychological and social wellbeing.

Table 2.2 WHO guidelines for physical activity

Age group	*WHO guidelines*		*Physical activity guidelines for Asian Indians*	
	Duration	*Intensity*	*Duration**	*Intensity*
0–5 years	None	None	None	None
5–17 years old	60 min daily	Moderate to vigorous intensity	60 min/ day	Moderate to vigorous intensity
18–64 years old	150 min per week/70 min week	Moderate/vigorous/ combination of both	60 min/ day	Moderate intensity
65 years and above	150 min per week/70 min week	Moderate/vigorous/ combination of both	60 min/ day	Moderate intensity

* 30 min moderate intensity aerobic activity, 15 min of work related activity and 15 min of muscle strengthening exercise.

Anaerobic Exercise

Anaerobic exercise or weight lifting exercise is performed mostly to build muscles and enhance their size, strength and endurance *i.e.*, to increase the muscular fitness. The benefits of performing exercise to increase muscular fitness are:

- Increased bone density and decreased risk of osteoporosis.
- Increased lean tissue and improved metabolic rate (calorie burning).
- Increased strength of ligaments and tendons, reducing injury risk.
- Improved posture and stability, reducing risk of low back pain.
- Improved ability to carry out daily activities (lifting, pushing, pressing, carrying) thus improving physical esteem.
- Improved glucose tolerance, reducing risk of type 2 diabetes.

Beneficial Level of Exercise

To build aerobic capacity, the level of exercise must raise the pulse rate to within 70 per cent of maximal heart rate. Determine cardiac rate by subtracting age from 220. This calculation estimates maximal heart rate and 70 per cent of this figure tells the rate to which one wants to raise pulse in the course of exercise. This rate should then be maintained for an uninterrupted period of at least 20 min. and be practiced at least three times a week to have aerobic benefits. Resting pulse before starting the exercise period, then again during and immediately afterward need to be monitored to know the progress in developing maximal exercising heart rate and aerobic capacity.

Table 2.3 Equations for calculating training heart rates at various exercise intensities (Example is for a 40-year old subject)

Equations	*Sample calculations*
HR max = 200 – age	HR max = 220 – 40 = 180 bpm
HR range = HR max – HR rest	HR range = 180 – 80 = 100 bpm
HR 60% = (HR range × 0.60) + HR rest	HR 60% = (100 × 0.60) + 80 = 140 bpm
HR 85% = (HR range × 0.85) + HR rest	HR 85% = (100 × 0.85) + 80 = 165 bpm

* Assuming maximum heart rate of 180 bpm and resting heart rate of 80 bpm.

Source: Jordan Peg (ed), 1997, *Fitness Theory and Practice*, Aerobics and Fitness Association of America, Sherman, Oaks, California.

Exercise and Oxidative Damage

Regular physical exercise enhances the antioxidant, defense system and protects against exercise induced free radical damage. On the other hand, intense exercise in untrained individuals results in increased free radical damage. Most of the data suggest that increased intake of vitamin E is protective against exercise induced oxidative damage.

Inadequate preparation can result in injuries, pulled muscles and stress fractures. Excessive exercise can lead to amenhorrea or cessation of menstruation, delayed menstruation (to as late as 18 years), oligomenhorrhea (infrequent or scanty menstrual period) and decreased bone mass.

Moderate exercise benefits during childhood, adolescence and adulthood by establishing life long health habits, by preventing and treating eating disorders and controlling weight in the respective stages. Physical exercise is the best way to enhance the immune system of people. Families that exercise together achieve better results.

Tracking Devices

Tracking devices like pedometer help in measuring the number of steps a person takes and in turn the energy expended. Many such devices as attachments to the wrist or waist are available in the market.

YOGA

Yoga is a psycho-somatic-spiritual discipline for achieving union and harmony between mind, body, and soul and the ultimate union of individual consciousness with the universal consciousness. Mind-body practices such as Yoga, which capitalize on the ability of the mind to enhance physical health (and vice versa), appear particularly suited for addressing multifactorial conditions. Asanas particularly have a positive effect on fitness and physical flexibility with a secondary effect on the mental state. Yoga may also boost confidence and reduce anxiety.

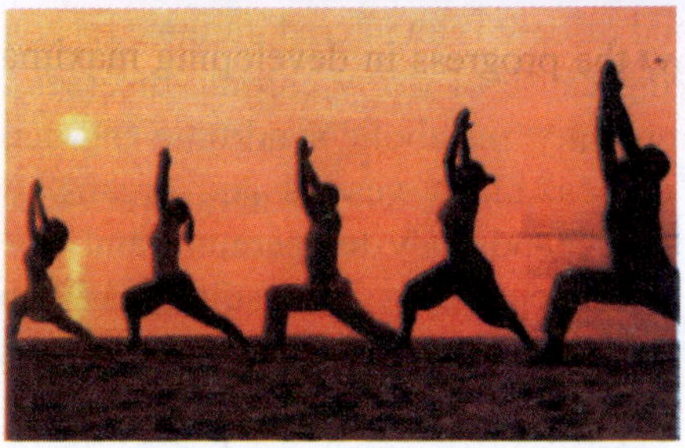

Fig. 2.2 **Asanas help to improve posture and to increase strength and flexibility.**

Benefits of Yoga

Physical

- Creates energy and improves stamina, fitness and concentration.
- Keeps the body flexible so that energy flows freely.
- Works on the internal organs and endocrine system, and regulates metabolism, improves digestive and elimination processes.
- Rejuvenates, decreases tension and teaches relaxation.
- Improves posture and delays the ageing processes.
- Helps reduce excess fat.
- Improves circulation and skin tone.
- Not expensive-needs no expensive equipments or gear.
- Postures provide a full balanced range of motion.

Mental

- Calms and disciplines the mind.
- Improves concentration and counteracts stress.
- Gives control over emotions, particularly anger.
- Creates a flexible mind where energy flows freely.
- Promotes a positive, happy attitude.

STRESS MANAGEMENT

Stress is a perceived state of disturbed harmony produced by a stimulus, condition or an event called the stressor. The disturbance results from the concerned person's inability to meet the threat posed by the stressor or from his inadequacy to satisfy the demands imposed by it. The disturbance produced by the stressor is generally unpleasant or painful. This is known as distress.

The organs most affected by stress are the adrenal glands that produce hormones which regulate many bodily functions. The thymus gland is also affected by stress. This master gland of immune system and digestive tract alter how foods are digested and absorbed and may alter immune function. All are subjected to accelerated wear and tear by stressful stimuli.

Physical stress can be caused by surgery, infection, burns and pain. Environmental stress is due to air and noise pollution and crowding. Psychological stress is due to death of a spouse, friend or loved one.

One link between stress and disease is an altered immune response that causes inflammation. Inflammation is an underlying cause of many chronic diseases like heart disease, diabetes, visceral type obesity, autoimmunity, metabolic syndrome and major depression.

Stress affects muscles, tissues, blood vessels and organs. It speeds up heart rate and respiration, raises blood pressure and body temperature and can interfere with metabolism, appetite, digestion, fertility and sleep. Stress can result in early menopause. Stress can impair memory. It can make a person obese or undernourished. Stress can be the cause of rheumatoid arthritis, osteoporosis, cancer, diabetes and heart disease. Stress is the cause of many diseases. Disease causes stress.

Stress Management Techniques

Physical activity reduces stress. Research shows that people who work out even once a week or for as little as 10 minutes a day tend to be more cheerful. Yoga and breathing exercises bring joy. Apart from regular physical activity, there are many other methods to reduce stress.

Meditation

Meditation is the most powerful tool to integrate all the six components of health, that is, physical, mental, social, emotional, environment and spiritual. Meditation is a part of the yogic tradition of India. It is a union of body, mind, soul, spirit and environment. This union is possible through meditation.

Meditation or contemplation simply means single-pointed attention on any given object, be it material or subtle. It is a process to internalize or observe oneself, a process to quiet or still the mind. In this process, one observes, understands and becomes aware of thoughts, mind and its activities. A constant, silent and passive observation of mind can bring about a peculiar state of mind called mindfulness, a state full of awareness, yet of total silence and stillness. It gives deep rest and relaxation to mind. By keeping still the mind, one conserves energy, eliminates negative attitudes and develops creativity. All meditation techniques call upon breathing discipline in one form or other to reach a thoughtless state of mind, a silence zone, pure conscience, a world of its own.

> It is not the stress but the reaction that kills.

Benefits of Meditation

- Brings in behaviour transformation.
- Increases willpower, tolerance, clarity in thinking and perception.
- Increases capacity for concentration and memory power.
- Sharpens power of judgement and decision making capability.
- Increases power of creativity and intuition.
- Develops positive attitude to the events of life overcoming bad habits and negative thought patterns.
- Relieves physical, mental and emotional stresses.
- Relaxes body-mind system.
- Increases bio-magnetism. This is achieved by alignment of all electrons in the body in the same direction like in a laser beam.
- Increases energy level by ten times.
- Brings in a state of supreme happiness, harmony or bliss.

Pranayama

The primary purpose of breathing is to deliver oxygen to every cell in every tissue and organ in the body, while removing carbon dioxide. Breath provides oxygen to the body and is responsible for:

- chemical and physiological processes that take place within the body.
- glandular secretion.
- all muscular secretions.
- motion and movement, and
- thought processes.

Prana is that vital force which pervades the whole cosmos and activates the whole human organism. Prana is a force or energy, which resonates throughout the physical system of man and makes the body machine work. Inhalation and exhalation processes are the obvious proofs of Prana Shakti. Yama means control or regulation. Thus, Pranayama means controlled rythmic breathing. Pranayama is voluntary controlled flow of breath in a firmly stabilized posture. Pranayama is a bridge between body and mind. If one controls the breath or prana, the mind is also controlled and vice versa.

Benefits of Pranayama

- With every inhalation, cosmic energy, vital power and internal peace are drawn and one should have the mental attitude (visualization or auto suggestion) that positivity is entering the body system with all body cells getting fresh oxygen and being energized.
- With every exhalation, one should have the mental attitude that negativity, tension, diseases and impurities/toxins are thrown out of the body system.
- Enhances bio-energy, buoyancy, and latent power within.
- Freedom from/control of physical and mental diseases/ailments.
- Purifies mind, calms mind and thoughts do not go astray.
- Strong base is formed for meditation and spiritual empowerment.

Slow and rhythmic breathing has also been shown to promote the release of prolactin and the hormone oxytocin, which can foster feelings of friendship, calmness and bonding to others.

Mind Training

Mind training is the strengthening of the mind. The following methods help to make mind strong.

Positive thinking: Positive thinking is the filling of the mind with positive, optimistic and happy thoughts and ridding it of the negative, pessimistic and the gloomy ones. It is associated with an upbeat attitude. The chief advantages of positive thinking are that it keeps a person away from despair, it acts as an antidote to self-criticism, and it enables one to succeed in all his endeavours.

Laughter: Laughter is a series of explosive inarticulate sounds produced in response to joy, fun, mirth, amusement or body tickling. Smile is its abridged soundless version. Regular indulgence in laughter acts as a foolproof shield against the harmful effect of stressors. Laughter has the following advantages:

- It relaxes muscles and rids them of tension.
- It expands lungs and helps them draw in oxygen to capacity.
- It upgrades the body's immune system.
- It lowers the catecholamine level in the blood and promotes the body's inflammatory response.

Relaxation: Relaxation is the reduction of tension in, and the rigidity of, the body. It acts as the antidote for fatigue and boredom. When a person who has been practicing relaxation faces a stressful situation, his body does not tense up but lets him deal with it coolly and confidently. Some methods of relaxation are:

1. **Muscular relaxation:** This is achieved by a technique called the progressive muscular relaxation or PMR. At a quiet place and a pleasant time, the person sits comfortably in a chair or lies flat on his back, keeping his legs slightly apart. Starting from feet muscles, and going step by step upwards to the facial muscles, he contracts the muscle groups and suddenly relaxes them.
2. **Sensory relaxation:** Following are some of the methods of sensory relaxation.
   - Use of a light and sound machine. This produces colourful light and pleasing sound. These have soothing effect on the sight and hearing of the person exposed to it. The soothing experience slowly diffuses to the entire body and even spills over into the mind.
   - Music therapy- Listening to music of one's choice produces auditory relaxation that radiates to muscles and the brain.

Table 2.4 Some Recommendations for reducing stress

Intervention	*Description*
Meditation	• Repetition of a sound, word, phrase, prayer, or muscular activity (*i.e.*, a mantra, minimizes distracting thoughts and invokes the relaxation response).
Guided imagery	• Using the mind's ability to imagine sights, sounds, smells or movements induced specific physical reactions in the body. • Imagining 'calm thoughts' triggers the relaxation response. It can change a person's emotional outlook, and relieve depression and anxiety.
Music therapy	• Designer music decreases cortisol, epinephrine, and norepinephrine. Listening results in significant increases in caring, relaxation, mental clarity and vigour.
Dance therapy	• Psychotherapeutic use of movement to further the emotional and physical integration of the individual. Can be used by patients with eating disorders to express feelings and release tension.
Aromatherapy	• Aroma of oils extracted from plants are applied via massage, baths, hot or cold compresses, or inhalation. Citronella, eucalyptus, and sage elicit relaxation response; lavender, chamomile, and sandalwood induce meditative state. • Nerves involved in smell linked to the limbic system; aromas are linked to 'emotional' memory.
Touch	• Systematic manipulation of soft tissue increases circulation and decreases muscle tension. • May help relieve anxiety, depression, insomnia, and emotional stress.
Humour	• Humour is life-affirming – we can laugh at ourselves. • Cognitive control – we can't control life, but we can control how we view things and our emotional response.
Sleep	• Deep sleep enables nervous system to function well. It helps to concentrate, remember or analyse.
Rearing a pet	• Keeps the person busy and the pet reciprocates affection.

- Listening to the wind chimes or the gurgling of a river has the same effect as music.
- Viewing the greenery of a meadow and the expanse of ocean against the setting sun has soothing effect on the eyes and the whole body.
- Aroma therapy- Burning the incense, mopping of floor with water to which a few drops of eucalyptus oil are added, smelling of essential oils extracted from herbs, leaves and stem soothes the sense of olfaction directly and the body indirectly, relieves pain and boosts the immune system.
- Touch therapy- Massage or systematic manipulation of soft tissue increases circulation and decreases muscle tension. It may also relieve anxiety, depression, insomnia and emotional stress.

3. **Distraction:** Continuous work produces mental tension and thus predisposes the individual engaged in it to stress-induced damage. Such tension therefore needs to be dissipated. The best way of doing so is to pause from time to time and do things that take the mind off work. These things are called distractions.

Some may get massaged, some may sing bhajans, some may visit friends or talk on the phone; some may follow religious rituals or visit temples and churches; some may give parties and assemble people in their houses; all these are stress busters. One has to find out the recipe of one's happiness.

Lifestyle Modifications

Police forces are taking first step in 2018 for healthier lifestyle by insisting on consuming millets and making spend more time on workouts focussing on physical, emotional, mental and spiritual fitness of the personnel.

Nutritious food, physical activity for all age groups maintaining muscle mass while reducing adiposity, a happy life style, a clean environment, hygienic habits and stress coping mechanisms promote long term health and wellness.

29th August is National Sports day.

SUGGESTED READINGS

- McArdle D. William et al., 2010, Exercise physiology, Wolters, Kluwer, USA.

QUESTIONS

1. Bring out importance of physical activity.
2. How is stress related to disease? Give five methods to overcome stress.
3. What are the benefits of Yoga and meditation?
4. Explain the following
   (*a*) Aerobic exercise
   (*b*) Pranayama
5. Give the classification of exercise and explain with examples.

TOPIC FOR DISCUSSION

- Discuss the advantages of walking over other methods of exercise/physical activity.

3

Nutritional Recommendations and Food Requirements of Adults

Man needs a wide range of nutrients which perform various functions in the body. During adulthood nutrients are required for energy, for replacement of worn out tissues and for maintenance of body functions. Though there is no growth during adulthood, protein is required for the replacement of worn out tissues. The nutritional requirement of other age groups is sometimes extrapolated from adult requirements.

NUTRITIONAL RECOMMENDATIONS

Table 3.1 gives RDA for an adult suggested by ICMR in 2020.

Table 3.1 ICMR Recommended Dietary Allowances for an adult man and woman–2020.

	Man			*Woman*		
Nutrient	*Sedentary*	*Moderate*	*Heavy*	*Sedentary*	*Moderate*	*Heavy*
Body weight kg	65	65	65	55	55	55
Energy kcal	2110	2710	3470	1660	2130	2720
Protein g	54	54	54	46	46	46
Dietary Fibre g	30	40	50	25	30	40
Calcium mg	1000	1000	1000	1000	1000	1000
Magnesium mg	440	440	440	370	370	370
Iron mg	19	19	19	29	29	29
Zinc mg	17	17	17	13.2	13.2	13.2
Iodine μg	140	140	140	140	140	140
Vitamin A μg Retinoal	1000	1000	1000	840	840	840
Vitamin D IU	600	600	600	600	600	600
Thiamine mg	1.4	1.8	2.3	1.4	1.7	2.2
Riboflavin mg	2.0	2.5	3.2	1.9	2.4	3.1
Niacin mg	14	18	23	11	14	18
Pyridoxine mg	1.9	2.4	3.1	1.9	1.9	2.4
Folate μg	300	300	300	220	220	220
Vitamin B_{12} μg	2.2	2.2	2.2	2.2	2.2	2.2
Vitamin C mg	80	80	80	65	65	65

Energy

Energy requirements are based on energy expenditure. There is no RDA for energy.

Energy requirements of an adult man and woman are based on Reference man and Reference woman. Energy requirements for other individuals of different body weights and age are extrapolated.

Indian Reference Man and Woman

Reference man is between 19–39 years of age and weighs 65 kg with a height of 1.77 m with a BMI of 20.75 and is free from disease and physically fit for active work; on each working day, he is engaged in 8 hours of occupation which usually involves moderate activity, while when not at work he spends 8 hours in bed, 4–6 hours in sitting and moving about, 2 hours in walking and in active recreation or in household duties.

Reference woman is between 19–39 years of age, non-pregnant non-lactating (NPNL) and weighs 55 kg with a height of 1.62 m and a BMI of 20.75, is free from disease and physically fit for active work; on each working day she is engaged in 8 hours of occupation which usually involves moderate activity, while when not at work she spends 8 hours in bed, 4–6 hours in sitting and moving about, 2 hours in walking and in active recreation or household duties.

An important factor which determines energy needs is the nature and duration of physical activity, whether moderate or heavy. For those whose occupation entails heavy work, allowances have to be higher than for those who are either sedentary or engaged in moderate work. The allowances are made under the assumption that the energy expenditure for non-occupational activities remains unchanged.

In adult men and non-pregnant non-lactating women, BMR multiplied by PAL (Physical Activity Level) is equal to Total Energy Expenditure.

Table 3.2 ICMR Classification of activities based on occupation

	Male	*Female*
Sedentary	Teacher, tailor, barber, executive, shoemaker, priest, retired personnel, landlord, peon, postman, computer professional	Teacher, tailor, executive, housewife, computer professional
Moderate	Fisherman, basket maker, potter, goldsmith, agricultural labour, carpenter, mason, rickshawpuller, electrician, fitter, turner, welder, industrial labour, coolie, weaver, driver, servant	Maid, coolie, basket maker, agricultural labour, beedi maker, brick maker
Heavy	Stone cutter, blacksmith, mineworker, wood cutter, gangman	Stone cutter

Protein

The value for protein requirement given by FAO/WHO/UNU consultation is 0.66 g/kg/day.

When corrected for marginally lower amino acid score and lower digestibility the protein requirement of healthy Indian adult on a well balanced cereal-legume-milk in the ratio be 3:1:2.5. According to ICMR 2020 safe protein requirements are 0.83 g/kg/d for healthy Indian adults.

Protein Energy Ratio of Diets

It is useful to consider together the protein and energy requirement on habitual Indian diets. The protein requirement can be expressed as the ratio of protein calories to total dietary calories (PE ratio).

This concept is useful because in many population groups enough diet is not consumed to meet energy needs resulting in energy deficits. Since protein requirement is constant at different levels of activity, while the energy requirement changes, the PE ratio also changes. It will be seen that a PE ratio between 6 and 12 would meet the protein requirement of any group provided its energy needs are met.

Fat

Recommended total fat calories is between 20–35 per cent E (energy). In the diets of adults in India, about 20 per cent energy is derived from fats. At all levels of calorie intake, invisible fat furnishes about 9 per cent energy and visible fat 10 per cent. This would come to 10–20 g of fat per day depending upon the level of calories consumed.

According to ICMR 2020 minimum intake levels for essential fatty acids to prevent deficiency symptoms are estimated to be 2.5% E linoleic acid plus 0.5% E alphalinolenic acid.

A higher level visible fat intake of 20–40 g/d is recommended in accordance with physical activity to provide energy density and palatability to the diet. A minimal intake of 12 g visible fat can meet linoleic acid requirement.

Saturated fatty acids, *cis*-monosaturated fatty acids, proteins and cholesterol can increase essential fatty acid requirement. It would appear prudent to choose the visible or cooking fat from unsaturated vegetable oils. Blend of two or more vegetable oils ensures the recommended intake of fatty acids.

Minerals

After examining the evidence for calcium nutrition status of the Indian population, the Expert Committee suggested an upward revision of calcium RDA from 400 mg to 600 mg.

The requirement of calcium prescribed by ICMR is same for both men and women. To meet this requirement an adult needs to take at least 300 ml of buffalo's milk on cereal legume diet. It is suggested that a Ca : P in the diet should remain 1 : 1. Hence the RDA of phosphorus is 1000 mg. During infancy the Ca : P ratio suggested is 1 : 1.5. Bone mass increases during childhood and adolescence and peaks between the ages of 20 and 30 years. Peak bone mass is influenced by calcium intake. Other factors like age, sex, genetic factors, hormonal status and exercise also influence. After 30, the rate of withdrawal exceeds the rate of deposit; therefore establishing healthy bone mass in childhood and early adulthood is crucial.

Iron requirement for woman is 10 mg higher than man. Iron loss through menstruation in women of reproductive age groups are 0.6 mg/day on an average, when spread over the whole month. Those who are taking vegetarian diets should ensure adequate amounts of vitamin C for enhancing iron absorption.

The requirement of zinc is 2.7 mg/d. To get this amount, the RDA (2020) suggested is 17 mg/d, correcting individual variation. In an Indian population the rate of absorption is 20–25 per cent.

Vitamins

The requirement of vitamin A is same for both men and women. The conversion ratio of retinol to β-carotene is 1 : 8. The requirement of B vitamins is based on calorie requirement (0.5 mg of thiamine, 0.6 mg of riboflavin and 6.6 mg of niacin per 1000 calories). Hence, requirements of B vitamins are higher for moderate and heavy workers. The previous recommendations of 2 mg/d of pyridoxine of adults is retained.

An intake of 20 mg of vitamin C may be sufficient to maintain the ascorbic acid levels in the adults. Taking into account that 50 percent of vitamin C is lost in cooking, 40 mg is suggested for all adults. The Expert Committee (2020), suggested conversion rate of 6:1 to convert canotemids to retinol. For adult man 1000 μg and for adult woman 840 μg of retinol are recommended. Where there is minimal exposure to sunlight, a specific recommendation of a daily supplement of 600 I. U. of vitamin D is made (2020). The requirement of vitamin E are suggested is 0.8 mg/g of essential fatty acids. This roughly works out to 8-10 mg tocopherol/d depending on the edible oil used. FAO/WHO suggested 55 μg of vitamin K for adults.

Dietary Fibre

Based on energy intake, the requirement of dietary fibre is recommended.

FOOD REQUIREMENTS

The foods to be included in the diet should meet nutritional requirement. Functional foods should be included in balanced diets of all age groups.

Dietary Guidelines

The diet should include foods from all the food groups. The foods chosen should be nutrient dense.

For all nutrients minimum RDA must be met. For energy, the total calorie requirement depends on energy expenditure. One should maintain healthy weight.

Cereals

Energy derived from cereals should not be more than 75 per cent. It is better to include two cereals in one meal like rice and wheat or millets and rice. Whole grain cereals, brown rice, hand pounded rice, unpolished or parboiled rice or malted grains give higher nutritive value and higher phytochemical value. They also contribute to fibre. At least half the grains should be whole grains. Refined cereals like maida, should be taken in minimum quantity. To improve the cereal and pulse protein quality, minimum ratio of cereal protein to pulse protein should be 4 : 1. In terms of grains, cereals and pulses should be in the proportion of 8 : 1.

Pulses

Two to three servings of pulses should be taken everyday. Whole grams and germinated pulses are more nutritious.

Animal foods

Eggs are very nutritious. Atleast one egg should be consumed per day. Inclusion of egg in the diet improves the quality of protein of other foods like cereals and pulses. Instead, one serving of poultry can also be included in the diet. Red meat should be taken in minimum quantity. Lean meat should be preferred. Fish, preferable oily fish, should be included in the diet at least twice a week.

Milk and milk products

A minimum quantity of 500 ml milk/day should be included. Two glasses of milk or curd should be included in a balanced diet. Curd provides probiotics. Low fat milk should be preferred.

Vegetables and fruits

Inclusion of salads or raita not only help in meeting the vitamin requirements but the meals would be attractive and have high satiety value due to the fibre content. Green leafy vegetables should be taken minimum of one serving per day. Five servings of colourful fruits and vegetables should be included in a day's diet to meet antioxidant requirement. Vegetables should be selected from green leafy vegetables like carrots, pumpkin, beet root, tomatoes and coloured vegetables, fresh legumes (peas, edamame) and other vegetables.

Every meal should contain at least one medium size fruit. It is better to serve the fruit as such. Taking juice out of it causes loss of vitamin C and fibre. Fruits should never be cooked.

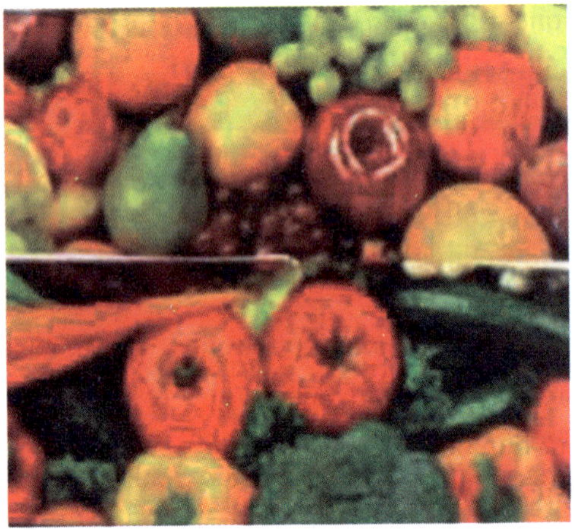

Fig. 3.1 **Balanced diet advocates minimum of five servings of colourful vegetables and fruits per day.**

Fats, Oils and Sugar

Energy derived from fats or oils should be 15–20 per cent and 5 per cent from sugar and jaggery of total calories. It is better to use more than one type of oil. Combination of oils give proper balance of n-3 and n-6 fatty acids. Most fats should come from PUFA and MUFA. Diet should be low in fat, saturated fat, *trans* fat and cholesterol. The World Health Organisation has recommended (2018) that adults should consume a maximum of 10 per cent of their calorie intake in the form of saturated fat and 1 per cent *trans* fats. Fried foods cannot be planned if oil allowance is less or in low calorie diets.

Antioxidants

There are two types of antioxidants. Preventive antioxidants will inhibit the initial production of free radicals. They are catalase, glutathione peroxidase, diethyl triamine penta-acetate and ethylene diamine tetra acetate. Chain breaking antioxidants can inhibit the propagative phase. They include superoxide dismutase, uric acid and vitamin E. β carotene can act as a chain breaking antioxidant but is less effective than α - tocopherol. Cysteine, glutathione and vitamin A are minor antioxidants.

ICMR (2020) recommended a minimum of 500 g/d of fruits and vegetables to obtain sufficient amounts of antioxidant nutrients such as β-carotene, vitamin C and certain non-nutrients like polyphenols and flavonoids which may protect against chronic diseases. This should be complemented with sufficient amount of vegetable oil so as to obtain vitamin E.

Water

The water required from beverages for adult man ranges from 32-58 ml/kg and for woman 27-52 ml/kg.

Dietary Guidelines suggested by ICMR

- Eat variety of foods to ensure a balanced diet.
- Ensure provision of extra food and healthcare to pregnant and lactating woman.
- Promote exclusive breastfeeding for six months and encourage breastfeeding till two years or as long as one can.
- Feed home based semi solid foods to the infant after six months.
- Ensure adequate and appropriate diets for children and adolescents, both in health and sickness.
- Eat plenty of vegetables and fruits.
- Ensure moderate use of edible oils and animal foods and very less use of *ghee*/butter/ *vanaspati*.
- Avoid overeating to prevent overweight and obesity.
- Exercise regularly and be physically active to maintain ideal body weight.
- Restrict salt intake to minimum.
- Ensure the use of safe and clean foods.
- Adopt right pre-cooking processes and appropriate cooking methods.
- Drink plenty of water and take beverages in moderation.
- Minimize the use of processed foods rich in salt, sugar and fats.
- Include micronutrient-rich foods in the diets of elderly people to enable them to be fit and active.

Table 3.3 Balanced diet for moderate active woman with nutrient content values- ICMR 2020

Food composition	*Amount (g/day)*	*Nutrient*	*Vegetarian diet*	*Non-vegetarian diet*	*EAR*	*RDA*
Cereals and Millets	300	Energy kcal Protein g	2135 74.2	2084 13.3	2130 36.0	– 46.0
Pulses (Legumes)/ flesh foods[1]	90	Visible fat g	20	20	25	20
Green leafy vegetables	100	Calcium mg	999	989	800	1000
Other vegetables	200	Iron mg	29.0	27.9	15.0	29.0

Roots and tubers (excluding potatoes)	100	Zinc mg	14.0	13.6	11.0	13.2
Fruits	150	Magnesium mg	841	806	310	370
Milk	300	Vitamin A μg*	1804	1741	390	840
Fats and oils	20	β-Carotene μg	1804	1741	390	840
Oil seeds and Nuts (gingely seeds and Pea nuts)	30	Thiamine mg	1.75	1.70	1.4	1.7
Spices	10	Riboflavin mg	1.65	1.64	2.0	2.4
		Niacin mg	16.3	16.8	12	14
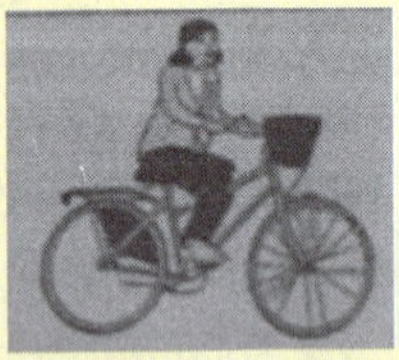		Vitamin B_6 mg	1.96	1.97	1.6	1.9
		Vitamin C mg	187	187	55	65
		Total Folates μg	191	459	180	220
		Vitamin B_{12} μg	1.5	2.0	2	2.2

Note: Total protein from the above diet = 76 g, Digestible protein = 62 g, PDCAAS = 85%

[1]Pulses can be replaced with animal foods (egg, meat, fish and chicken) for non-vegetarians.

* Retinol derived from β caroterne from diet was also added to the total Vitamin A.

For cereals and millets, it is recommended to consume 50% as whole grains.

DIET FOR SHIFT WORKERS

Irregular working hours have an impact on health because the internal circadian biological clock is connected not only to core body temperature, blood pressure and alertness but also to the synthesis and secretion of many hormones including cortisol, growth hormones and metabolism.

Research indicates that shift work may alter body natural rhythm enough to lead to chronic sleep disturbances, weight changes and even heart and gastrointestinal disturbances.

Shift work influences the frequency and regularity of eating. Irregular eating habits and skipping meals can occur. Small regular meals with balance of protein, healthy fats and carbohydrates should be taken. Atleast one half of carbohydrates should be whole grains and/or these with a lower glycemic index.

On the night shift, a light meal should be eaten before 1 am and another light meal should be taken before sleep. Main meal should be taken after a day's sleep, with protein rich snack in- between as desired.

To enhance alertness, it may be helpful to have more protein at the beginning of the shift and then shift the balance to more carbohydrates by the end. If possible, a meal break should be taken at work. It may be beneficial to avoid eating for a couple of hours before going to sleep and limit alcohol consumption.

A 20 minute aerobic workout or walk can delay by three to four hours the energy/alertness drop which shift workers experience during their circadian law and can help workers sleep when the shift is over.

A 20 minute power nap has been shown to provide a four hour boost in alertness and productivity.

LOW COST BALANCED DIETS

Diets of economically weaker sections can be improved nutritionally by (1) replacing a single cereal with mixed cereals, one of them being a millet, (2) inclusion of at least 50 g green leafy vegetables to improve the intake of Vitamin A, iron and calcium, (3) inclusion of inexpensive yellow fruits like papaya or mango and greens to increase vitamin A and C intake, (4) inclusion of at least 150 ml of milk improves intakes of riboflavin and calcium besides improving protein quality of diet, (5) Oil consumption increases energy and essential fatty acid intake. An example of low cost improved diet by modifying the existing diet as suggested by ICMR is given in Table 3.4.

Table 3.4 Low cost Indian vegetarian diet

Food composition	*Amount g*	*Protein content g*	*Other nutrients*	
Cereals and Millets	460	46.0	Calories kcal	2736
Pulses (legumes)	40	9.5	Proteins g[b]	65
Green leafy vegetables	50		Calcium mg	781
Other vegetables	60	4.0	Iron mg	17
Roots and tubers	50		Vitamin A µg	715
Fruits[a]	30		Riboflavin mg	1.15
Milk	150	5.7	Thiamine mg	2.45
Fats and oils	40		Vitamin C mg	74.8
Sugar and jaggery	30		Niacin mg	15.7
			Total fat g	67

[a]Additionally included [b]Protein content depends on the type of protein-containing foods.

Source: Nutrient requirements and recommended dietary allowances for Indians 2010. ICMR.

Dietary Guidelines to Reduce the Cost of a Meal

- Cereals, which are less expensive, can be increased to more than the normal amount present in a balanced diet.
- Inclusion of millets like, ragi, jowar and bajra can reduce the cost of meal.
- Big and thick rotis can be prepared to save time and fuel.
- Combination of cereals and pulses improve the quality of cereal as well as pulse protein.
- Pulses like horse gram and cow-pea can be included to reduce the cost of a meal.
- Fermenting, malting and sprouting can enhance the nutritive value without increasing the cost.
- Greens particularly from trees like drumstick or agathi are cheaper.
- Locally available or kitchen garden produce can be used.

- Leaves of cauliflower, carrots, knol khol and beet root which are highly nutritious can become part of a meal. Curry leaves can be used in consumable form like chutneys, chutney powder or in ground form. Greens can be used in all recipes.
- Inexpensive and nutritious fruits like papaya and guava can be included in the diet.
- Inclusion of dry fish (like nethili) may supply good amount of nutrients.
- Broken rice, broken eggs (fresh), left over vegetables and fruits (in the shop at the end of the day), and cheaper cuts of meat can be bought.
- Jaggery can be used instead of sugar.
- Toned milk with low fat is less expensive but gives all the nutrients except fat.
- Steamed foods are less expensive than fried foods. Low cost diets have less amount of fats, oil and sugars.
- Low priced biscuits or buns can be used as snacks in the diet.
- Natural foods are less expensive compared to processed and preserved foods.
- Foodstuffs that are distributed through public distribution system (Ration shops) can be used. In PDS staple cereals and millets are distributed with no cost or little cost.

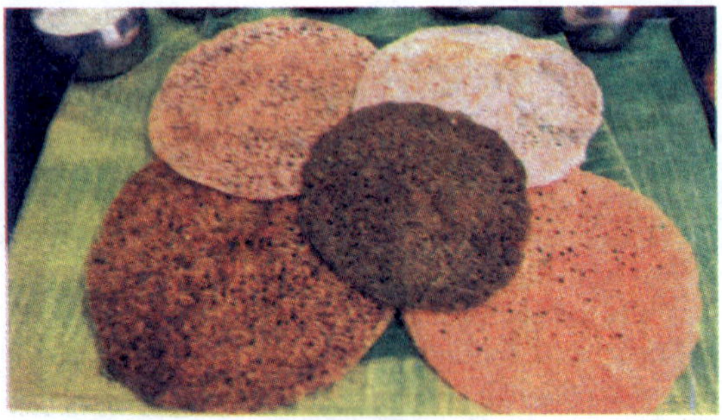

Fig. 3.2 **Millets can not only be incorporated in all indigenous recipes but also in bread biscuits and snacks. Inclusion of millets like ragi, bajra and jowar in the diet helps in meeting the nutritional requirement of protein, fibre and B vitamins. Millets add variety, give satiety, locally available and contribute to the health of an individual. They are less expensive than rice and wheat.**

- Children should participate in Government programmes like midday meal.
- Pregnant and lactating mothers can use 'Sathumavu' (health mix) given at Anganwadis.
- Recipes made at home are cheaper than bought. Home made food can be carried to the workplace instead of buying from the canteen.
- Unbranded foods can be included.
- Inclusion of locally available ingredients and seasonal foods reduce the cost of a meal.

VEGETARIAN DIETS

Vegetarian diets consist of foods of plant origin. The two classic variants are lacto-vegetarian and strict vegetarian or vegan. Vegetarians should include variety of plant foods like whole grains, legumes, nuts and seeds to meet the nutritional requirement. Those whose nutrient needs are especially high due to growth, pregnancy, lactation, or recovery from illness can generally meet their nutrient requirements on well planned vegetarian diet containing dairy products. Vegetarian diet is nutrient dense.

Table 3.5 Classification of vegetarianism

Classification	Foods included	Foods excluded	Limiting nutrients
Semi-vegetarian	Fruits, grains, legumes, nuts, seeds, vegetables, milk, milk products, eggs, chicken, fish	Meat	—
Pesco-vegetarian	Fruits, grains, legumes, nuts, seeds, vegetables, milk, milk products, eggs and fish	Meat	—
Lacto-ovo-vegetarian	Fruits, grains, legumes, nuts, seeds, vegetables, milk, milk products and eggs	Meat	Iron
Lacto-vegetarian	Fruits, grains, legumes, nuts, seeds, vegetables, milk, milk products	Meat and eggs	Iron
Ovo-vegetarian	Fruits, grains, legumes, nuts, seeds, vegetables, and eggs	Meat, milk and milk products	Vitamin D, calcium, riboflavin, iron
Vegan	Fruits, grains, legumes, nuts, seeds, vegetables	Animal food	High quality protein, calories, vitamin D, B-12, and riboflavin, iron and calcium
Macrobiotic	Unrefined/unprocessed grains with smaller amounts of fruits, vegetables and legumes; milk and milk products optional. Some include fish	Meat, eggs, processed foods	Iron, calcium
Fruitarians	Raw fruits, avocado, nuts, seeds and berries	All other foods	Calories, protein, calcium, iron B.vitamins
Raw food diet	Similar to vegan diet and uncooked and unprocessed foods	All cooked and processed foods	Difficult to take for long time and may not meet all nutrient requirements

Recent surveys show that about 30 per cent of Indians are lacto vegetarians, 10 per cent are ovo vegetarians and 60 per cent are nonvegetarians. These surveys have also shown that women are more likely to be vegetarians than men and so are those above the age of 55. In reality in India, most of the population are vegetarians due to economic reasons. There are a number of dietary, religious and moral considerations that may make individuals to follow vegetarian diet.

Vegetarianism is an inherited cultural practice rather than individual belief. Rajasthan, Haryana, Punjab, Uttar Pradesh, Madhya Pradesh and Gujarat have higher percentage of vegetarians. Lowest proportion of vegetarian families are in coastal states such as Kerala, Tamil Nadu, Andhra Pradesh, Orissa and Bengal.

Classifications of vegetarian diet and nutritional adequacy is given in Table 3.5.

Nutritional Considerations

In nature though nutrients are widely distributed, certain nutrients are present only in foods of plant origin and certain other nutrients are present only in animal foods. Table 3.6 gives occurrence of nutrients in plant and animal foods.

Table 3.6 Occurrence of Nutrients in foods of plant and animal origin

Nutrients present only in plant foods	*Nutrients present only in animal foods*
Vitamin C	Good quality protein
Fibre	Good quality calcium
	Haeme iron
	Retinol
	Vitamin D
	Vitamin B_{12}

Energy: Vegetarian diets are low in fat and therefore, often are lower in calories. In addition, these diets are frequently high in fibre and low in energy value. Low-fat vegetarian diets may be too high in bulk. Children on vegetarian diets get satiety before consuming adequate calories. Encouraging frequent meals and snacks and including full fat milk may provide additional calories.

Protein: Essential amino acid requirements can be met by consuming a variety of plant protein sources with the optimal addition of dairy products or eggs. Cereals are low in lysine, threonine and some in tryptophan. Pulses are limited in sulphur containing amino acids like methionine. Nuts like peanuts are low in methionine, lysine and threonine.

Over the course of a day, consumption of various protein rich plant foods create a pool of essential amino acids that can be used for protein synthesis. Vegans can include soya products and nuts to increase calorie and protein value.

Vegetarian athletes should consume adequate calories to prevent protein being used for energy. Plant based protein requirements for athletes are estimated to be 1.0–1.7 g per kg body weight, with a little more during the training period. The increased requirements can be met by plant proteins.

ω-3 fatty acids: α-linolenic acid is present in eggs, fish and algae but also found in green leafy vegetables, flax seeds, rape seed, soybean and walnuts. In vegetarian diets, the primary source of ω-3 fatty acids is from the conversion of the essential fatty acid α-linolenic acid to eicosapentaenoic acid (EPA) and docosahexaenoic acid (DHA). But this conversion efficiency is low. DHA and EPA may reduce risk of developing cardiovascular diseases. Pregnant and lactating mothers need more ω-3 fatty acids. Vegeterians should include in their diet flax seed, walnuts and soybean.

Calcium: Lacto vegetarians get calcium from milk and milk products. Vegans, those who do not use dairy products, should include nondairy calcium sources. Foods like ragi, greens and gingelly seeds are good in calcium but bioavailability of calcium is less due to the presence of oxalates and phytates. Pregnant women, lactating mothers, children and post menopausal women need to take dairy products to meet increased requirements of calcium. Vegans may need to take calcium supplements.

Though calcium intakes of many vegetarians are below the Daily Recommended Intake, this may not necessarily result in health problems. This may be attributed to enhanced absorption and retention of calcium, in addition, the lower protein intakes of vegetarians are associated with decreased urinary excretion of calcium.

Iron: Vegetarian diets are generally higher in iron content than nonvegetarian diets. But iron stores are lower in vegetarians because the iron from plant foods is poorly absorbed. Inorganic iron binds to phytates, tannins and phosphates in plant foods and these may have an inhibitory effect on iron absorption. Soaking, sprouting and fermenting diminish phytate levels and thereby enhance iron absoption. Fibre binds iron and reduce the amount absorbed. Fibre also stimulates the passage of food through the GI tract, further reducing the absorption. Haeme iron which is more easily absorbed by the body is found in animal tissues. On the other hand, vegetarian diets provide ample quantities of vitamin C which is known to enhance the absorption of iron.

There is evidence that adaptation to low quality intake of iron takes place over the long term. Adaptation involves both the increased absorption and decreased losses. Incidence of iron deficiency anaemeia among vegetarians is similar to that of nonvegetarians.

Zinc: The best dietary sources of zinc are animal products like meat, poultry, eggs and oysters. Plant foods like nuts, seeds and whole cereals also contain zinc. The bioavailability of zinc may be diminished by the presence of phytic acid, oxalates and fibre. Soaking, sprouting and fermenting increase bioavailability of zinc. Although slightly lower levels of plasma zinc have been found in those following vegetarian diets, there is no significant effect on the health and growth of individuals. The vegan diet has the potential to be low in zinc.

Iodine: Plant based diets are typically low in iodine. Vegetarians who do not consume sea food, should take iodized salt.

Vitamin A: Only foods of animal origin have retinol. Plant foods contain carotene which can be converted to vitamin A in the body. The conversion efficiency is better with β-carotene. β-carotene also acts as phytochemical. It is present in yellow orange fruits and vegetables.

Vitamin D: Vitamin D is present only in foods of animal origin. Vegetarians need to expose themselves to sunlight or need to take supplementation of vitamin D. The requirement can be met by fortified foods like milk and oil. Vitamin D is essential for the absorption of calcium.

Folic acid: Folate is higher in vegetarian diets due to greater use of greens, vegetables and fruits.

Vitamin B_{12}: Plant sources do not contain vitamin B_{12}. Vitamin B_{12} is produced by micro-organisms and the requirement is met by fermented foods and by contamination. Vegans should ensure that they meet the requirement of vitamin B_{12} by taking fermented foods or fortified foods. Absorption of vitamin B_{12} decreases with age. Elderly vegetarians should take vitamin B_{12} supplement orally or intramuscularly. Deficiency causes pernicious anaemia.

Vitamin C: Ascorbic acid occurs in plant foods particularly in fruits and vegetables. Foods of animal origin do not contain vitamin C.

Fibre: Vegetarian diets are rich in fibre and low in energy. Vegetarians consume greater amounts of fibre from whole grains, fruits and vegetables. Vegetarian diets result in less gastrointestinal transit time, bulkier stools and low serum cholesterol levels. Fibre also reduces the absorption of trace minerals and other nutrients. Fibre is present only in foods of plant origin.

Vegetarians diet can be healthful and nutritionally adequate if a variety of foods are consumed. Vegetarian diets require special consideration for energy, iron, calcium, zinc, vitamin D, vitamin B_{12} and the ω-3 fatty acids.

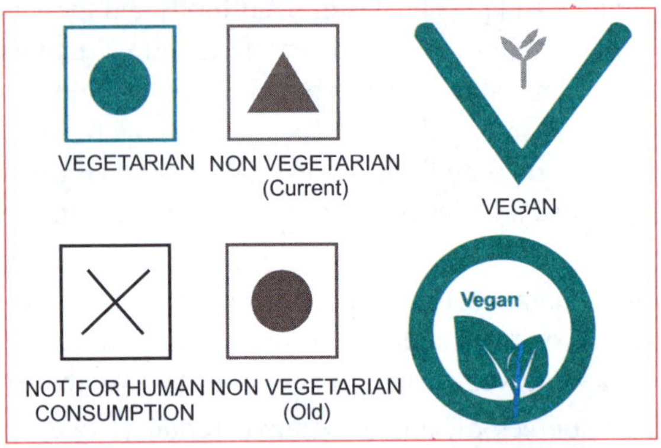

Fig. 3.3 All packed foods should have prescribed logos.

> ***His last meal***
>
> A combination of medical care and self care is the only route to health. On the day of death, Mahatma Gandhi was 5.5′ tall and weighed 109 pounds. His BMI was ideal.
>
> His last meal comprised of a bowl of cooked vegetables, 350 ml of goat's milk, four ripe tomatoes, four oranges, one glass of raw carrot juice and finally a small glass of decoction of ginger, sour lime and aloe.

Health Benefits

In the past 30 years, scientific endeavours found that there exists relationship between vegetarian diet and various medical conditions particularly in the prevention of degenerative diseases. Populations of vegetarians living in affluent countries appear to enjoy unusually good health, characterized by low rates of cancer, cardiovascular disease and mortality.

Although the dietary sources of vegetarians are not necessarily unique, the removal of meat as a major source of energy does create an opportunity for larger consumption of plant foods.

Obesity: Since vegetarian diets are low in calories and high in fibre, there is less chance to become obese. Usually BMI is low for vegetarians.

Heart diseases: In addition to being devoid of cholesterol, a vegetarian diet is usually low in fat. Most of the vegetarian diets can be prepared palatably with very little oil. Vegetarians tend to have lower rate of hypertension than nonvegetarians. The incidence of heart disease and related deaths is much lower among vegetarians than meat eaters.

A low fat vegetarian diet free from animal products reduces serum cholesterol, blood pressure and risk of cardiovascular disease. An unrefined plant-based diet may be effective for reducing risk factors for cardiovascular disease. In lactovegetarian diet the legumes namely red gram and black gram, wheat, parboiled rice and milk provide selenium, an antioxidant which decreases the risk of CHD. Intake of vitamin E from food sources protect against nonfatal coronary heart disease. Vegetarians tend to have lower BMI and have normal blood pressure.

Table 3.7 Lacto-vegetarian diet - Limitations and solutions.

Nutrient	*Limitations*	*Solutions*
Protein	Generally biological value of plant protein is not high.	Protein requirement can be met by including a variety of plant foods. Energy requirement should be met so that protein need not be used for energy purpose. Quality of protein can be improved by adding good quality protein like milk or by complementary value of protein. Cereals tend to be low in lysine by including soya bean and legumes the quality of protein can be improved.
	Lacto-vegetarians require more protein as they are less well digested and absorbed.	Quality and quantity of protein should be improved.
ω-3 fatty acids	Present only in limited foods like walnuts, flax seeds and soya bean.	DHA supplements derived from microalgae or ω-3 fatty acids are taken when the requirements are increased like in pregnancy and lactation.
Calcium	Lacto vegetarians get similar amount as nonvegetarians. A high sodium intake can increase urinary calcium losses.	Sodium content of the diet is to be reduced.
	Diet rich in meat, fish dairy products, nuts and grains produce high renal acid load increasing bone resorption and urinary losses.	Fruits and vegetables rich in potassium and magnesium produce a high alkaline load and slows bone resorption.
	In lacto vegetarian diet the ratio of dietary calcium to protein is better predictor of bone health than calcium intake alone.	Oxalate and phylate for rich-foods should be restricted.
Iron	Vegetarian diet has inhibitors of iron absorption like phytates, calcium and polyphenolics in tea coffee and cocoa.	Soaking sprouting beans and seeds diminish phytate levels and thereby enhance iron absorption. Inclusion of vitamin C rich fruits increases iron absorption.
Zinc	Bioavailability is low due to higher phytic acid content	Soya products, legumes, grains, cheese and nuts to be included in the diet. Soaking and sprouting beans, grains and seeds reduce binding capacity of zinc to phytic acid.
Vitamin D	Plant origin foods do not contain vitamin D.	By exposing to ultra violet rays one can get vitamin D. Fortified foods like milk, fruit juice and oils contribute to vitamin requirement.
Vitamin B_{12}	No plant food contains vitamin B_{12}	Fermented foods and B_{12} fortified foods should be consumed.

Vegetarian diets contain phytochemical like flavonoids which have protective effects as antioxidants. They reduce platelet aggregation and blood clotting as anti-inflammatory agents and improve endothelial function.

Increased fruit consumption has been associated with reduced risk of both coronary artery disease and cerebrovascular disease.

Cancer: Vegetarians have a significantly lower rate of cancer than the general population. Lactovegetarian diet is a low risk diet for colon and oesophageal cancer. Capsaicin, the principal component of capsicum possess chemo preventive properties that may be antimutagenic and anticarcinogenic. High consumption of tomato is protective for both prostate enlargement and prostate cancer.

Studies conducted at Tata Memorial Hospital, Mumbai showed that a vegetarian is found to be protective for oesophageal cancer. There is a positive association of prostate cancer with animal but not vegetable fat consumption.

Red meat consumption, particularly in high amounts is associated with colon cancer and possibly prostate cancer. People with colon cancer seem to eat more meat, more saturated fat and fewer vegetables than others without cancer. Instead of red meat, white meat and legumes can be consumed.

One of the most consistent observations has been an association between consumption of dairy products and prostate cancer.

Other diseases: In general, the incidence of, or the death rate from type 2 diabetes tends to be lower among vegetarians who consume unrefined grains.

Reduced risk of macular degeneration and cataract have been observed with increased intakes of certain vegetables. Folic acid deficiency causing neural tube defect is common among western population due to lack of consumption of fruits and vegetables.

Potential health-promoting benefits of vegetarian diet is due to the presence of nutrients and phytochemicals.

Research also suggests that vegetarians have lowered risk of type 2 diabetes, gallstones, atonic constipation, dementia and stroke. Disease protection may be due to lowered intake of sodium, saturated fat, cholesterol and animal protein. They also consume usually high amounts of fibre, folic acid, antioxidants such as vitamin C and E. carotenoids and phytochemicals. Enhanced health in vegetarians may be due to better life style including increased physical activity, lower Body Mass Index (BMI) and abstinence from alcohol and decreased use of tobacco products.

Both plant based and meat based diets can be detrimental to health when overloaded with fat, sugar and salt.

Vegan diets

Vegan diet is plant based diet excluding all animal products like milk, curd and meat. Vegan diet is taken for religious reasons or to reduce weight. Vegan diet can be healthful if proper choices are made.

Vegan diets are typically higher in dietary fibre, folic acid, vitamin C and E, iron and phytochemicals and tend to be lower in calories, saturated fat, ω-3 fatty acids, vitamin D, calcium and zinc and lack cholestrol and vitamin B_{12} as these two nutrients are found only in animal foods. The low saturated fat content of vegan diet might contribute to lower risk of cardiovascular diseases.

Vegans should aim to consume 80 to 100 grams of good quality vegetable proteins from foods such as soya, nuts, legumes and cereals.

The body mass index of vegans is considerably lower than that of non-vegetarians and lacto ovo-vegetarians. Vegan diet is an important protective factor for lowering cancer risk.

To avoid B_{12} deficiency, all vegans must regularly consume vitamin B_{12} fortified foods or should take B_{12} supplements. Foods like green leafy vegetables and gingelly seeds contain calcium but calcium present in them is not bio available. Vitamin D supplementation should be taken regularly during winter season.

Vegan diet must contain whole grains, brown rice, quinoa, millets, and beans. Soya bean can be consumed in the form of tofu, textured vegetable protein like soya chunks, okara, soya cheese, soya sauce, soya yoghurt, tempeh.

Vegans have a relatively high intake of dietary iron and their mean ferritin concentrations are significantly lower than those of nonvegetarians. Lower ferritin concentrations are associated with a lower risk of heart disease.

In conclusion, one needs to understand that by eating a particular food or by not eating a food, one cannot balance the diet. There is no substitute for balanced diet. One needs to follow the principles of balanced diet throughout life. The advantage of proven phytochemicals can be felt only when all the principles of life style are followed.

The diet which is not good for health:

- too high in total fat, saturated fat, *trans* fat and cholesterol
- too high in sodium and sugar
- too high in processed foods and food that give only empty calories
- too high in snack foods, junk foods and refined flours
- too low in antioxidants
- too low in fibre and fluid
- too low in α linolenic acid and
- too low in protein, minerals and vitamins.

Thus diet planning needs to follow the principles of adequacy, balance and moderation.

Food and nutrition professionals must continue to educate the public about the importance of balanced diets, eating a nourishing breakfast, including variety of foods promoting family meals and home availability of healthful foods.

November 1st is World Vegan day.

The United Nations has declared 2023 as the International year of millets.

SUGGESTED READINGS

- Arlappa N, *et al.*, "Consumption Pattern of Pulses, Vegetables and Nutrients Among Rural Population in India". Nutrition News. National Institute of Nutrition 2011; 32.
- Craig John Winston Nutrition concerns and health effects among vegetarian diets. Nutrition in Clinical Practice 2010; 25.
- Sharon Palmer, "No meat no problem", Today's Dietitian, 2010.
- 5 a Day for Better Health, www.5aday.com.

CHAPTER 3

QUESTIONS

1. Define Indian reference man and reference woman and bring out the importance of it.
2. Give RDA suggested by ICMR (2020) for a male executive.
3. Give RDA suggested by ICMR for female servant.
4. Why a balanced diet should contain functional foods?
5. Give ICMR dietary guidelines for an adult man.
6. Bring out importance of including millets in the diet.
7. Calculate the cost and nutritive value of low cost balanced diet suggested by ICMR and give your comments.
8. Describe any five methods to reduce the cost of a meal.
9. Give the classification of vegetarian diets.
10. Discuss advantages and disadvantages of taking lacto vegetarian diet and ovo-lactovegetarian diet.
11. Describe special advantages of taking nonvegetarian diet.
12. What is vegan diet? Explain the limitations of this diet.
13. Explain diet for shift workers.

TOPICS FOR ACTIVITY

- Plan and prepare a low cost balanced diet for an adult woman who is moderately active.
- Plan and prepare a millet based balanced diet for adult man who is doing heavy work.
- Plan and prepare non vegetarian diet for an adult man doing sedentary work.
- Plan and prepare vegan diet for a middle aged woman.

4

Nutritional Recommendations and Food Requirements of Infants

GROWTH AND DEVELOPMENT DURING INFANCY

Next to foetal period, the infant's first year is the time of most rapid growth. According to WHO figures the average weight of most healthy new born babies is around 3.2 kg. Healthy child doubles his birth weight by six months. His weight becomes three times by the time the child is one year old. The normal birth length of 50 to 55 cm increases by another 23 to 25 cm during the first year. With increase in length the body proportions also change.

At birth the child has 75 per cent water and 12–15 per cent fat. By the end of one year the water content decreases to 60 per cent and fat increases to 24 per cent. Muscles would be comparatively well developed at the end of the year.

Infants have rapid heart rate, 120–140 per minute. At birth the haemoglobin level of a well nourished infant is 17–20 g per 100 ml. This provides a reserve for expansion of the blood circulation and adequate oxygen-carrying capacity to the growing tissues during the first 4–6 months.

The full-term infant is able to digest protein, emulsified fats and simple carbohydrates such as lactose. Salivary secretion and gastric acidity are low in infants under three months.

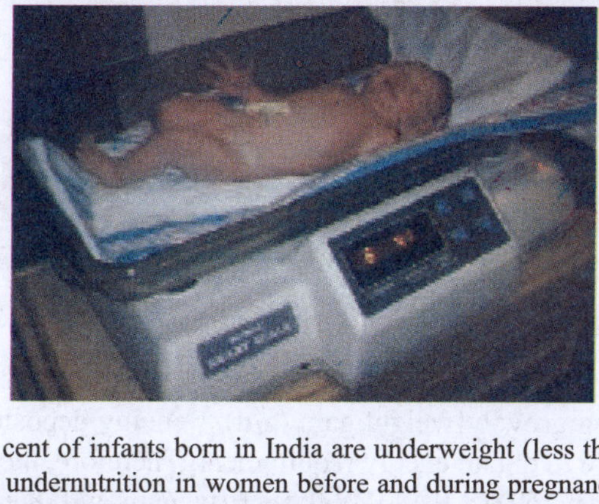

Nearly 30 per cent of infants born in India are underweight (less than 2.5 kg) due to undernutrition in women before and during pregnancy.

Fig. 4.1 Average weight of healthy new born baby is around 3.2 kg.

Kidneys reach their full functional capacity by the end of first year. During the first few months the glomerular filtration rate is somewhat lower and therefore the excretion of high concentration of solutes is more difficult. The increase in the number of brain cells is most rapid during foetal life and in the first 5-6 months after birth.

As per Barker's hypothesis, most of the chronic adult diseases have origins in foetal stages or in early life.

NUTRITIONAL RECOMMENDATIONS

As growth during infancy is very rapid, dietary adaptation is required. During early infancy, much of the nutrient requirements are met by breast feeding and the RDA of an infant is based on composition of breast milk. Growth standards are established based on the growth of children who are fed breast milk. Table 4.1 gives the RDA for infant suggested by ICMR in 2020.

Table 4.1 ICMR Recommended Dietary Allowances for infants–2020

Nutrient	*Months*	
	0–6	*6–12*
Body weight kg	5.8	8.5
Energy kcal	530	680
Protein g	8.0	10.5
Dietary Fibre g	–	–
Calcium mg	–	300 AI*
Magnesium mg	30	75
Iron mg	–	3
Zinc mg	–	2.5
Iodine μg	100	130
Vitamin A retinol μg	350	350
Vitamin D IU	400	400
Thiamine mg	0.2	0.4
Riboflavin mg	0.4	0.6
Niacin mg	2	5
Pyridoxine mg	0.1	0.6
Folate μg	25	85
Vitamin B_{12} μg	1.2	1.2
Vitamin C mg	20	30

*AI-Adequate Intake.

Energy

Energy deposition during growth [weight gain (g/d) × energy deposited/g] has to be added to Total Energy Expenditure to obtain energy requirement. Therefore, the total energy requirement during infancy (kcal/d) = [–152.0 + 92.8 BW (kg)] + [wt gain (g/d) × energy deposited (kcal/g)]. Using the new child growth standards, the energy requirements for infants are 98 kcal/kg/d for 0-6 months and 80 kcal/kg/d for 6-12 months. The adult requires 32 kcal/kg/d.

Protein

Protein intake of healthy infants is about 1.16 g/kg body weight. The recommendations for infants are based on the total protein content and amino acid pattern of the average daily intake of human milk. Like calories, infants' protein requirements per kg body weight are higher compared to adults due to increased demands for skeletal and muscle growth. Human milk provides all the amino acids more than the required amount needed for proper growth. Histidine, which is a non-essential amino acid for adults, is necessary for growth and maintenance of an infant. The requirement for essential amino acids are affected by the amounts of protein sparing nutrients and the ratio of essential and non-essential amino acids in the diet. Human milk protein is 100 per cent utilised. Protein content of human milk is 1.1 g/100 ml or 6 per cent total energy. Protein requirement per kg body weight decreases gradually during the first 12 months as do energy requirements.

Excess protein is harmful as it needs to be deaminated. Since the infant has a limited capacity to concentrate waste metabolites, such as urea in the urine, the excretion of more wastes requires a larger volume of water. If the necessary water is not available, urea gets accumulated and ironically the infant will suffer from protein oedema. Higher rate of infection is common in infants fed on cow's milk because the mechanism related to formation of antibodies to protect against infections are diverted to take care of excess milk protein.

Fat and Essential Fatty Acids

The adequate intake of α linolenic acid for infants 0–6 months is 0.2–0.3% and 6–12 months is 0.4–0.6%.

Fat content of human milk is relatively constant at 3–4 per cent by weight and delivers 50–60% E.

Fat intake should be reduced to 35% E gradually, depending on the physical activity of the child from the age 6 months to 2 years. The mix of fat from breast milk and complementary foods should provide infants with at least 3–4% E from LA and 0.4 to 0.6% E ALA. Twenty five grams visible fat is recommended in diet of young children assumming 10% E fat from breast milk and infant formula + fat from complementary foods (except visible fat). It would also ensure adequate supply and absorption of fat soluble vitamins.

Calcium and Phosphorus

With mean intake of breast milk at 700 ml for first six months and 600 ml for the next six months, the recommended adequate intake of 300 mg of calcium and 450 of phosphorus is enough to meet the requirement of both age groups of infants.

Rapid growth requires 300 mg of calcium and 450 mg of phosphorus with a ratio 1 : 1.5. Adequate prenatal nutrition supplies a store of bone minerals to prevent rickets provided post-natal care furnishes a liberal supply of calcium and phosphorus. Large percentage of calcium from breast milk is retained by the infant. Bones are poorly calcified at birth. Rapid rate of calcification of bone is needed to support the weight of body by the time the baby walks. When sufficient calcium is not supplied to the infant, his motor development is delayed. Ca : P ratio of 1.2 : 1 as in cow's milk is lower compared to 2 : 1 in human milk. High phosphorus can lead to hypocalcaemic neonatal tetany.

Iron

RDA of iron for an infant is 3 mg for 6–12 months. At birth, body contains 80 mg/kg. This is about three times that of an adult. During the first four months, the baby's blood volume doubles and concentration of iron in haemoglobin falls to about half that present at birth. That is why infant doubles his birth weight by six months without depending on dietary iron. There is no reserve store of iron after 6 months. Iron requirements increase markedly especially in relation to body size and energy intake during latter 6 months of life. Therefore iron-enriched solid foods should complement breast milk from 7–12 months of age. There is no reserve store of iron. Low birth weight infant requires dietary iron earlier in life. Premature infants are susceptible to anaemia as there is not enough storage of iron.

Zinc

High levels are present in colostrum and it promotes normal growth. Zinc is necessary for normal brain development. ICMR Expert Group (2020) has suggested 2.5 mg of RDA of zinc for infants. 6–12 months.

Sodium

Mature human milk, contains 7 mmol/L. Cow's milk contains 21 mmol/L. Infant needs 4–8 mmol/d. Intake of sodium by breast fed infant is less than 1/3rd that of one fed on cow's milk. The smaller amount present in human milk is considered adequate.

Iodine

Infants from 0.6 months require 100 μg of iodine. Breast milk gives 90 μg/d. And 6–12 months infants require 130 μg/day.

Vitamin A

The RDA for retinol is 350 μg. The amount of vitamin A content of breast milk is sufficient, provided mothers' diet is rich in vitamin A. Daily intake of vitamin A by Indian infants through breast milk is about 140 μg during the first six months of life. Rest of the requirement is met by reserves. A healthy infant has sufficient store of vitamin A in liver at birth which may last for six months. After six months egg yolk is supplemented in the infants'diet.

Vitamin D

It is essential for utilization and retention of calcium and phosphorus. Neither human nor cow's milk provides enough vitamin D to prevent rickets. A good supply of vitamin D during pregnancy benefits the mother and helps satisfactory development of the infant. The requirement may be obtained in great measure in tropical countries through exposure to adequate sunlight.

ICMR-20 20 has suggested 400 IU or 10 μg vitamin D for infants.

Vitamin K

The newborns are susceptible to haemorrhage caused by lack of vitamin K. Breast-fed baby is more susceptible than artificially fed. Deficiency of vitamin K in children can occur if mothers have received anticoagulants. A single dose of 1 mg of water miscible form of vitamin K immediately after birth is considered adequate in premature newborn infants to prevent haemorrhage. Excess dosage is harmful.

Vitamin B Complex

Thiamine requirement of infants less than 6 months of age is generally computed from the quantity available through breast milk of healthy well nourished mothers. Assuming thiamine content 20 μg/100 ml and secretion of breast milk 700 ml, the RDA for infants 0–6 months is 0.3 mg/1000 kcal or 0.2 mg/day.

ICMR 2020 has suggested an adequate intake of riboflavin 0.4 mg/d for 0-6 months and 0.6 mg/d for 6-12 months. It has recommended adequate intake of niacin 2 mg and 5 mg for 0-6 months and 6-12 months children respectively.

The vitamin B_6 content of Indian mothers' milk is 60–80 μg/l. At this level, no deficiency of B_6 is found in children.

Vitamin C

The RDA prescribed by ICMR (2020) is 20–30 mg. Human milk contains twice the ascorbic acid in comparison to cow's milk though both are not good sources of vitamin C. Deficiency in mothers during pregnancy and lactation results in very little reserve of vitamin C in body. If less vitamin C is present in breast milk the infant may develop scurvy. Suddenly the body swells due to internal bleeding and the condition is fatal.

Fruit juice should be introduced in sufficient amounts in the diet from the 4th month onwards to prevent vitamin C deficiency.

Nutritional Assessment

Each individual serves as his or her own control in the measurement of progress. Weight, length, head circumference, skin fold thickness and haemoglobin level can be used to assess the nutritional status. Eruption of teeth is complete by the end of first year. Healthy child has normal elimination and is active and sleeps well.

Studies conducted at National Institute of Nutrition showed that growth rate of infants upto one year is influenced to a large extent by the birth weight.

FOOD REQUIREMENTS

The word Nutrition is derived from 'nutricus' which means to 'suckle at the breast'. Breast milk is the natural food for the infant. Successful breast feeding is an important child rearing skill to be learnt and practiced. Breast feeding is a biological norm.

BREAST FEEDING

The infant should be put to breast within half an hour after normal delivery and within four hours after caesarian sections. Prelacteal foods like honey, distilled water or glucose should not be given. These foods will satisfy the thirst and will reduce the vigour to suck and may lead to diarrhoea and helminthic infestation. Breast feeding can be initiated even when the mother is sedated or on IV fluids. Sucking reflex is most active at birth.

Colostrum: During the first two or three days after delivery, thick and yellowish fluid is secreted from the mammary gland. This differs from the mature milk and is called colostrum. It is secreted in small quantity of about 10–40 ml. It is rich in protein. The total fat content of colostrum is less than mature milk. Concentration of arachidonic acid and docosahexaenoic acid (DHA) as per cent of total fatty acids is higher in colostrum than mature milk. It has more amount of vitamin A and K. The concentration of lactose is less. The levels of niacin, pantothenic acid, biotin and riboflavin are also low. Vitamin C is secreted at about the same level as in mature milk. Zinc content of colostrum is 20 mg/l whereas mature milk has 2.6 mg/l. The composition of colostrum is given in Table 4.2.

Table 4.2 Nutritive value of colostrum, transitional milk and mature milk g 100 ml

	Fat	*Protein*	*Lactose*
Colostrum	1.83 to 4.49	1.54 to 8.36	4.5 to 6.47
Transitional milk	2.6 to 5.59	1.08 to 2.38	4.8 to 7.37
Mature milk	2.77 to 4.78	0.87 to 2.33	6.78 to 7.7

Apart from methodological factors, human milk is known to be influenced by maternal nutritional status, dietary intake, socioeconomic status and regional variation.

Source: Khanna Deepti et al. Century wide changes in macronutrient levels in Indian mother's milk: A systematic reviews MDPI Nutrients 2022; **14**.

Colostrum is the first immunisation to the infant. It contains an interferon like substance which possesses strong antiviral activity. Colostrum contains B_{12} binding protein which renders B_{12} unavailable for the growth of E. Coli and other bacteria. It also contains antibodies against viral diseases such as small pox, polio, measles and influenza. Enzymes like lysozyme, peroxidase and xanthine oxidase that promote cell maturation are found to be more in colostrum. Colostrum contains large quantities of protective substances and enhances the development and maturation of the baby's gastrointestinal tract. Colostrum helps a baby pass his or her first stool and help in the excretion of excess bilirubin and prevent jaundice.

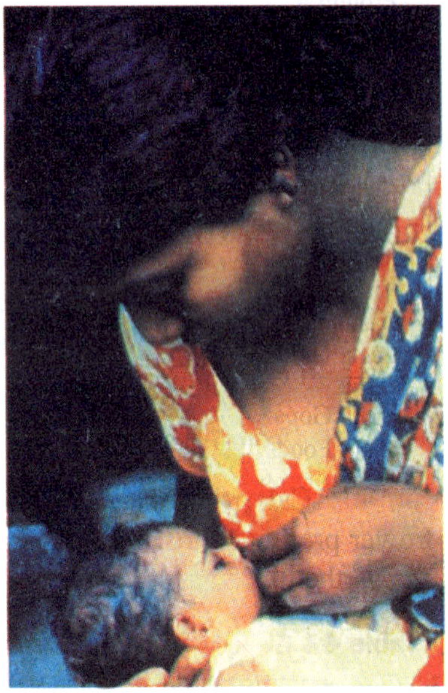

Fig. 4.2 Colostrum should be given within half an hour of birth. Swabbing inside of the infant's cheeks with colostrum helps to bring down infections.

Transition milk: During the next two weeks, the milk increases in quantity and changes in appearance and composition. This is called transition milk. The immunoglobulin and protein content decreases while the fat and sugar content increases. Exclusive breast feeding of colostrum and transition milk minimises infection related to neonatal deaths.

The composition of milk changes even during the length of a single feed to exactly suit the need of a particular baby.

Foremilk: The milk that comes at the start of a feed is called foremilk. Foremilk which is watery has a low level of fat and is high in lactose sugar, protein, vitamins, minerals and water. It satisfies the baby's thirst.

Hindmilk: Hindmilk which comes later in a feed, is richer in fat. It satisfies the baby's hunger and supplies more energy than foremilk. Babies who are fed fore and hind milk sleep well and grow healthy.

There is no tailor made schedule for breast feeding, as milk production, sucking habits and stomach capacity vary from infant to infant. A few days after the initiation of breast feeding, the length of each feed and the interval between two feeds will automatically get regularised. Exclusive breast feeding for the first six months gives a baby best start to life. No water or supplementary food is given during this period.

Advantages of Breast Feeding

Breast feeding is not only beneficial to the infant but also to the mother. The advantages of breast feeding can be considered under nutritional, immunological, psychological, economical and physiological and other factors.

Nutritional benefits

The composition of human milk is best suited to the infants and provides nutrients in easily digestible and bioavailable form. Table 4.3 shows the comparative data of human milk with cow's and buffalo's milk.

Table 4.3 Comparison of human milk with cow's and buffalo's milk (Values per 100 g)

Nutrient	*Human milk*	*Cow's milk*	*Buffalo's milk*
Water g	88	87.5	81
Energy kcal	65	67	117
Protein g	1.1	3.2	4.3
Carbohydrate g	7.4	4.4	5
Fat g	3.4	4.1	6.5
Calcium mg	28	120	210
Phosphorus mg	11	90	130
Iron mg	—	0.2	0.2
β-Carotene/Carotene μg	41	53	48
Thiamine mg	0.02	0.05	0.04
Riboflavin mg	0.02	0.19	0.1
Vitamin C mg	3	2	1
Caseinogen and Lactalbumin ratio	1:2	3:1	—

Source: Gopalan C., B.V. Ramasastri and S.C. Balasubramanian (Reprinted 2011), Nutritive Value of Indian Foods, National Institute of Nutrition, ICMR, Hyderabad, India.

Energy: Calorie value of human milk and cow's milk are similar as is the total fat content. Lower protein content of human milk is compensated by higher amount of lactose. Table 4.4 shows the percentage calories from protein, fat and carbohydrate in human and cow's milk.

Table 4.4 Calorie percentage from protein, fat and carbohydrate in human and cow's milk

Nutrient	*Human milk*	*Cow's milk*
Total energy (per 100 ml)	65	67
Protein	7	19
Fat	47	55
Carbohydrates	31	26

From Table 4.4 it is clear that human milk protein calorie per cent is less than cow's milk whereas carbohydrate calorie per cent is higher in human milk. Ideally for an infant 6 per cent of calories should come from protein. Fat content in human milk is comparatively less. It is advantageous, as it is absorbed easily.

In first 24 hours, glycogen is used for energy. Later on, glucose and fatty acid from the diet or from body fat stores are used up. Free fatty acids are released from triglycerides by lipase which is present in human milk. These are preferred source of energy for the infant's heart, throughout the sucking period. The switch over to fatty acid calls for a source of carnitine to transport fatty acid within the cell. Newborns do not have a fully developed ability to synthesise carnitine and they must obtain it from breast milk or from formulas where carnitine is added. Carnitine is absent in cow's milk.

Carbohydrate: Human milk is the sweetest milk due to the high amount of lactose. Lactose which is present in higher levels in human milk facilitates the absorption of magnesium and calcium and favours amino acid absorption and nitrogen retention. Galactose is present only in milk and is essential for the formation of myelin, which in turn is essential for the normal nerve function. Myelin is a protective sheath that surrounds the nerve fibre and protects their ability to transmit nerve messages. High content of galacto lipids promotes rapid brain growth of infant. Lactose promotes synthesis of cerebrosides in the brain. Lactose which is least soluble cannot be added to milk at home. Lactose is added in commercial formulas. Sucrose if added may cause gastrointestinal distress in infants. Human milk contains a salivary enzyme-like amylase which helps in digesting lactose at a stage in life when little or no pancreatic amylase is produced.

Protein: Human milk contains 1.1 g per cent protein. The protein content in cow's milk is three times more than that in human milk. However, it is biochemically different and less digestible.

Human milk has 20 per cent β-casein and 80 per cent whey proteins which constitute lactalbumin and lactoferrin. Cow's milk has 80 per cent α-casein and 20 per cent whey proteins which constitute lactoglobulin. This lactoglobulin is one of the causes of intolerance to cow's milk. β-lactoglobulin which is an allergen is absent in human milk.

Lactalbumin has an amino acid pattern that mainly approaches that of body protein and provides more essential aminoacids than does casein. Among the amino acids, glutamic acid is maximum and glycine is absent in human milk.

Casein forms a firm curd with rennin and lactalbumin forms a soft flocculent curd that is most rapidly digested and absorbed by the infant.

Human milk with its low protein and solute load is suitable for immature kidney, for the slower somatic growth in the baby and for rapid brain growth in the first year of life. Breast milk contains amino acids specific for brain development. It is rich in sulphur containing amino acids and cysteine to methionine ratio is high. This compensates for low cysteine methionine conversion which is essential for central nervous system development. Taurine is an important neurotransmitter and neuromodulator for brain and retina. Taurine is present in large amounts in human milk compared to cow's milk.

Human milk offers a high tryptophan to neutral amino acids ratio which controls brain serotonin synthesis. Human milk also contains binding proteins of thyroxine, corticosterol, vitamin D, folate and B_{12}.

Even though protein content is low in human milk, non-protein nitrogen content is high and net nitrogen content is comparable to cow's milk. The non-protein nitrogens in human milk are urea, amino acids, peptides, nucleic acids, N-acetyl glutamine and N-acetyl neuraminic acid.

Presence of protein splitting enzymes in breast milk reduces protein to the less complex peptone stage, on which digestive enzymes act more effectively. These enzymes in cow's milk are destroyed by the heat of pasteurisation.

Lipids: Lipids present in human milk are unsaturated fat, essential fatty acids, prostaglandin precursors, fat soluble vitamins, steroids, phospholipid and cholesterol.

Infants have only a limited ability to convert α-linolenic acid to eicosapentaenoic acid (EPA) and docosahexaenoic acid (DHA) but these are present in human milk. Human milk has arachidonic acid content of about 0.5 per cent and DHA content of about 0.3 per cent of

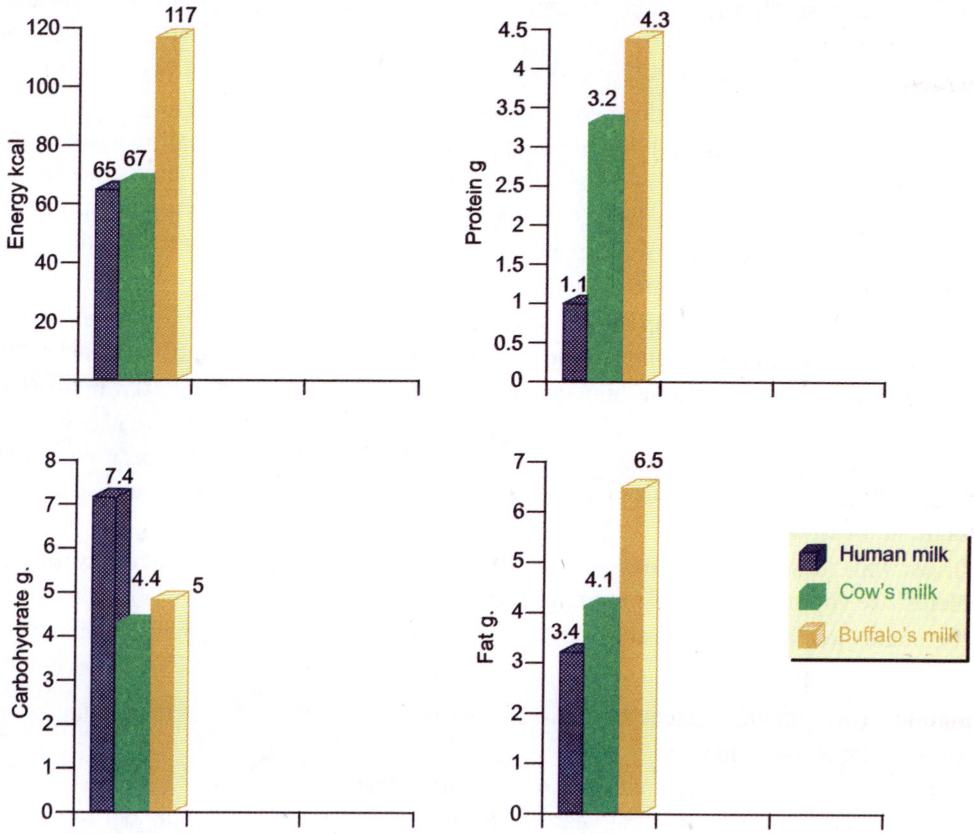

Fig. 4.3 Comparison of nutrients of human, cow's and buffalo's milk

total fatty acids. In cow's milk and infant formula, on the other hand, EPA and DHA are either absent or present at low levels.

Lipids involved in the development of brain are mostly long chain polyunsaturated fatty acids. These are abundant in breast milk. DHA is important for neural division. Breast fed infants may have an enhanced mental development with 5–6 IQ point difference, improved visual acuity and attention and a better neural development during childhood and adolescence in comparison to those fed formula devoid of long chain PUFAs. If mother's intake of fish is increased, the level of EPA and DHA in milk can be increased. Type of fat present in human milk depends on dietary fat of the mother.

Human milk also has high carnitine content which increases metabolism by mitochondrial oxidation and transport of essential fatty acid. Human milk contains cholesterol and is essential for the synthesis of myelin of the nervous system. Presence of choline, acetylcholine, phospholipid precursors and carnitine ensure optimum metabolism and brain development. Carnitine levels are low in pre-term babies.

Breast milk meets the essential fatty acid needs of infants which is about 6 en%. The polyunsaturated to saturated fat ratio is 1.2 : 1 in breast milk, compared to 1:2 in cow's milk.

The increase in the fat content of human milk from the beginning of feeding to the end is believed to increase its satiety value. This makes the breast fed infant to regulate caloric intake and weight gain.

Minerals: Unlike vitamins, mineral content of human milk is minimally influenced by the mother's stores and immediate intake of calcium, magnesium, phosphorus, iron, copper, zinc, sodium and potassium. Minerals in breast milk are largely protein bound and balanced to enhance bioavailability.

Calcium content in human milk is 28 mg and in cow's milk 120 mg. Though the calcium content of human milk is 1/4th of cow's milk, calcium phosphorus ratio of 2:1 in human milk is favourable. Infantile tetany rarely occurs in breast-fed infants.

Low sodium content of human milk is advantageous to the infant as kidneys have difficulty in handling excess sodium. Sodium content of milk is influenced by diet of the mother.

Though iron content is low in human milk a full-term infant needs only 0.3 mg/day and human milk meets this requirement. Iron is more available in the presence of lactoferrin in human milk. Human milk enhances zinc absorption. Human milk has high Cu:Zn ratio of 1:5 and cow's milk has 1:15 ratio. Copper content of human milk is more. No copper deficiency is found in breast-fed infants.

Breast milk ensures better oxygen saturation and increases the bioavailability of trace elements like copper, cobalt, selenium, iron and zinc.

It contains less poisonous residues than cow's milk which are neurotoxic like chromium, aluminum and manganese.

Vitamins: The vitamin content of human milk generally reflects the vitamin intake and nutritional status of the mother.

Breast milk contains more vitamin A, C and E than cow's milk. Xerophthalmia and keratomalacia can occur in the first year of life among artificially fed infants but rare among breast fed. Breast milk contains water soluble vitamin D along with fat soluble fraction which protects against rickets. Vitamin D content of human milk reflects maternal intakes and nutritional status of the mother. Human milk may be low in vitamin K and all infants should receive vitamin K supplement soon after birth.

Riboflavin, pyridoxine and B_{12} content of human milk are also related to the dietary intake of mother. Heat labile vitamins like thiamine and ascorbic acid are completely available in human milk. Cow's milk is heated before consumption and these heat labile vitamins may be lost.

Breast-fed infants receive about 25–30 μg of folate daily, most of which is available for absorption.

Hormones and growth factor benefits

Breast milk is a rich source of hormones like thyroid stimulating hormone (TSH), thyroxine, parathyroid hormone, corticosteroids, calcitonin, erythropoietin, oxytocin, growth hormone releasing factor, insulin and prolactin. It contains growth regulating factors, growth promoting factors and growth modulators. Epidermal growth factor enhances maturation of the infant gastrointestinal tract.

Immunological benefits

These factors are present in colostrum as well as in matured milk. Colostrum particles which have anti-infective properties of human milk are stable in acid medium of the stomach and resistant to the digestive enzymes. Human milk provides cellular components and humoral factors. With different factors bestow passive immunity, that is, they provide a form of immunity that does not require the activation of the infant's own immune defenses.

Macrophages: Human milk contains macrophages. They contribute immunity in two ways:

(*a*) They engulf and digest bacteria.

(*b*) These cells synthesize complement, a protein involved in establishing immunity to infectious organism.

The bacteria and viruses that are responsible for diseases such as poliomyelitis, influenza and diphtheria can be destroyed by this way.

Lymphocytes: Lymphocytes are the white blood cells responsible for mediating most aspects of the immune system, with its ability to attack a wide range of infectious microorganisms. Human milk contains T and B lymphocytes. T. lymphocytes are responsible for transfer of immunological memory. Transfer of maternal antibodies and T. lymphocytes may offer some protection against malaria.

Lymphocytes produce lymphokynes and other growth factors which stimulate proliferation and differentiation in lymphoid tissue and its capacity to react antigens. Lymphocytes also produce an antiviral substance called interferon.

These cells in breast milk may therefore play an important role in the infant's transition from passive to active immunity.

Immunoglobulins: Immunoglobulins are the defensive proteins that include all types of antibodies. Secretary IgA plays a major role in defending an infant against viruses, bacteria and other pathogens and harmful food components in the first few days of life. It acts within the gastrointestinal tract and is especially effective against pathogens to which the mother has been exposed such as polio virus, streptococcus and pneumococcus. Infants with a strong family history of allergic disease benefit from this protection particularly through extended breast feeding.

Human milk also contains IgG and IgM immunoglobulins but at a much lower level than that of IgA. It is interesting that the infant makes relatively low levels of its own IgA immunoglobulin and high levels of its own IgG and IgM immunoglobulin during the first year of life. This is an example of the functional development of the infant working in harmony with the composition of the milk it receives from its mother. Immunoglobulins are resistant to the acidity of the stomach.

Research indicates that breast feeding must be maintained until the infant is atleast 3 months of age in order to get this protection.

Lactoferrin and vitamin B_{12} binding protein: Lactoferrin is an iron containing protein found both in colostrum and mature milk. It inhibits the growth of *staphylococcus* organism and *E. Coli* by tying iron that is needed for growth. By removing free iron and thus preventing bacterial proliferation and free radical generation, lactoferrin has a protective effect. If excess of iron is provided in the diet the infant is susceptible for infection. Similarly vitamin B_{12}

binding protein present in breast milk makes vitamin B_{12} unavailable to pathogens that require B_{12} to survive in the infant's gastrointestinal tract.

Lactobacillus Bifidus Factor: The bifidus factor as Gyorgy called it, is present in human milk in a concentration 40 times greater than in cow's milk. It is an amino sugar and contains N-acetyl neuraminic acid, a substance that has a very wide biological role. It is a nitrogen containing carbohydrate in human milk. It encourages the growth of microorganism, *lactobacillus bifidus* and produces acetic acid or lactic acid from lactose and depresses the growth of pathogenic or disease producing organisms like *Escherichia coli.* Growth of *lactobacillus bifidus* is enhanced on a high lactose and low protein diet. Lactose/protein ratio in human milk is 7:1 compared to cow's milk which is 4:1.

Table 4.5 Protective and other bioactive factors unique to human milk

Factor in milk	*Target or function*
IgG	*E coli., B. pertussis, H influenza type b, S pneumonia, N meningitidis* and more.
Secretory IgA	Protects intestinal epithelium. Targets enteric and respiratory pathogens, *e.g., Salmonella* spp, *G lamblia, S pneumonia, Influenza virus*
IgM and IgD	*V cholerae, E coli, S flexneri*
Cytokines	Activate T cells, enhance IgA production, induce proliferation of macrophages, decrease inflammatory cytokine synthesis
Anti-inflammatory components, such as histaminase, antiproteases, prostaglandins	Histaminase degrades hydrogen peroxide, antiproteases neutralize enzymes that act in inflammation, and prostaglandins are cytoprotective.
Bifidobacterium bifidum, growth factors oligosaccharides, glycopeptides, alpha-lactoglobulin, lactoferrin, sialyllactose	Enteric bacteria, lactoferrin competes with bacteria for nonprotein-bound iron.
Macrophages	Engulf bacteria
Interferon	Antiviral agent
Oligosaccharides	Inhibit bacteria adhesion to epithelium
B-12 and folate-binding proteins	Compete with bacteria for these vitamins
Anti-*Giardia* factor	Lipid with anti-*Giardia* action
Trophic factors	Accelerate gut development
Growth factors in colostrum and milk	Insulin, EGF, NGF, IGF-I, IGF-II* for continued rapid growth of infant, especially important for gut development.
Bile-salt-stimulated lipase	Improves fat digestion in the neonates
Docosahexaenoic and arachidonic acids	Constituents of cell membranes in brain and neural tissue
Lysozyme	An antibacterial enzyme, lyses cell walls.

*EGF – Epidermal Growth Factor; NGF – Nerve Growth Factor.

IGF – I and II. Insulin like growth Factor I and II.

Source: Cited from Levin - Folino Nancy 2008, Nutrition for the full term infant, Pediatric manual of clinical dietetics, American Dietetic Association.

Human milk contains probiotics, specially from the genera *bifidobacteria* and *lactobacilli*. It also contains prebiotics. Human milk is ideal synbiotic. It has oligosaccharides that passed undigested to a large intestine where they are fermented by colonic bacteria, Prebiotics stimulate growth of probiotics.

Enzymes: Breast milk supplies enzymes like amylase, lipoprotein lipase, bile salt stimulated lipases, oxidases, lacto peroxidase and leucocyte myeloperioxidase. These enzymes increase digestibility and also act as defence against microbes. Lipases kill bacteria. Bile salt stimulated lipase kills amoeba and giardia. Lysozyme digests the cell wall of bacteria after the bacteria have been inactivated by the peroxide and vitamin C. Lactoperoxidase attacks the streptococcus organism.

Enzymes like lysozyme, peroxidase and xanthine oxidase promote cell maturation.

Fatty acids and Monoglycerides: These are present in human milk and are able to penetrate the membranes of viruses and bacteria and destroy them. They contribute for passive immunity and provide protection without the use of medicines or vaccines.

Para Amino Benzoic acid: Para amino benzoic acid is absolutely essential for erythrocytic stages of malarial parasite. Lack of PABA in human milk inhibits malaria.

Human milk may be useful in the treatment of protracted diarrhoea presumably through local effects in the gut. More generally, the ability of the mother to secrete antibodies directed against specific antigens in her environment, imparts to human milk an environmental specificity with significant protective potential.

Psychological benefits

An infant derives a sense of security and belonging in the mother and child relationship from the comfort of being held than from feeding process. Mother also feels that she is involved in a unique process for which there is no substitute.

Economic benefits

It is economical to breast-feed an infant, even though mother's requirements are increased. Commercial preparations are expensive. In artificial feeding money has to be spent not only for milk or milk powder but also for sterilising the equipment. Also there is no wastage of human milk. By breast feeding the child, one can save money spent on gastrointestinal and respiratory diseases for children. Breast feeding is capable of saving 13 per cent of all under 5 child deaths. Breast feeding is associated with reduced need for hospitalisation and improved child survival.

Infant and child morbidity

Infants fed human milk substitutes have five fold more gastrointestinal illnesses, three fold more respiratory illnesses and double the episodes of otitis media—inflammation of the middle ear cavity. Studies confirm that the relationship between breast feeding and reduced risk for childhood asthma, childhood leukemia, childhood obesity and malalignment of teeth and Sudden Infant Death Syndrome (SIDS).

Mental development

Breast milk contains specific substances involved in brain development. It is rich in sulphur containing amino acids. Cysteine methionine ratio is high and this compensates for low cysteine methionine conversion which is essential for CNS development. It is rich in taurine which is an important neurotransmitter and neuromodulator for brain and retina. It offers high tryptophan to neutral amino acid ratio which controls brain serotonin synthesis.

The arachidonic acid and DHA present in breast milk are essential for neural division. The linoleic acid and α linolenic acids are required for myelination. Arachidonic acid acts as precursor for prostaglandins. Presence of choline, acetyl choline, phospholipid precursors and carnitine ensure optimum metabolism and brain development.

Exclusive breast fed preterms have shown higher IQ scores and better cognitive abilities.

Other advantages to the infant

- Infant's jaw is more fully developed and teeth are less crowded as he works harder to extract mother's milk.
- Microbiologically it is sterile and less danger of contamination and gastrointestinal problems. Mortality rate is lower in children who are breastfed.
- Reduced risk for otitis, severe lower respiratory tract infections and asthma.
- Low danger of incorrect formula and overfeeding.
- Reduced chances of allergic reactions, as human milk protein do not cause allergies.
- Lower rate of sudden infant death or cot death, as infant is not sensitive to human milk and less possibility of aspiration following regurgitation or higher vitamin E content in human milk that protects the membrane in the lungs.
- Less renal solute load as there is less urea and sodium to excrete.
- Less colic as fats and protein in human milk are more easily digested and less likely to create gastric and intestinal distress.
- Human milk is always fresh and at the right temperature. It has optimum fluidity.
- Breast feeding can be continued during illness of the infant like diarrhoea and also can be given after vaccinating the infant.
- There is evidence to suggest that breast fed babies are less likely to develop obesity, hypertension, diabetes mellitus and atherosclerosis in later life. Perhaps adiponectin, the protein present in human milk may have some influence. Late onset tetany, metabolic acidosis and acrodermatitis enteropathica are limited to top fed babies.
- There is evidence to suggest that breast fed babies have better cognition and IQ score later in life.
- It is one food that makes a complete meal. Food is always ready; no need of any preparation and there are no leftovers.
- Breast milk is a renewable resource. It cannot be adulterated. It cannot be diluted nor concentrated. It is organic.

Advantages to the mother

- Breast feeding creates strong bonding with infant.
- Breast feeding is an important birth control method. Prolactin which stimulates milk production, decreases the synthesis of ovarian hormones. It is the most cost effective method of family planning.
- It reduces postpartum bleeding and delays the menstrual cycle. When the mother feeds the infant, the uterus comes back to normal size and arrests bleeding due to the secretion of oxytocin.
- Breast feeding enables the mother to shed extra weight accumulated during pregnancy under the effect of various hormones.
- It is convenient to administer for the mother at any place and time. It saves time, money and energy.
- Risk of breast and ovarian cancer is higher in women who have not breastfed their children. It decreases the risk of type 2 diabetes. By breast feeding, the requirement of insulin decreases for a diabetic mother. Less chance of getting rheumatoid arthritis. There is improved cardiovascular health.
- Breast feeding provides in a mother a sense of calm and satisfaction which favours the production of required hormones.
- Breast feeding improves bone density and decreases the risk of fractures.
- It decreases the risk of postpartum depression.
- Enhances self-esteem in the maternal role.

Environmental benefits

Breast feeding is a natural resource that is renewable with each pregnancy. Breast feeding requires no packaging and no shipping or disposal is needed. By delaying the return of menses, breast feeding suppresses fertility and increases birth spacing, improving maternal and child health while limiting population growth.

Breast feeding is cost effective and socially beneficial health practice.

Breast feeding during illness

Breast feeding is possible with appropriate medication, treatment and support in diseases like insulin dependent diabetes mellitus, multiple sclerosis, systemic lupus erythematosis, hypothyroidism, hypertension, Crohn's disease and ulcerative colitis.

Breast feeding can be continued during most of the maternal illnesses including mastitis, breast abscess, TB and hepatitis B. Breast feeding can be given during infections, rhinitis, viral fever, respiratory infections and asthma. Human milk has been successfully used for infants with cleft palate, inborn errors of metabolism, especially phenylketonuria, cystic fibrosis and down's syndrome. It should be discontinued only if there are gastrointestinal contraindications to oral feedings. In AIDS, as long as there is no caretaker or agency to take up the feeding and care of the baby, breast feeding may be continued. This is the only possible option in many cases even though there is a chance of HIV transmission through breast milk.

Breast feeding can be done during illness of the child because

- breast milk is the most easily digestible food for the sick baby
- breast feeding is the best pacifier to the sick baby

- breast milk satisfies the nutritional and fluid demands
- breast milk offers anti-infective and immunological factors.

> **Determinants of Adequacy of Breast Milk**
>
> - Infant passes a light coloured urine more than 6 times in 24 hours on exclusive breast feeding.
> - Infant gains weight and grows normally.

Recommendations for promotion of successful breast feeding by WHO and UNICEF

- Foster the establishment of breast feeding support group and leader.
- Have a written breast feeding policy that is routinely communicated to all health care staff.
- Train all health care staff in skills necessary to implement this policy.
- Practice rooming in—allow the mother and infant to remain together 24 hours a day.
- Education and advice must be given to every mother in the antenatal clinic. Retracted and crackled nipples must be managed before delivery.
- The first feed should be breast milk (no water, honey, glucose water or tea should be given).
- Give no artificial pacifier.
- Breast feeding should preferably be started in the first hour of life.
- Bottle feeds should never be introduced.
- A breast fed baby does not require supplementation with water.
- Frequent suckling, complete emptying of the breast, correct positioning and supportive care are the cornerstones of successful lactation.
- Encourage breast feeding on demand.

A full term appropriate for gestational age baby who is thriving well does not need multivitamin drops as well.

Mothers' need counselling and family support. It is the lack of these that become missing links for early initiation of breast feeding and exclusive breast feeding for six months. In addition to family support, physical and mental well being of mothers are the key. Breast feeding needs social support.

Infant Milk Substitute (IMS) Act 1992

Aggressive marketing of infant foods and feeding bottles leads to a decline in breast feeding, hence the World Health Assembly in 1981 passed an International code of Marketing of Breast milk substitutes. In 1992, the government of India passed the Infant Milk Substitutes, feeding bottles and Infant Foods Act 1992, which came into force on 1st August 1993.

The IMS, feeding bottles and infant foods (Regulation, production, supply and distribution) Act 1992, amended in 2003, was passed to protect, promote and support breast feeding. The salient features of the act are the following:

- There should be no promotion of infant feeding products in health care facilities.
- Booklets, leaflets, brochures, posters, feeding bottles, cot tags, stickers, clinic cards, prescription pads and similar materials which advertise infant feeding products should not be permitted.
- There should be no display of artificial infant feeding products in health care facilities.
- Company marketing personnel, no matter what they are called, should not be permitted to have contact with mothers.
- Artificial infant feeding should be the exception and not the rule. Only parents who need to artificially feed their infants should be instructed. Instruction should be given only by health or community workers. The instructions should include a clear warning about the health hazards of artificial feeding.
- Bans financial inducement to any person, commission on sales to employees, gifts and samples to health workers.

The Maternity Benefit (Amendment) Act 2016

Under this new law, maternity leave is raised from current 12 weeks to 26 weeks. The prenatal leave is also extended from 6 to 8 weeks.

This period is based on the advocacy of breast feeding for six months by the mother.

This promotes breastfeeding and increases immunity of newborn.

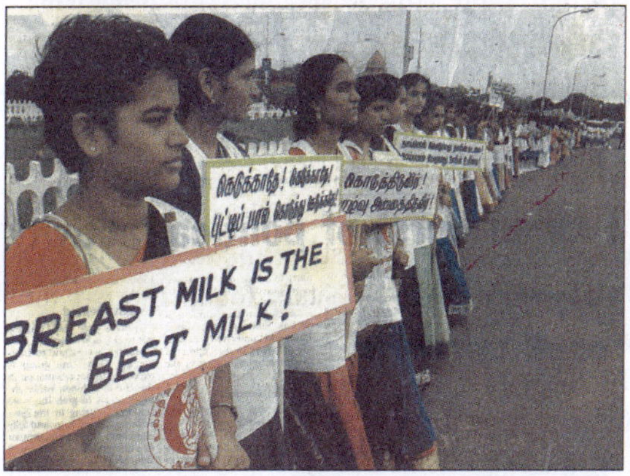

Fig. 4.4 **Forming a human chain to propagate the virtues of breast feeding. Breast milk is not only the best but it is a must for the infant.**

Low Milk Production

One of the commonest reasons mothers give up feeding breast milk or supplement their milk with breast milk substitutes, is because they think that they do not have enough milk. Most often, the mother has enough milk and all she needs is reassurance. At other times, her milk production may be increased by adopting feeding practices that enhance milk production. Very rarely mother is physiologically unable to produce enough milk.

It is important to distinguish between a mother whose milk production is low and a mother who feels that her milk production is low but whose baby is receiving enough milk. This is usually because she lacks confidence. The mother may believe that she does not have enough milk because the child cries often, wakes up frequently, demands for feeds frequently and is irritable, breasts are soft and feel empty. Low prevalence of breast feeding among adolescents also may be the result of their lack of emotional and cognitive development.

Delayed start, infrequent feeds, no night feeds, short feeds, poor attachment, bottle feeding, pacifiers, complementary feeds, lack of confidence, worry, stress, dislike of breast feeding, rejection of baby, tiredness, contraceptive pills, diuretics, and severe malnutrition are some of the causes of low milk production.

The Institute of Child Health and Hospital for Children, Chennai, has a department called "Lactation failure". Here mothers are encouraged breast feeding and avoid formula feeding as part of treatment.

Factors like lack of suitable information, inappropriate health practices, biased health professionals and aggressive promotion of milk substitutes discourage breast feeding. Accurate knowledge, a supportive environment and confidence are major factors which enable mothers to breast feed successfully.

Breast milk bank

It is in operation in many hospitals for infants who cannot get their mother's milk. Institute of child health, Chennai has one such bank. Kolkata, Udaipur and Pune have established milk banks. Vijaya Health Centre, Chennai has come up with one. If the need arises, expressed colostrum can be fed to the child. Milk is screened for organisms, pasteurised and stored at 62.5°C temperature. This milk is charged nominally and given to babies admitted to the intensive care units and preterm babies. Expressed milk can be stored 8 hours at room temperature, 24 hours in refrigerator and if frozen can be kept for 6 months.

According to Breast feeding Promotion Network of India (BPNI) studies there was a decline in breast feeding during the last decade, especially during first four months of life. BPNI recommends exclusive breast feeding for first six months, continued breast feeding upto two years and beyond and addition of complementary foods after six months of age as optimum infant feeding practices.

UNICEF and WHO have initiated a scheme called "The Baby friendly Hospital Initiative" to impart health education which includes breast feeding to rural women who deliver at home and who are unaware of the modern health care system. World Alliance for Breast feeding Action, WABA, is a network of organisations and individuals in collaboration with the WHO and UNICEF to protect, promote and support breast feeding as natural and inherent right of all newborn babies and mothers.

ARTIFICIAL FEEDING

Though no milk can be a real substitute for mother's milk, sometimes it is necessary to give artificial feeding. Circumstances under which artificial feeding is essential are: (1) The mother is suffering from serious illness, fever or infection, (2) Another pregnancy intervenes during lactation, (3) The child is too weak to nurse or cannot because of harelip or cleft palate, (4) Breast milk has completely stopped or insufficient for the child, (5) Mother is not available to feed the child, (6) The mother is on anticoagulants, steroids and radioactive drugs, (7) Death of the mother.

Advantages of Bottle Feeding

- Creates no additional requirements in the mother.
- No problems in establishing the milk supply.
- The volume of milk given is visible.
- Feeding in public is acceptable.
- Other members of the family can feed the baby.
- Creates no problems for the working mother.
- Provided the correct amount is given it is nutritionally adequate.

Modification of the Formula

Cow's milk is diluted to provide a concentration of protein similar to that of human milk. And also this leads to the formation of a softer, more flocculent curd that can be more easily digested by the infant's enzymes. The dilution of milk has the advantage of creating a calcium concentration more near to human milk but reduces caloric concentration. Sucrose can be added to increase the calories.

During the first two weeks about 15 g of sugar is added to the day's formula. Thereafter, 30 g is sufficient. Sugar is discontinued at the time the baby is taking appreciable amounts of other foods.

At two months the infants take about 120 ml of formula. This is increased by 30 ml every month until the infant is taking a maximum of 240 ml at approximately 6 months of age. Formula fed babies should not, as a rule, be fed at less than 3 hour intervals since the cow's milk remains in the stomach for a longer time.

Technique of Feeding

Milk, bottle and other equipment should be sterilised before use. The feeding is usually warmed to body temperature or can be fed cold. As with breast feeding the baby should be held in a semireclining position. The hole in the nipple should not be too large or too small. The nipple should be filled with fluid and not air. The baby should not be expected to finish the entire amount of formula in the bottle at each feeding. Proprietary formulas are available in dry form. Specified quantity of water is added to make up the volume.

Growth failure due to repeated infections or over diluting the formula, infantile obesity, iron deficiency anaemia, hypernatremia, neonatal hypocalcaemia, amino acidaemias in premature infants and acrodermatitis and enteropathica have all been reported in artificially fed infants. There is a higher prevalence of allergic disorders, infective morbidity, emotional instability and sudden death syndrome in bottle fed than in breast-fed infants.

Table 4.6 gives undesirable effect of cow's milk on human infant.

Table 4.6 Undesirable effects of cow's milk on human infant

Composition	*Undesirable effect*
• Low level of lactose	• Reduced calcium absorption.
• High protein	• In small infants as the gut is not mature enough, there is chance for unsplit protein to escape into the circulation and cause sensitisation.
• Cow's milk protein intolerance	• Lactoglobulin or alpha casein may cause diarrhoea, respiratory allergy and eczema.
• Low osmolarity	• There is an increased additional load on immature kidney. Due to increased demand for water to excrete this solute load, there is a chance for dehydration and constipation.
• High levels of tyrosine and aromatic amino acids that are not utilised	• Lead to azotemia and acidosis.
• SDA high	• Increased energy waste
• High fat	• Infantile obesity
• Low amount of iron and poor availability, enteric loss of blood, low vitamin C	• Iron deficiency anaemia.
• High Phosphate	• Decreased iron and calcium absorption

LOW BIRTH WEIGHT

Low birth weight babies are born with birth weight less than 2500 g. The incidence of low birth weight babies in India is 30 per cent. LBW neonates are susceptible for recurrent infections and have neuro developmental handicaps. India accounts for 10 lakh neonatal deaths every year due to low birth weight.

A pre-pregnancy weight of less than 40 kg serves as a useful cut off to predict women who will deliver low birth weight babies. Infants who start with the initial handicap of low birth weight in spite of their being full term (Small for Gestational Age, SGA) may continue to be malnourished later in life. If the baby is less than 1.5 kg, it cannot such mother's milk.

The possible reasons for low birth weight of babies are low maternal body mass index, low age at marriage, high parity, small stature, low gain in weight during pregnancy, low maternal nutritional status with respect to iron and folic acid and shorter duration of full term gestation.

PRETERM BABY

The preterm babies are those who are born before 37 weeks of gestation and are underweight due to shorter duration of full term gestation.

Feeding is one of the major challenges in the care of the low birth weight babies. Goal of feeding the preterm is to achieve a growth rate that approaches the normal growth rate of foetus in utero.

The preterm is at a disadvantage in many aspects of nutrition. The problems facing the preterm babies are poor sucking and swallowing reflexes, relatively high caloric requirement with small stomach capacity, poor gag reflex and incompetent cardio esophageal sphincter leading to aspiration, decreased absorption of essential nutrients.

The preterm babies lack adequate stores of brown fat and are therefore vulnerable to become hypothermic.

Nutritional Requirements

In critically ill infants, it is common to initiate parenteral nutrition with minimal macronutrients and to advance as tolerated to meet estimated needs for growth. Initially premature infants require parenteral nutrition and take several days to reach enteral feedings.

Calories: The caloric need of non-growing preterm babies during the first week of life are 60 kcal/kg/day. After first one or two weeks of life, most preterm babies require 120–150 kcal/kg/day to maintain satisfactory growth. High calories may be necessary in babies who are not gaining weight, post-operative patients and extreme preterms.

Table 4.7 Energy and protein requirements of preterm baby who is on enteral feeding and parenteral nutrition

	Enteral feeding		*Parenteral nutrition*	
Body weight, g	*Protein, g/kg/d*	*Energy, kcal/kg/d*	*Protein, g/kg/d*	*Energy, kcal/kg/d*
500–700	4.0	105	3.5	89
700–900	4.0	118	3.5	92
900–1200	4.0	119	3.5	101
1200–1500	3.9	127	3.4	108
1500–1800	3.6	128	3.2	109
1800–2200	3.4	131	3.0	111

Fluid: Fluid needs of the preterm babies are relatively high during the first week of life. The intake of fluids varies from 90-100 ml/kg/day for 7–10 days. Additional fluids may be required when the baby is under the phototherapy or a radiant warmer.

Carbohydrate: Preterm babies can tolerate 50 per cent of the calories in the form of carbohydrates. Very low birth weight babies may have difficulty in tolerating the lactose, the first few days. Glucose polymers are well tolerated.

Protein: Preterm babies require 3–4 g of protein per kilogram of body weight for rapid growth. Excess of protein may lead to metabolic problems of acidosis and hyperammonemia. Human milk contains mainly whey protein which are better utilised. Certain amino acids essential for the preterm are cystine, taurine, alanine and arginine. Carnitine levels are found to be low in preterm babies. These are present in breast milk.

Fat: Fat malabsorption and steatorrhea can occur in preterms due to reduced amounts of pancreatic lipase, carboxylic ester hydrolase, bile acids and lingual lipase.

Preterm infants have a higher requirement for arachidonic acid and decosahexaeneric acid to allow rapid brain and body growth.

About 40–50 per cent of calories in diet of the preterm should be available from fats. Very low birth weight babies poorly digest and absorb saturated triglycerides. Vegetable oils containing unsaturated long chain fatty acids are better absorbed. Better still are medium chain triglycerides because their digestion and absorption are not dependent on bile salts level.

Premature babies are given polyunsaturated fats and high levels of iron. Iron promotes peroxidation of polyunsaturated fatty acids and this might imply that vitamin E requirements are higher in such infants. They may develop haemolytic anaemia, characteristic of vitamin E deficiency.

Minerals and Vitamins: Calcium and phosphorus supplements may be needed to prevent rickets or osteopenia in preterms. Iron deficiency can occur by 6–12 weeks and hence 2.5 mg/kg/day of iron starting from 6-8 weeks of age may be given. Zinc supplementation increases weight gain. Mineral and vitamin supplements required by preterm babies are as follows

- Calcium: 120-160 mg/kg/day
- Phosphorus: 60-90 mg/kg/day
- Magnesium: 8-15 mg/kg/day
- Copper: 150-200 μg/kg/day
- Zinc: 2-2.25 mg/kg/day
- Iron: 2-3 mg/kg/day (birth weight < 1500 g); 2 mg/kg/day (birth weight 1500-2500 g).
- Vitamin D: 400-1000 IU/day.

All low birth weight babies should receive vitamin supplementation in addition to the amount present in human milk. This is because (*a*) Premature infants are born with low body stores of vitamins, (*b*) Their growth rates are rapid, (*c*) Their gastrointestinal absorption is low, and (*d*) Their daily intake of milk feedings is initially low. Table 4.7 shows the nutritional supplements required for preterm babies.

Feeding the preterm baby

Studies conducted at Sooriya Hospital, Chennai in 2017 on premature babies showed that swabbing the insides of cheeks with colostrum several times a day helps to bring down the incidence of hospital-acquired infections and speeds up overall recovery.

The preterm babies are best fed with unprocessed human milk obtained from their mothers. It has been shown that milk of mothers delivering prematurely has higher protein chloride and sodium content which is suitable for the nutritional needs of low birth weight babies. Antimicrobial property of breast milk is of great importance to the preterm baby and the incidence of infectious sepsis and meningitis are greatly reduced. If the baby does not gain weight satisfactorily with breast milk alone, dietary supplements like vegetable oils (corn oil, groundnut oil) may be used which increase the caloric value without increasing its volume.

The advantages of feeding breast milk to preterm babies are availability of easily digestible protein and fat and feeding tolerance. Factors in human milk may stimulate GI growth, motility and maturation. Enzymes naturally present in human milk help in the absorption and utilisation of nutrients.

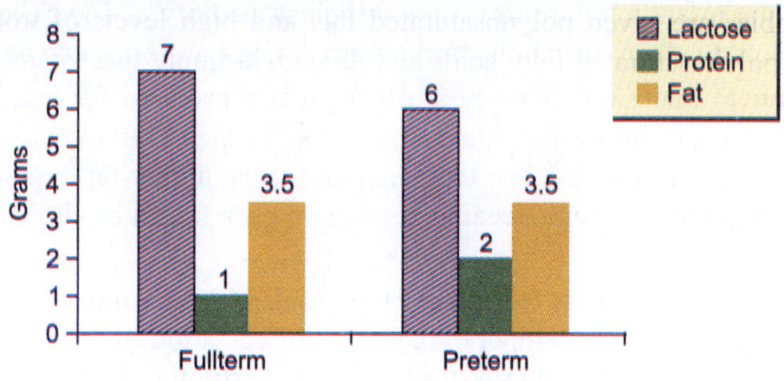

Fig. 4.5 Composition of breast milk–full term versus pre-term

The decision whether a baby is to be breast fed or through a gavage is guided by maturity, birth weight and general condition of the baby. The infant can be started with expressed mother's milk. Bolus, intermittent, naso-gastric tube feeds every 2 hours in small babies and every 3 hours in larger babies can be done. Initial volume used will be as low as 1–2 ml for feeding infants of 1000 g or less or as much as 4–5 ml per feed for an infant of 1500 g. If oral feeds are tolerated, then increase the volume of feeding by 1 ml/day in smaller infants or by as much as 3–5 ml in the larger infants. Feeding must be reduced, withheld or even omitted entirely when there is gastric retention or abdominal distension. Ultimately the volume of intake should be 150–170 ml/kg/day and caloric value 110–120 ml/kg/day. If the rate of weight gain is low, the caloric intake is increased by adding vegetable oil (coconut oil or peanut oil, 0.5 ml every other feed). Most infants begin to gain more rapidly as their postnatal weight approaches 1400–1500 g and their caloric intake increases.

The preterm infant's poor nutritional reserves, high requirements for normal growth and development, and gastrointestinal immaturity pose a particularly challenging nutritional problem. Human milk is most suitable for preterm infant due to its protein and lipid composition, easy digestibility, feeding tolerance, maturation of the gastrointestinal tract and neurologic development. Human milk reduces the incidence of infection and sepsis/meningitis and necrotising enterocolitis. Nutritional programme should be given a high priority in the overall care of preterm infants.

Preterm babies have higher risk of chronic respiratory diseases. There is emerging evidence that low birth weight or growth retarded neonates are prone to manifest diabetes mellitus, hypertension and coronary artery disease in later life. Therefore low birth weight is a key risk factor for adverse outcome in life.

Feeding Problems of Infants

Tooth decay: A pattern of tooth decay that involves the upper anterior and sometimes lower posterior teeth is common among infants and children who are given sugar-sweetened beverages or fruit juice in a bottle at bed time. Infants should be fed, burped and put to bed without milk or juice bottle.

Underfeeding: Underfeeding is suggested by restlessness and crying and by failure to gain weight adequately, despite complete emptying of the breast or bottle. Underfeeding may also result from the infant's failure to take a sufficient quantity of food even when offered. Constipation, failure to sleep, irritability and excess crying can result due to underfeeding.

Lactose intolerance: Lactase deficiency is usually not a problem for infants. Slow weight gain or failure to thrive in breast fed infants may be associated with excessive lactose intake. This results when feeding does not last long enough for the higher-fat hind milk to let down. Mothers should lengthen the breast-feeding session on each breast or allow an entire feeding to be taken at one breast.

Diarrhoea: Diarrhoea in a breast fed infant is unusual. Mild diarrhoeal disturbances due to over feeding respond quickly to temporary decrease or cessation of feeding. Withholding all solid food as well as one or several milk feedings and substituting boiled water or a balanced electrolyte solution are usually all that is required.

Constipation: Constipation in the artificially fed infant may be caused by insufficient amount of food or fluid. In other cases, it may result from diets too high in fat or protein or deficient in bulk. Simply increasing the amount of fluid or sugar in the formula may be corrective in the first few months of life. After this age, better results are obtained by adding or increasing the amounts of cereal, vegetables and fruits.

Colic: The term colic describes a frequent symptom complex of paroxysmal abdominal pain, presumably of intestinal origin and of severe crying. It occurs usually in infants younger than 3 months. Prevention of attacks should be sought by improving feeding techniques, including burping, providing a stable emotional environment, identifying possibly allergenic foods in the infant's or nursing mother's diet and avoiding underfeeding or overfeeding.

WEANING

The term 'weaning' comes from the word 'wemian' which means to accustom. Weaning begins from the moment supplementary food is started and continues till the child is taken off the breast completely. Solid food added to an infant's diet is called beikost. There is an increase in activities of enzymes at the time of weaning.

The ideal time to start introducing semisolid food is when a baby is ready to sit up, swallow and eat and taste other foods, the baby's stomach is ready to digest food and the baby has good appetite and accepts food readily and there is more activity in the child.

Need for weaning

Infants in our country thrive on breast milk alone up to six months of life and their growth rate during this period is satisfactory. After six months, increasing needs of calories and protein of growing children cannot be met by diminishing output of mother's milk. Milk is also a poor source of vitamin C and supplementation with fruit juice is essential. Iron stores in liver of the infant would last only upto 4–6 months. Hence iron-rich foods should be given at least from six months onwards. Milk is deficient in vitamin D.

If the baby is to maintain the expected rate of growth, remain healthy and well nourished, supplementary feeding has to be resorted around 6th month.

Investigations conducted at National Institute of Nutrition, Hyderabad, suggest that early introduction of supplements before six months of age is not associated with any beneficial effect on infant's growth. The supply of breast milk decreases because the baby suckles less frequently, less vigorously and less effectively at the breast. The baby runs the risk of recurrent infection which is likely to result in malnutrition, diarrhoea and respiratory infection. Shorter duration of lactation and shorter duration of lactational amenorrhoea can reduce inter-pregnancy interval.

Introduction of weaning food too late can lead to undernutrition and increased diarrhoeal morbidity. The child may be unwilling to accept new food.

Though Indian babies are given supplementary foods, either they are introduced very late or given adult form of diet. The age of introduction of supplementation is 3–5 months in the urban elite and middle income group. The supplementation is delayed in urban poor by 7–9 months and rural poor by 9–11 months.

Bulky adult diet, when given to infants, usually does not meet the nutritional requirement, particularly calories. Nutrient density of weaning foods of western diet is 1.0 kcal/g of food whereas in Asia, the nutrient density is 0.25 kcal to 0.4 kcal/g. Hence calorie dense foods like malted food should be given to infants. Weaning food should provide at least 10 per cent of the energy as protein.

According to NNMB (2000–2001) survey about 43 per cent of mothers started complementary feeding such as milk or biscuits in addition to the breast milk during 4–6 months of age.

Types of Supplementary Foods

Liquid supplements

Milk: At about the sixth month of life the frequency of breast feeding is reduced to 3 or 4 times per day and animal milk is substituted. Since the proportion of nutrients in animal milk differs from that of human milk, the cow's milk is diluted with boiled and cooled water in the proportion of 2:1 for the first feeds. The amount of water is gradually reduced so that in the course of a few weeks the baby receives undiluted animal milk. Two feeds, with 225 ml of milk per feed is an ideal replacement. Sugar can be added for taste and to increase calories.

Juice of fresh fruits: Oranges, tomatoes, sweet lime, grapes serve to supplement the protective nutrients not present in sufficient amounts in breast milk as well as in animal milk. It is advantageous to start feeding small quantities of fresh fruit juice even in the 3rd or 4th month of life.

In the early stages, the fruit juice is diluted with an equal amount of boiled water and only a couple of teaspoonfuls are fed. The amount of fruit juice fed is gradually increased and at the same time the dilution with water is cut down. In a week's time the baby receives 85 ml orange juice or about 170 ml fresh tomato juice. Since tomato juice does not contain the same proportion of nutrients as orange juice, double the quantity is required.

Soup from green leafy vegetables: In case fresh fruits are not available, green leafy vegetables may be used as an alternative. Strained soup can be given in the beginning with unstrained soup later on.

Fish liver oil: Fish liver oils are good source of vitamin A and D. Infants should be given a few drops to 1/2 tsp per day mixed in small quantity of milk.

Solid supplements mashed well before feeding

Mashed food is started around the 7th or 8th month of life. Around this time, the infant is already receiving animal milk, fruit juice or vegetable soup and fish liver oil.

Cereal and starchy gruels: To meet the increasing demands of calories and protein, well cooked mashed cereals like rice, rice flour, rice flakes, and ragi flour mixed with milk and sugar can be given. Addition of a small amount of vegetable oil to the porridge makes it less glutinous increasing the energy density.

Calorie dense cereals can be prepared using malted wheat or ragi. To prepare amylase rich food, the cereal is soaked overnight. Water is removed and the cereal is tied in a moist cloth and kept in a warm place. After 48 hours or so sprouts come out. It should be dried in the sun or can be roasted. The malted cereal is powdered after removing the sprouts. During the process of malting, starch is converted to maltose due to increased production of enzyme amylase. This is also called Amylase Rich Food. Due to the conversion of starch into amylose, thinner gruels are made. With this either the infant can consume more gruel or more flour can be added to make thick gruel. This way calorie consumption can be increased. Fig. 4.6 gives steps involved in making amylase rich food.

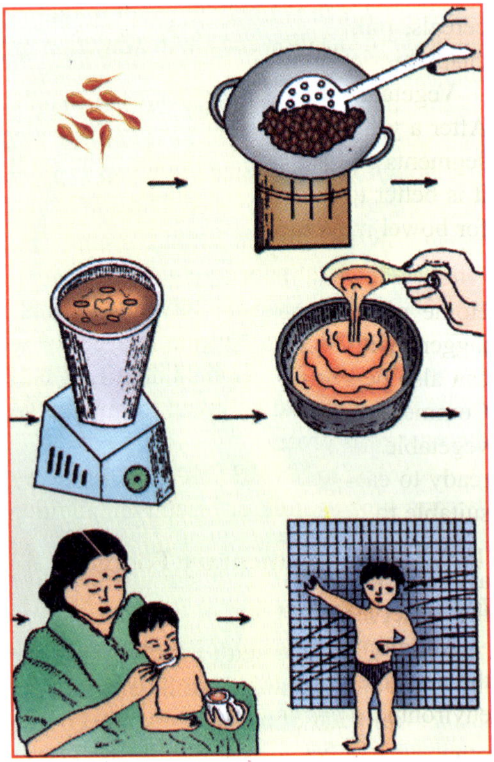

Fig. 4.6 Preparation of amylase rich food. Weaning food can be prepared at home easily

Vegetables: Cooked, mashed vegetables like potato, green leafy vegetables and carrots can be introduced to get vitamins and minerals and different flavours in the diet.

Fruits: All fruits, with the exception of banana which is mashed, must be stewed and sieved for one year old baby. Thereafter, it is given simply stewed, with the addition of a little sugar and lime juice for favour.

Non-vegetarian foods: A small amount of hard boiled yolk of egg is given to start with and if the infant tolerates, the amount may be gradually increased to a complete yolk of an egg. Yolk is a good source of vitamin A, iron and protein. Soft custard is also a suitable way in which to introduce egg yolk. Egg white, because of the frequency of allergic manifestations, is not given until the infant is 8 to 10 months old and then it is given very cautiously. The whole egg may be poached or soft boiled and fed by the time the baby reaches the age of one year.

Finally, minced and cooked meat or boiled fish may be fed after suitably flavouring with salt, 3 to 4 times a week.

Pulses: Well cooked pulses along with cereals in the form of kichidi/pongal can be given or can be made into porridge. Pulse and meat preparations can be given in alternate days.

Solid supplements unmashed

When the baby starts cutting his teeth, it is time to start chopped and lumpy foods. Cooked cereals, pulses and vegetables can be given to the child. Solids like idli, idiappam, bread, chapathi, rice and dal can be given after the child gets used to semi-solids.

Vegetables may be chopped into small pieces, and boiled. Cooked potato can be given. After a year, leafy vegetables can be given well boiled and soft. A slice of raw carrot or fruit segments with all skin and seeds removed is a good exercise for the gums. As the child grows, it is better to give fruit segments instead of juice. Fruit provides bulk in the diet and is good for bowel movement.

Processed Foods: Home made or commercial processed foods can be given as weaning foods. Home made processed weaning foods can be prepared by using cereals, pulses, nuts and jaggery with or without milk products. Processed foods like bread, pasta, rusks and biscuits can also be given. Commercially available weaning foods are predigested but are expensive. Commercially available weaning foods like vegetable soups and fruit desserts, puddings and vegetable juices and fruit juices can be given as part of weaning food. Weaning foods can be ready to eat or ready to reconstitute foods. Processed foods are standardised, convenient and suitable to the infant.

A spray dried milk based infant formula containing 0.5 per cent lactulose or carrot juice is available in the market. It stimulates bifidobacterial growth in human infants comparable with that observed in breast fed babies.

Addition of foods to the infants results in slight changes in the gut flora. By 2 years of age the intestine is thought to be colonised, known as the Microbiodata Finger print. Genetics and environment contribute for the type of flora present.

Points to be considered in introducing weaning foods

- Introduce only one food at a time.
- Allow the infant to become familiar with the food before trying to give another.
- Give very small amounts of any new food at the beginning, for example, one teaspoon full or less.
- At first strained fruits, vegetables and cereals are given.
- Fruit juice should be fed only by cup not by bottle.
- When the baby is able to chew, gradually substitute finely chopped fruits and vegetables usually at 8 to 9 months.
- Variety in choice of foods is important.
- Infants may object to taking some foods by themselves but will take them willingly if one is mixed with another, e.g., egg may be mixed with formula, cereal or vegetable. Vegetables may sometimes be made into soup with little milk until the baby becomes accustomed to the new flavour.
- If, after several trials, the baby has an acute dislike for a particular food, omit that item for a week or two and then try again. If the dislike persists it is better to forget about the food for a while and substitute another.

- The mother or anyone feeding the infant must be careful to avoid showing in any way a dislike for a food which is being given.
- A baby's appetite varies a lot from meal to meal and day to day. During hot weather or when the child is teething or suffering from cold the child's appetite may be less.
- Use a very thin consistency when starting solid foods. Gradually the consistency is made more solid as the infant learns to propel the food back with the help of tongue.
- The child can be fed with a katori and spoon and the baby gets used to an adult method of feeding.
- To make the food calorie dense add oil, butter or ghee to the infant's diet.
- Food should be given between breast feeds.
- Give freshly prepared food.
- Food should be only slightly seasoned. The addition of salt or sugar is not necessary in all foods. Water can be given in between the feedings with a cup and spoon.

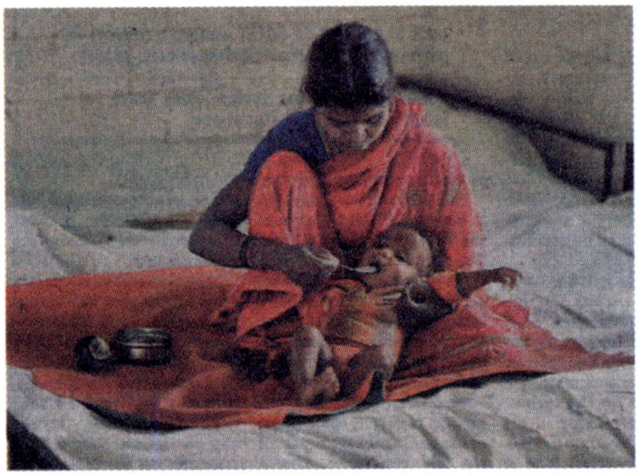

Fig. 4.7 Feeding supplementary food to an infant demands greater skills

Feeding an infant with supplementary foods demands greater skill and ingenuity on the part of the mother than the mere selection of suitable foods and cooking them in suitable ways. To guide the child to learn to eat and enjoy foods, the mother must be patient, resourceful and not too serious.

By one year, the infant can be given family diet, modified, in small quantities but at frequent intervals in addition to milk. The best indication of adequacy of the diet is the growth pattern of the child.

Low cost supplementary food

Indian mothers wean their infants into the traditional adult diet because of their ignorance of low cost weaning foods and also because of incapacity to buy expensive commercial foods. Table 4.8 gives a list of some of the low cost nutritious supplementary foods.

Table 4.8 Low cost supplementary foods developed in India

Name of the product	*Composition*
• Indian multipurpose food (C.F.T.R.I.)	Low fat groundnut flour and bengal gram flour (75:25) fortified with vitamins A and D, B_1, B_2 and calcium carbonate. Contains 42 per cent protein.
• Malt food (C.F.T.R.I.)	Cereal malt, low fat groundnut flour, roasted bengal gram flour (40:40:20) fortified with vitamins and calcium salts. Contains 28 per cent protein.
• Balahar (C.F.T.R.I.)	Whole wheat flour, groundnut flour and roasted bengal gram flour (70:20:10) fortified with calcium salts and vitamins. Contains 20 per cent protein.

• Supplementary food (N.I.N.)	Roasted wheat flour, green gram flour, groundnut and sugar or jaggery. (30:20:8:20). Contains 12.5 per cent proteins.
• Supplementary food (A.H.S.C.W.) Kuzhandai Amudhu	Roasted maize flour, green gram flour, roasted groundnut and jaggery (30:20:10:20). Contains 14.4 per cent proteins.
• Win food (Gandhigram Rural Institute)	Pearl millet, green gram dal, groundnut flour, and jaggery (50:15:25:25). Contains 20 per cent proteins.
• Amutham	Rice flour, ragi flour, bengal gram flour, sesame flour, groundnut flour and jaggery (15:15:15:10:10:25). Contains 14 per cent proteins.
• Poshak	Cereal (wheat, maize, rice or jowar) pulse (chana dal or green gram dal) and oil seed (groundnut) and jaggery (4:2:1:2).
• Poshak (least cost weaning mix)	Same ingredients as poshak but in the proportion of 60:17:14:9
• Kerala Indigenous Food (KIF)	Tapioca, Bulgar wheat and groundnut (25:50:25)

Low cost supplementary foods can be made at home by dry roasting with the above mentioned combinations or equal quantities of sprouted ragi, green gram, whole wheat, roasted channa, red rice few almonds and making into powder.

Problems in weaning

Obesity: Many infants are overfed by overzealous parents who mistake acceptance of food for appetite. Too early and too much quantity of feeding or too concentrated food can lead to overweight of the infant. Commercially available processed foods when overfed may lead to obesity.

Underweight: Too less quantity of food and less concentrated foods can lead to underweight. Bulky adult food when consumed by an infant gives satiety without meeting calorie requirement. This results in underweight of the child. Frequent illness and repeated diarrhoeas can also result in underweight of the child. Malnutrition in early childhood results in impaired cognitive and social development, poor school performance and reduced productivity in later life.

Food Allergy: Food sensitive enteropathis occur principally during first six months of life and mostly limited to early childhood. Predisposing factors may be malnutrition, infection and genetic background. Increased gut permeability, low level of secretory IgA and enzymatic immaturity put the infant at higher risk for allergy.

The foods most frequently implicated in infant allergies are wheat, milk, egg and citrus juices. Rice is probably the most safe food of the commonly eaten cereals. The consumption of wheat is best delayed until after the 6th month. Egg white, which is a potent sensitiser is usually deferred until the 10th month. Egg yolk is less allergenic and heat denaturation renders egg yolks nonreactive. Pure orange juice does not give rise to allergic reactions in infants or children. Improperly prepared orange juice may contain excessive amounts of peel oil or of seed proteins which have leached into the juice from broken seeds and may therefore cause reactions in susceptible children.

Allergy to milk is the most serious of the commonly encountered food allergies since milk supplies the basic nutritional requirements in early infancy. In most cases the allergic reaction is due to the presence of lactoglobulins and to some extent lactoalbumin. The infant can be fed evaporated milk in which these proteins are denatured. Artificial flavours and colours have been associated with respiratory allergic disorder.

In most cases, food protein allergy is transitory. Tolerance is achieved in 50 per cent by the end of first year and 80 per cent after three years.

Refusal to take new food: If the child refuses to take new food, form of the food can be modified or should be mixed with the food he likes and should be tried again after a week or so. Frequently a child may spit out the first spoon of food but usually this means that he does not know how to swallow the nonliquid food.

Choking: Choking and aspiration can be caused as the child is trying to eat, run and breathe at the same time. Choking can be caused by peanuts, seeds, small hard sweets, crisps and raisins. Hard and big pieces of fruit like apple or vegetable or popcorn should be avoided for children under 3 years of age since they can cause choking which can lead to death. Choking can be prevented by cutting or breaking into bite-sized pieces. Conversation and motor activity should be discouraged during eating. Foods sticky like peanut butter should be avoided. Children need to be supervised while eating.

Diarrhoea: Infections due to lack of proper hygiene and inappropriate complementary feeding can cause diarrhoea in infants.

Table 4.9 Some suggested recipes during infancy

Recipe	*Reason*
Fruit juice (6 months)	Provides vitamin C which is lacking in milk. Tomato and orange juice also supply some amount of β carotene.
Greens soup (6 months)/Mixed vegetable soup	Child gets used to new taste, provides iron, calcium, beta carotene, riboflavin and vitamin C.
Stewed apple (8 months)/Mashed vegetables	Gives calories and should not be given in raw pieces since it may choke the child.
Soft custard with egg yolk (8 months)	Provides vitamin A, iron, protein and B vitamins. Egg white should be introduced later as it may cause allergy.
Kichdi (pongal), idli, chapathi + milk, (10-12 months)	Easily digestible and gives calories and good quality protein.
Malted cereals and gruels made out of rice, rice flour, rice flakes, corn flakes and milk.	Meets increased demands of calories and protein.

January 19th is National Immunisation day.
August 1-7 is World breast feeding week

SUGGESTED READINGS

- The efficacy of an integrated feeding and care intervention among 3–15 month old infants in Andhra Pradesh. Annual report 2010–2011, NIN, Hyderabad.
- Assessment of nutritional status under five year rural children in the districts of Madhya Pradesh state. Annual report 2011–2012, NIN, Hyderabad.
- Breast Feeding Promotion Network of India. (BPNI) – www.bpni.org.

QUESTIONS

1. Give the RDA of an infant aged 8 months.
2. Explain the nutritional importance during infancy.
3. Write a note on colostrum. Bring out the difference between fore milk and hindmilk.
4. Compare the nutritive value of human milk with cow's milk.
5. 'Breast milk is the best milk'—explain.
6. Explain 'Lactobacillus Bifidus factor'.
7. Describe the disadvantages of artificial feeding.
8. Give the nutritional importance for preterm baby and explain problems involved in feeding them.
9. State the need for introducing weaning foods to an infant's diet. Give the method of preparing any one low cost weaning food.
10. Define weaning and give the schedule for it.
11. List the problems of weaning and explain any one in detail.

TOPICS FOR ACTIVITY

- Log on to www.akshayaposhan.gov.in and www.poshan.nic.in.

  Discuss the golden rules promoted by Ministry of Women and Child development for preventing malnutrition in infants.
- Plan and prepare low cost weaning foods.
- Plan and prepare weaning foods for 6 months, 9 months and 12 months old infants.
- From the market survey list the commercial weaning foods available and critically evaluate them.

5

Nutritional Recommendations and Food Requirements of Preschool Children —1 to 6 Years

Children under six years of age make up nearly 20 per cent of India's population. The years between 1 and 6, growth is generally slower than in the first year of life but continues gradually. The child may gain in weight 150–200 g per month between one and two years. Activity also increases markedly during the second year of life as the child becomes increasingly mobile. Development of a full dentition by about the age of 2 years also increases the range of foods that can safely be eaten. There is an increased need for all nutrients, but the pattern of increase varies for different nutrients in relation to their role in growth of specific tissues.

Establishing healthy childhood feeding practice is often a challenge for many parents and caregivers. Dietary patterns and eating behaviours formed during this period have lasting influence on preference, energy balance and health in later life.

NUTRITIONAL RECOMMENDATIONS

Energy

The RDA for energy suggested by ICMR in 2020 is 1110 kcal for 1–3 years, 1360 kcal for 4–6 years. Energy is required for growth and activity. Insufficient food will not only result in undernutrition in terms of inadequate weight gain but will also hinder growth. The rate of growth fluctuates from one age to another. Up to 10 years of age there is no difference in sex for RDA. Due to improper weaning practices, the child may not meet calorie and protein requirement leading to Severe Acute Malnutrition. Insufficient calorie intake can lead to protein deficiency.

Protein

The increase in the muscle mass that must accompany bone growth requires positive nitrogen balance that is met by protein intake of 0.8–0.9 g/kg body weight. The increase in total body size necessitates a larger vascular system to transport nutrients to the tissues and waste products away from the tissues. Thus there is an increase in demand for nutrients needed in blood formation like protein, iron, folacin and pyridoxine. Bone growth also creates a need for protein. Protein recommendations for 1–3 years is 12.5 g and for 4–6 years old children it is 16 g.

Fat and Essential Fatty Acids

Fat energy including invisible fat for children should be 25 per cent of total energy. To provide 25 per cent fat calories, the minimum level of visible fat in the diet of children should range between 25–30 g/day. Saturated fats should be less than 10 per cent of total energy.

Studies showed that infants consuming infant formula supplemented with DHA and ARA improved visual activity, brain development and verbal intelligence quotient.

Calcium

Calcium requirements of children are calculated on the basis of the amount of calcium accretion in the body. This deposition is not uniform throughout growing period, but would be relatively greater during early childhood and during adolescence than during the other periods of growth. Since, all dietary calcium is not absorbed 500–550 mg/day is prescribed though the actual requirement may be less. The RDA of phosphorus is 500–550 mg/day. Deficiency of calcium can affect the bones of growing children. Milk is the best source of calcium. Hence the diet of preschool child should include 1–2 glasses of milk per day.

The RDA of preschool children (1–6 years) is given in Table 5.1.

Table 5.1 ICMR Recommended Dietary Allowances for preschool children-2020

Nutrient	*Years*	
	1–3	*4–6*
Body weight kg	12.9	18.3
Energy kcal	1110	1360
Protein g	12.5	16.0
Dietary fibre g	15	20
Calcium mg	500	550
Magnesium mg	90	125
Iron mg	8	11
Zinc mg	3.3	4.5
Iodine µg	90	90
Vitamin A Retinol µg	390	510
Vitamin D IU	600	600
Thiamine mg	0.7	0.9
Riboflavin mg	1.1	1.3
Niacin mg	7	9
Pyridoxine mg	0.9	1.2
Folate µg	120	135
Vitamin B_{12} µg	1.2	2.2
Vitamin C mg	30	35

Iron

During growth, for an increase in each kilogram in body weight 30 mg of iron is required and since the increase in body weight during childhood is 2 kg/year on an average, the daily requirement of iron for growth will be 0.2 mg. The physiological requirement can vary markedly for 1–2 years from 0.2–0.5 mg per kg of body weight per day.

Children 6–24 months old are at the greatest risk of the irreversible long-term consequences of iron deficiency namely impaired physical and mental development. Under Reproductive and Child Health Programme Government is providing 20 mg of elemental iron and 100 μg of folic acid in syrup form to 6–24 months old children to prevent anaemia. Dietary lack of iron accompanied by hookworm infestation can lead to anaemia. The ICMR 2020 RDA recommends 8 mg and 11 mg for 1–3 years and 4 to 6 years of iron respectively.

To meet this increased demand for iron, iron-rich foods like egg yolk and greens should be included in the diet.

Vitamin A

Vitamin A requirements of children have been computed from the requirement figures of infants (50 μg/kg) and adults (9.3 μg/kg) taking into account growth rates at different ages. The incidence of vitamin A deficiency signs are high and serum vitamin A levels are generally low among Indian children whose dietary intake is less than 100 μg. According to the studies conducted by ICMR, children receiving food supplements which provided a total of 300 μg of vitamin A per day over a period of 6 months, serum vitamin A levels were found to be around 30 mg/dl and no clinical signs of vitamin A deficiency. Based on this data 390–510 μg have been suggested including the safety allowances for 1–3 years and 4–6 years. Deficiency of vitamin A in children can cause Bitot's spots, night blindness or in severe cases total blindness also. Milk, eggs, carrots and green leafy vegetables should be included in the diet.

B Vitamins

The daily allowances of B-vitamin requirements are based on energy intake. The allowances per 1000 kcals are (same as an adult) 0.5 mg thiamine, 0.6 mg riboflavin and 6.6 mg niacin equivalents. Dietary folate requirement for 1–3 and 4–6 year old is 120 and 135 μg/d respectively.

Vitamin D

Vitamin D is more a pro-hormone than a vitamin. It can be synthesised in the body in adequate amounts by simple exposure to bright sunlight even for 5 min per day. Habitual Indian diets do not provide even 10 per cent of the requirement.

The expert committee suggested that outdoor physical activity is a means of achieving adeqate vitamin D status. RDA recommendations 2020 are 600 IU eqivalent to 15 μg.

Infections and Nutritional Status

Nearly two out of three preschool children in India are malnourished. Incidence of severe acute malnutrition and vitamin A deficiency are high among this age group.

Growth is influenced by nutrition. Frequent attacks of infectious diseases affect their growth and increase the requirements of various nutrients.

Repeated illnesses—especially the common illnesses such as diarrhoea, measles, whooping cough and other respiratory infections—are the principal underlying causes of malnutrition.

The mechanisms by which infections worsen nutritional status are anorexia, malabsorption, catabolic losses, fever, additional intestinal losses, reduced growth, weight loss and above all superstitious and improper feeding methods used during infection.

FOOD REQUIREMENTS

Parents are responsible for choosing the type of foods offered (nutritious), when they are offered (at regular scheduled times) and where they are offered (at home or outside) and children are responsible for how much they eat.

Children are born with the ability to self-regulate their energy needs. Studies have found that when parents try to force or bribe their children into eating or if they feed their kids extremely large portions, they actually are teaching them to over eat.

The child should be given foods from all the groups. Fruits and nuts which are health foods can be added to the diet. Parents should be role models and the child should observe the parents enjoying balanced diet with Basic Five Food Groups. Parents should offer new and appealing foods constantly to the child. Children should be encouraged to help in preparing foods.

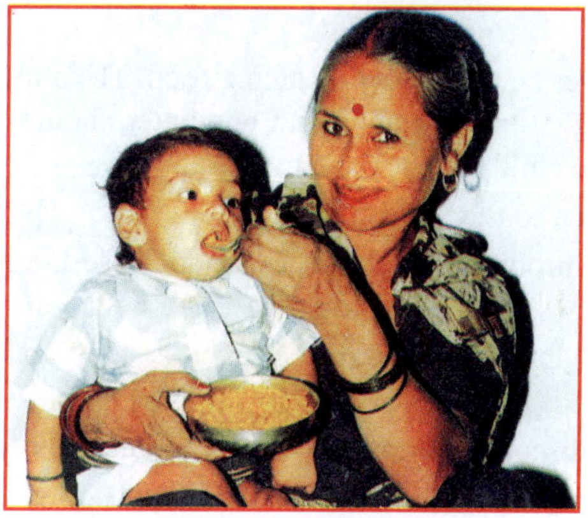

Fig. 5.1 After one year the child takes the same food as the family takes with little modification.

Good eating habits begin at infancy. Transition from infant diet to regular adult diet should be smooth and gradual. If solid foods have been gradually introduced before the age of one year, feeding the child should be no problem in the subsequent years. But some preschoolers are difficult eaters at times. Some children less than 5–6 years of age are finicky eaters. Moreover, many tend to use eating (or not eating) to exert control over parents.

Dietary Guidelines

- The diet should be adequate in quantity and quality of different nutrients. In addition to the amount of milk recommended, the preschool child should have two small servings of protein-rich foods like eggs and other nonvegetarian foods, pulses, paneer or cheese. When the child is about 18 months old, finger foods such as carrots can be given.
- Proper elimination is usually maintained by a daily diet of fruits, vegetables and whole grain products. Fruits and vegetables not only supply vitamins and minerals but also are rich sources of antioxidants.
- The diet should include a variety of foods. The child who is taught to eat everything on his plate is much more likely to enjoy optimal health than the one who picks and chooses. The child should have access to items from all food groups on a regular basis.

- Food intake of children improve if the food is interesting and attractive, e.g., chapathis, puris can be made into different colours with incorporation of greens and vegetables or can be served in attractive plates. Flavour or colour of the milk can be changed to encourage the child to drink milk.
- Foods should be slightly seasoned so that they taste better and the child takes it well.
- Child should never be forced to eat more than he can take.
- The person feeding the child with the food should not show any dislike of that food in front of the child. This may lead to the rejection of food by the child.
- Disliked food should be mixed with favourite food.
- Food preferences of the child should be taken into consideration.
- Regularity of meal times is essential. This leads to the development of good eating habits.
- Different cooking methods and new attractive combinations encourage the child to eat more.
- The child should never be hurried while taking food. The atmosphere should be pleasant, peaceful and lacking distraction. T.V. and computer should be turned off during meal time. This allows the child to enjoy the meal.
- Water should be given to the child frequently.
- Inclusion of curd, a probiotic, in the diet can decrease the incidence of diarrhoea and cold.
- Unripe bananas and apples should not be given as they are difficult to chew and may choke the child.
- Children should be discouraged to take processed and junk food.
- Most of the food served must be from the family pot.

The surveys of the National Nutrition Monitoring Bureau indicate that the average cereal intake is 106 g/day among 1–3 year old children. The energy density should be 1.0 to 1.2 kcal/ml. This can be achieved by adding milk and oil to the diet. Malted foods can also be included in the diet to increase calorie density.

Home based diets provide adequately for growth and development of the child provided they are calorie dense and given in small feeds frequently.

Even if there is enough food in the house to provide an adequate diet, growth can be faltered due to feeding a young child with bulky staple foods which fill the child's stomach and assuage its hunger without meeting its energy needs. Also feeding a child's small stomach infrequently (only twice instead of four times) can affect the growth of the child.

Protein present in foods of plant origin is not complete, that is, lack in certain essential amino acids. But judicious combination like cereals and pulses make the protein quality of both foodstuffs better and may be equivalent to animal protein quality. Addition of milk to vegetarian diet not only improves quality and quantity of protein but also supplies calcium in best absorbable form. It is also good source of B-vitamins.

Overall need for nutrients increases throughout the growth period but there will be periods when growth is slow and the need for certain nutrients will be reduced proportionately. Children reflect these changes in need, by fluctuations in appetite. This may cause anxiety to parents. Unless such period is prolonged or is accompanied by signs of undernutrition such as lethargy, fatigue and increased susceptibility to infection, should not cause concern. Special care is needed for feeding children below two years of age, since they cannot ask for food and have not yet learnt to eat by themselves. Preschoolers who are overweight have an increased risk of health problems. Parents play an important role in the availability of quantity and quality of food and schedule of eating. They should provide an opportunity for physical activity of the child.

Feeding Problems

Dental Decay

Tooth decay can be caused by caries. This can occur in children who are susceptible and whose integrity of tooth structure may be affected by the nutritional deficiency. Vitamin A is necessary for enamel and vitamin C is essential for dentine. Calcium, phosphorous and vitamin D are needed for the process of calcification. Flourine decreases susceptibility to caries. It protects against caries by preventing demineralisation aiding reminerilisation and interferning with bacterial enzymatic activity.

Fermentable carbohydrate which adheres to the tooth surface is the major dietary factor influencing tooth decay. The acids produced by bacteria which grow on this carbohydrate dissolve the mineral phase of the enamel of the tooth, leading to dental caries. Stickier the carbohydrate and longer the sugar in the mouth, greater is the cariogenic effect. Intake of sodas, juices and sweets increase both calories and caries risk. This effect can be reduced by eating cheese at the end of the meal. Cheese increases the pH of mouth. Brushing the teeth after eating chocolates/sticky sugar can reduce the incidence of caries.

To prevent dental decay regular brushing of teeth, twice daily, in the morning and before going to bed is essential. During night salivary secretion is reduced. On the food particles which remain in teeth the microorganisms grow and can cause dental decay. Hence there is need to brush teeth before going to bed. Only water should be given in the bottle for night time feedings. Tooth brushing disrupts the oral biofilm at the tooth surface, limiting development of plaque.

Pica

This disorder involves repeated or chronic ingestion of non-nutrient substances which may include plaster of paris, charcoal, clay, wool, ashes, metal (pins, nails or blades), paint and earth. The age of onset is usually 1–2 years. Psychological theories of pica have found evidence for mental deprivation, high frequency of maternal and paternal deprivation, family disorganisation, poor supervision and low socioeconomic status.

Pica can be treated with a combination of education and guidance, family counselling and behaviour modification. Children with pica are at increased risk for lead poisoning, iron deficiency anaemia and parasitic infections.

Feeding Disorders

Feeding problems become feeding disorders. These children who are not consistently hungry at mealtimes or they may end mealtimes after a brief amount of time or they may be picky eaters. Some common feeding disorders in children include adipsia—absence of thirst—dysphagia, food refusal, self feeding inadequacy, food refusal by volume, excessive meal duration, choking, gagging or emesis, inappropriate mealtime behaviour and food selectivity by type and texture.

Food reluctantance tend to have poorer vegetable consumption and lower protein and fat intake. These children are often associated with nutritional deficiencies and inadequate weight gain.

Nutrition deficiencies at a young age put young children at higher risk of suffering from stunted growth, malnutrition psycho social problems and the emergence of chronic health diseases such as metabolic syndrome, osteoporosis and diabetes later in life.

Picky Eating

Picky eater is the one who

- accepts only limited number of food choices.
- is unwilling to try new foods.
- avoid some food groups such as vegetables.
- exhibit strong food preferences including presentation and preparation styles.

Picky eater phenomenon is independent of social status. Psychological and physiological problems need to be corrected.

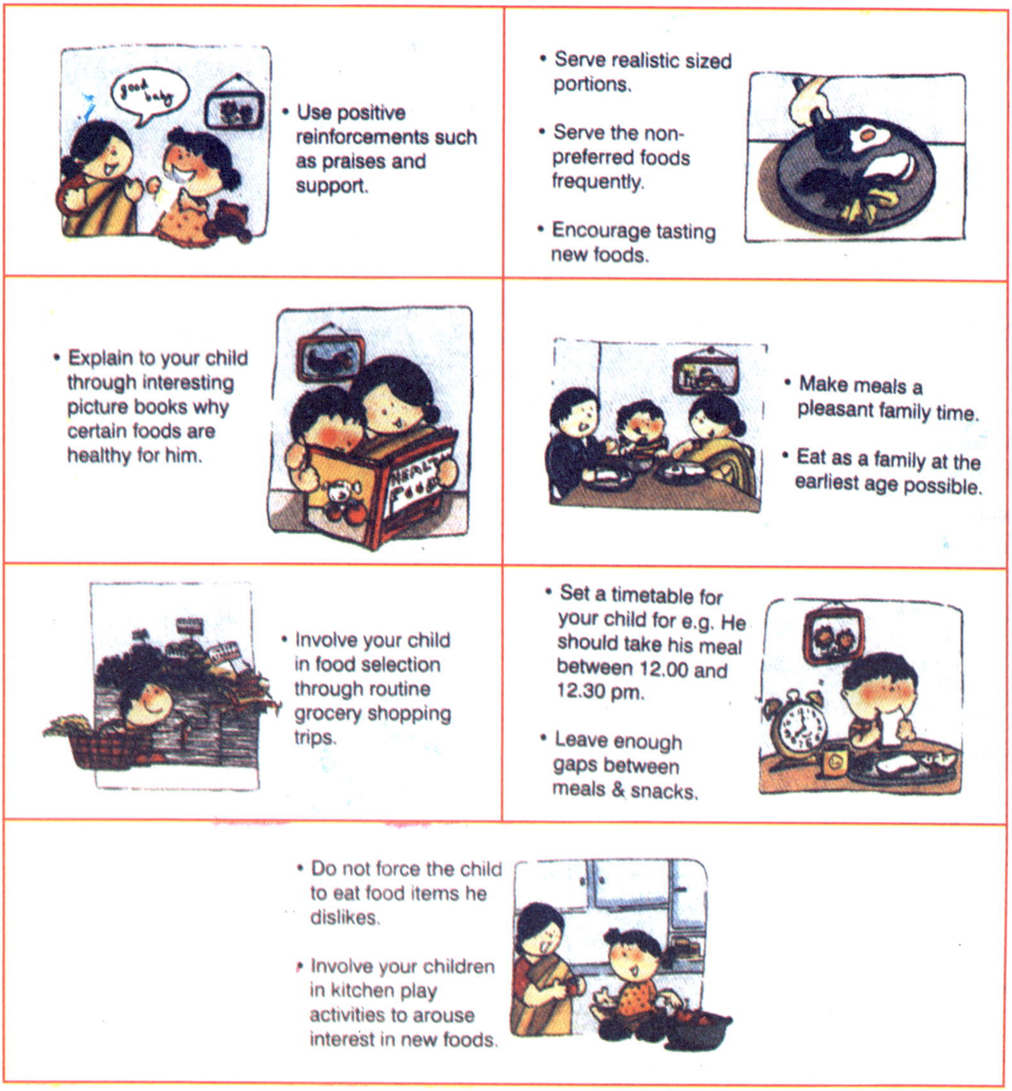
good baby
• Use positive reinforcements such as praises and support.
• Serve realistic sized portions.
• Serve the non-preferred foods frequently.
• Encourage tasting new foods.
• Explain to your child through interesting picture books why certain foods are healthy for him.
• Make meals a pleasant family time.
• Eat as a family at the earliest age possible.
• Involve your child in food selection through routine grocery shopping trips.
• Set a timetable for your child for e.g. He should take his meal between 12.00 and 12.30 pm.
• Leave enough gaps between meals & snacks.
• Do not force the child to eat food items he dislikes.
• Involve your children in kitchen play activities to arouse interest in new foods.

Fig. 5.2 Some solutions for picky eating

Source: Abbott Healthcare Pvt. Ltd. Mumbai.

Picky eating is a common childhood behaviour and the habit will wear with time. Children need variety as they get bored with same kind of food.

They must be encouraged to eat along with adults. Eating habits are taught better by example than formal explanation. Parents should be role models—as children pick up on the food habits of their parents. Children should be given home cooked food rather than outside food.

Preschool years could be the best age to implement interventions aiming to rectify problematic eating behaviours and encourage appropriate weight gain.

Age appropriate food should be offered for the children and new eatables should be introduced regularly. It is common to see mothers offering quick bites when the children refuse to eat meals. Mother should be firm and should not substitute snacks for meals.

Small portion of food given at regular intervals can help picky eaters to meet their requirement of nutrition. Mother should limit feeding duration of meals. If it extends beyond half an hour, the child is not interested in that food. Mother should stop feeding and should feed only when the child is hungry. Mother should understand that there is nothing wrong with the child if he skips the meal once in a while.

Conducive environment and the attitude of parents are crucial when feeding the children.

Table 5.2 Suggested recipes for preschool children

Recipe	*Reasons*
Idli, vada, khuzhi paniyaram, dhokla, poha.	Supply good quantity and quality of protein. Easily digestible.
Noodles made with whole wheat flour and pulses. Served with vegetables and homemade masalas.	Give calories and the child enjoys the shape of it. Commercial masalas may have additives.
Tricolour sandwich (mint chutney, tomato sauce or jam) with vegetables Bread is made from whole wheat flour	Attractive, tempting to the child. Gives calories and vitamins.
Biscuits (different types and shapes)	Preschool child identifies and enjoys in eating. Provides calories and proteins.
Milk shakes, fruit shakes, ice creams fruit salad smoothies	Indirect form of consuming milk and fruits as the child may get bored to take plain milk.
Chikki	The child willingly consumes crisp foods. It is rich in calories, protein and B-vitamins.
Papads made with dals as accompaniment for sambar rice, curd rice or pulao	Child likes to eat the main dish.

NUTRITION RELATED PROBLEMS OF PRE-SCHOOLERS

According to United Nations report (2007), 46 per cent of children under the age of five suffer from under nutrition. Around 35 per cent of the world's undernourished children live in India. Malnutrition is the direct or indirect cause for 50 per cent of total deaths among children.

Obesity

Children are overfed by mothers due to wrong perception of healthy and obesity. Mothers force feed children with high calorie foods like processed food, sweets and ghee and make the child obese. Development of over weight begins in early childhood by increasing the number adipocells resulting in hyper plasia. Preschool and elementary school aged children who are overweight are five times more likely to become overweight adolescents.

Parents should encourage self feeding and should not do forced feeding. Parents play an important role in the quality and quantity of food consumed by children. Parents should encourage physical activity of children.

Severe Acute Malnutrition

Severe Acute Malnutrition-SAM or severe wasting is defined by very low weight for height. According to The Indian Academy of Pediatrics weight for height/length below 70 per cent or ≤ 3 SD of NCHS median and/or visible severe wasting and/or bipedal oedema.

Malnutrition can be in the form of underweight (weight/age), stunting or (height/age) wasting (weight/height). Severely Acute Malnourished child is deficient not only in protein and calories but also in micro nutrients.

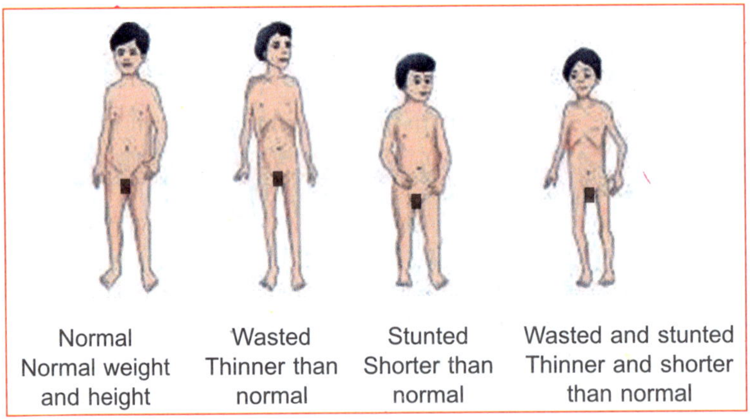

Fig. 5.3 Malnutrition in children

Ecology of SAM is given in Fig. 5.4.

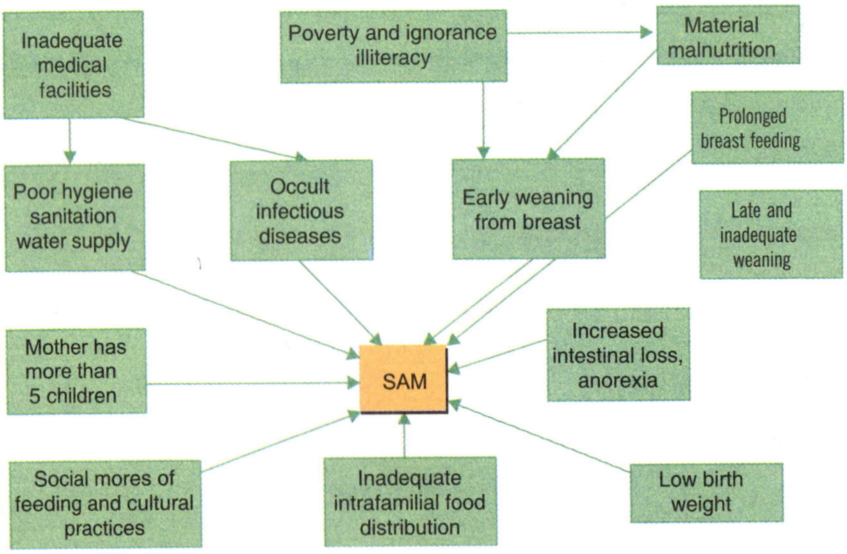

Fig. 5.4 Ecology of Severe Acute Malnutrition

The following are the causes for underweight for age which may precipitate into SAM:

(a) Due to poverty, mother is not able to provide sufficient food to the child resulting in undernutrition. **(b)** The starchy gruels made from local staple food like rice, wheat, bajra, ragi, jowar or maize would result in "dietary bulk with a low caloric density". Hence the child may not be able to meet calorie requirement. Malted foods meet calorie requirement as they increase the caloric density. **(c)** Abrupt weaning, late weaning due to ignorance of importance of weaning can lead to undernutrition. **(d)** Malnutrition can result in less enzymes synthesis and less appetite leading to less consumption of food. **(e)** Chronic infections like primary complex may result in anorexia. **(f)** Infestation like ascariasis particularly giardiasis may lead to anorexia.

Symptoms of Different Types of SAM

Kwashiorkor: In kwashiorkor the usual history is of prolonged breast feeding, late and inadequate weaning leading to low intakes of energy but relatively better biological value. Hence the child with kwashiorkor faces compromising growth and preservation of most of the organ function. The problem is compounded by sudden episodes of infections like measles, gastroenteritis or pneumonia which increases requirements and intakes remain reduced. This situation can precipitate disadaptation and the child may present with oedema of the face and lower limbs, failure to thrive, anorexia, diarrhoea, apathy, dermatosis (hypo and hyper pigmentation) flaky paint appearance, sparse, soft and thin hair, angular stomatitis, cheilosis, and anaemia.

Marasmus: In Marasmus the children are usually born full term low birth weight or pre term followed by early weaning, inadequate feeding and live in unhygienic conditions and suffer from infections. There is chronic energy deficiency and failure to thrive—means children are not able to gain weight. Irritability, fretfulness and apathy are common among them. Their weight is persistently below the third percentile for age or less than 80 per cent of ideal weight for age. Diarrhoea is frequent. Many are hungry but some may be anorexic. The child is shrunk and there is little or no subcutaneous fat. There is often dehydration. The temperature is subnormal. Watery diarrhoea and acid stools may be present. The muscles are weak and atrophic and this together with the lack of subcutaneous fat, makes the limbs appear as skin and bones.

Figure 5.5 shows the typical sign of PEM.

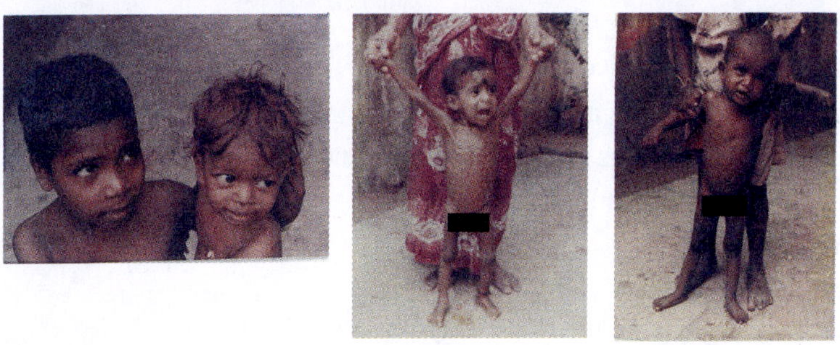

Fig. 5.5 **Marasmic children with minimum subcutaneous fat. Observe changes in hair like sparseness, thinness and depigmentation.**

Nutritional Requirement

The diet should be rich in proteins of good quality and high in calories. The other nutritional requirements also must be met.

Energy

The extra energy requirement for catch.up. growth, to support weight gain in the nutritional treatment of severe acute malnutition, is based on the desired composition of weight gain and the desired rate of catch up growth.

According to WHO the child should be given 100–135 kcal/kg body weight/d for the existing weight. For children less than 2 years 135 kcal/kg body weight should be given and for older children 100 to 175 kcal/kg body weight. This meets normal energy requirement and catch-up requirement. It is very important that there should be enough calories in the diet, otherwise proteins will be utilised for energy purposes and not for building the tissues.

Typically, the normal diets of young children would have an energy density of 1-2 kcal/g food. During SAM it should be increased marginally.

Malted cereals can also be given to increase calorie density. Fifty per cent of total calories can be from carbohydrate. If needed milk can be fortified with cooking oil (5–10 ml/1000 ml) to increase energy density.

Protein

Five grams of protein/kg body weight/day should be given for the existing weight (e.g., weight of the child 5 kg. requirement of protein is 25 g). The calories derived from protein should be 10 per cent of the total calculated calories per day if the main source is animal protein. If the main and the only source is from cereal and pulse then the percentage of calories derived from protein can be 13 to 14 per cent of the total calories because of the net protein utilisation of cereal and pulses is around 60 per cent whereas milk or egg is around 90 per cent. Though vegetable protein is as good as milk protein in reversing the acute manifestations of kwashiorkor, they are inferior in their ability to promote regeneration of serum albumin. This can be overcome by giving 3 parts of vegetable protein to one part of animal protein like skim milk.

Fats

Forty per cent of total calories can be from fat which can be tolerated by children. Foods containing short and medium chain fatty acids such as butter, milk and coconut oil are preferred to long chain unsaturated fatty acids in case the child has diarrhoea.

Vitamins and minerals

Supplementation of vitamins and minerals is mandatory.

Treatment

Treatment strategy can be divided into three stages:

- Resolving life-threatening conditions
- Restoring nutritional status without disrupting homeostasis
- Ensuring nutritional rehabilitation

Criteria for improvement

- Disappearance of mental apathy in 4 to 5 days.
- Disappearance of oedema in 7 to 10 days.
- Weight gain in 3 to 4 weeks.
- Rise in serum albumin level in about 2 weeks time.

WHO and UNICEF recommend two major approaches to the treatment.

1. Facility/hospital-based approach for clinical management using the WHO protocol.
2. Home/community-based approach, an integrated public health response to acute malnutrition without medical complications.

There are three stages of treatment—hospital treatment, dietary management and rehabilitation.

I. Hospital Treatment

Malnutrition contributes to an estimated 60 per cent deaths in children under 5 years. Most deaths occur during the first few days of treatment. This is mainly due to failure to prevent hypoglycaemia, hypothermia (rectal temperature 35.5°C) management of dehydration, missed infections and severe anaemia. To reduce deaths it is recommended that treatment be divided into an initial stabilisation phase during which acute medical conditions are addressed including severe anaemia and infections. Cautious feeding is initiated followed by longer rehabilitation phase. The reduction in mortality to 5 per cent in severely malnourished children can be achieved by applying WHO guidelines.

The WHO manual presents 10 essential steps to treat severe malnutrition.

Hypoglycaemia

Ten per cent dextrose solution should be given 2–4 ml per kg body weight intravenously. Oral feeding should be initiated as early as possible.

Hypothermia

Hypothermia, hypoglycaemia and gram negative sepsis often go together. The child should be kept warm and practised "bedding in" with the mother.

Dehydration and Electrolyte imbalance

- In children with diarrhoea, if there is no dehydration, half to one glass of Oral Rehydration Solution or Oral Rehydration Therapy is given after each stool.
- In mild to moderate dehydration, 70 ml/kg ORS in 4 hours, sip by sip or as intragastric drip should be given.
- In severe dehydration 100 ml/kg sodium saline or Ringer Lactate (RL) in 3 to 6 hours should be given.
- In oedematous children 70 ml/kg should be given as a slow ration. Half the calculated fluid can be given as sodium saline or Ringer Lactate and the rest as 10 per cent glucose. This will tackle hypoglycaemia and will reduce sodium intake.
- Potassium supplement, 2–4 mEq/kg/day may be continued for 1–2 weeks in kwashiorkor. Fruit juice can be encouraged to supplement potassium.
- Sodium should be restricted to 2–3 mEq/day.
- If there is evidence of acidosis, sodium bicarbonate 2 ml/kg intravenous fluid diluted with equal quantity of distilled water should be given.

Septicaemia/Infections

Broad spectrum antibiotics, crystalline penicillin or ampicillin with an aminoglycoside should be given. Staphylococcal infections should also be treated.

Vitamin and mineral deficiencies

The WHO manual recommends vitamin A administration on admission in standard age-related doses (50,000 IU, 1,00,000 IU or 2,00,000 IU) and repeat doses on days 2 and 14 with clinical deficiency. There is preliminary evidence suggesting a need to modify the current single high-dose regime to a lower daily dose (5000 IU) for children with severe malnutrition. The possibility of the single high dose on admission increasing the risk of respiratory infection and leading to poor absorption are concerns. Later the child is initiated to vitamin A prophylaxis programme.

About 2–5 mg IM/IV of vitamin K per day may be given for 2–3 days in florid PEM and in those with persistent diarrhoea. Vitamin B complex, C, D, and minerals like zinc and calcium need to be supplemented.

Severe anaemia should be corrected by small packed cell transfusion, 5–10 ml/kg slowly along with furosemide. In mild to moderate anaemia, 6 mg/kg of elemental iron is given after the patient has been stabilised and after deworming. As per recommendations of WHO iron therapy should be delayed until rehabilitation phase. Magnesium is given if there is seizure due to tetany or apathy. Up to 0.8 mEq/kg/day is given in 2 divided doses for 1–3 days. Malnourished children should receive zinc supplementation. A total daily dose of 20 mg of zinc is safe and beneficial.

Initiate refeeding and facilitate catch-up growth

This phase is for restoration of weight for height. This is the second and often the first step in those with mild to moderate SAM.

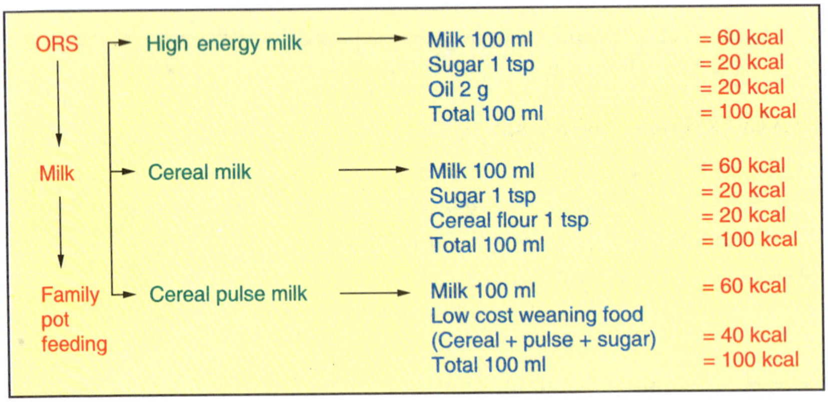

Fig. 5.6 Nutritional therapy in SAM

Source: Elizabeth, K.E., 2005, Nutrition and Child Development. Paras Publishers, Hyderabad.

ORS is followed by dilute milk, whole milk, high energy milk and high energy cereal milk as the patient improves. To make high energy milk 1 tsp sugar and ½ tsp coconut oil are added to 100 ml milk in order to give 100 kcal/100 ml. Cereal flour or cereal+pulse flour may be added to 100 ml of high energy milk. A precooked, ready to mix cereal pulse combination can be easily prepared at home by roasting and powdering rice, wheat, black gram and adding powdered sugar in the ratio 1 : 1 : 1 : 2. This mix can be given as a semisolid with hot water or hot milk. Or any other low cost weaning food can be given to the child. Coconut oil is preferred as it contains medium chain triglycerides, MCT, which are absorbed even during fat malabsorption.

Multivitamins and micronutrient should be started early. Iron therapy is not initiated till carrier proteins are synthesised. Otherwise *E. Coli* will thrive on the unbound iron in the gut.

If the child is very sick, milk, bread and sugar can be started from the hospital diet for 1 to 2 days.

The WHO recommends 4 hourly feeds night and day during initial treatment and during rehabilitation. Although continuous nasogastric tube-feeding may result in more rapid weight gain, it demands close nursing supervision.

Table 5.3 Formula of F75 and F100

Food	*F75*	*F100*
Dried skimmed milk g	25	80
Sugar g	70	50
Cereal flour g	35	–
Vegetable oil g	27	60
Mineral mix ml	20	20
Vitamin mix mg	140	140
Water ml	1000	1000

The treatment is initiated with WHO-F-75 milk formula which gives 75 kcal/100 ml with low protein. Once a child with severe malnutrition is clinically stable (e.g., resolution of oedema, diarrhoea and sepsis) a high energy milk formula. WHO-F-100 milk oil formula is given. Ready to use therapeutic food which can replace F-100 formula contains lactoserum and groundnut paste and can be used for rapid catch-up growth.

According to WHO after facilitating catch-up growth, child needs to provide sensory stimulation and emotional support and prepare for follow-up after recovery.

II. Dietary Management

Dietary management is the same for all clinical types of SAM (marasmus, kwashiorkor, marasmic kwashiorkor or undernutrition). The diet should be

- from locally available staple foods
- inexpensive
- easily digestible
- consisting of minimum of 100 ml of milk per day. If the patient can afford, more milk as well as eggs can be given.
- of cereal and pulse combination 5 : 1 proportion
- evenly distributed throughout the day
- consisting of all the food groups
- of increased quantity of food which the child is already used to
- of many number of feedings to increase the quantity of food
- high in calories by adding oil and banana. Banana is also a bowel binder.

Traditional food items such as rice, idli, uppuma, tubers, legumers, payasam, egg, fish, green leafy vegetables and seasonal fruits should be introduced gradually. "Family pot feeding" should be ensured as early as possible. Groundnuts can be given to older children. There will be improvement in mental apathy in 3 to 4 days. There will be increase in appetite and the child gains weight for age. Oedema disappears by 7–10 days and diarrhoea and respiratory infection disappear in about 2 weeks. After clinically and biochemically improving in 3 to 4 weeks the child is discharged from the hospital. Nutrition education should be given at home at the time of discharge to prevent recurrence.

Studies have shown that not only with skimmed milk but also by giving cereal and pulse combination there can be improvement in PEM children clinically and biochemically.

III. Rehabilitation

As soon as children are able to take normal food and infection is under-control, it is economical for medical services to discharge them to a centre where their nutritional rehabilitation can be supervised. Follow up studies done at the Institute of Child Health and Hospital for Children

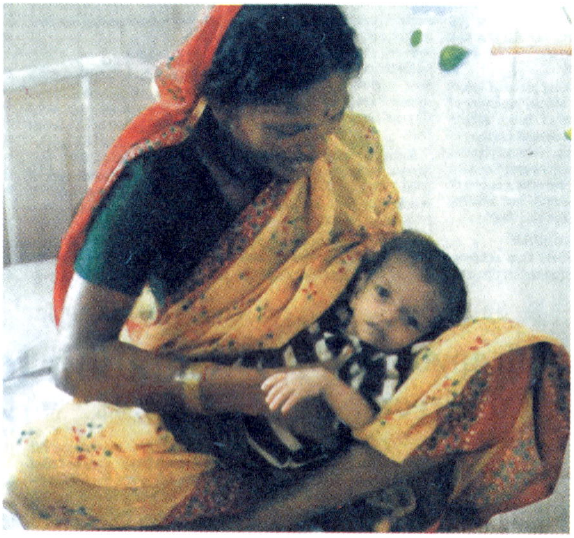

Fig. 5.7 **Mother and her 21 month old daughter in Nutrition Rehabilitation Centre at Gondia.**

at Chennai revealed that one-third of the children who had been treated in hospital for PEM were dead within a year from the disease for which they had been successfully treated and still others were malnourished. Causes can be attributed to poverty or failure to involve parents particularly mother in treatment and recovery. The concept of nutritional rehabilitation is based on practical nutritional training for mothers in which they learn by feeding their children back to health, under supervision and using local foods.

During rehabilitation rapid catch up growth in weight > 10g/kg/day needs to be attained as it facilitates early discharge and prevents secondary infections.

NIN suggested rehabilitation maintenance diet, using local foods. The diet increases to 170–220 kcal/kg/day from 100 kcal/kg/day, and provides 3–4g of proteins/kg/day.

A typical diet of a child weighing 7 kg

Milk fortified with oil	– 350 ml
Kichidi (rice and dhal in 2 : 1 ratio with added oil)	– 250g
Bread	– 1–2 slices
Eggs	– 2
Banana	– 1

Micronutrients are provided in the form of multivitamin-multimineral syrups containing thiamine hydrochloride, riboflavin, nicotinamide, pyridoxine, cyanocobalamine, vitamin A, cholecalciferol, calcium, copper sulphate, zinc sulphate, selenium and potassium iodide.

Folic acid is given regularly but iron is withheld during the initial phase of rehabilitation. Iron supplementation is started once the child starts gaining weight. Children are fed every 2 hours initially and once appetite improves they are fed adlibitum.

WHO recommendations help in improving the rate of weight gain > 10g/kg/day during nutrition rehabilitation of severely malnourished children.

Residential units

In residential units mothers are admitted with their children. Under the guidance of nutrition demonstrator they work as a group and prepare a suitable therapeutic diet with available foods and feed their children.

Day-care centres

In these centres mothers help in cooking and feeding in one or two days a week, though the children attend daily. It therefore takes longer for mothers to appreciate the essential messages about better feeding.

Domiciliary rehabilitation

This is done at home and is more personal, as nutritional advice and help is given on one to one basis by a nutrition demonstrator or specially trained health worker.

Successful nutritional rehabilitation require detailed knowledge about local foods, cooking and feeding practices. Based on this knowledge a diet should be designed which can be practised even by poor families. Mothers who take active part in preparation of food and feeding their children and watching them recover to their health and vitality are more likely to retain ideas and continue with a similar regime at home.

Home/Community based management of SAM

Evidence suggests that large numbers of children with SAM and with no medical complications can be treated in their communities without being admitted to a health facility or a therapeutic feeding centre. Community-based management of SAM is based on early detection and assessment of children with SAM in the community and home based care of those without complications.

Suggested diet during convalescence

- Increasing the quantity of existing food (like idlis, rice, chapathis).
- Increasing the number of meals to satisfy calorie and protein requirement.
- Addition of oil or ghee 1 to 2 tsp to increase calories without increasing bulk.
- Consumption of sugar can be increased to increase calories in the diet.
- The child can be given cereal and pulse mixture.
- If the patient can afford milk, egg and skim milk can be included in the diet.

Low cost recipes for children recovering from SAM

- Ragi, green gram, jaggery: puttu
- Ragi, bengal gram, wheat: puttu
- Bengal gram, milk, jaggery: payasam
- Rice, bengal gram: porridge

- Redgram, spinach, dal
- Wheat rava, green gram dal, vegetable upma
- Malted wheat, green gram and groundnut powder (can be made as chapathi, gruel or laddu with jaggery)
- Rice, green gram dal: pongal/kichidi
- Idli with sugar and ghee

Concentrated food supplements

For rapid replacement of lost tissues and to catch up with growth, children need a high energy diet with ample protein. It is often difficult when the energy density of the family is low. Malnourished children need supplements of vegetable oil to increase the energy density. Concentrated foods like malted cereal in combination with pulses can be given. If the child can afford, commercial weaning mixes or egg custard can be given.

Ready-to-Use Therapeutic Food (RUTF), a high energy food is used in the acute phase of rehabilitation and is prescribed as a therapeutic item and not as a food. It does not require additional processing before feeding. It is alternative to F100 formula.

The RUTF is produced by mixing together ground roasted peanut powder, milk powder and sugar in a ratio of 30 : 28 : 25 (grams) along with 15 g of gingelly oil. This mixture gives 5.5 kcal per g of total energy 10–12 per cent calories is from protein and 45–60 per cent is from fat. The child can be given 50 g/day of RUTF. Sometimes it is fortified with micronutrients or oral multivitamin supplements can also be given to the child.

This RUTF is given in addition to normal diet.

Not many peanut allergies are noted in developing countries and the RUTF ingredients can be substituted with locally available foods. And there is experimental evidence that the RUTF is effective in treating severe acute malnutrition.

RUTF can be stored without refrigeration and without the high risk of contamination like liquid milk. Its use made easier for the rapid catch-up growth phase to occur out of hospital at lower cost and without the risk of nosocomial infections.

RUTF is an important development in the management of severe malnutrition.

RUTF is designed to be consumed without the addition of water hence eliminating the risk of bacterial contamination. It is energy dense without any clinically significant osmolarity problems.

Prevention

SAM is a consequence not only of inadequate food intake, but also of poor living conditions, unhygienic environment and lack of health care. It is primarily a disease of socioeconomic inequalities and maldistribution of food and health.

There is no simple solution to the problem of SAM. The following steps are suggested by FAO/WHO Nutrition Expert Committee:

Health Promotion

- Measures directed to pregnant and lactating women (education, distribution of supplements).
- Promotion of breast-feeding.
- Development of low cost weaning foods. The child should be made to eat more food at frequent intervals.
- Measures to improve family diet.

- Nutrition education, promotion of correct feeding practices.
- Home economics.
- Family planning and spacing of births.
- Improving family environment.

Specific Protection

- The child's diet must contain protein and energy rich foods. Milk, eggs, fresh fruits should be given if possible.
- Immunisation schedule should be followed.
- Food fortification may help the child in meeting micronutrient requirements.

Early Diagnosis and Treatment

- Periodic surveillance.
- Early diagnosis of any lag in growth.
- Early diagnosis and treatment of infections and diarrhoea.
- Development of programmes for early rehydration of children with diarrhoea.
- Development of supplementary feeding programmes during epidemics.
- Deworming of heavily infested children.

Integrated Child Development Services

Isolated feeding programmes will not be effective unless efforts are made simultaneously to improve the environment and to control infections. Supplementary nutrition is therefore integrated with other health activities like immunisation, treatment of minor illnesses, growth monitoring and health education under the ICDS.

Nutrition Education

Education programmes to improve child nutrition should stress the importance of breast-feeding and timely introduction of supplements. Mothers should be advised to give supplements based on the household foods like cereals and pulses. Addition of oil/sugar increases calorie density. Amylase rich food prepared from wheat or maize can be used to reduce the bulk of the cereal mixture.

UNICEF recommended GOBI that is Growth monitoring, Oral rehydration, Breast feeding and Immunisation an inexpensive measure to prevent SAM.

Deficiency of Vitamin A

Surveys carried out by the National Nutrition Monitoring Bureau (NNMB) and Integrated Child Development Services (ICDS) indicate that prevalence of Bitot's spots in preschool children (1–5 years) ranges between 1–5 per cent in different parts of India. The corneal xerophthalmia has been reported to be 0.05–0.1 per 100 preschool children in South India. It is estimated that over 50,000 children become blind every year in India due to vitamin A deficiency. According to NNMB survey 0.04 per cent of blindness in India is due to vitamin A deficiency which can be prevented. Figure 5.7 shows prevalence of Bitot's spots in some States of India.

The NIN study (2005–2006) found that the magnitude of prevalence of subclinical vitamin A deficiency was as high as 62 per cent in preschool children in all the States.

According to the studies conducted at National Institute of Nutrition, Hyderabad (2003–2004) the overall prevalence of night blindness among preschool children was 0.3 per cent and that of Bitot's spots was 0.8 per cent. The prevalence of Bitot's spots was > 0.5 per cent, a cut off level recommended by WHO to indicate public health significance, in all the States, except Kerala and Orissa.

Epidemiology

Age: Vitamin A deficiency is preponderant in children. While it is rare during infancy, preschool children are at a greater risk. The corneal lesions, however, are rarely seen in the children above the age of 6 years. A great majority of the cases of corneal xerophthalmia occur between 1 and 3 years, coinciding with the peak-prevalence of severe protein energy malnutrition.

Socioeconomic factors: Children from rural and tribal families belonging to low-income group are more vulnerable to vitamin A deficiency. Cases are common in remote villages. The mothers of vitamin A deficient children are generally illiterate and unaware of the importance of diet in disease. Due to food fads and false beliefs, foods like colostrum, green leafy vegetables and papaya which are rich in vitamin A are avoided. The poor families cannot afford animal foods like eggs which are rich in preformed vitamin A.

Aetiology

Inadequate dietary intake of vitamin A or its precursor (β-carotene) is the most contributory factor for vitamin A deficiency. Vitamin A deficient diets are consumed by pregnant and lactating mothers, as a result the off-spring is born with poor liver stores of vitamin A. Though during infancy, mother's milk protects the child from vitamin A deficiency, the intake of vitamin A by the children either during the weaning period or at later ages is woefully inadequate and provides only 25–30 per cent of recommended intake. Consequently the hepatic stores to vitamin A in children are depleted gradually leading to hypovitaminosis A. Due to female illiteracy and consequently ignorance, supplementation with vitamin A rich foods is delayed and certain rich sources of β-carotene like green leafy vegetables and papaya are avoided with the belief that these are deleterious to the health of children.

Animal foods like eggs, milk and liver provide preformed vitamin A. But these are expensive and the poor communities cannot afford. Consequently they depend on plant foods which provide only provitamin A.

In addition to inadequate dietary intake, other factors such as the poor nutritional status of the mother during pregnancy and lactation, delayed supplementary feeding, are also causes of vitamin A deficiency.

The common childhood infections like measles, diarrhoea, respiratory tract infections and infestations like ascariasis and giardiasis interfere with the absorption of vitamin A.

Due to lack of awareness, the community does not make use of primary health care services like diarrhoea-control, immunisation, vitamin A supplementation and other basic health services.

Symptoms

Deficiency symptoms show up after liver reserves of the vitamin have been depleted. These symptoms can also be the result of a deficiency of protein or zinc, either of which reduce the amount of vitamin A released from liver stores. Symptoms may result from low dietary intakes, interference with absorption and storage or interference with the conversion of carotene to vitamin A.

Nutritional blindness due to xerophthalmia is an important public health problem among young children in India. The term xerophthalmia encompasses all ocular manifestations of vitamin A deficiency. It includes the structural changes affecting conjunctiva, cornea and occasionally retina and also the biophysical disorders of retinol rod and cone functions.

Clinical Signs

The WHO gives the following classification of xerophthalmia:

Night Blindness (XN): The speed with which the eye recovers its full powers after exposure to bright light is directly related to the amount of vitamin A that is available to form rhodopsin. The recovery process is known as dark adaptation because it allows the eye to adapt to vision in dim light after exposure to bright light.

When vitamin A is deficient, the formation of rhodopsin is impaired giving rise to night blindness. Night blindness is an early symptom of vitamin A deficiency and is often present without any signs of xerophthalmia. It responds well to treatment. It is a useful screening tool and correlates closely with other evidence of vitamin A deficiency.

Conjunctival Xerosis (XIA): It manifests as dry patches of non-wettable conjunctiva. It may be associated with various degreses of thickening, wrinkling and pigmentation (muddy colouring) of the conjunctiva. The pigmentation gives the conjunctiva a peculiar 'smoky' appearance. This symptom in children under 5 years is more likely to be due to dietary deficiency.

Bitot's Spots (XIB): It is more an extension of the xerotic process. These spots are raised, muddy and dry triangular patches. Bitot's spots are not only easily diagnosable but are also of considerable diagnostic value in young children. Typical symptoms of vitamin A is given in Fig. 5.8.

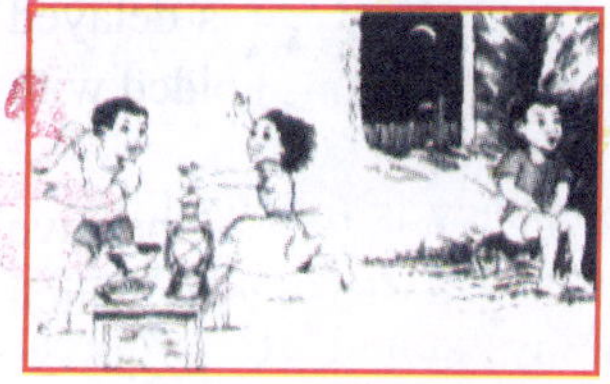

Night blindness

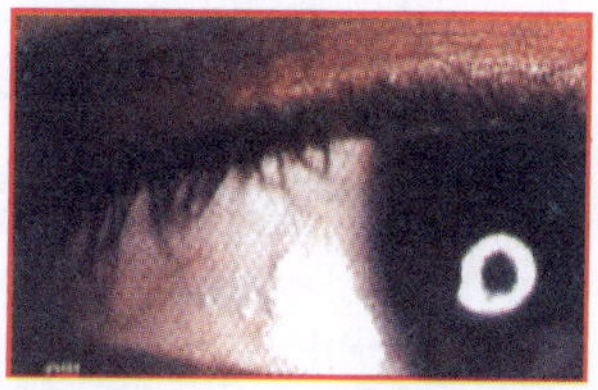

Bitot's spots

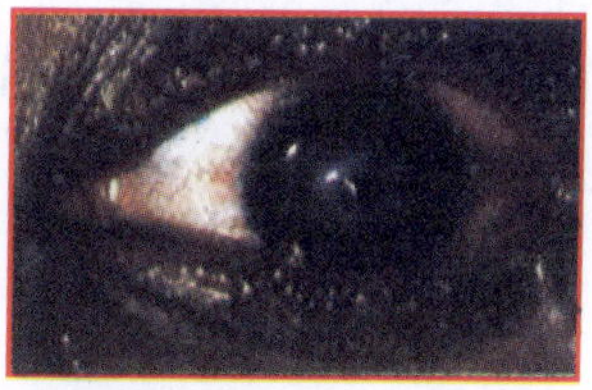

Corneal xerosis/ulceration

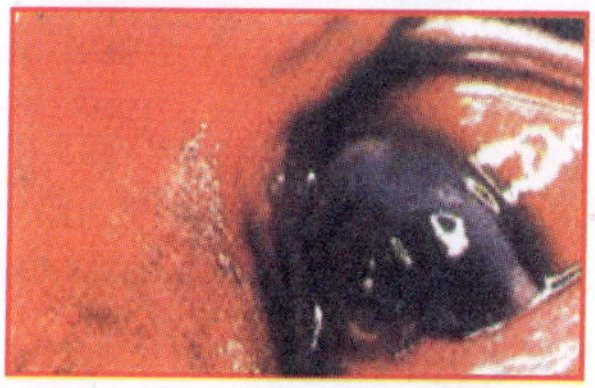

Keratomalacia

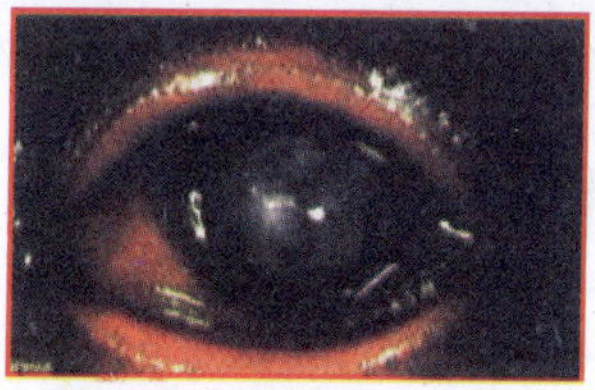

Corneal scar

Fig. 5.8 Typical symptoms of vitamin A deficiency.

Source: Prevention and treatment of vitamin A deficiency. 1991, Ministry of Health and Family welfare, Government of India.

Corneal Xerosis (X2): When dryness spreads to the cornea there is a dull hazy lack lustre appearance. This is due to the keratinisation which is the result of vitamin A deficiency on all epithelial surfaces. The characteristic feature is a loss of substance (erosion) of a part or the whole of the corneal thickness. If there is secondary infection there is inflammation. The lesion only heals by scarring. If properly managed the corneal changes usually heal leaving useful vision. Corneal xerosis may progress suddenly and rapidly to keratomalacia.

Keratomalacia (X3B): In this condition softening and dissolution of the cornea occurs. If the process is not stopped by treatment, perforation of the cornea leads to prolapse of the iris, extrusion of the lens and infection of the whole eyeball which almost invariably occurs. Healing results in scarring of the whole eye and frequently in total blindness.

Increased Susceptibility to Infection: The action of the cilia of the epithelial cells is involved in protecting the body against infection by sweeping the cell surfaces clear of invading microorganisms. In vitamin A deficient keratinised cells, the cilia are lost and the body is more vulnerable to infection.

Vitamin A is known to be required for the proper activity of the immune system, which defends us against infection. Once an infection has taken hold, it can aggravate a pre-existing vitamin A deficiency, placing the individual at even greater risk of further infections and perhaps eventual death. Carotenoids, which do not act as a source of vitamin A also stimulate immune response. This may be due to their role as antioxidants.

Children with mild xerophthalmia are known to be at increased risk of respiratory infections and diarrhoea. Supplementation of vitamin A has been shown to reduce the prevalence of the infections and diarrhoea and lead to increased growth rates. It is also known that vitamin A deficiency is a significant factor in the course and severity of measles in developing countries. The presence of measles virus infection probably causes a depletion of the body's stores of vitamin A by increasing the use of vitamin A and so compounding the problems caused by decreased dietary intake and absorption of the vitamin.

The WHO and UNICEF have jointly recommended that high oral doses of vitamin A should be given to all children suffering from measles in communities that are known to be at risk of vitamin A deficiency.

Administering vitamin A to individuals with a vitamin A deficiency is followed by a rise in serum iron levels, increased saturation of transferrin and increased haemoglobin levels. Vitamin A deficiency may be associated with a failure to mobilise stored iron properly or could directly prevent normal differentiation of red blood cells. Infections brought on by the impaired immunity of individuals with vitamin A deficiency could also interfere with the normal functioning of the bone marrow tissue responsible for generating red blood cells.

Public Health Significance

If the per cent prevalence of symptoms of vitamin A deficiency is more than the value as given in Table 5.4, then it is considered as a public health problem.

Table 5.4 Prevalence rates of xerophthalmia and vitamin A deficiency defining public health significance

Sign/Symptom/Biochemical indicators	*% prevalence*
Night blindness (XN)	> 1.0
Bitot's spots (X1B)	> 0.5
Corneal xerosis (X2, X3A & X3B)	> 0.01
Corneal scar related to xerophthalmia (XS)	> 0.05
Serum retinol level less than 10 ug/dl	> 5.0

Source: Bhaskaram, P., 1999, *Programmes for Preventing Vitamin A Deficiency—Indian Status*. Heinz Nutrition Foundation of India. In Touch 1,2.

Treatment

Table 5.5 gives treatment schedule.

Table 5.5 Treatment schedules for xerophthalmia—Oil miscible oral vitamin A

	< 1 year of age	*> 1 year of age*
Immediately	100,000 IU	200,000 IU
Next day	100,000 IU	200,000 IU
2–4 weeks later	100,000 IU	200,000 IU
Severe Protein Energy Malnutrition (PEM)		
Additional monthly dose until PEM resolves	100,000 IU	200,000 IU

Source: WHO/ UNICEF/ IVACG Task Force.

Immediately on diagnosis, an oral dose of 200,000 IU if oil miscible vitamin A should be given to children in the age of 1–6 years. In the case of those with persistent vomiting and diarrhoea an intramuscular injection of 1,00,000 IU of water miscible vitamin A can be substituted for the oral dose.

This is followed by another dose of 2,00,000 IU one to four weeks later. In the case of infants and children weighing less than 8 kg, the same schedule may be followed using half the dose of vitamin A. Acute corneal lesions should be considered as medical emergency and should be referred to the nearest hospital for treatment of the general condition in addition to the treatment of the eye disease.

Prevention

Under the MCH services and the ICDS programme, record of vitamin A administration of all 9 doses is maintained for under fives that is 2,00,000 IU of vitamin A for every six months.

A comprehensive strategy simultaneously addressing the following issues is crucial to achieve the goals of elimination of vitamin A deficiency.

Nutrition education

The education of the people to promote dietary intake of vitamin A and β-carotene rich foods is the foremost requirement for alleviating the problem of vitamin A deficiency in all age groups. The strategy though it sounds simple is a complex one needing inputs from various sectors of the Government, Research Institutions, Home Science Colleges, NGOs and the private sector.

National programmes like Integrated Child Development Services (ICDS) and Child Survival and Safe Motherhood (CSSM) need to promote the following activities:

- Ensuring adequate intake of vitamin A and carotene rich foods by pregnant mothers for building up vitamin A stores in mothers and the foetus.
- Early initiation of breast feeding (within one hour of delivery) to establish good lactation.
- Feeding of colostrum to build up vitamin A stores in infants.
- Exclusive breast feeding for first 4–6 months.

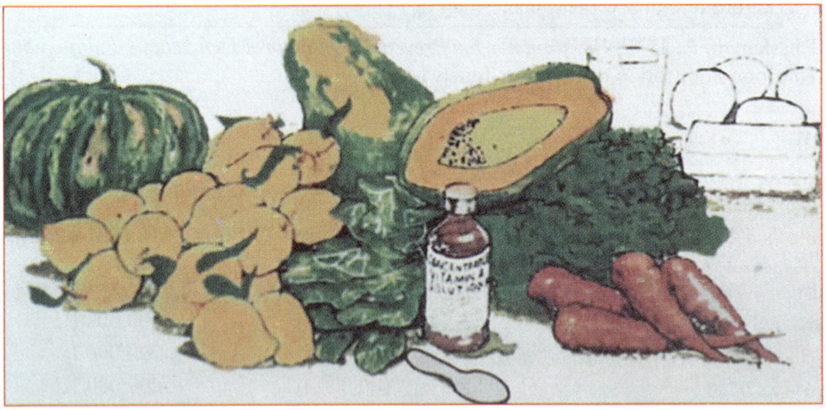

Fig. 5.9 **Foods rich in Vitamin A and carotenoids.**

- Supplements of vitamin A and β-carotene rich foods like carrots, pumpkin, spinach and other dark green leafy vegetables to be given in puree form (boiled and mashed) with addition of a little ghee or oil and fruits like papaya, mango are to be given to the infants from 4–6 months onwards atleast once daily.
- Ensuring regular intake of vitamin A and β-carotene rich food by preschool children.
- School children to be used as "change agents" for communicating the information on vitamin A to their families and the community. For this purpose, adequate information on various aspects of vitamin A deficiency and its prevention and control is to be incorporated in their existing curriculum.
- Nutrition information on vitamin A is to be communicated extensively to all sections of population by all concerned sectors, NGOs, extension agencies and the food industry.

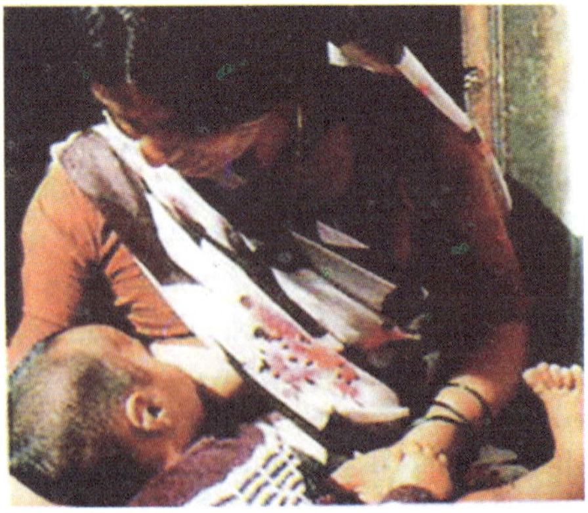

Fig. 5.10 **Breast feeding the child is the first measure to prevent vitamin A deficiency.**

According to NIN annual report 2009–2010 despite the vast expenditure in India on programmes for improving young children's nutrition and health poor dietary intakes by under three-year olds, was observed even in families where the adults met their daily dietary requirements. Parents and caregivers need to be educated about the kind of food to be given and how to give nutritious food to children.

Horticultural interventions including home gardening

Ensuring an adequate supply of β-carotene rich foods for the population is one of the most important prerequisites for promoting the dietary intake of vitamin A.

- Specifying annual requirements of β-carotene rich plant foods at production level for the country.
- Department of Horticulture and Social Forestry should encourage production of green leafy vegetables, fruits and vegetables which are rich in micronutrients like vitamin A, iron and vitamin C.
- Development of village level community nurseries.
- Distribution of seeds, saplings and plant materials of species known to be rich in β-carotene.
- Identifying less familiar local fruits and vegetables with high β-carotene content and promoting them.
- Promoting production and consumption of non-conventional foods like red palm oil for combating vitamin A deficiency.
- Krishi Vigyan Kendras to emphasise on the production and consumption of fruits and vegetables, through demonstration, vocational training, in-service training and on-farm research.
- School gardens and kitchen gardens to be encouraged.
- Strengthening linkages between the infrastructures of Agriculture (Horticulture), Nutrition (ICDS, FNB) and Maternal Child Health (MCH) with a view to ensure nutrition oriented horticultural activities at the village level.

Nutrient supplementation

"The National Prophylaxis Programme Against Nutritional Blindness" is being implemented in the country since 1970 through Health and family infrastructure. This involves oral administration of a massive dose of 2,00,000 IU of vitamin A in oil every six months to preschool children.

Since, vitamin A can be stored in the liver for a prolonged period, it is possible to build up adequate stores of vitamin A through periodic administration of massive doses of vitamin A. This approach has been found to be feasible in extensive field studies carried out at the National Institute of Nutrition. Studies in preschool children have shown that following a massive dose of 2,00,000 IU of vitamin A, there is significant reduction in the prevalence of ocular signs of vitamin A deficiency.

Since 1992, the programme is included in the 'Package of services' provided to children under the Child Survival and Safe Motherhood (CSSM) programme and it addresses children in the age group of 9 months to 3 years only. The first dose of 1,00,000 IU of vitamin A is administered at nine months of age along with measles vaccine. The subsequent doses of 2,00,000 IU are given at 18 months along with DPT Booster dose, at 24, 30 and 36 months. Children in the age group of 3–6 years are also covered under the vitamin A deficiency control programme.

Prevention of infection

Vitamin A deficiency is often precipitated by a range of infections including measles, diarrhoea and acute respiratory infection. Studies have documented corneal xerophthalmia, following episodes of these common infections of childhood. Frequent infections in children lead to greater requirement for vitamin A. These infections need to be prevented through immunisation and intensification of programmes on supply of safe drinking water and improved sanitation.

Selective fortification

The first food fortified with vitamin A in India was vanaspati. All hydrogenated fats, by legislation are expected to be fortified with vitamins A and D. The general fortification of common foods with high levels of vitamin A is not recommended in view of the risk of toxicity caused by excess of vitamin A. Selective fortification of food with vitamin A is recommended.

- Foods meant for identified high risk areas of vitamin A deficiency such as tribal areas should be fortified with vitamin A.
- Low cost processed foods for supplementary feeding of infants, preschool children and school children (ICDS and Mid Day Meal Programme) to be fortified with vitamin A.
- All special foods meant for children to be fortified with vitamin A.
- All toned and double toned milk to be fortified with vitamin A so as to replace the amount of vitamin A lost during the process of toning.
- The legislation of fortification of vanaspati with vitamin A to be extended to include all vegetable oils in view of the greater consumption of vegetable oils than the hydrogenated fat in recent years.
- The scope of fortifying sugar with vitamin A needs to be explored.

The strategy to prevent vitamin A deficiency should be a combination of long-term programme of nutrition education and improvement in house-hold food security and a short-term periodic massive dose of vitamin A. There is also a need for intensification of research and development activities to identify technologies to increase the production and consumption of less familiar β-carotene rich foods such as red palm oil and spirulina, a blue-green algae. Involvement, motivation and mobilisation of community are essential for achieving the goal of prevention of vitamin A deficiency.

Better implementation of the Union Government's food based programme would help to improve nutrition levels. The plan calls for universalising the Public Distribution System, a life-cycle approach for nutrition programmes to address different nutrition requirements and a "Food Guarantee Act" that would combine the features of the food-for-work and national rural employment guarantee schemes.

Suggested recipes for vitamin A deficiency

Recipe	*Reasons*
Boiled egg, egg custard	Rich in vitamin A and good quality protein
Coriander and mint chutney with bread/ chapathi	Not only rich in β-carotene but also rich in iron and vitamin C.
Carrot halwa, carrot salad, carrot kheer, carrot juice	Rich in β-carotene
Papaya	Rich in β-carotene
Orange, tomato, and mango fruit	Rich in β-carotene and Vitamin C
Palak dal, Palak paneer	Rich in β-carotene and protein

National nutrition programmes have contributed in raising the nutritional status of the population. Various nutrition programmes in the country beginning with the Applied Nutrition Programme in sixties the Special Nutrition Programme in seventies and Integrated Child Development Services Scheme from the eighties and noon meal programme have been effective in alleviating SAM and vitamin A deficiency.

SUGGESTED READINGS

- Cooper C. Christen, Preschool nutrition, Today's Dietitian, 2011.
- Batada Ameena *et al.*, Nine out of 10 food advertisements shown during Saturday morning children's television programming are foods high in fat, sodium or added sugars or low in nutrients. J Am Diet. Assoc. 2008; **108**.
- Nekitsing Chandani *et al.*, Taste exposure increases intake and nutrition education increases willingness to try an unfamiliar vegetable in pre school children J Acad Nutr Diet 2019; **119**.
- Indian Academy of Paediatrics. www.iapindia.org.

QUESTIONS

1. Give the RDA for a 5 year old child.
2. Explain the nutritional importance during pre-school.
3. Discuss the factors affecting the nutritional status of children.
4. Describe the factors to be considered in planning a diet for a pre-schooler.
5. Poverty may not be the only reason for malnutrition during pre-school age. What are the other reasons?
6. How can you prevent dental problems in children?
7. Write in detail about nutrition related problems of pre-schoolers.
8. Describe in detail the stages of treatment of SAM.
9. Describe the nutritional requirement of SAM child and explain the sequence of dietary treatment.
10. Plan a day's diet for a 4-year-old child from a low income group.

11. Explain prevalence of vitamin A deficiency in India and discuss the prophylactic measures used in India.
12. Suggest five recipes rich in vitamin A suitable for a pre-school child.
13. Give the clinical symptoms of vitamin A deficiency.
14. How can one modify the food habits of children?
15. Explain RUFT.
16. Give details of ARFID.

TOPICS FOR ACTIVITY

- Plan and prepare a diet for a child recovering from SAM.
- Plan and prepare four low cost vitamin A rich recipes.
- Discuss the different aspects of 'table manners' to be taught to preschool children.
- Find out the nutritional status of children in an anganwadi.

6

Nutritional Recommendtions and Food Requirements of School Children — 7 to 12 Years

During the pre-adolescent period the child grows, on an average, 6–7 cm in height and 1.5 to 3 kg in weight every year and simultaneously development and maturation of various tissues and organs take place. Adolescent growth spurt starts at about 10–12 years in girls.

NUTRITIONAL RECOMMENDATIONS

The RDA of school children aged 7–12 years suggested by ICMR is given in Table 6.1.

Table 6.1 ICMR Recommended Dietary Allowances for children 7-12 years – 2020

Nutrient	*Years*		
	7–9	*10–12*	
		Boys	*Girls*
Body weight kg	25.3	34.9	36.4
Energy kcal	1700	2220	2060
Protein g	23	32	33
Dietary Fibre g	26	33	30
Calcium mg	650	850	850
Magnesium mg	175	240	250
Iron mg	15	16	28
Zinc mg	5.9	8.5	8.5
Iodine μg	90	100	100
Vitamin A Retinol μg	630	770	790
Vitamin D IU	600	600	600
Thiamine mg	1.1	1.5	1.4
Riboflavin mg	1.6	2.1	1.9
Niacin mg	11	15	14
Pyridoxine mg	1.5	2.0	1.9
Folate μg	170	220	225
Vitamin B_{12} μg	2.2	2.2	2.2
Vitamin C mg	45	55	50

Nutritional requirements of boys and girls are more or less the same till the first 9 years. After that, there is a variation in the requirement. Nutritional requirement supports optimal growth, development and activity.

Calories and Protein

Energy needs vary with the child's growth rate, body size and physical activity. To be healthy, children need to be engaged moderately in intense physical activity at least for one hour per day. This fact is taken into consideration by the Nutrition Expert Committee (2010) in prescribing the energy needs of children. Body requirements of calories are increased steadily for this age group.

Same amount of energy requirement –1700 kcal- is required for 7–9 year old boys and girls. There is gradual increase in need because reserves are being laid down for the demands of the approaching adolescent period. Younger school-age children (7–9 years old) require more energy per kilogram of body weight compared to 10–12 years old. The increased requirements of protein would meet demands of growth.

In children protein energy ratio is low owing to high energy needs. Protein requirement is constant at different levels of activity, while the energy requirement changes, the PE ratio becomes higher requirements of boys differ from girls. The protein requirements of girls aged 10–12 years is higher than boys due to rapid growth in pubertal age.

Fat

Total fat intake below 25% E is considered to affect growth in children. To provide 25 per cent total fat calories, a minimum level of visible fat in children should range between 25–35 g/day.

Minerals

Calcium: Ten to twelve-year old children require in purberital age 850 mg of calcium and 850 mg of phosphorus to meet skeletal growth demands. They need to take 2–3 glasses of milk to meet the requirement of calcium and improve bone density.

Iron: In childhood, the mean increase in body weight is 2.8 kg/y, which necessitates an iron requirement of 0.7 mg/d. The average iron requirement for growth would be about 17 μg/kg/d. During childhood (4 to 9 + 4) body store of iron builds up to 5 mg/kg, which is maintained in girls until menarche. The RDA of iron for 7–9 year old is 15 mg. The requirements of iron for 10-12 year old girls is 28 mg and for boys 16 mg.

Iron deficiency anaemia is a risk factor for poor educational performance in school-age children.

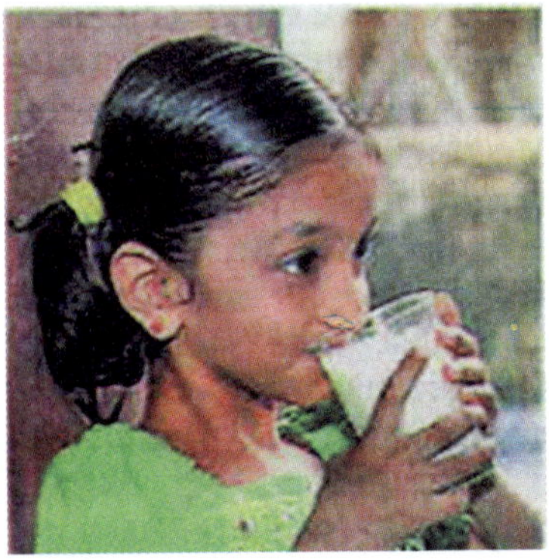

Fig. 6.1 In addition to supplying calcium, milk satisfies appetite and prevents overeating.

Iodine: The RDA suggested by ICMR for iodine is 90 μg and 100 μg for 7-9 year old and 10-12 year old respectively.

Zinc: Zinc supplementation improves linear growth in stunted and underweight children at young age. WHO/UNICEF recommend zinc supplementation during diarrhoeal infection and for treatment of severe malnutrition.

The RDA suggested by ICMR 2020 for Zinc is 5.9 mg and 8.5 mg for 7–9 year old and 10–12 year old respectively.

Vitamins

Vitamin A: Vitamin A requirements of the children have been computed from the requirement figures for infants (50 μg/kg) and adults 9.3 μg/kg taking into account growth rates at different ages. The RDA of vitamin A for 7–9 years is 630 μg. For 10–12 year old the RDA for boys is 770 μg and for girls 790 μg.

Vitamin D: From the age of one year to 18 years the RDA of vitamin D is 600 I.U.

B-Vitamins: The RDA of B-vitamins is based on calorie requirement.

Vitamin C: In general, Indian diets have iron inhibitors. Hence a minimum of 40 mg of vitamin C is needed. For children the RDA of vitamin C is 40 mg.

Dietary fibre

ICMR (2020) has suggested dietary fibre requirement of children aged 7-9 year is 26 g. Higher requirement of fibre is suggested 33 g and 30 g for 10–12 year old boys and girls respectively.

FOOD REQUIREMENTS

The school age period is one of steady growth, usually with fewer feeding problems than during toddler and preschool years. A natural increase in appetite is responsible for an increase in food consumption. The child's growing independence leads to a gradual transfer of control of food selection from the parent to the child.

Parents or caretakers should provide nutrition education for their children as being role models. Parents should encourage the child to eat appropriate portion size, eating a variety of foods and trying new foods. Negative behaviours such as using food as an emotional coping mechanism or as a reward, should be discouraged. Parents should establish in children healthy eating habits for lowering the risks for nutrition-related chronic diseases.

Between the ages of 8 to 11, some girls may be at risk for developing eating disorders.

Snacks remain an important part of the diet. The meal taken on return from school is important to meet the nutritional requirement and to have interaction with parents. Children who do not eat breakfast at home are more likely to buy junk food. Parents should give healthful breakfast at home before sending children to school.

Though media influences diet choices of children, parents should know nutritional facts and suggest to their children. Government should regulate advertisements aimed at children.

There is an increasing interest and participation in other activities which compete with meal times. The important relationship of sound nutrition and learning has long been established.

The diet should contain all Basic Five Food Groups. If the child does not have access to items from all food groups on a regular basis, self-selection of a balanced diet either within a day or over several days is impossible.

Unrefined cereals, whole grams, soya and vegetables can be incorporated in regular foods to make the food more nutritious.

Family Meals

Family dinner has been identified as a foundation of healthful food choices. This is due to the higher quality of food served and the family conversations at the dinner table about healthful eating and possibly control the weight of the family members. Family dinner creates a relaxed atmosphere and members are receptive for the suggestions. During the family dinner time, TV should be switched off so that the members can concentrate on the food and the conversation. Family meals not only help dietary pattern of children and adolescents but also adults who are supposed to be role models. Adults while eating family dinners help children and adolescents in consuming balanced diets by giving explanation or being role models. Incidental advantages are the children learn not to waste food, to clean up the place and eating neatly.

Importance of Breakfast

Breakfast is important particularly for a school child. It breaks the fast of the sleep hours and prepares a child for problem solving and memory spans in the learning period at school. Children who skip breakfast do not make up for nutrient and energy deficits later in the day and tend to perform more poorly on tests of cognition than those who eat breakfast. Study conducted by NIN confirmed that eating breakfast regularly is a significant factor influencing better academic performance. Eating breakfast at home is a healthy habit. It is not enough for children to have just a glass of milk. An ideal breakfast should have all basic five food groups.

Liquids like porridges are absorbed quickly. Solids like idlis and rotis are preferred. It is better to include eggs in breakfast as they are rich in protein, vitamins and minerals. A good mix of low and high glycaemic index foods release energy continuously. Ready to eat cereals provide calcium, protein, iron and vitamins due to the added substances such as milk, fruits, dry fruits and nuts.

Benefits of breakfast eating include

- improved cognitive function and academic performance in school.
- improved school attendance
- improved micronutrent profile
- reduced body mass index
- improvement in psychosocial well being, discipline and social behaviour.
- less aggression and fewer suspensions.

Government of Tamil Nadu is planning to introduce breakfast for school children in addition to mid-day meal.

Dietary Guidelines

- Nutritional requirement should meet their increasing activity and growth and additional requirement for sickness or injury.
- Every meal should include all five food groups including lunch taken at school.
- Growing children drink 2–3 glasses of milk or equivalent milk products like curds.

- If the child does not like salads, vegetables can be incorporated, in recipes like sandwiches. Food should include green leafy and other coloured vegetables.
- Snacks and food eaten on returning from school make negative or positive contribution to diets. Fruits, nuts and dry fruits can be served as snack item.
- The climatic and weather conditions are important consideration too. In hot weather extra liquids and salts are to be given because children do not generally like to drink plain water.
- Children have varying appetites and often prefer snacky meals at frequent intervals to a few large ones.
- Children also tend to be bored with foods easily. So menus need to provide variety in colour, texture, taste and flavour.
- Children are generally restless and do not like to spend too much time at the table for eating. Besides, they feel rushed in the morning because they must reach their classes on time. So menus have to provide dishes that are quick to eat and yet satisfying nutritionally.
- New foods are likely to be accepted if it is given in a form which can be easily handled and they should be offered at regular intervals until the child learns to accept it.

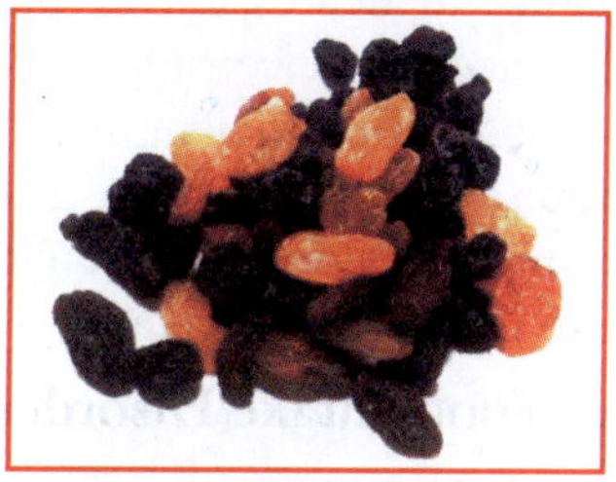

Fig. 6.2 Raisins are good for children as snacks since they are rich in calories and iron. Brown raisins contain 4.2 mg and black raisins contain 6.8 mg of iron per 100 g.

- The young child should be encouraged to eat with the rest of the family as he is ready to take the family meals and also because the interactions between family members are a part of normal development.
- The child should develop liking for home food. Intake of processed food should be discouraged.

Making Healthful Choices: As children grow up, they become more independent about choosing their food. Children can be made to make healthful choices by

- being a role model
- making them plant vegetables or fruit trees (children take pride in eating foods they have grown)
- taking them to farmer's or vegetable market
- allowing them to plan the dinner menu with the help of food guide pyramid
- encouraging them to prepare simple recipes (They are more likely to eat foods they have prepared)
- pre-portioning can help in preventing over eating or under eating
- appreciating when children make healthful food choices
- nutritious ready to eat snacks only to be stocked at home

DIET RELATED PROBLEMS

Feeding Problems

School children take more fatty foods as their lives grow stressful. They eat less fruits and vegetables and do not eat breakfast. Stress appears to be consistently harmful to children in terms of steering their food choices away from the healthy and towards the unhealthy. With the right guidance and nutrition education children learn to prefer healthy foods such as milk, eggs, carrots, greens, fruits, whole grams and unrefined cereals.

Underweight

Many school children consume inadequate diet and so they are malnourished. Malnutrition can be due to poverty. Parents may not be able to provide nutritious food to their children. Sometimes ignorance on the part of parents to know the requirements of children quantitatively or qualitatively may lead to malnutrition of children. When the child is in a hurry to go to school, he may miss breakfast or may not carry proper lunch to school or may become too tired after school activities and sleep off without taking night meal and thus skip the meals. Emotional disturbances at school due to poor academic performance or problems with siblings at home may reflect on the consumption of food.

Psychological factors contributing to depression or poor motivation to eat should be identified. Child's likes and dislikes need to be considered while feeding. The diets of school going Indian children have been found to be deficient in energy, protein, vitamin A and iron.

In order to overcome malnutrition in school children, government through ICDS provides school lunch so that at least one-third of calorie and protein requirements are met. Children should be encouraged to participate in such programmes.

ARFID: Avoidant/Restrictive Food Intake Disorder

ARFID Avoidant/Restrictive Food Intake Disorder is an eating disorder. It is not picky eating. Children with ARFID symptoms will not eat when they are hungry if their extremely limited preferred foods are not available.

The child persistently fail to meet nutritional or energy needs through the oral intake of food. Lack of intake of food leads to significant weight loss or failure to grow along the expected development trajectory in children; significant nutritional deficiency depending on oral supplements or tube feeding or significant interference with psychological functioning such as ability to eat with others.

Lack of interest in eating is related to interoceptive differences, sensory sensitivities and food avoidance due to averse consequences such as GI distress. ARFID is a fairly frequent presenting feature of autism spectrum disorder and extreme and narrow food preferences may pesist.

Etiology of all eating disorders is that they are the result of a combination of genesis, environment, personality characteristics and neurobiology.

Constipation

Consumption of less quantity of food can lead to constipation. Children need 3 basic small meals and two snacks. Early morning hurry to go to school and lack of sleep and activity can also lead to constipation. Children may not relish vegetables and fruits particularly green leafy vegetables. Parents should make an effort to motivate the child to eat by serving in different forms. Processed food should be avoided as they are usually low in fibre.

Dental Caries

Total sugar consumption is not the critical factor for caries development; the oral contact time of cariogenic foods is the major dietary concern. Consumption of sticky sweets can result in dental caries. Chocolates and sugar sweetened beverages are most commonly associated with caries.

Brushing teeth before going to bed and after a meal should become a habit in children. Children should be encouraged to eat hard raw crisp foods, like carrots and cucumbers.

Obesity

Parent-obesity is a prominent factor for childhood obesity. Psychological factors and the child's body type right from the birth also matters. Childhood obesity leads to adult obesity. It can be prevented by avoiding

- forced feeding.
- not instilling in the child's mind that all the food in the plate has to be completed.
- psychological stress at home or stress at school.
- avoiding junk food.
- reducing eating in front of the television or computer.
- skipping breakfast.
- not using food as the reward.

Urbanization, increased income, availability of fast foods, educational demands, television viewing and gaming have led to a rise in the consumption of foods high in fats, sugar and salt and low physical activity. Low activity, excess energy intake and dietary patterns high in fat and low in fibre increase the risk of obesity.

Most obese children develop early puberty, joint pain and find it difficult to exercise. This in turn results in metabolic syndrome and they end up with type-2 diabetes. Childhood is an important time to establish both healthful eating and physical activity habits.

Hormonal imbalance sometimes can also lead to obesity.

Clinicians should involve the family and all caregivers in the treatment programme. It should institute permanent changes in the dietary habits and physical activity. The change should be brought out gradually.

Infections

Common infections and malnutrition contribute significantly to child morbidity and mortality. Infections are prevented by good hygiene practices and developing immunity in the child. A child needs to eat more during and after episodes of infections to maintain good nutritional status.

PACKED LUNCHES

Packed lunches have become a necessity for school going children as schools are either away or the lunch period is too short for the children to go home and have food. The packed lunch is a lunch that is packed in a tiffin box to be eaten by the child while away from home. The packed lunches carried by them are usually not adequate both in quantity and quality.

Taking lunch from home needs a little effort, but helps in maintaining good health. Carrying food from home is less expensive, more convenient, more hygienic and meets the individual requirements.

Points to be considered in planning a packed lunch

- The packed lunch should meet one-third daily requirement of calories, protein and other nutrients of the child, to boost concentration and energy for the rest of the school day.
- Preferably, the packed lunch should consist of all five food groups, though the number of dishes may be less.
- Inclusion of one serving of green leafy vegetables would take care of one-third requirement of many vitamins and minerals.
- Some amount of good quality protein like milk or milk product like curd or paneer would improve vegetable protein. Or combination of vegetable proteins like cereals and pulses can be given for better utilisation. Addition of egg would also improve the quality of protein besides meeting many protective nutrient needs.
- To make the food appetising, whole fruit or butter milk in a bottle or crispies in a polythene bag can be taken.
- Monotony should be avoided in packed lunches. There should be variety.
- It is sensible to have a different food in packed lunch than what one had for breakfast.

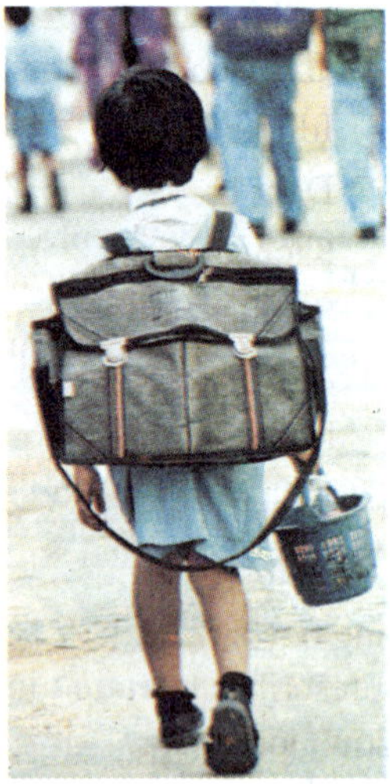

Fig. 6.3 Packed lunch should contain balanced diet which should be completed by the child at school.

- The food should have the correct consistency. Too watery things may leak and too dry food may not be appetising to the child. Chapathis can be covered in cloth to retain moisture. Curd rice should be made with cold rice. Hot rice makes the water to separate from the curd.
- Containers should be cleaned and dried immediately after returning from school.
- Non-perishable items should be included in the lunch box.
- The different items should be packed separately or a tiffin box with compartment should be used.

Packing lunch for the child does not guarantee that he consumes it. Suggestions that encourages the child to eat

- Involve the child in planning, preparing or packing the lunch box.
- Make the lunch simple. Most children eat lunch quickly so that they can spend more time socialising or playing with friends.
- Send easy-to-open packages, cut-up fruits and vegetables, rolled chapathis with stuffing or sandwiches.
- Send portions which can be completed during lunch period.

Suggested packed lunches

- Vegetable pulao, boiled egg, tomato raita and orange fruit.
- Fenugreek leaves stuffed chapathi, thick dal and buttermilk.
- Chapathi stuffed with dal (thikada) with green leafy vegetables sag.
- Chapathi, usual and carrot salad.
- Cheese sandwiches or paneer sandwiches, guava.
- Idli and kurma.
- Dahi bhat, tomato or cucumber slices and lemon pickle.
- Kichidi, buttermilk, coriander chutney.
- Sambar rice, amaranth porial, buttermilk.
- Adai with drumstick leaves and coconut chutney.
- Home made granola (oats, nuts, kismis, sugar).

PHYSICAL ACTIVITY

Going beyond academics, the new syllabus aims to inculcate a healthy lifestyle among students by prescribing a range of physical activities as well as nutritional choices. In this connection, yellow book, an interactive and illustrated book is brought out by Food Safety and Standards Authority of India (FSSAI). Yellow book contains:

- Good food safety practices
- Personal hygiene and cleanliness habits
- Consuming a balanced diet
- Packing a wholesome lunchbox
- Preventing nutritional deficiencies and making healthy choices

FSSAI has prescribed the following physical activities to three different age groups.

Primary Classes (I–V)	*Middle and Secondary School (VI–X)*	*Senior Secondary School (XI–XII)*
• Locomotor activities such as sitting, standing, walking, running, jumping and throwing	• Body awareness – includes learning about BMI and anthopometry measurements	• Basic and floor aerobics
• Calisthenics	• Physical fitness and movement eduction – includes calisthenics and indigenous exercises, such as dands and baithak	• Yoga – pranayama, asanas and meditation
• Breathing exercises	• Kho-kho, kabaddi, throwball, basketball and track and field events	• Sports and track and field events.
• Recreational and traditional games	• Breathing exercises and yoga	• Training methods, including interval training, weight training and polymetric training
• Healthy habits and safety education	• Safety education and first aid	• Introduction to the foundation of physical education
• Yogasanas	• Gymnastics	
• Chess		

After getting approval from school education department the principles of yellow book would be incorporated into school syllabus. This helps in inculcating wholesome food habits, personal hygiene and safe food choices. It has also suggested activities for indoor and outdoor games keeping in mind overall development of the child. Schools should see that no junk food is available nearby.

Appropriate diet and physical activity during childhood is essential for optimum body composition, BMI and to reduce the risk of diet-related chronic diseases in later life.

School health day is on 16th July
Children's day is on 14th November

SUGGESTED READINGS

- Au E. Lauren, *et al.*, Eating schools meals daily is associated with healthier dietary intakes: The healthy communities study, J. Acad. Nutr. Diet 2018: **118**.
- Childhood obesity: A multicentric study on its measurement and determinants. Annual report 2014–15, NIN, Hyderabad.
- Richie D. Lorren *et al.*, School Breakfast policy is associated with dietary intake of 4th and 5th grade students J Acad. Nutr. Diet 2016, **116**.
- Trof holz C. Amanda *et al.*, watching television while eating. Association with dietary intake and weight stands among a diverse sample of young children J Acal Nutr Diet. 2018; 119 (9).
- Dept. of Women and Child Development, Ministry of Human Resource Development, Govt. of India. www.wcd.nic.in.

QUESTIONS

1. Give the RDA for a 11-year-old girl.
2. Compare the nutritional requirements of 7–9 year old and 10–12 year old and discuss the causes for the differences.
3. Describe the points to be considered in planning diets for school children.
4. 20–35 per cent Indian school children are underweight. What are the reasons for this?
5. Plan a packed lunch for a 12 years old boy.
6. Write a note on packed lunch.
7. Explain the causes of obesity in school going children.
8. What is 'Yellow Book'? Explain its importance.
9. Discuss the importance of physical activity in children.
10. What is ARFID?
11. Bring out the importance of breakfast for school going children.
12. What are the feeding problem of school going children.

TOPICS FOR ACTIVITY

- Plan and prepare a packed lunch for a nine year old child.
- Plan and prepare a breakfast for 11 year old who does not like milk.
- Topics to be discussed at family meal time. Do's and don'ts.

7

Nutritional Recommendations and Food Requirements of Adolescents

According to WHO, individuals between 10 and 19 years are considered adolescents. The period of transition from childhood to adulthood is called adolescence with accelerated physical, biochemical and emotional development. There are many physical and mental changes which result due to the influence of hormones. It is during this period that the final growth spurt occurs with increase in height and weight. The growth spurt of boys is slower than that of girls.

The growth spurt signals the onset of critical body composition of 10 per cent body fat. However, 22 per cent of body fat is required to maintain regular ovulation. Growth velocity is maximum for boys between 12–15 years and for girls 10–13 years. They attain their adult stature between 18–20 but bone mass continues to increase up to age of 25. With the profound growth of adolescence there is increased demands for energy, protein, minerals and vitamins. Body composition also changes during puberty. Lean body mass doubles in boys between 10–17 years of age. The per cent of body fat decreases in boys during their height spurt but increases thereafter to about 12 per cent of body weight by late puberty. In contrast girls gain proportionately more fat than boys and have a continuous increase in body fat during puberty.

Growth velocity pattern of adolescents is given in Fig. 7.1.

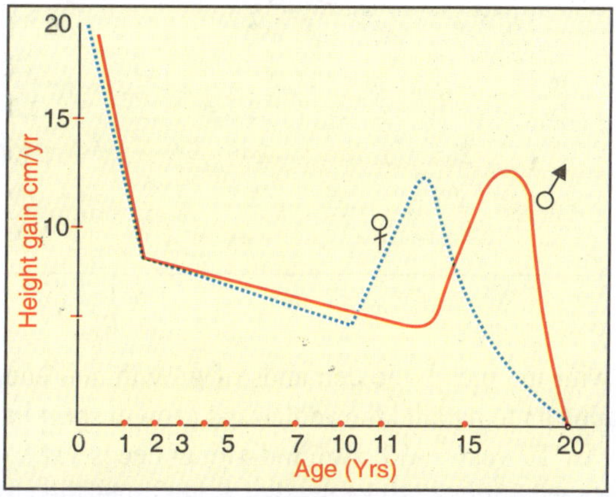

Fig. 7.1 Comparison of growth velocity pattern in boys and girls

The dimensional changes and changes in maturational timing over the generations are called secular changes, the term secular referring to successive periods of time. There is an increase in the intake of cereals and millets over the past 25 years among the adolescents. Secular changes in heights and weights are observed with increase of about 2.5 to 3.5 cm and 1 to 1.5 kg in mean heights and weights respectively. Magnitude of secular trend in stature which may approximate 1 cm/decade and the inverse secular trend in menarcheal timing, which may approximate 0.2 yr/decade. Adolescent anorexia may lead to diminution of the secular trend. Malnutrition delays menarche. The mean age of menarche for Indian girls is 13.5 ± 0.8 years.

NUTRITIONAL RECOMMENDATIONS

The RDA of adolescents suggested by ICMR is given in Table 7.1.

Table 7.1 ICMR Recommended Dietary Allowances of adolescents – 2020

Nutrient	*Years*			
	13–15		*16–17*	
	Boys	*Girls*	*Boys*	*Girls*
Body weight kg	50.5	49.6	64.4	55.7
Energy kcal	2860	2400	3320	2500
Protein g	45.0	43.0	55.0	46.0
Dietary Fibre g	43	36	50	38
Calcium mg	1000	1000	1050	1050
Magnesium mg	345	340	440	380
Iron mg	22	30	26	3.2
Zinc mg	14.3	12.8	17.6	14.2
Iodine µg	140	140	140	140
Vitamin A Retinol µg	930	890	1000	860
Vitamin D IU	600	600	600	600
Thiamine mg	1.9	1.6	2.2	1.7
Riboflavin mg	2.7	2.2	3.1	2.3
Niacin mg	19	16	22	17
Pyridoxine mg	2.6	2.2	3.0	2.3
Folate µg	285	245	340	270
Vitamin B_{12} µg	2.2	2.2	2.2	2.2
Vitamin C mg	70	65	85	70

Energy

Caloric needs increase with the metabolic demands of growth and energy expenditure. In boys the peak calorie intake appears to parallel the adolescent growth spurt increasing until 16 years of age and then decreasing by 19 years. Although individual needs vary, girls consume fewer kilo calories than boys. Boys need 2860–3320 kcal a day. Sometimes the large appetite characteristic of this growth period leads adolescents to satisfy their hunger with snack foods that are high in sugar and fat and low in protein.

From the age of 10 years, there is a marked difference in the caloric needs of boys and girls. As seen from the Fig. 7.2 the needs of boys are higher than those of girls which continues till the adult stage. Adults, both female and male require less calories compared to 18–19 year old. Growth and physical activity contribute significantly to the total energy requirement.

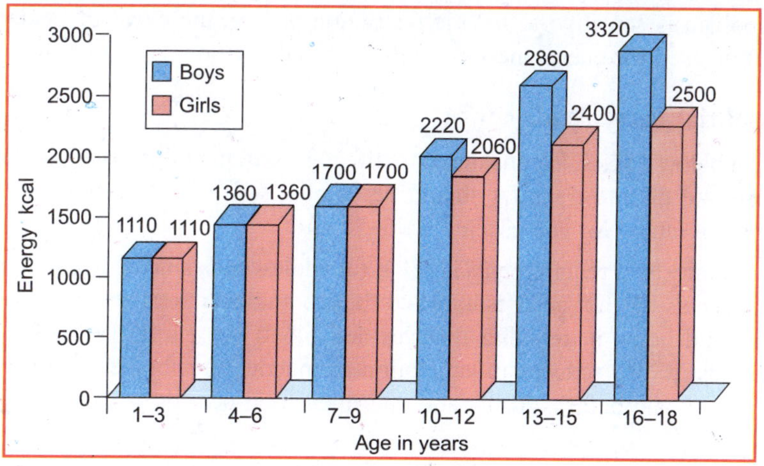

Fig. 7.2 **Comparison of RDA (2020) for energy of different age groups**

Proteins

For most adolescents, eating to satisfy appetite offers a reasonably sensitive indicator of energy needs. Protein needs represent 11–12 per cent of energy intake. The protein intake usually exceeds 1 g/kg body weight. This meets growth needs and for the pubertal changes in both sexes and for the developing muscle mass in boys.

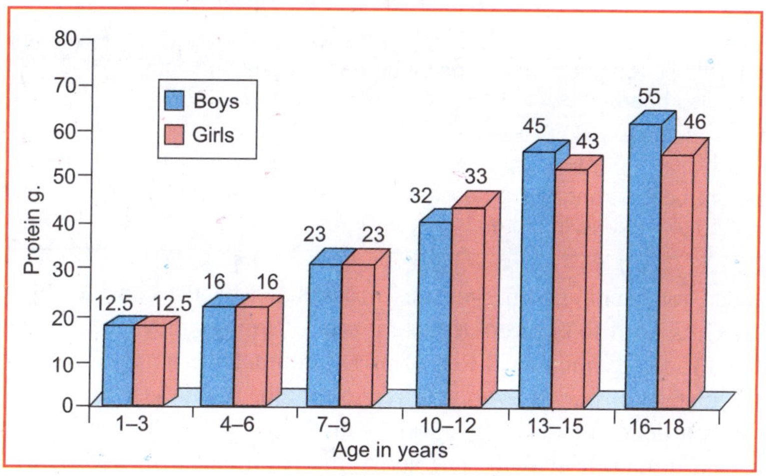

Fig. 7.3 **Comparison of protein RDA (2020) of different age groups**

As is evident from the Fig. 7.3 the protein requirements for both boys and girls are the same up to the age of ten years. But there is a gradual difference in their requirements from the age of 13 years where the boys have a higher requirement compared to girls. This pattern is similar to calorie requirement. Between 10–12 years the requirement of protein for girls is higher compared to boys. Both for boys and girls, the total protein requirement increases, as the age increases during adolescence. But per kilogram of body weight the requirement decreases. Peak requirement of protein coincides with peak energy needs. In rapidly growing adolescents protein metabolism is sensitive to calorie restriction, *i.e.*, in the event of inadequate energy intake, protein is used for energy needs resulting in malnutrition.

Fat and Essential Fatty Acids

Total fat intake below 25% E is considered to affect growth in children and adolescents. Food low in fat, saturate fat and trans fat should be emphasised in meal planning. The desirable level of visible fat intake for adolescents is 35–50 g/d.

The essential fatty acid requirements is 3% E for adolescents; since the requirements of fatty acids for adolescents has not been established the recommendations are same as in adults.

α-linolenic acid helps in relaxing muscles and blood vessels of the uterus and reduces menstrual cramps. It also reduces inflammation of mucous membrane of the uterus. Thus it reduces abdominal pain before, during and after menstrual periods.

Minerals

ICMR 2020 determined calcium EAR and RDA based on bone accretion of healthy population.

During adolescence, 1000–1050 mg of calcium and 1000–1050 mg of phosphorus per day is needed. Bone growth demands calcium. About 150 mg of calcium must be retained every day to allow for the increase in bone mass. Adolescents who have less bone mineral density are susceptible for osteoporosis later in their life. Elemental Ca : P ratio of 1 : 1 should be maintained.

> ***Adolescence and bone health***
>
> While calcium and vitamin D are the primary nutrients required for bone health other nutrients such as protein, zinc, magnesium and phosphorus also play an important role. Vitamin C and vitamin K are also needed for the health of bones.
>
> Physical activity is essential for bone health.
>
> Oestrogen prevents bone loss, whereas progesterone promotes bone formation. The best way to measure bone strength is by assessing bone mineral density. The lower the density, the greater the risk of bone fractures.

Iron is needed for haemoglobin synthesis necessitated by the considerable expansion of blood volume. Girls need to ensure adequate intake of iron as they lose 0.5 mg/day by way of menstruation. The daily menstrual loss of iron is computed from the iron content of blood lost during the menstrual period averaged over a month. If this lost iron is not replaced, it predisposes to iron deficiency anaemia. Iron is also needed for the synthesis of myoglobin which is involved in muscle growth. The additional requirement of iron during adolescence for the growth spurt, expansion of blood volume and increase in Hb concentration would be 12 μg/kg for boys and 8 μg/kg for girls. Girls would require an additional 8 μg/kg to compensate for menstrual blood loss.

During adolescence there is an increase in body mass corresponding to about 4.3 kg/year in the male and 4 kg/year in the female. With a further increase in haemoglobin by 2 g/dl in the male and 1 g/dl in the female, the respective requirement for growth alone is 0.7 mg/day in males and 0.45 mg/day in females. The obligatory losses also increase with age. Body iron stores continue to increase during adolescence.

Frank zinc deficiency is not normally seen in adolescents. Zinc supplements have been shown to increase pubertal growth in adolescents suffering from pubertal delay.

Vitamins

Skeletal growth requires vitamin D while the structural and functional integrity of newly formed cells depends on the availability of vitamins A, C and E. The Expert Committee recommended a daily allowance of 860–1000 μg of retinol for adolescents. When there is minimal exposure to sunlight 600 IU or 15 μg of vitamin D is recommended.

The need for thiamine, riboflavin and niacin increases directly with increased caloric intake.

Tissue growth involves amino acid metabolism particularly transamination to synthesise nonessential amino acids. So the requirement for B_6 is increased. Premenstrual tension can be reduced if adolescent girls consume vitamin B_6 100 mg/day.

Folacin and B_{12} are essential for DNA synthesis and needed in higher amounts when tissue synthesis is occurring rapidly. The neurological symptoms of B_{12} deficiency include depression, confusion, cognitive decline and demensia. For all adolescents 2.2 μg have been prescribed.

Water

Adolescent usually drink less water. Low water intake may be due to frequent consumption of snacks/soda while watching T.V./movies. Best way of meeting the requirement of water is drinking plain water. Intake of 100 per cent fruit juice (without the addition of sugar); butter milk and milk should be encouraged among the adolescents.

FOOD REQUIREMENTS

Physical and psychosocial pressures influence adolescents' eating habits. Boy fares better than girl in that his large appetite and sheer volume of food leads him to consume adequate nutrients. The adolescent girl may gain weight easily due to her physiologic sex differences associated with fat deposits during this period and comparative lack of physical activity. Social pressures and personal tensions concerning figure control may make her follow unwise, self-imposed crash diets for weight loss. Self starvation may result in complex and far reaching eating disorders like anorexia nervosa and bulimia.

Teenagers have the reputation of having the worst eating habits. They may skip a meal particularly breakfast. There are more skippers among girls than boys. Those who take breakfast may consume foods which are nutritionally inadequate. Missing breakfast may be due to eating disorders, peer pressure, lack of time and no nutritional awareness. They may eat fast foods which are generally inadequate in calcium and vitamin A but high in calories, saturate fat and sodium.

Dieting places adolescents at risk for unhealthful eating and physical activity behaviours. People "go on a diet" often have a time-limited behaviour. Instead they should plan for long-term behaviour changes such as avoiding eating binges, eating more fruits and vegetables, starting the day with breakfast and engaging in physical activity.

Food habits of adolescents were studied by NIN in 2013. Data from Food Frequency Questionnaires indicated less consumption of millets like jowar and more consumption of carbonated beverages, instant foods and bakery items among the adolescent girls. Bakery items contain trans fatty acids which are not good for health.

Eating patterns of adolescents are characterized by an increased tendency to skip meals, enjoying meals outside the home, frequent snacking, heavy reliance on convenience foods, dieting, vegan or vegetarian diets, fad diets and frequent changes in eating habits.

Benefits of home food

There is complete control over what goes into the food and how it is prepared. Food can be prepared sugar free or gluten free or with less salt or less fat. Food can be prepared with high fibre and with plenty of antioxidant rich vegetables.

Fresh ingredients can be included as per the choice of the individual. Healthy food can be prepared hygienically. Spices and herbs can be added as per the taste of the family.

There is satisfaction in preparing and consuming the food.

Home food is desirable, less expensive helps in forming good eating habits.

Dietary Guidelines

Diet in adolescents is very significant because it influences the nutritional status later in life.

- Adequate well balanced nutritious foods should be taken to prevent obesity or undernutrition.
- An adolescent girl should take enough calcium rich foods in her diet to increase bone density. This helps in delaying the onset of osteoporosis.
- No meal of the day should be missed, as adolescence represents a period of active life. Junk food should be avoided.
- Food should be colourful and attractive.
- Empty calorie foods such as carbonated beverages should be avoided.
- Iron rich foods like non vegetarian foods and green leafy vegetables may be included in the diet to prevent anaemia.
- Calorie and protein rich foods should be taken to support the growth spurt.
- Inclusion of fruits and vegetables in the diet meet the vitamins, minerals and fibre requirement.
- Eating habits should be independent of emotions.
- Parents should encourage the adolescents (both boys and girls) to cook at home nutritious and tasty food.
- Home based diets are best for children.
- Adolescents need to be encouraged to do physical activity particularly outdoor games. Physical activity regulates appetite.

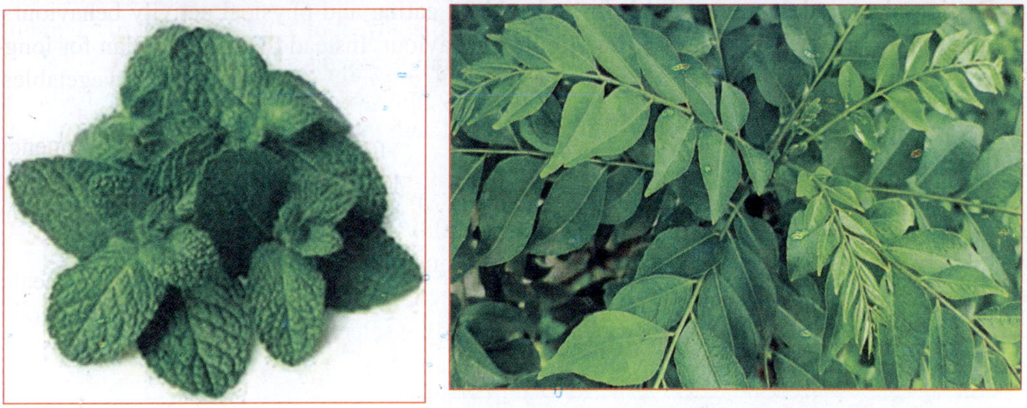

Fig. 7.4 Mint leaves and curry leaves contain more than 8 mg of iron per 100 g. Ground mint and curry leaves can be used in different recipes.

Junk Food

Foods that are high in salt, sugar, fat or calories and low in nutrient content are called junk foods. Children, specially adolescents influenced by advertisements consume foods which are high in fat, sugar and salt. These foods are high in calories but not nutrient dense. Junk foods give generally 'empty calories'.

One of the important reasons for the rise in obesity among children is consuming junk foods.

Fast Food may cause excessive weight gain and obesity. This is due to massive portion size high energy density, palatability (preference for fat, sugar and salt), high intake of saturated and *trans* fat high glycaemic load and low content of fibre.

Research findings reveal that overuse of processed food leads to a rise in polycystic ovarian disease and anaemia. It may impair cognitive development.

Functional food keeps cells active delaying the onset of degenerative disease.

Salted snack foods like chips, candies, french fries and sweetened carbonated beverages with added sugars are considered as junk foods. Bakery products like cakes with icing and biscuits are mostly made with maida, saturated fat and sugar also come under the category of junk foods. Puffs and kari biscuits, get the characteristic layers due to the addition of *trans* and saturated fat. Increase in serving size of foods like pop corn in theatres is not desirable.

Idli, vada and dosa contribute protein and vitamin requirements in addition to calories. These foods are not junk foods.

Junk food should be restricted in the diets and occasionally consuming them may not harm the body. Pizzas are nowadays made with whole wheat flour. Addition of more vegetables make it more nutritious. Cheese present in pizzas contribute to protein requirement.

Indian sweets like jalebi made with maida and sugar can also be considered as junk food. All sweets should be consumed in limited quantities due to high content of sugar and trans fats and occasional consumption may not imbalance nutrient intake.

Foods like vadas and bhajjis can be consumed occasionally though they are rich in calories.

Milk based beverages like milk shakes and lassi either sweet or salt contain lot of sugar and salt. One need to appreciate those foods with no or limited sugar and salt.

Most of the junk foods are processed. Limiting processed foods and outside foods, is desirable. Appreciating natural foods like fruits and nuts as snacks would pave the way to good health.

High school students are less likely to select milk, whole fruit and water when sweetened fruit juice is available, decreasing the nutritional quality of food.

In 2016 the Central Board of Secondary Education had sent out a circular to its affiliated schools stating that junk food should not be sold in campuses. Many organizations over the last few years have been calling for a blanket ban for the sale of junk food across schools and colleges.

Guidelines for Eating Out

Eating out is an enjoyable occasion. Following points should be considered while eating out.

- Balance the menu with low fat and high fat foods (Idli and vada)
- Have 'thali meal' than Ala carte menu
- Avoid foods where unpermitted colours are added
- Enjoy salad buffets
- Have cut fruits for dessert
- Avoid having only empty calories (like chips and carbonated beverages)
- Do not order too much quantity lest one may end up eating forcely
- Do not yield for external cues
- Enjoy recipes which are not usually made at home
- Avoid junk food (rich in saturated fat, sugar or salt)
- One should not get addicted to eating out.

NUTRITIONAL PROBLEMS

Obesity

In adolescence, obesity is due to defective thyroid fun chon, eating disorders and childhood obesity.

Poor dietary habits combined with decreased physical activity would lead to an increase in over-weight and obesity. Studies revealed that in South India, 22 per cent of boys and 18 per cent girls in the age group of 13–18 are either over-weight or obese.

Adolescents who eat high calorie and high fat foods become overweight and obese. Skipping meals at home and consuming foods that are junk (very salty, high sugar and fat) also contribute to overweight. They may snack between meals. Studies have shown that one of the important contributing factor for obesity is frequent consumption of sweetened beverages in adolescents. They may consume sweetened beverages too many. They may not include fruits and vegetables in their diets. Consumption of high glycaemic foods may lead to hormonal and metabolic changes promoting excessive food intake.

An excessive intake of calories is less often the cause than lack of exercise. Concern about personal appearance may make the adolescent more reluctant to participate in activities like dance or sports that control weight. Adolescents may not do exercise, watch TV for long times and commute to school by vehicles. Other causes of obesity may be family habits, emotional stress and hormonal imbalance. Sometimes adolescents spend all their time on studies, leading a sedentary life. And they do not spend time for physical activity. As mental activity requires very little energy, they may tend to put on weight.

The prevalence of adolescent obesity can be reduced by initiating programmes of health and nutrition education for school children, encouraging physical activity and healthy food habits.

Parents play an important role in promoting healthful dietary intake, eating behaviours and strategies to control weight among children and adolescents. Excessively restricting food access, encouraging youth to diet for weight control and engaging in weight talk and teasing have been associated with the use of maladaptive weight control and disordered eating behaviours as well as higher weight among adolescents. Parents should be role models. Adolescents should focus on studies and physical activity.

Eating Disorders

Adolescent girls perceived their diets in the light of appearance and body shape while boys are more concerned by fitness and general well being. There are three recognised eating disorders—anorexia nervosa, bulimia nervosa and binge eating disorder.

They do not chose to do this to themselves. It is a copying mechanism, a means to deal with depression, stress and self-hate which have been building for years.

In addition to psychological factors, interpersonal relationship in families, cultural norms that value people on the basis of physical appearance and not inner qualities and strengths and possible biochemical or biological causes of eating disorders.

Anorexia Nervosa

Physical signs

- Onset in early to middle adolescence
- Extremely thin or emaciated (less than 85 per cent of normal or ideal body weight)
- Rapid loss of weight
- Loss of menstrual periods
- Development of lanugo-a fine, downy hair on arms, legs, and sometimes cheeks
- Complaints of nausea, bloating, or constipation after eating normal amounts of food.

Food and exercise habits

- Cooking for others or obsessed about food but not eating
- Rigidly avoiding specific foods or whole categories of food (dairy, meats, fats, etc.)
- Refusing to eat, denying hunger, eating tiny portions of food
- Exercising excessively
- Possessing in-depth knowledge of calories and fat in foods
- Consuming odd food combinations or large amounts of low-calorie condiments (*e.g.*, mustard, vinegars)

- Exhibiting ritualistic eating behaviors, such as cutting foods into tiny bits or using special utensils or plates each time when eating
- Avoiding social invitations because of food that might be served.

Psychological signs

- Feeling 'fat' even when emaciated, intense fear of gaining weight, distorted body image
- Excessive preoccupation with weight, food, exercise, and dieting
- Social withdrawal, depression, moodiness
- Emotional withdrawal
- Perfectionism
- Refusal to admit eating patterns are abnormal
- Low self-esteem
- Fatigue or weakness due to malnutrition.

Bulimia Nervosa

Physical signs

- Onset in late teens or early twenties, often after weight loss or dieting attempts
- Usually near ideal body weight, but often with weight fluctuations
- Eats large meals, but without gaining weight
- Calluses–calcified tissue—on back of hands
- Dental enamel erosion, cavities
- Fatigue or weakness due to malnutrition
- Irregular menstrual periods.

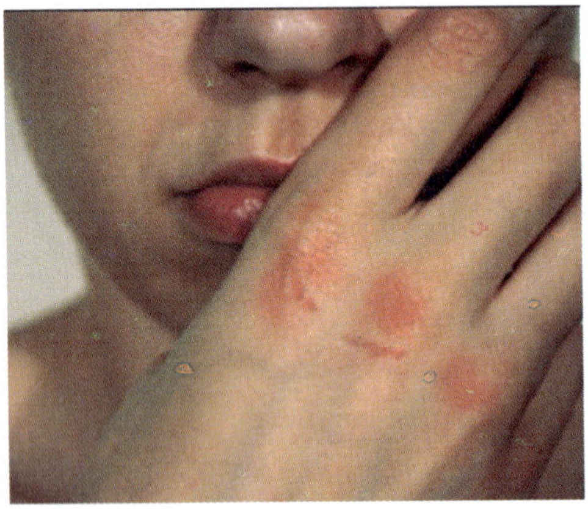

Fig. 7.5 The Russell sign in bulimia nervosa. Calluses are developed on the dorsal aspect of the hand. This is due to self-induced vomiting by traumatic irritation of the hand. Repeated insertion of the hand into the mouth to provoke vomiting causes calluses

Source: Nitsch Allison *et al.*, Medical complications of bulimia nervosa, Cleveland Clinic journal of medicine 2021; **88**.

Food and exercise habits

- Frequent binge eating
- Strict dieting followed by bingeing
- Leaving room after eating, often to bathroom
- Purging via diuretics, laxatives, emetics, or enemas, overexercising, fasting, or vomiting
- Hiding eating from others
- Avoiding social invitations because of food that might be served.

Psychological signs

- Excessive preoccupation with weight, food, exercise, and dieting
- Feeling uncomfortable eating in front of others
- Feeling out of control when eating and unable to stop binges
- Depression, loneliness, shame, and feeling of emptiness (although may pretend to be cheerful)
- Alcohol or drug use, personal problems
- Realization that eating patterns are abnormal
- Low self-esteem.

Binge Eating Disorder

More common among females.

Physical signs

- Onset at any age, often not recognized until adulthood
- Usually overweight or obese
- May have obesity-related diseases, such as type II diabetes, high blood pressure, high cholesterol.

Food and exercise habits

- Frequent dieting
- Losing and regaining weight (weight cycling) or chronically dieting without losing weight
- Frequent binge eating or eating when not hungry
- Eating to point of extreme discomfort
- Frequently eating large amounts in short time
- Hiding eating or eating only small amounts when with others
- Avoiding social invitations because of food that might be served
- Having difficulty exercising because of excess weight
- Trying to avoid physical activity or anything that might call attention to or increase own awareness of one's body.

Psychological signs

- Depression, loneliness, shame, guilt, and emotional emptiness.
- Feeling out of control when eating and unable to stop binges.
- Eating to espace from emotions (anxiety, worry, or emotional pain)
- Feeling uncomfortable eating in front of others
- Being preoccupied with food, dieting, body weight
- Feeling irritable when withdrawing from binge or trying to diet, and depressed and sleepy immediately after overeating
- Realizing that eating patterns are abnormal
- Having low self-esteem.

Treatment

The incidence of eating disorders among adolescent Indians is less compared to adolescents in developed countries–though not free from it. Eating disorders are complex problems that are best treated by a team of health care specialists including medical, psychological and nutrition professionals.

Contrary to popular belief, eating disorders are not just about weight, food or even being thin or fat. They are usually about self-esteem, self expression, depression, power and communication. Eating disorders are difficult to understand as well as treat and cure.

A standard model of effective team treatment includes a physician, psychiatrist, psychotherapist and dietician.

For all eating disorders, establishing a weight goal is essential. For anorexia nervosa, establishing a healthy weight loss is the first step. Establishing a healthy weight range with a gain of 1.5 to 3 pounds per week for 8-12 weeks is ideal for preventing cardiac complications with inpatient treatment. For outpatients a weight gain of 0.5 to 2 pounds per week is acceptable.

Weight goals of bulimia nervosa and binge eating disorder are usually higher than these patients would like but it is important to avoid weight cycling. Weight loss is secondary to breaking cycles of chaotic eating, binge eating and fluctuating weight. Initially, weight maintenance is encouraged since dieting may restart the cycles and more weight may be gained.

Only weight restoration can help to increase bone density.

Supplementation with multivitamin and minerals should be given to eating disorder patients.

Nutrition therapy starts with a diet history that provides material for future sessions. The assessment consists of a weight history, eating behaviours, history of binge-eating or purging behaviour, dieting history, use of diet aids or substances, exercise pattern, body image and menstrual history.

Nutrition instruction may include food guidelines, meal plans, calories and weight goals.

Oestrogen supplement is given to reinitiate menses.

Underlying psychological issues need to be addressed for all disordered eating problems. Psychotherapy for both individual and family is essential.

The Plate-by-Plate approach

It is a visual, no-numbers, no counting approach used in the nutritional rehabilitation and treatment of those with eating disorders across all diagnoses.

The approach can be used along side Family Based Treatment as well as other treatment modalities. It is customizable to meet individual nutrition needs. It guides individuals and families to plate full and cohesive plates while challenging eating disorder and with exposure and variety.

Using the Plate by Plate Approach there is a focus on balance, variety and 'what looks normal' rather than numbers, measuring and counting.

The approach offers simplicity, normalizes eating from the start and can be used long after recovery is achieved.

The Plate by Plate Approach is different than other treatment models

- The Plate by Plate Approach is purely visual
- Family, parents and caregivers are included in the process
- It's simple and easy to use
- It can be used anywhere in any eating setting
- It focuses on establishing normalcy in eating
- It is customizable to meet individual nutrition needs
- It is endorsed by leading experts in eating disorder treatment.

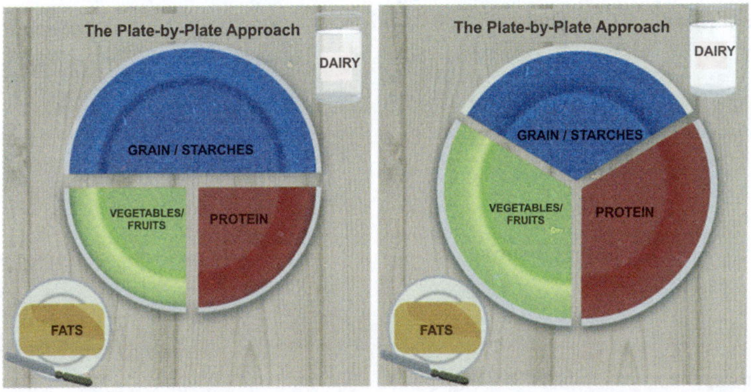

Fig. 7.6 The Plate-by-Plate Approach Visual Guide. On the left is the plate with 50% of the content coming from grains/starches. This plate, is designed for someone undergoing weight restoration, such as someone with anorexia nervosa or amenorrhea. It is also used for individuals with higher caloric demands because of age, growth, and activity level. The plate on the right represents a plate with 33% of the content coming from grains/starches. This plate is appropriate for someone who does not need to gain weight but is looking for help in achieving balanced eating, such as someone with bulimia nervosa or binge eating disorders. The plate on the right, the 33% plate, can also used to help transition someone back to weight maintenance.

Source: Sterling wendy The use of the Plate-by-Plate approach for adolescents undergoing family based treatment. J Acad Nutr Diet. 2019; **119.**

Predisposition to Osteoporosis

A protective factor is the maximisation of peak bone mass at skeletal maturity. Skeletal maturity is achieved during the late stage of pubertal development. Peak bone mass attained by the second decade of life and bone growth during adolescence accounting for about 45 per cent of this attainment.

Excessive exercise, high fibre, low fat intake lead to low circulating estrogen levels, irregular menses and low bone mass. Predisposition to osteoporosis is in part atleast the result of dietary deficiency and exercise patterns during the developmental years. Low dietary intake of calcium rich foods such as milk in teenagers could be because of the misunderstanding about the amount of fat provided by the milk and substitution of milk with soft drinks. Soft drink consumption reduces calcium intake and due to the presence of phosphoric acid which may lead to bone resorption. Bone density can be increased by including in the diet calcium rich foods.

The Female Athlete Triad

The characteristics of female athlete triad are disordered eating, amenorrhea and osteoporosis. Eating disorder leads to amenorrhea and osteoporosis. Or amenorrhea can directly lead to osteoporosis.

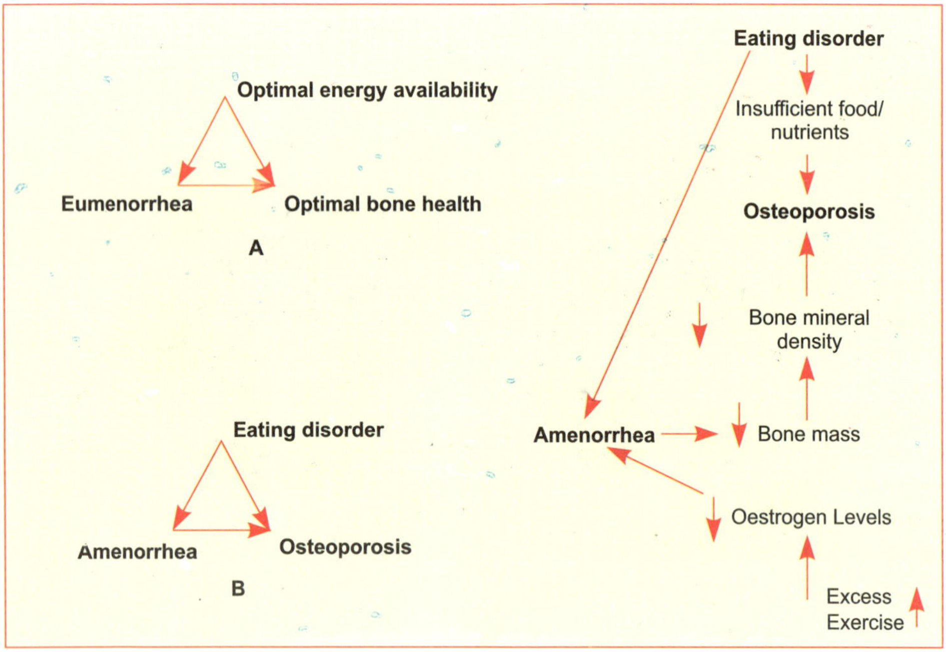

Fig 7.7 Female athlete triad

A - Normal health condition **B** - Relationship of eating disorder, amenorrhea and osteoporosis. Excessive exercise affects estrogen levels and causes amenorrhea leading to osteoporosis.

Anaemia

According to NFHS-3, 2006 surveys 55.3 per cent are anaemic and 1.8 per cent are severely anaemic among women aged 15–49 years. There does seem to be a trend towards a decrease in the age at menarche over the decades both in the rural and urban situations, not only in the affluent upper classes but also among the poor classes and making adolescent girl susceptible to anaemia. With the practice of early marriages in rural India, the adolescent girls are at risk of anaemia.

Anaemia is most common in all the groups of adolescent girls irrespective of the social class. Anaemia is common in low socioeconomic class since intake is poor mainly due to the non-availability of healthy foods. In higher classes personal likes and dislikes and food taboos lead to anaemia. Supplementation of 100 mg iron and 0.5 mg of folic acid is given in primary health centres to 'mothers to be' under Nutrition and Health Services.

Undernutrition

Studies have shown that pre-pregnant material size and weight gain during pregnancy seem to be emerging as important determinants of the birth weigh of children.

Undernutrition during adolescence, confounded by childhood marriages, leads to higher mortality and morbidity among women and young children, thus perpetuating the vicious cycle of undernutrition.

Low female literacy (14.5 per cent against 47 per cent) high maternal (992 against 195) and infant mortality (85 against 64) have been reported among tribal population as compared to their rural counterparts. The study among the tribal adolescents indicates that the food and nutrient intake was low compared to RDA as well as that of their rural counterparts. The extent of deficit was relatively more with respect to micronutrients such as iron, vitamin A, riboflavin and free folic acid. Higher prevalence of undernutrition among boys could be attributed to the fact that a higher proportion of them have energy intakes of < 70 per cent RDA (NIN, 2007).

Results of the studies conducted at National Institute of Nutrition Hyderabad showed a higher percentage of upper-middle class girls (36 per cent) had deficit in BMI indicating that the weight deficit is a major factor, possibly related to the poor energy intake of this group of population. While among the urban poor and rural girls, this is mainly due to their getting lower priority for the food over the boys in the family. In the upper class, the weight deficit is related to the personal likes and dislikes and also a conscious attempt towards maintaining a low weight in the fear of becoming overweight. Avoiding milk, peer influence, eating outside the home with poor selections, skipping meals, food faddism and emotional disturbance may all contribute to under nutrition in adolescence.

Micronutrient deficiency disorders in the adolescent phase result in growth retardation, low immunity and impaired reproductive functions. At times this may affect pregnancy related complications or results in low birth weight. Thus perpetuating the trans-generational cycle of malnutrition.

Iodine is one of the essential micronutrients required for normal growth and development of the human brain and body. Adolescent girls should ensure to meet iodine requirement through fortified salt. Iodine deficiency causes hypothyroidism or goitre as shown in Fig. 7.8.

Premenstrual Syndrome

This is not so uncommon in adolescence and is characterised by physical and psychological symptoms which occur 7–10 days prior to the onset of periods and disappear within the first day or two of menstrual flow. These include weight gain, abdominal bloating, breast engorgement and pain, constipation, peripheral oedema, headache, irritability, anxiety, depression, tension, fatigue, lack of concentration, increased appetite, craving for sweet and salty foods. The etiology and pathophysiology have not been identified. Management includes reassurance, exercise and dietary modifications to meet all the nutritional requirements.

Studies suggest that inadequate vitamin D status may be associated with increased severity of some but not all premenstrual symptoms.

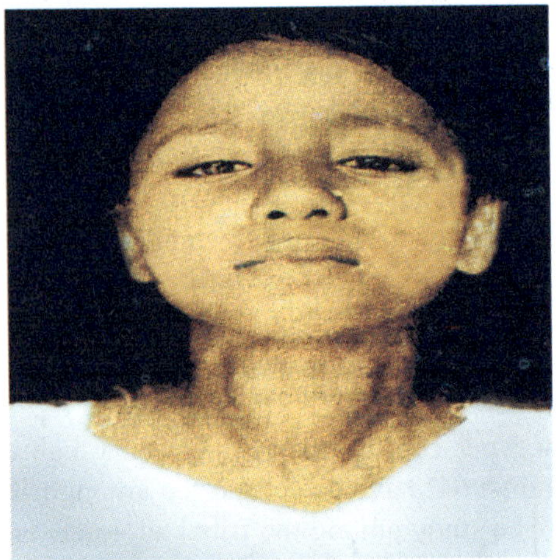

Fig. 7.8 In endemic areas goitre is observed at the time of puberty, particularly in girls

Malnutrition due to Early Marriage

Often a significant proportion of Indian girls get married soon after menarche and bear a child when she herself is still a child. These child-mothers are considered 'high risk' as maternal and perinatal death rates and infant mortality rates are higher among them. In India almost 40 per cent of girls are married and have the first child before 18 years of age. Pregnancy is optimal when the mother is biologically mature. A biologically mature female is a young woman who is atleast 5 years post menarchal and this has greater impact on pregnancy than her chronological age.

Nutritional deficiency signs get aggravated if the adolescent girl conceives immediately after menarche since she has to meet the demands of not only her growth, but also that of conceptus. The incidence of both preclampsia and eclampsia have been found to be higher and so also the incidence of pregnancy wastages.

In the poorer section of the society, complications are more common in adolescents, which have a direct bearing on the outcome of pregnancy.

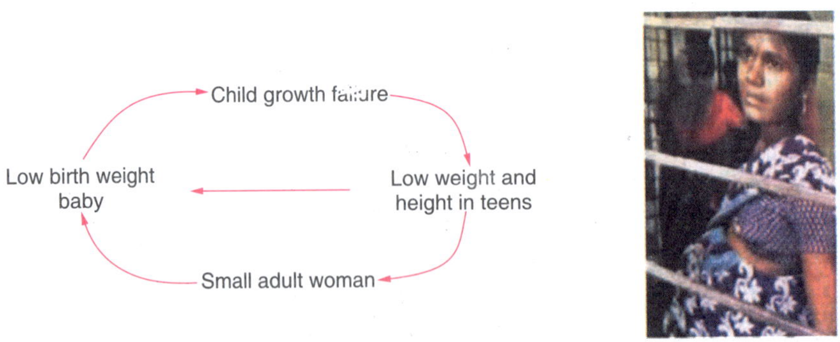

Fig. 7.9 Early marriage and consequent early pregnancy is detrimental to the health of the mother and the baby

Studies on age-related infant mortality in various parts of the country have shown that early neonatal deaths are almost double in the adolescent age group. Maternal mortality again is high due to eclampsia and haemorrhage.

There is a close association between the maternal body weight and the incidence of low birth weight. The lactation failure is also a more common occurrence among the adolescents, resulting in high infant mortality and morbidity due to earlier introduction of supplements. Due to small size of the pelvis, there is increase in the rate of premature deliveries and also high incidence of low birth weight.

Pregnancy and child birth are safest not at 15 but between 25 and 30 years. There is a need to bring about behavioural changes in the community to prevent early marriages and provide opportunities for adolescents to achieve their maximum growth potential.

PHYSICAL ACTIVITY

Regular exercise and participating in school games adolescents can prevent obesity. Physical activity can also prevent premenstrual dysphoric disorder (PMDD) in adolescent girls. Exercise helps adolescent boys to develop muscles.

Children and adolescents should take part in a total of 60 minutes of physical activity every day; 20 to 30 minutes of that should be vigorous, high-impact activity such as running, jumping rope or participating in sports.

Suggested recipes during adolescence

Recipe	*Reasons*
Samosa with channa, uthapam (cereal + pulse)	To meet increased needs of calories and protein
Bajji, bonda, vada, spring rolls	Adolescents are fascinated by junk foods but one can select these. Rich in calories.
Basundi, ladoos	Protein rich foods meet growth needs
Instead of carbonated cool drinks, fresh juices can be given	Vitamin C requirement can be met.
Rice and rajmah, vegetable fried rice, pav bhaji omelette	Nutritious and give variety
Kathi rolls, Bhelpuri, Roasted Groundnuts	Nutritional

The nutritional concerns of adolescents have largely been neglected. They constitute one of the nutritionally vulnerable group who have not received the attention they deserved. Only healthy adolescent girl can become healthy mother who in turn can give birth to healthy child.

January 12th is National Youth Day.

SUGGESTED READINGS

- Marshall A: Teresa *et al.*, Beverage consumption patterns at age 13 to 17 years are associated with weight, height and body mass index at age 17 years, J Acad. Nutr. Diet. 2017; **117**.
- Savoie-Roskos R., Mateja *et al.*, Increasing fruit and vegetable intake among children and youth through gardening-based interventions: A systematic review J Acad. Nutr. Diet. 2017; **117**.
- Jarosz c. Alicia and Ahmed EL-Sohemy, Association between vitamin D status and premenstrual symptoms. J Acad Nutr Diet, 2019; **119**.
- Hasan Kulik Bruna *et al.*, Breakfast consumption, family breakfast and adiposily trajectory in adolescence, J Acad Nutr Diet, 2019; **119**.
- Eating Disorders. www.aedweb.org.

QUESTIONS

1. Give the RDA of a 16-year-old boy.
2. Discuss the common nutrient deficiencies in adolescents.
3. Plan a day's diet of an adolescent girl suffering from nutritional anaemia.
4. Give the nutritional importance in adolescence.
5. Write a note on "Anaemia in adolescence".
6. Explain anorexia nervosa and bulimia.
7. Distinguish the nutritional problems of Indian and western adolescents.
8. Discuss the eating disorders of adolescent girls.
9. Explain the nutritional problems of adolescent boys.
10. Explain female athlete triad.
11. Define 'Junk Food'. Why is it not good for health?

TOPICS FOR ACTIVITY

- Make innovative meals for adolescents on the basis of 'My healthy plate'.
- Make recipes using ground curry leaves as main ingredient.
- Discuss pros and cons of street food.

8

Nutritional Recommendations and Food Requirements of Expectant Mothers

Adequate nutrition before and during pregnancy has greater potential for a long-term health impact than it does at any other time. Maternal health is a complex, influenced by various genetic, social and economic factors, infections and environmental conditions, many of which may affect the foetal growth. Physiological adaptations result in improved utilisation of nutrients either through increased absorption, decreased excretion or alternations in metabolism.

PHYSIOLOGICAL CHANGES

Total plasma volume in a nonpregnant woman averages 2600 ml. By 34 weeks it is about 50 per cent greater than it was at conception. If the plasma volume does not increase up to the standard value, there is risk for still birth, abortion and low birth weight babies.

The expansion of blood volume is required to allow the circulation of blood through the placenta and allow it carry nutrients and oxygen to the fetus and metabolic wastes away from the foetus. Blood volume expands by 50 per cent resulting in a decrease in haemoglobin levels, blood glucose values and serum levels of albumin, other serum proteins and water-soluble vitamins. The decline in serum albumin levels contributes to a tendency for extracellular water to accumulate during pregnancy. The decrease in water soluble vitamin concentration makes determination of an inadequate intake or a deficient nutrient state difficult. By contrast, serum concentrations of fat soluble vitamins and other lipid fractions, such as triglycerides, cholesterol and free fatty acids increase.

There is a decreased ability to taste saltiness. This may infact, be a physiologic mechanism for increasing salt intake. Increased progesterone level relaxes the uterine muscle to allow expansion with fetal growth. Gastrointestinal motility diminishes, to allow for increased absorption of nutrients. This often results in constipation. Additionally, a relaxed lower oesophageal sphincter can cause regurgitation and heart burns.

During pregnancy appetite increases and nausea and vomiting may occur. Motility is diminished and intestinal secretion is reduced absorption of nutrients is enhanced. Increased progesterone production causes decreased tone and motility of smooth muscles of the gastrointestinal tract. This leads to oesophageal regurgitation, decreased emptying time of the stomach and reverse peristalisis. As a result pregnant woman may experience heart burn and constipation.

Increased blood volume produces a high glomerular filtration rate. It appears that the renal tubules are unable to adjust completely and a percentage of nutrients that would have been reabsorbed in the nonpregnant women are excreted in the urine. Increased amounts of amino acids, glucose and water soluble vitamins may appear in the urine. This may be a reason for the increased number of urinary tract infections seen in pregnant women.

The ability to excrete water is lowered and oedema in the legs and ankles is common and normal.

Less than half of the total weight gain resides in the fetus, placenta and amniotic fluid; the remainder is found in maternal reproductive tissues, fluid, blood and maternal stores, a component composed largely of body fat. Gradually increasing subcutaneous fat in the abdomen, back and upper thigh serves as an energy reserve for pregnancy and lactation.

Increased weight gain during pregnancy is associated with increased birth weight and a progressive decrease in the number of low birth weight infants. High estrogen levels during pregnancy promote a gynecoid type of fat distribution.

Role of Placenta

Placenta forms a vital link between the mother and the growing baby. It enables three generations of genomes of the mother, foetus and foetal ovaries to interact. Adverse influences during the lifetime of the mother can thus impact three generations. Placental size is compromised in the small pelvis of a woman who grew up as an undernourished girl child in pecuniary or prejudicial when she has a nutritionally deprived pregnancy it affects her unborn daughter as well as her yet-to-be conceived grand children.

The placenta is the principal site of production for several hormones responsible for regulation of fetal growth and development of maternal support tissues. It is also involved for exchange of nutrients, oxygen and waste products. Any derange to or inadequacy in the placenta compromises its ability to nourish the fetus, regardless of how well nourished the mother is or how optimal her dietary intake. Most of the nutrients for growth are derived through the placenta although some are provided by the portion of amniotic fluid the infant swallows during the latter part of pregnancy.

PRECONCEPTUAL NUTRITION

A woman who has been well nourished before conception begins her pregnancy with reserves of several nutrients so that the needs of the growing foetus can be met without affecting her health. Infants who are well nourished in the womb, have an enhanced chance of entering life in good physical and mental health. The effects of undernutrition during reproduction will vary depending upon the nutrients involved, the length of time it is lacking and the stage of gestation at which it occurs.

A woman whose diet is adequate before pregnancy is usually able to bear a full term viable infant, without extensive modifications of her diet. Mother's diet should produce adequate nutrients so that maternal stores do not get depleted and produce sufficient milk to nourish her child after birth. The nutritional demands are highly increased in an adolescent mother.

Women with low body weight and poor nutritional status prior to pregnancy have more low birth weight infants, premature spontaneous rupture of membranes, infection and anaemia. A pre-pregnancy weight of less than 40 kg serves as a useful cut off to predict women who will deliver low birth weight babies and who are small for gestational age (SGA).

Maternal nutrition plays a role in certain types of fetal malformations or spontaneous abortion. Because these abnormalities occur so early in pregnancy (during organogenesis) modifications must be made before pregnancy begins. In diabetes, incidence of congenital defects can be reduced almost to normal by bringing the blood glucose under good control prior to pregnancy. Administration of folic acid 220 μg per day around and during conception and early gestation can reduce the incidence of neural tube defects.

On the other end of the spectrum, overweight women are more likely to have fetal death, diabetes, hypertensive disorders and labour abnormalities. Because these maladies are difficult to correct once pregnancy begins, a woman should achieve a body mass within 90–120 per cent of ideal weight prior to conception.

Major Prenatal Nutrition Alterations

↓	Haematologic status
↑	White blood cells
↓↓	Serum albumin
↓	Serum vitamin C, folic acid and B_{12}
↑	Serum carotene
→	Vitamin A
↑	Serum tocopherol
↑	Urinary N′-methylnicotinamide
↑	Urinary riboflavin
↑	Urinary xanthuric-acid excretion

Globally, there is an emphasis on the importance of children's growth and development starting early, particularly during the first 1000 days beginning at conception and through the child's second birth day. Preconception is also critical for initiating development of the embryo, placenta and course of pregnancy in an optimal fashion.

Mother's cardiopathic environment during preconception can adversely affect her offspring's health and subsequently into childhood and beyond.

NUTRITIONAL RECOMMENDATIONS

Importance of Nutrition During Pregnancy

Undernutrition of the mother, preceding and during pregnancy affects the growing foetus in the womb. If the semi starved foetus is to escape still birth, it has to programme itself to survive on limited nutrition. The growing brain and nervous system are prioritized for nutrition because they are the key to survival. Muscles grow insulin-resistant to spare glucose for the brain. The child is born malnourished, metabolically compromised and suffering some loss of cognitive potential.

Diet is one of the main factors influencing pregnancy outcomes. An unhealthy diet rich in saturated fats, sodium and sugar and poor in fibre, vitamins and minerals impair the metabolic profile, increasing oxidative stress and insulin resistance and consequently increasing fat and glucose transfer to the fetus.

The mismatch between early programming for extreme frugality and later availability of more nutrients as the child grows, leads to accumulation of body fat in the preference to lean muscle mass. This is associated with metabolic abnormalities that lead to early on set of diabetes and

Table 8.1 ICMR–2020 Recommended Dietary Allowances for a pregnant mother

Nutrient	*Normal adult woman*	*Pregnant woman (For second and third trimester)*
Body weight kg	55	55 + 10
Energy kcal		
Sedentary	1600	
Moderate	2130	+350
Heavy	2720	
Protein g	46	+ 9.5 (2nd trimester)
Dietary fibre g		+ 22.0 (3rd trimester)
Sedentary	25	
Moderate	30	–
Heavy	40	
Visible fat g		
Sedentary	20	30
Moderate	25	30
Heavy	30	30
Calcium mg	1000	1000
Magnesium mg	370	440
Iron mg	29	27
Zinc mg	13.2	14.5
Iodine µg	140	220
Vitamin A		
Retinol µg	840	900
Vitamin D IU	600	600
Thiamine mg		
Sedentary	1.4	
Moderate	1.7	2.0
Heavy	2.2	
Riboflavin mg		
Sedentary	1.9	
Moderate	2.4	2.7
Heavy	3.1	
Niacin mg		
Sedentary	11	
Moderate	14	+2.0
Heavy	18	
Pyridoxine mg		
Sedentary	1.9	
Moderate	1.9	2.3
Heavy	2.4	
Folate µg	220	570
Vitamin B_{12} µg	2.2	+0.25
Vitamin C mg	65	+15

a higher risk of heart disease. This link between early life malnutrition and chronic diseases in adulthood described as the Barker hypothesis, is now known to be due to epigenetic changes in gene expression. While the basic genetic structure of the child's genome remains unaltered the functional effects of some genes may vary because their expressions modified induced by an adverse environment.

Such epigenetic changes can also occur due to other adverse intrauterine or early childhood influences.

Increase in nutritional requirements is due to metabolic changes of pregnancy and the nutrition reserves of the mother. The RDA of the expectant mother suggested by ICMR is given in Table 8.1.

Energy

Energy needs during pregnancy increase because of the

- growth and physical activity of the foetus,
- growth of the placenta and maternal tissue,
- normal increase in maternal body size, and deposition of fat,
- additional work involved in carrying the weight of the foetus and extra maternal tissues and
- slow but steady rise in basal metabolic rate during pregnancy.

BMR increases by about 5 per cent during the first trimester and increases by about 12 per cent during the third trimester. The total weight gain during 9 months of pregnancy may range from 10–12 kg.

For reference Indian woman whose body weight is 55 kg. the following additional energy requirements are recommended by ICMR (2020).

The caloric requirements of a pregnant woman is mostly increased in the latter half of pregnancy. Expert committee recommended an additional intake of 350 kcal/day during the second and third trimester.

Hence ICMR 2020 recommended energy requirement of pregnant woman as follows:

Sedentary worker	:	1660 + 350 = 2010 kcal
Moderate worker	:	2130 + 350 = 2480 kcal
Heavy worker	:	2720 + 350 = 3070 kcal

Energy requirement during pregnancy comprises the normal requirement for an adult woman and an additional requirement needed for gestational weight gain associated with protein and fat accretion in maternal, foetal and placental tissues and increase in BMR.

For a 12 kg weight gain, basal metabolism would increase by about 35000 kcal.

Protein

The normal protein requirement of an adult woman is 46 g/day. ICMR (2020) prescribed an amount of 46 + 9.5 for second trimester and 46 + 22.0 for third trimester for a pregnant woman. Additional protein is essential for:

- rapid growth of the foetus.
- the enlargement of the uterus, mammary glands and placenta.
- increase in maternal circulating blood volume and subsequent demand of increased plasma protein to maintain colloidal osmotic pressure and circulation of tissue fluids.

- formation of amniotic fluid and storage reserves for labour, delivery and lactation.
- the transfer of amino acids from the mother to foetus (up to 20 weeks all amino acids must be provided to the foetus as it cannot oxidise amino acids as a source of energy).

Protein requirement during pregnancy has been computed on the basis of N accretion. By factorial approach protein deposition values calculated to be 2.7 g/d in the second trimester 5.7 g/d in the third trimester.

Nutrition expert committee has prescribed an additional safe intake of protein 26.3 g/d in the third trimester.

If protein requirements are not met during pregnancy

- there is increased risk of pregnancy.
- the foetus may grow at the expense of mother.
- maximum growth of the baby cannot be obtained.
- number of cells in tissues particularly in brain may be less.

Protein and calorie deficiency during gestation may result in poor utilisation of food by the off-spring after birth and a failure to even compensate for early food deprivation. When amino acids are transferred, some big protein molecules also cross the placental barrier which give immunity to the infants. In the total weight gain during pregnancy there is 1 kg of protein and half of which is foetal tissue.

Milk, meat, egg and cheese are complete proteins and of high biological value. A pregnant woman requires 600 ml of milk per day. Additional protein may be obtained from legumes and whole grains, nuts and oil seeds. Pulse: Cereal intake ratio should be 1 : 5. Protein supplements are not required.

Visible Fat and Essential Fatty Acids

ω-3 fatty acids are required for normal conception, growth and development of an embryo. The minimum level of total fat should be 20%E. To meet this, diets of pregnant women should contain 30 g of visible fat. A pregnant woman should consume at least 200 mg/d DHA, docosahexaenoic acid, for optimal health and fetal development. During the third trimester, 50–60 mg/day of maternal DHA stores are transferred to the foetus via placenta.

DHA plays a critical role in both vision and cognitive function acuity. DHA is particularly highly concentrated in the brain and retinal membranes especially in photoreceptors and is therefore assumed to play a critical role in both vision and cognitive function. A positive association has been observed between red blood cell DHA content and improved visual acuity and brain development in human infants.

ω-3 fatty acid supplementation may further enhance DHA content in maternal plasma potentially offering added benefits to infants. Clinical studies have also reported improved visual acuity and hand eye coordination in infants receiving greater DHA in the womb and/or during lactation.

DHA at the early stages of development is critical and subsequent deficiency could result in irreversible functional limitations. Essential fatty acids relax muscles and blood vessels of the uterus and makes delivery easier. Essential fatty acid deficiency adversely affects pregnancy outcome.

Increased intake of ω-3 fatty acids should be encouraged for pregnant and lactating mothers for optimal health of the infant.

Corn, cotton seed, safflower and soyabean oils are good sources of linoleic acid. α-linolenic acid is present not only in fish oils but also found in green leaf vegetables, flax seeds, rape seed, soyabean and walnuts.

Calcium

Calcium requirement suggested by ICMR for an adult woman is 1000 mg/day. Requirement during pregnancy is also 1000 mg.

Although the infant bones are poorly calcified at the time of birth an appreciable amount of calcium is involved in foetal development. A full term foetal body is made up of 30 g of calcium.

Increased intake of calcium by the mother is highly essential, not only for the calcification of foetal bones and teeth but also for protection of calcium resources of the mother to meet the high demands during lactation.

The pregnant woman routinely exhibits extensive adjustments in calcium metabolism, largely as a result of the influence of hormonal factors. Human chorionic somato mammotropin from the placenta progressively increases the rate of bone turnover. Estrogen also largely derived from the placenta, inhibits bone resorption, provoking a compensatory release of parathyroid hormone, which maintains the serum calcium level while enhancing intestinal absorption. The net effect of these changes is the promotion of progressive calcium retention to meet progressively increasing foetal skeletal demands for mineralisation.

Two-thirds of foetal calcium is transferred from the mother to the foetus after 30th week of pregnancy at the rate of 300 mg per day. Radioisotopic studies revealed that nearly 80 per cent calcium of the foetal skeleton and mother were obtained from the mother's diet, and the rest was obtained from maternal reserves. Pregnant woman usually absorbs not less than 40 per cent of the calcium available in their diet. Calcium retention by pregnant woman is of 2 to 5 times the amount needed by the foetus in the 6th and 7th months of pregnancy indicating that maternal reserves are being built up at this stage. The amount of dietary calcium needed is reduced when vitamin D is available. Use of vitamin D and calcium reduces muscular cramps of pregnancy.

Physical activity also influences bone density of the mother.

Maternal skeleton acts as a reservoir of minerals that potentially can be mobilized to buffer short falls in mineral supply.

Young women who had not attained their peak bone mass when there is extra demands imposed by fetal skeletal mineralization, supplementation of calcium and vitamin D should be given.

To prevent 'osteomalacia' mother's diet should contain less of phytic acid, adequate amounts of vitamin D and sufficient amount of calcium. Mothers should avoid repeated pregnancies.

Dairy products are a primary source of calcium. Green leafy vegetables like agathi and gingelly seeds also contribute to calcium.

Iron

Normal iron requirement of an adult woman is 29 mg/day. ICMR 2020 requirements during pregnancy is 27 mg/day.

- It is also required for the formation of haemoglobin as there is 40–50 per cent increased maternal blood volume. For this 400 mg of iron is required.
- Loss of maternal iron through skin and sweat is about 170 mg of iron.

Table 8.2 Iron requirement during entire pregnancy with a weight gain of 10 kg and 12 kg

	Weight gain 10 kg	*Weight gain 10 kg*
Foetus	179 mg	179 mg
Expansion of maternal red cell mass	246 mg	295 mg
Obligatory loss	14 µg/kg	14 µg/kg

The iron requirement for the entire period of pregnancy is 425–474 mg of obligatory loss.

The actual increase in requirement of iron is only in second and third trimester. But a single large dose of iron at the beginning of pregnancy is an effective way to build up iron stores and to protect against depletion of reserves. To avoid iron deficiency a woman should enter pregnancy with a store of atleast 300 mg of iron. Iron requirement in first trimester is similar to the normal requirement of 0.70 mg. During second and third trimester, the daily requirement is 3.3 mg and 5 mg respectively.

Liver, dried beans, dried fruits, green leafy vegetables, eggs, enriched cereals and iron fortified salt provide additional sources of iron.

Sodium

In early pregnancy there is an increase in the glomerular filtration and filtered sodium loss. An increase in progesterone also can inhibit sodium reabsorption. However, an intact renin-angiotensin-aldosterone system, with an increase in aldosterone in pregnancy increases sodium reabsorption. Further as the extra-cellular fluid volume increases and osmotic pressure falls additional increase in production of renin and aldosterone accelerates sodium reabsorption. The regulatory mechanisms are not exhausted until the sodium intake is severely restricted.

On the basis of average weight gain of 11 kg of which 70 percent is water the sodium requirement in pregnancy is calculated to be about 75 mmol which is only 3 mmol of sodium above the non pregnant requirement and is usually met by the diet of pregnant woman. No need to take extra sodium during pregnancy.

Uses of diuretics should be discouraged during pregnancy as they can cause loss of sodium. Sodium is restricted when there is oedema or hypertension.

Iodine

According to ICMR, 2020 iodine requirement for a pregnant woman is 220 µg which is close to FAO/WHO recommendations. Iodine deficiency in mother can lead to abortion, still births, congenital anomalies, increased perinatal mortality, cretinism and psychomotor defects. Mothers who are residing in goitre endemic areas should ensure that they get enough iodine through iodised salt and other means.

Zinc

The zinc requirement is increased from 13.2 mg to 14.5 mg during pregnancy. Zinc deficiency during the antenatal period leads to adverse effects on the newborn including foetal mortality, foetal malformations including CNS teratogenecity and reduced intrauterine growth rate. Low zinc during pregnancy doubles the risk of low birth weight and trebles the risk of preterm delivery.

Fat Soluble Vitamins

Vitamin A: Normal requirements of retinol for an adult woman is 840 μg and during pregnancy it is increased to 900 μg of retinol. Vitamin A requirements during pregnancy have been calculated on the basis of the vitamin content of livers of the newborn.

Vitamin A requirement during pregnancy has been calculated considering the additional requirement of 14 μg, for gestational weight gain. For an adult woman with 55 kg weight RDA during pregnancy is 900 μg/d.

The importance of vitamin A deficiency during pregnancy on maternal and child health has been recognised by the studies conducted by NIN as shown in Fig. 8.1. Night blindness is associated with malnutrition, severe anaemia and preterm deliveries in the mother and birth asphyxia in the new-born. Serum retinol < 20 μg/dl was found to be associated with preterm deliveries and higher risk of systolic hypertension.

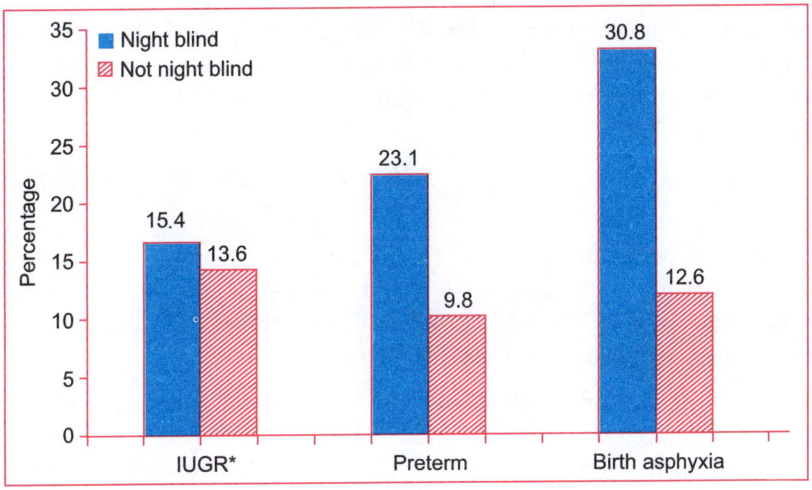

*Intra uterine growth restriction

Fig. 8.1 Neonatal complications of infants of mothers with and without night blindness – ICMR study

Liver, egg yolk, butter, dark green and yellow vegetables and fruits are good source of vitamin A.

A daily supplementation of 6000 I.U. for about 12 weeks appears to improve serum vitamin A levels and correct vitamin A deficiency in the pregnant women. Improving vitamin A status of pregnant women reduces maternal mortality.

Excess vitamin A should not be taken during pregnancy.

Vitamin D: The RDA of vitamin D prescribed by ICMR-2020 is 600 IU. Vitamin D is highly essential as it enhances the maternal calcium absorption. Its active form calcidiol and calcitriol cross the placenta with ease and play an important role in calcium metabolism of the foetus. Maternal deficiency of vitamin D results in neonatal hypocalcaemia and hypoplasia. Research suggests an association between vitamin D status and pregnancy complications such as preclampsia, gestational diabetes and risk of cesarian section. Low maternal vitamin D status may impact off spring, length of gestation and potentially fetal growth.

Excessive vitamin D can also result in complications such as atherosclerosis, hypercalcaemia, calcium deposits in various vital organs and mental retardation in the infants.

Vitamin E: In animals vitamin E has an important role to play in the reproductive process and reduces the number of spontaneous abortions and still births. In women it has not been evidently proved that vitamin E deficiency can cause pregnancy failure although it may prove beneficial to those who have had repeated spontaneous abortion or failure to conceive. Very little vitamin E crosses the placenta, so infant has low tissue concentrations that persist up to at least 6 years. Requirement of vitamin E increases with increased intake of PUFA.

Vitamin K: Vitamin K is essential for synthesis of prothrombin that is necessary for normal coagulation of blood. It is highly essential for preventing neonatal haemorrhage. An oral dosage of menadione (synthetic form of vitamin K) during the last weeks of pregnancy or an injection during labour is essential to stimulate prothrombin synthesis. But care should be taken to see that the dosage is given at an average level to prevent adverse effects.

Water Soluble Vitamins

As water soluble vitamins are not stored much, the pregnant woman must rely on her daily intakes that is high enough to meet the added requirements of pregnancy. Generally maternal blood levels for water soluble vitamins tend to fall and foetal blood levels tend to exceed those of mother by 50 to 100 per cent during pregnancy.

Thiamine: The ICMR recommendations in 2020 for thiamine RDA for pregnant woman is 2.0 mg.

The relationship between thiamine and caloric intake remains the same as normal adult during pregnancy i.e., for 1000 calories 0.5 mg of thiamine is required. The normal urinary excretion of thiamine drops indicating that more is being retained and used by tissues. In some cases thiamine helps to relieve the nausea of pregnancy.

Riboflavin: The ICMR recommendations of riboflavin RDA for a pregnant woman is 2.7 mg. For 1000 calorie intake, 0.6 mg of riboflavin is required.

Requirements are increased due to increase in maternal body size and growth of foetus and accessory tissues. Riboflavin is present in higher amounts in the foetal blood than in maternal blood.

Niacin Equivalent: The ICMR recommendations of niacin equivalent RDA for an adult woman is 11 mg for sedentary worker, 14 mg for moderate worker and 18 mg, for heavy worker. For a pregnant woman the RDA is increased by 2 mg, corresponding to the increase in calories. The conversion of amino acid tryptophan into niacin is more efficient during pregnancy.

Vitamin B_6: Normal requirement of pyridoxine in an adult woman is 1.9–2.4 mg. ICMR suggested for pregnancy 2.3 mg/day. In hypertrophy, when the cells are growing in size, B_6 and amino acids are required. During 'toxaemia of pregnancy' (high B.P., oedema, proteinuria) the B_6 levels are lower. Women who used oral contraceptives prior to conception often enter pregnancy with low tissue levels of vitamin B_6. There is no satisfactory theory to explain that these low levels affect the outcome of pregnancy but they do reduce the amount of pyridoxine in breast milk during lactation. Vitamin B_6 is said to be used to control nausea of pregnancy.

Dietary Folate: Normal adult woman requirement of folate is 220 μg/day. ICMR recommendations during pregnancy are 570 μg/day. The recommended intake of folacin is based on its role in promoting normal foetal growth and preventing macrocytic anaemia of pregnancy. Folic acid is needed for the synthesis of essential components of DNA and RNA which increase rapidly during growth thereby increasing the requirements. Also folic acid is essential for the development of RBCs which increase as the mother's blood volume increases.

Malformations have been noted in the offspring of women using folate antagonist drugs such as methotrexate and valproic acid. There is some evidence in humans to suggest that deficiency of folic acid may be associated with spontaneous abortion and obstetric complications such as preterm labour and low birth weight.

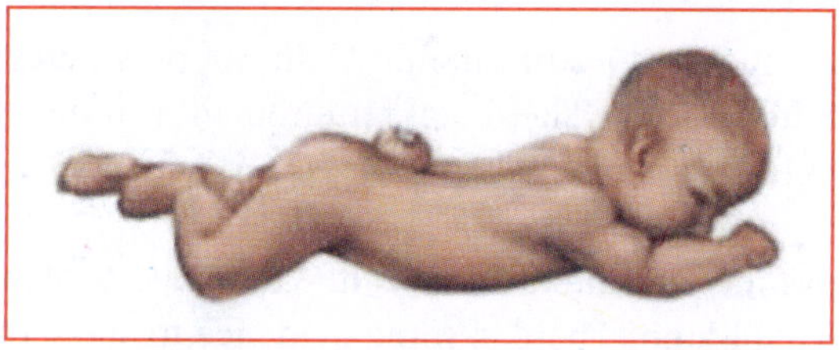

Fig. 8.2 Congenital anomaly—Spina bifida

In spina bifida, defective development of vertebrae allows a portion of the spinal cord and meninges to protrude through the defect, causing outpouching. Neurologic dysfunction is caused by this anomaly. Folic acid deficiency at the time of conception can cause spina bifida.

The greatest significance of folic acid and its potential influence on pregnancy outcome is its role in preventing neural tube defects, such as spina bifida. In this condition there is a congenital defect in which the vertebral neural arches fail to close, so exposing the contents of the spinal canal posteriorly.

Folic acid deficiency can lead to anencephaly—absence of brain. Folic acid deficiency has also been implicated in pregnancy induced hypertension.

All women of child bearing years should take folic acid supplementation. It is crucial to note that, because the neural tube closes by 28 days of gestation (before most women realise that they are pregnant) supplementation with folic acid should ideally occur prior to conception. Studies have shown that red cell folate levels exceeding 400 ng/ml are best for preventing neural tube defects. This can be achieved only with folic acid supplementation. Studies have shown that folic acid acts through an unusual mechanism—terathanasia—the selective promotion of spontaneous abortion of defective fetuses.

Women of child bearing age should be encouraged to take generous amounts of folic acid. In addition women planning pregnancy should begin periconceptional supplementation with folic acid at levels of 400 to 800 μg per day. New research suggests that women who take folic acid supplements for at least one year before they become pregnant can cut their risk of having a premature baby by one half. It is difficult to provide 300 μg of additional amount of folic acid during pregnancy through food and can be met through supplements of medicinal folate.

Green leafy vegetables like gogu leaves and tamarind leaves and legumes like moth bean, red gram, rajamah and soya beans are good sources of folic acid. Nuts (ground nuts), vegetables (beet root, lady's finger, capsicum) and fruits (mango) also contribute to folic acid.

Vitamin B_{12}: Normal adult woman's requirement of vitamin B_{12} is 2.2 μg and this requirement is increased by 0.25 μg during pregnancy. The foetus has priority over the mother in B_{12}, and foetal blood has twice the amount of B_{12} than does maternal blood, even when maternal levels are depleted. Low maternal levels are associated with prematurity. The capacity of a woman to absorb B_{12} is increased during pregnancy and a large amount is transferred to the foetus. Vegan mothers have more chances of getting B_{12} deficiency as vitamin B_{12} is present in foods of animal origin. Serum levels drop during pregnancy and return to normal without supplementation after delivery. On the basis of B_{12} content of foetuses, it has been estimated that foetal demands may be of the order of 0.3 µg per day.

Vitamin C: ICMR recommendations of vitamin C during pregnancy is 15 mg higher than normal woman requirement 65 mg. The foetal requirement is too small and sufficient safety margin is given for an adult woman and extra allowance may not be necessary during pregnancy. In pregnancy
vitamin C can fully cross the placental barrier. The vitamin C content of foetal blood is thrice as much as maternal blood. There is some evidence to show that the placenta can synthesize vitamin C. This may account for higher levels in foetal tissue. Low maternal intake of vitamin C is associated with premature rupture of foetal membranes and increased neonatal death rates.

A few studies have suggested an association between low plasma levels of vitamin C and preeclampsia.

Share of Nutrients

- Nutrients given to foetus at the expense of mother—folic acid, vitamin C, vitamin B_{12}, iron and calcium
- Nutrients for which mother and foetus compete—vitamin B_1, B_2, B_6 and D
- Nutrients for which mother has priority over foetus—vitamin A and Iodine
- Nutrients stored in foetus—vitamin A and iron
- Nutrients not stored in foetus—vitamin C, D and calcium

Largely because of assisted reproduction, the rate of multifoetal pregnancy is rising rapidly. Women with multifetal pregnancy have an increased need for weight gain, energy, essential fatty acids, iron, calcium and other nutrients compared with women with single fetus pregnancy. Total weight gain in twin pregnancy is 16–20 kg.

Fibre

Consuming a healthy diet rich in fibre during pregnancy may promote the well being of both the mother and child. It reduces the risk of preeclampsia. The mother's gut bacteria and diet appear to be crucial to promote a healthy pregnancy. A study found that reduced levels of acetate, which is mainly produced by fibre fermentation in the gut is associated with preeclampsia.

The study also found that preeclampsia affected the development of an important foetal immune organ the thymus. These results showed that promoting specific metabolic products of gut bacteria during pregnancy might be an effective way to maintain a healthy pregnancy and prevent allergies and autoimmune conditions later in life.

Relationship between Maternal and Foetal Nutrition

Studies from NIN have indicated that maternal lean body mass is the most important determinant of infant's birth weight.

Nutritional deficiencies during the growth period in the womb and after birth tend to cause low weight and small size rather than deficiency abnormalities at earlier times.

Due to undernourishment of the mother the baby is at an increased risk of being premature with low birth weight and developmental irregularities. Intrauterine nutrition is highly important for the growth of the central nervous system and kidneys of the foetus which mature during the latter part of pregnancy. Therefore nutrition deficits before birth can never be wholly reversed after birth.

Schematic diagram, Fig. 8.3 shows the relationship between maternal and foetal nutrition.

Inadequate food intake and poor nutrient utilisation
↓
Maternal malnutrition
↓
Reduced blood volume expansion
↓
Inadequate increase in cardiac output
↓
Decreased blood and nutrient supply to the foetus
↓
Reduced placental size
↓
Reduced nutrient transfer
↓
Foetal growth retardation

Fig. 8.3 Relationship between maternal and foetal nutrition

Intrauterine growth retardation can occur due to deficiency of energy, dietary folate, vitamin A, zinc, vitamin B_{12}, riboflavin and iodine.

Table 8.3 Impact of nutritional deficiency on the outcome of pregnancy

Nutrient	*Impact of deficiency on the*	
	Mother	*Infant*
Energy and Protein	• Abortion • Complications during delivery • Ketosis • May not gain enough weight to have normal lactation. • PIH	• Premature infant • Low birth weight infant • Less brain cells
Linoleic Acid	—	• Retarded foetal growth
Calcium	• Muscular cramps • Repeated pregnancy with poor diet can result in osteomalacia • During lactation breast milk may be deficient in calcium	• Calcification of bones and teeth is decreased • Underweight due to the decreased foetal bone growth

Iron	• Hypochromic microcytic anaemia. Complications during delivery	• Born with less stores of iron and susceptible for anaemia
Iodine	• Goitre • Increased risk of miscarriage and still birth	• Chance of getting goitre • Cretinism
Zinc	• Foetal mortality • Foetal malformations including central nervous system and teratogenicity	• Reduced intrauterine growth rate • Low birth weight • Preterm baby
Vitamin A	• Mortality • PIH	• Decreased levels in foetus so more susceptible for vitamin A deficiency
Vitamin D	• Decreased calcium absorption	• Calcium metabolism of foetus is affected
Vitamin K	• Decreased prothrombin synthesis • Increased loss of blood during delivery	• Increased risk of neonatal haemorrhage
Thiamin, Riboflavin and Niacin	• Deficiency symptoms	—
Folic acid	• Megaloblastic anaemia • Abruptio placentae • PIH	• Foetal malformation • Neural tube defects, spina bifida, congenital abnormalities like hare lip, cleft palate, hydrocephalus • Low birth weight
Vitamin B_{12}	• Pernicious anaemia	• Premature baby
Vitamin C	• Premature rupture of foetal membranes	• Increased neonatal death rate.

FOOD REQUIREMENTS

For a pregnant woman whose diet has conformed to the 'Basic Five Food' pattern, it is merely a matter of emphasising the more nutrient dense foods within each of the five food groups. Nutrient dense foods are those that give the most nutrients per calorie consumed. Most mothers are concerned enough about the health of their offspring and have a high motivation to eat right food. Pregnancy is perhaps the most effective time to attempt nutrition education.

Usually a daily diet containing 3 cups of milk or its equivalent, 2 servings of meat, fish, poultry, eggs, or a source of complete protein, a dark green or yellow vegetables and a generous serving of citrus fruits will provide a foundation for a nutritionally adequate diet. Between the 6th to 14th week of pregnancy 75 per cent women suffer from nausea which in turn affects their appetite. The consumption of small and frequent meals at regular intervals are helpful to many women. This pattern is also very helpful in the later part of pregnancy when discomfort is experienced after large meals due to over crowding by foetus in the abdominal cavity.

Eating a small meal just before hunger sensations usually become most severe, has been a useful method of controlling total intake. Intake must be maintained at steady levels so that the weight gain is not more than 400 g/week, in the 2nd and 3rd trimesters of pregnancy. An erratic weight gain during pregnancy is associated with toxaemia and prematurity.

The selection of diet is also quite complicated because many women experience strong food dislikes and cravings. They often crave for foods they do not take ordinarily and develop strong distastes for foods they previously liked. In certain cases the aroma or sight to certain foods may evoke strong reactions. Mostly dislikes are oriented towards food that have no nutritional consequences. But if the dislike is for foods such as milk, which has good amounts of calcium then attention should be directed towards such an issue.

Plenty of water at least four to six glasses in addition to what is contained in the form of milk and other beverages should be taken daily throughout pregnancy. This will help keep the bowels regular. It has been found that infection of the tube connecting the kidney and bladder is less common among pregnant women who drink a lot of water. It is recommended that pregnant women limit their intake to 2 cups of caffeine containing beverages per day like tea, coffee and chocolate.

Faulty beliefs and wrong food habits need to be corrected during pregnancy. This is the best period when mother is willing to practice the principles of balanced diet. Stress, anxiety, fatigue and other psycho social characteristics may influence the food choice of pregnant woman.

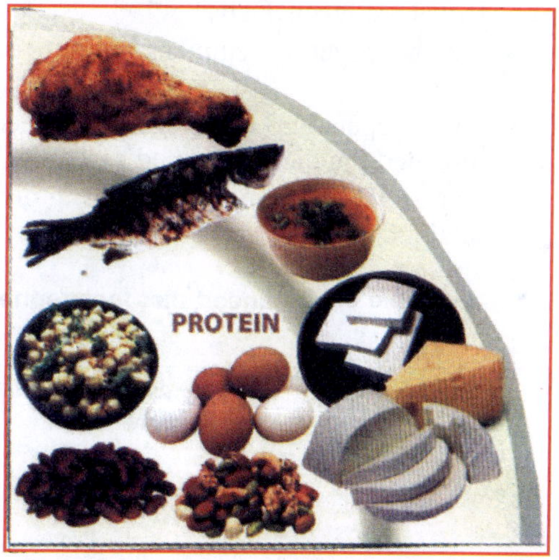

Fig. 8.4 **Increased requirements of protein during pregnancy can be met by inclusion of protein rich foods. These foods are also good sources of minerals and vitamins and supply calories.**

Dietary Guidelines

- Small and frequent feedings should be taken. Fasting or missing meal should be avoided.
- Consumption of eggs and other nonvegetarian foods help in meeting increased protein requirement.
- More fibre should be included in the diet to prevent constipation which is a common problem during pregnancy. About 5-6 Servings of fruits and vegetables should be included in the daily diet.
- Diet should be rich in calcium to prevent osteomalacia. Calcium supplements may also be taken. A minimum of 3 glasses of milk should be taken.
- Iron rich foods should be taken to prevent anaemia and to build up iron stores in the foetal body. Iron supplements may be taken. Haeme iron is better absorbed. Inclusion of green leafy vegetables ensures minerals like calcium and iron.
- Diet should contain optimum amount of sodium. In case of oedema or hypertension, sodium is restricted.
- Raw fruits and vegetables are to be included in the diet to meet vitamin C and fibre requirement.
- Plenty of water should be taken to keep the bowels regular.
- Fatty rich foods, fried foods, excessive seasoning, strongly flavoured vegetables may be restricted in case of nausea and gastric distress.
- Too much of coffee or tea is to be avoided.

- The diet should include fish, flax seed and soyabean to meet the requirement of ω-3 fatty acids.
- Fluids should be taken between meals rather than along with the meals.
- Adequate amount of calories should be taken so that enough fat is deposited during pregnancy which is used for lactation.
- Sugar substitute should be used in moderation during pregnancy as the effects on the foetus are inconclusive.
- Weight reduction regimens are not recommended because the effect of ketosis on the foetus.
- Lacto vegetarians and vegans can meet the nutritional requirements during pregnancy provided the diet is planned carefully.
- Vitamin D supplementation during pregnancy may play a role in insulin resistance and fetal growth.

Table 8.4 Balanced diet for pregnant woman with nutrient content values suggested by ICMR - 2020

Food Composition	*Amount (g/day)*	*Nutrient*	*Vegetarian diet*	*Non-Vegetarian diet*	*EAR*	*RDA*
Cereals and Millets	325	Energy kcal	2060	2040	2480	–
		Protein g	71.7	71.6	54	68
Pulses (Legumes)[1]	90	Visible fat g	15	15	30	30
Green leafy vegetables	100	Calcium mg	980	970	800	1000
Other vegetables	200	Iron mg	27.2	26.0	21	27
Roots and Tubers (excluding potatoes)	100	Zinc mg	13.1	12.8	12.0	14.5
Fruits	150	Magnesium mg	786	747	370	440
Milk	400	Vitamin A µg*	1821	1818	406	900
Fats and Oils	25	B-carotene µg	9634	9597	–	–
Oil seeds and Nuts (gingely seeds and Pea nuts)	40	Thiamine mg	1.64	1.60	1.6	2.0
Spices	10	Riboflavin mg	1.8	1.84	2.3	2.7
		Niacin mg	16.0	16.7	14	16
		Vitamin B_6 mg	2.0	2.0	1.9	2.3
		Vitamin C mg	210	210	65	80
		Total Folates µg	484	447	480	570
		Vitamin B_{12} µg	2.0	2.4	2.2	2.5

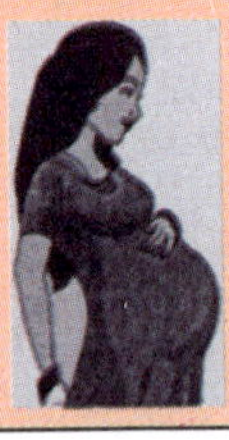

Note: Total protein from the above diet = 78.8 g, Digestible protein = 70 g, PDCAAS = 88%

[1]Pulses can be replaced with animal foods (egg, meat, fish and chicken) for non-vegetarians.

* Retinol derived from β carotene from diet was also added to the total Vitamin A.

For cereals and millets, it is recommended to consume 50% as whole grains.

GENERAL DIETARY PROBLEMS

Nausea and Vomiting

Nausea in pregnancy may be due to nervous disturbances, placental protein intoxication or due to derangement in carbohydrate metabolism.

Morning sickness of early pregnancy can be improved by small and frequent meals. Fairly dry and consisting chiefly of easily digested energy foods such as carbohydrates are more readily tolerated. Liquids may best be taken between meals instead of with food. If the condition develops to hyperemesis gravidarum, a severe prolonged persistent vomiting, peripheral parenteral nutrition and careful oral feeding is essential. Skim milk is better tolerated than whole milk. Fruits and vegetables can be given. Fatty rich foods, fried foods, excessive seasoning, coffee in large amounts and strongly flavoured vegetables may be restricted or eliminated if the nausea persists. She should avoid becoming too hungry. Small and frequent meals should be given.

In pregnancy 1g/day of supplemental ginger taken for 4 days to one week may decrease nausea without the drowsiness associated with antiemitics. Eliminating iron supplements for sometime may also reduce the symptoms.

Leg Cramps

The common occurrence of cramps during pregnancy, manifested nocturnally by sudden contractions of the muscle, is thought to be related to a decline in serum calcium levels related to calcium phosphorus imbalance. Prevention or relief of these leg cramps has been reported with reduction of milk (a high phosphorus, high calcium beverage) intake and supplementation with nonphosphate calcium salts. Magnesium is another mineral with the potential for relieving leg cramps.

Heart Burn

Increased progesterone production causes decreased tone and mobility of the smooth muscles of the gastrointestinal tract. This leads to regurgitation. In most cases, this is an effect of pressure of the enlarged uterus on the stomach which in combination with the relaxation of the oesophageal sphincter, results in occasional regurgitation of the stomach contents into the esophagus. Heart burn is a common complaint during the latter part of pregnancy. This can usually be relieved by small and frequent meals limiting the amount of food consumed at one time and drinking fluids between meals. Sitting upright after meals for at least 3 hours before lying down may also help.

Beliefs, Avoidances, Cravings and Aversions

Food avoidances reflect mother's conscious choice not to consume certain foods during pregnancy e.g., heat producing foods like papaya and gingelly seeds. Some consume saffron during pregnancy with the belief that they would get fair babies. Pregnant mother should understand the scientific basis and avoid superstitious beliefs. Consumption of papaya and saffron do not have any negative or positive effect on the foetus.

Cravings and aversions are powerful urges toward or away from foods which pregnant women experience. The most commonly craved foods are sweets and dairy products. The most common aversions reported are alcohol, coffee, other caffeinated drinks, meats and strongly spiced foods.

Consumption of non-food items like laundry starch, ice cubes or clay is called pica. It occurs more often during pregnancy than at any other time. The etiology of pica is poorly understood and one theory suggests that the ingestion of non-food substances relieves nausea and vomiting. It has also been hypothesised that a deficiency for essential nutrient, such as calcium or iron, results in the eating of non-food substances that contain these nutrients. Much of this behaviour appears to be based on superstitions, customs and traditions that one often passes from mother to daughter.

Weight Gain during Pregnancy

All pregnancies should be started with BMI of 20–26 because maternal and foetal consequences occur at both extremes. Optimal weight gain is about 11 to 13 kg. About 900 to 1800 g is an average gain during the first trimester. Thereafter 450 g/week during the remainder of the pregnancy is usual. Sharp sudden increase in weight after the 20th week of pregnancy, which may indicate excessive, abnormal water retention should be watched. Weight reduction should never be undertaken during pregnancy. Excessive weight gain places an extra strain on the organs and increases the incidence to toxaemia. It is not correct for the mother to think that low gain in weight results in smaller baby which is easy to deliver.

Excess gestational weight gain among women with overweight or obesity synergistically increases their already elevated risk of having gestational diabetes, a caesarean delivery, a large for gestational age infant and post-partum weight retention and increases their child's risk of obesity.

Pregorexia

Pregorexia means that pregnant woman who will reduce calories and exercise in excess in an effort to control weight gain. The term indicates an unhealthy restriction on food intake and an obsession with minimising weight gain during pregnancy.

Tables 8.5 and 8.6 give the components of weight gain during pregnancy and recommended weight gain based on body mass index.

Table 8.5 Components of weight gain during pregnancy (28–40 weeks)

Component	*Weight g*
Foetus	3000
Placenta and amniotic fluid	1500
Maternal tissues and blood	7000
Total	11500

Table 8.6 Recommended weight gain for pregnant woman based on body mass index

Weight category based on BMI	*Total weight gain (kg)*
Under weight (BMI < 19.8)	12.5–18
Normal weight (19.8–26)	11.5–16
Overweight BMI > 26–29	7–11.5
Obese > 29	6.0

Undernutrition during pregnancy is associated with low birth weight, CHD, type 2 diabetes, stroke and hypertension.

Research shows that continuing a regular exercise regimen throughout pregnancy is helpful in maintaining the desirable weight, improved fitness, prevention of gestational diabetes, facilitation of labour and reduced stress.

COMPLICATIONS

About 1,25,000 women die in India every year from causes related to pregnancy and child birth. The main causes are anaemia, haemorrhage and toxemia which are often preventable (2006).

Anaemia

According to WHO/UNICEF/UNO, a pregnant woman is anaemic if the haemoglobin level is below 11.0 g/dl or haematocrit per cent is below 33 per cent. Anaemia in pregnancy accounts for 1/5th of the maternal deaths worldwide and is a major factor responsible for low birth weight.

The demand for folate during pregnancy is increased because of increased cellular proliferation. Megaloblastic anaemia results in intensified nausea, vomiting and anorexia.

Aetiology: Factors implicated in the etiopathogenesis of anaemia during pregnancy and low birth weight are maternal age, weight, height, parity, literacy, income, infections, pregnancy related complications, nutritional stress, cultural beliefs, taboos and inappropriate food practice. Too little space between births or too many infections and too little intake of nutrients involved in erythropoiesis during pregnancy leads to anaemia. Open air defaecation, literacy status and trimester of pregnancy are found to be significantly associated with the prevalence of anaemia.

Physiological changes in the blood occur progressively during normal pregnancy. Haemoglobin mass increases, red blood cell volume increases, plasma volume rises and haemoglobin concentration drops from 13.4 to 11.6 g per 100 ml. Severe anaemia in pregnant women increases maternal morbidity and mortality and involves a higher risk of the foetus.

Symptoms: A significant fall in birth weight due to increase in prematurity rate and intrauterine growth retardation has been reported to occur when maternal haemoglobin level falls below 8 g/dl. Anaemic pregnant women are prone to urinary infections. The effect of anaemia and urinary tract infection in pregnancy could also be the cause of low birth weight infant.

Iron deficiency anaemia in the mother may also produce alterations in brain function and impaired schooling later. Low birth weight infants have a high mortality rate and those that survive have greater rates of morbidity and poorer neurological development.

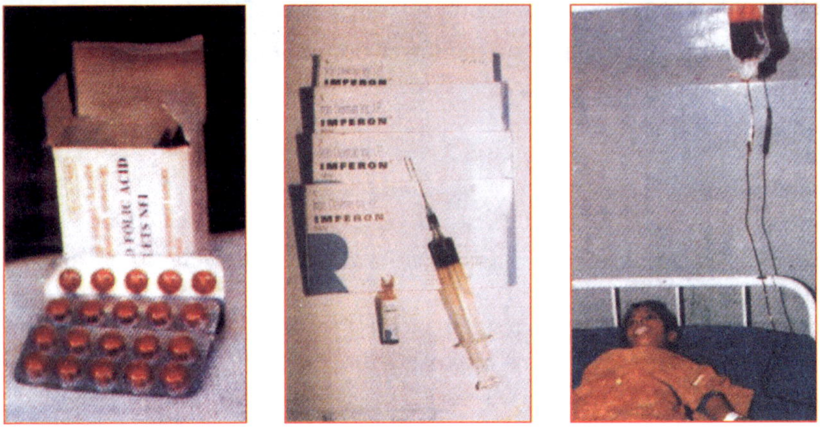

A B C

Fig. 8.5 Prevention and treatment of anaemia

A. Anaemia can be prevented by taking iron and folic acid tablets.

B & C In severe anaemia iron injections or blood transfusion should be given.

Source: Health of mother and child UNICF.

Treatment: Women with haemoglobin levels below 7 g/dl are considered to be severely anaemic and parenteral iron can be given by 20 weeks. Recommended therapeutic dose for women in the reproductive age group is one tablet of iron thrice daily for a minimum of 100 days. This will provide equivalent to 180 mg elemental iron and 1500 μg of folic acid per day.

Anaemia due to B_{12} deficiency in pregnancy is uncommon. A single injection of 40 mcg of B_{12} is enough to produce a maximum response in 10 days in B_{12} deficient mothers.

Pregnant mothers should take iron and folic acid rich foods. Regular consumption of iron rich foods such as green leafy vegetables, cereals such as wheat, ragi, jowar and bajra, pulses and jaggery. In addition, wherever culturally and economically feasible, consumption of animal flesh foods such as meat and liver must be encouraged. Vitamin C promotes absorption of iron. Regular consumption of vitamin C rich food such as lemon, orange, guava, amla, mango along with iron rich food must be promoted.

Prevention: The iron requirement of a pregnant woman is around 27 mg/day as against the dietary intake of Indian pregnant woman is 18 mg/day. Through the PHC or ICDS distribution channel 60 mg elemental iron and 500 μg of folic acid per day are distributed in the last trimester of pregnancy to prevent anaemia under National Anaemia Prophylaxis Programme.

Recent surveys carried out by Indian Council of Medical Research indicates that the beneficiaries covered are only about 25 per cent of the pregnant women. Consequently the prevalence of anaemia remained still high. The treatment of anaemia envisaged in the National Anaemia Control Programme had not been operationalized and coverage and compliance with oral iron folic acid supplementation is poor.

Universal cash transfer of Rs. 6000 to pregnant women was legislated by the 2013 National Food Security Act. This would allow the pregnant woman to access an adequate quantity and quality of nutritious food.

Some of the recent studies have indicated that vitamin B_{12} deficiency may play an important role in anaemia.

Constipation

The pressure of the enlarging uterus on the lower portion of the intestine, in addition to the hormonal muscle relaxant effect of placental hormones on the gastrointestinal tract may result in constipation. Increased progesterone production causes decreased tone and motility of the smooth muscles of the gastrointestinal tract. Physical inactivity may also make elimination difficult. Increased fluid intake and use of natural laxative foods such as whole grains, dried fruits and other fruits, vegetables that are rich in fibre and juices usually induce regularity. Laxatives should be avoided. Regular habits of exercise and sleep are essential for proper elimination.

Oedema

Mild, physiologic oedema is usually present in the extremities in the third trimester. The swelling of the lower extremities may be caused by the pressure of the enlarging uterus on the veins returning fluid from the legs. This normal oedema requires no sodium restriction or other dietary changes.

Pregnancy Induced Hypertension

Studies conducted at National Institute of Nutrition indicate that pregnancy induced hypertension (eclampsia) is associated with higher incidence of vitamin A and protein deficiencies resulting in poor pregnancy outcome.

It is common among women subsisting on inadequate diets with little or no prenatal care. The symptoms of PIH include hypertension, abnormal and excessive oedema, albuminuria, convulsions or coma. Optimal nutrition is a fundamental aspect of therapy. Emphasis is given to adequate dietary protein. Correction of plasma protein deficits stimulates normal operation of the capillary fluid shift mechanism and circulation of fluid tissue with subsequent correction of the hypovolaemia (abnormal reduction in volume of circulatory plasma). In addition, adequate salt and sources of vitamins and minerals are needed for correction and maintenance of metabolic balance.

In severe preeclampsia, oral feeding is suspended in favour of intravenous infusion with 10 per cent dextrose drip during which the patient remains in sedation. Then oral feeding with 10 per cent dextrose, barley and fruit juice is allowed. Bed rest is advocated.

Pregnancy induced hypertension is seen in 10–20 per cent of all pregnant women in India. It is associated with increased maternal morbidity and mortality, related to intrauterine growth retardation, premature delivery and perinatal asphyxia. Pregnant women with preeclampsia are at increased risk for abruptio placenta, intracerebral haemorrhage and hepatic and renal failure.

Preeclampsia is associated with oxidative stress, imbalance between prooxidants and antioxidants leads to potential cell or tissue damage. Vascular endothelial damage is known to play a key role in the patho physiological mechanism of preeclampsia. Free radical mediated lipid peroxidation may be involved in the endothelial damage.

Excess free radical disturbances are associated with increased utilisation of antioxidants resulting in decrease in the concentration of ascorbic acid, α-tocopherol and β-carotene. Antioxidant supplementation in primigravida may be helpful in preventing preeclampsia.

Hypertension

This can cause considerable maternal and foetal consequences. Nutritional therapy will centre on (1) prevention of weight extremes, underweight or obesity (2) correction of any dietary deficiencies and maintenance of optimal nutritional status during pregnancy and (3) management of any related preexisting disease such as diabetes mellitus. Sodium intake may be moderate but should not be unduly restricted.

Gestational Diabetes Mellitus

During pregnancy glycosuria is not uncommon, because of the increased circulating blood volume and its load of metabolites. Insulin antagonism is due to the combined effect of human placental lactogen, oestrogen, progesterone, free cortisol and degradation of the insulin by the placenta. Most of these women revert to normal glucose tolerance after delivery.

Several studies have shown that elevated glycosylated haemoglobin levels early in pregnancy correlate with increased incidence of malformations. Hence the management and counsellings of women with diabetes in the reproductive age group should begin prior to conception, with efforts aimed at achieving HbA1c concentration around 6.5 per cent. Glycosylated haemoglobin measurements are used to aid in the timing of conception. Among diabetic women with poor control, perinatal mortality ranges from 3–5 per cent and major congenital defects from 6–12 per cent.

NIN studies have indicated that the prevalence of insulin resistance around 50 per cent from early pregnancy. Insulin resistance during pregnancy has been shown to be associated with various complications in addition to impact on pregnancy outcome and birth weight of infants.

Strategies to reduce the occurrence of neonatal macrosomia and maternal prepregnancy obesity may help lower the rate of recurrence of gestational diabetes mellitus.

EXERCISE/PHYSICAL ACTIVITY

Physical activity during pregnancy improves or maintains physical fitness. It may help prevent gestational diabetes, support healthy gestational weight gain and improve mental health. Incidence of cesarean and operative vaginal delivery and postpartum recovery time is decreased. Exercise also helps in preventing preclampsia. Walking is the most common leisure time physical activity.

Normal pregnant mother can do regular mild to moderate physical activity. This does not affect the foetus and can benefit the pregnant mother. Strenuous activity should be avoided during the first trimester.

According to United States Department of Health and Human Services, physical activity guidelines, a healthy pregnant and post partum women should do at least 150 minutes per week of moderate intensity (brisk walking) aerobic activity. This activity should be spread throughout the week.

Woman who engages in physical activity during pregnancy should consume sufficient calories to meet increased demands of pregnancy and physical activity. They should drink liquids before, during and after physical activity to ensure adequate hydration. They should not overexert.

Exercise is contraindicated for pregnant women with risk factors for adverse maternal or prenatal outcomes and chronic diseases like cardiovascular disease. Such mothers should be evaluated by their physicians for exercise recommendations.

Maternal dietary imbalance in critical periods of intrauterine life can trigger a redistribution of foetal resources. This can affect a fetus's structure and metabolism in ways that predispose the individual to later cardiovascular and endocrine diseases. A good start in life is important.

Pregnancy is optimal when the mother is biologically mature. A biologically mature female is a young woman who is atleast 5 years post menarchial and this has greater impact on pregnancy than her chronological age.

Infrastructures of health services in the rural areas should be strengthened to provide primary health care to the mother. Social stature of women needs to be elevated so that they are not deprived or unfavourably discriminated for allocation of scarce food resources.

WHO and UNICF have repeatedly emphasised that too early pregnancies (teenager), too late (35 and over), too close (less than two years) and too many (four and over) are not safe or conducive to the health of either the mother or her infant.

International women's day is on 8th of March

SOME SUGGESTED RECIPES DURING PREGNANCY

Recipes	*Reason*
Mint and paneer pulao.	To meet the requirements of protein, calcium and vitamins
Fruit salad, vegetable salad	Appetising and provide many nutrients and also fibre.
Omlette, boiled egg, scrambled egg, liver curry	Good quality protein, iron, and vitamin A
Rice flakes upma, puffed rice ball	Easy to digest
Green gram, dal, pakoda, bread pudding, carrot halwa	Nutrient dense foods to be given to meet increased requirements.
Pickles, rasam, sour foods	These foods may give relief from nausea.
Kathi rolls, frankies.	Convenient to consume.
Homemade granola (oats, nuts and sugar)	Rich in calories and protein.

SUGGESTED READINGS

- Alves-Santos Helma Nadya *et al.*, Prepregnancy dietary palterns and their association with perinatal outcomes J Acad Nutr Diet., 2019; **119**.
- Gailo Sina *et al.*, Vitamin D supplementation during pregnancy J Acad Nutr Diet., 2020; **120**.
- Siega-Riz Anna Maria *et al.*, Preconception diet quality is associated with birth weight for gestational age J Acad Nutr Diet., 2021; **120**.
- Ashman M. Amy *et al.*, Factors associated with effective nutrition interventions for pregnant indigenous women, J. Acad. Nutr. Diet, 2017; **117.**
- Evaluation of the routine management of anaemia in pregnancy and effect on outcome Annual report 2009–2010, NIN, Hyderabad.

QUESTIONS

1. Give the ICMR allowance for protein, energy and calcium for a pregnant woman.
2. Give the complete RDA for a pregnant woman who is in last trimester of pregnancy.
3. Explain the reasons for increased nutrient requirement during pregnancy.
4. What modifications in diet would you suggest for a pregnant woman?
5. Describe the complications of pregnancy.
6. Why anaemia is common during pregnancy? What measures should be taken to prevent it?
7. Explain the impact of malnutrition during pregnancy.
8. Explain the role of Government in prevention of anaemia during pregnancy.

TOPICS FOR ACTIVITY

- Plan and prepare a diet for a woman who is pregnant 7 months. Give list of additional requirements required during pregnancy.
- Conduct a survey to find out the myths prevailing in the diets of pregnant women.

9

Nutritional Recommendations and Food Requirements of Lactating Women

The nutritional link between the mother and the child continues even after birth. The newborn baby depends for some period solely on breast milk for his existence.

ROLE OF HORMONES IN MILK PRODUCTION

Sucking by infant initiates hormonal changes that lead to milk production and let down reflex, which releases milk as shown in Fig. 9.1.

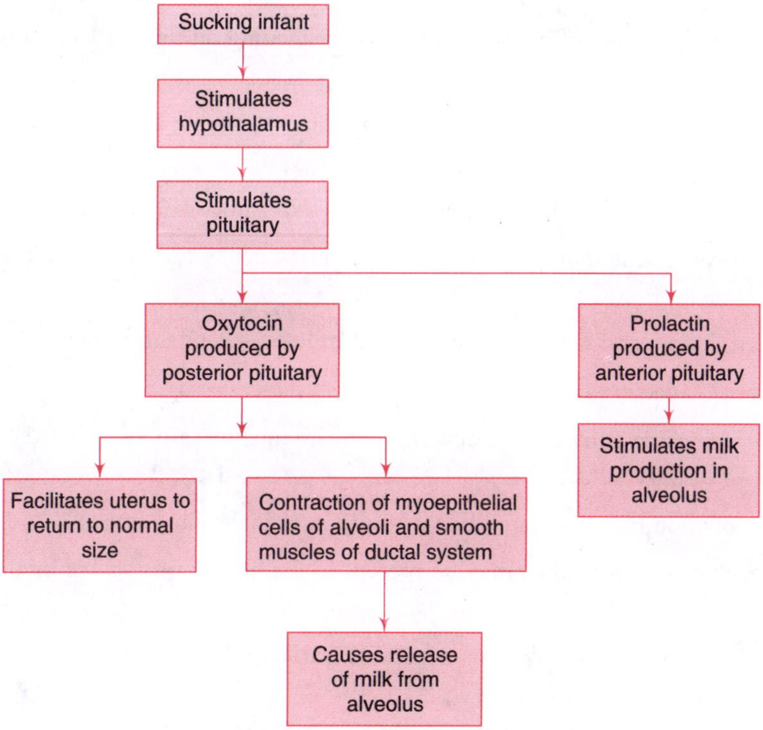

Fig. 9.1 Process of stimulation of milk production

The process of lactation is controlled by various hormones. The source of these hormones and their function is summarised in Table 9.1.

Table 9.1 Hormonal control of lactation

Hormone	*Source*	*Activity*
Oestrogen	Ovary and placenta	Stimulates breast development during pregnancy
Progesterone	Ovary and placenta	Stimulates breast development during pregnancy
Prolactin	Anterior pituitary gland	Stimulates milk production
Oxytocin	Posterior pituitary gland	"Let down" reflex: Smooth muscles surrounding the alveoli of the nipples contract to allow the release of milk. In pain, emotions or embarrassment the let-down reflex may sometimes be inhibited. Doubting about the ability to produce enough milk can interfere with the "let down" reflex. Oxytocin counteracts this.

Factors Affecting the Volume and Composition of Breast Milk

- Fat and energy concentration in milk are significantly related to maternal fat stores.
- Milk of primiparae has a higher fat concentration than that of multiparae.
- There is no significant effect of supplementary feeding on the production of milk.
- The frequency of milk removal is an important determinant of the volume of milk secreted. Sucking stimulates the release of hormones that stimulate milk production. Frequent feeding removes the locally active inhibitor.
- Undernourished mother produces less quantity but same quality of milk.
- Lactose, protein, calcium, iron, copper and flourine content of milk is independent of the mother's diet.
- Selenium, iodine and B vitamins content of milk is dependent on mother's diet.
- Lactational capacity is a function of genetic heritage.
- Maternal physical activity and maternal and infant illness may affect the amount and content of milk secreted.
- Milk production may also be affected by the inadequate fluid intake.
- Unusual flavour compounds may be present in the breast milk, if the mother consumes strong flavoured foods.

Analysis of has milk has shown considerable variation in composition, not only among women but also in the same women over a time.

Figure 9.2 shows the causes of failure to thrive while breast fed.

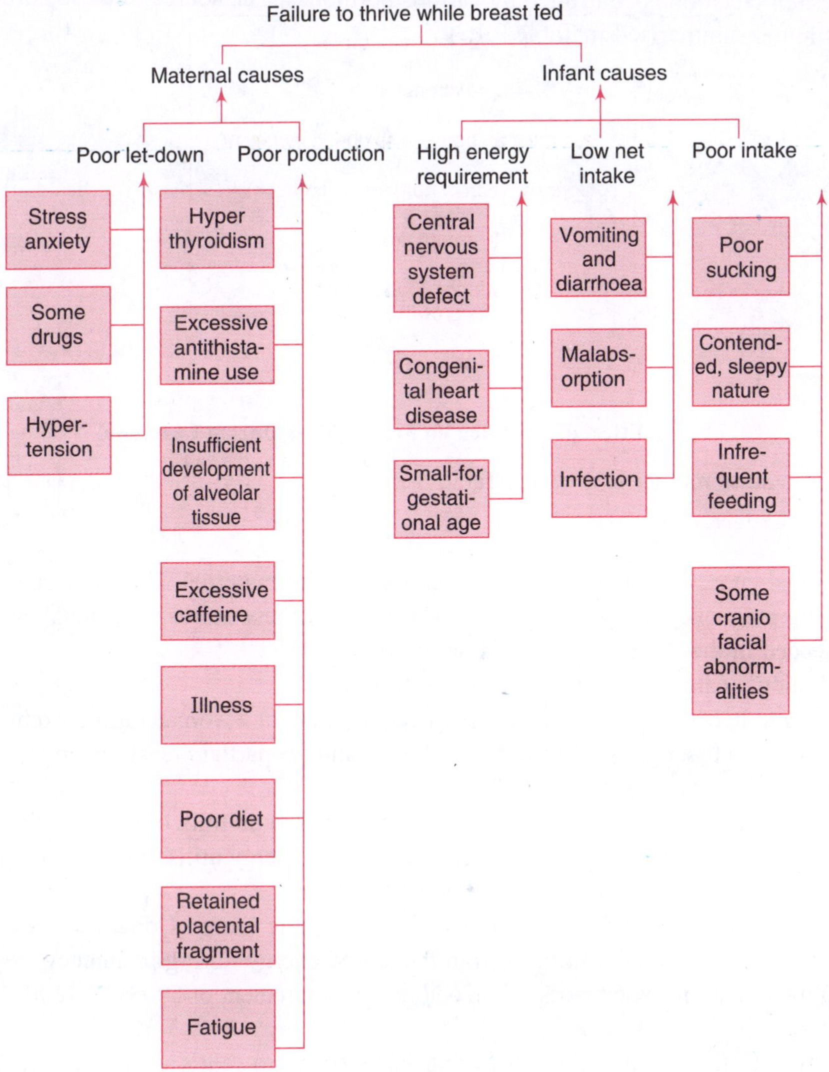

Fig. 9.2 Diagnostic flow chart for failure to thrive while breast fed

Source: (Modified) Mahan Kathleen K and Sylvia Escott-Stump (edited), 2000, Krause's Food, Nutrition and Diet therapy, W.B. Saunders Company, Philadelphia.

NUTRITIONAL RECOMMENDATIONS

Lactating mother's nutritional requirements should meet (1) her own daily needs (2) provide enough nutrients in milk for the growing infant and (3) furnish the energy for the mechanics of milk production. Diet of lactating mother and her nutritional status during pregnancy affect to a certain extent quality and quantity of breast milk.

Nutritional needs exceed during lactation compared to pregnancy. In six months a normally developing infant doubles the birth weight equivalent of which is accumulated in 9 months of pregnancy.

Better intake of protein
+
Micronutrients
↓
Accrue lean body mass during lactation
↓
↑ Concentration of nutrients in breast milk
↓
↑ Infant growth
↓
↑ Growth hormone and insulin like growth factor-1
↓
↑ Muscle mass

Fig. 9.3 **Effect of Nutrition on Muscle Mass During Lactation.**

RDA of a lactating mother is given in Table 9.2.

Energy

The additional energy needed for lactation is drawn from maternal adipose tissue stores laid down during pregnancy. Depending on the adequacy of these stores, additional energy input may be needed in the lactating woman's daily diet.

The additional calories are required for the following:

According to ICMR daily additional energy requirement of a woman during exclusive breast feeding during the first 6 months would be 600 kcal and for partial breast feeding during 7–12 months, it would be approximately 520 kcal.

A study of energy requirement of lactating women based on milk output and energy output computed from actual measurement showed that average energy utilisation for milk production of 722 ml the energy utilisation would be 594 kcal (600).

An additional amount of 600 kcals are suggested by the Expert Committee, as the rest of the calories required are to be utilised from the stored energy during pregnancy.

If lactating mother is undernourished an additional requirement of 500 kcals (600 + 500 kcal) are required.

In addition to the energy required during lactation extra requirements are needed if the mother is a teenager, feeding more than one child, underweight, or if she is also pregnant.

The increased energy demand during lactation is usually met through multiple strategies such as increased energy intake, energy sparing through decreased physical activity or possible energy sparing adaptations as well as mobilization of fat from maternal reserves developed during pregnancy.

Protein

During lactation, protein requirement has been computed on the basis of secretion of protein in milk. The protein content of human milk is 1.15 g/100 ml. On an average a mother secretes 680 ml and 580 ml during 0–6 months and 7–12 months of lactation period.

Assuming a 47 per cent efficiency of conversion of dietary protein into milk protein and 25 per cent of individual variation, the safe daily intake is calculated. The Nutrition Expert Committee (2020) has recommended, during lactation an additional daily intake of 19 g for the first 6 months and 13 g during 7–12 months of lactation taking into consideration a balanced diet with dietary protein is of PE ratio 5–15 per cent.

Table 9.2 ICMR Recommended Dietary Allowances of a Lactating Mother – 2020

Nutrient	Normal adult woman	Lactating mother	
		0–6	7–12
Energy kcal			
Sedentary	1660	+ 600	+520
Moderate	2130		
Heavy	2720		
Protein g	46	+ 17	+13
Dietary Fibre g			
Sedentary	25		
Moderate	30	–	–
Heavy	40		
Calcium mg	1000	1200	1200
Magnesium mg	370	400	400
Iron mg	29	23	23
Zinc mg	13.2	14.1	14.1
Iodine µg	140	280	280
Vitamin A µg Retinol	840	950	950
Vitamin D IU	600	600	600
Thiamine mg			
Sedentary	1.4		
Moderate	1.7	2.1	2.1
Heavy	2.2		
Riboflavin mg			
Sedentary	1.9		
Moderate	2.4	3.0	2.9
Heavy	3.1		
Niacin mg			
Sedentary	11		+3
Moderate	14	+5	+5
Heavy	18	18	
Pyridoxine mg			
Sedentary	1.9		
Moderate	1.9	+0.26	+ 0.17
Heavy	2.4		
Folate µg	220	330	330
Vitamin B_{12} µg	2.2	+1.0	+1.0
Vitamin C mg	65	+50	+50

CHAPTER 9

If energy or protein is lacking, there will be a reduction in milk volume rather than in milk quality. At very low protein intakes the proportion of casein may be reduced. The availability of more protein or more energy will not enhance the amount of protein in the milk nor increase the volume of milk.

Fat

The minimum level of total fat should be 20% E. Although the total amount of fat in breast milk is not influenced by the mother's diet, the composition of the milk fat reflects the composition of the mother's diet. ω-3 fatty acid content in milk can be improved in mother's milk by giving high amount in maternal diet.

The requirements of linoleic acid during lactation is 5–10% E. After taking into account the contribution from invisible fat, the visible fat requirement of lactating woman is 10% E and ω–3 fatty acid is 0.5–1% E. This supplies a high level of EFA needed. This would correspond to a daily intake of 30 g of visible fat. Lactating mother should consume 200 mg/d DHA for optimal health and infant development. The level of fat in the diet would provide adequate energy to enable a nursing woman to meet her higher energy needs.

The concentration of long-chain fatty acids, which are critical for growing foetal and infant brain is higher in lower-body fat than in abdominal fat. Mobilization of lower-body fat during lactation may be a mechanism to ensure that the fatty acids necessary for the brain development of the infant are available.

Calcium

Breast feeding is associated with transfer of approximately 200 mg/day of calcium from mother to the infant. Studies have demonstrated that the increased calcium demand leads to mobilisation of this important mineral from the mother's skeleton, leading to transient reduction in Bone Mineral Density (BMD) of lumbar spine and femoral neck regions (4–7 per cent) during 3–6 months of lactation.

Inspite of low intake and prolonged drain of calcium through breast milk, LS-BMD (Lumbar Spine-Bone Mineral Density) continued to rise in better nourished mothers. It is possible that conservation of calcium occurred through either increased absorption or reduced excretion or both. But these compensatory mechanisms could offset the breast milk calcium loss only in mothers with better nutritional status.

Inspite of low calcium intake, the negative effect of lactation may be spontaneously compensated provided the mothers have better body weights and BMIs.

The increased amount of calcium that is required during gestation for mineralisation of the foetal skeleton is now diverted into the mother's milk production. Both during pregnancy and lactation 1200 mg has been prescribed by ICMR 2020. The retention of dietary calcium in lactating woman is about 30 per cent, hence an extra amount of 200 mg is prescribed. About one litre of milk or milk products should be given to lactating mother to meet 1200 mg of calcium.

Iron

Normal adult woman requires 29 mg of iron. The iron requirement during lactation is 23 mg/day. This is due to amenorrhea during lactation and the basal requirement is 14 μg/kg same as normal adult woman. The baby is born with a relatively larger reserve of iron since milk is not a good source of iron. A good allowance of iron in the mother's diet during lactation does not convey additional iron to the infant. Iron requirement during lactation is the sum of the requirement of the mother and that required to make up the iron lost in breast milk.

Zinc

Assuming average milk volume is around 700 ml/d the amount of zinc needed works out to be 1 mg/d. Therefore an additional 1 mg/d zinc is suggested to normal requirement of 13.2 mg amounting to 14.1 mg during lactation.

Iodine

Normal mother requires 140 µg/d and it is increased to 280 µg/during lactation. The amount present in milk 102 µg/d from 700 ml of human milk. The estimated average requirement is 200 micro grams per day. Considering coefficient of variation of 20 percent the RDA is prescribed as 280 micrograms per day.

Vitamin A

The quantity of retinol present in of human milk is 46.4 µg 1100 ml, so the ICMR 2020 recommends an additional allowance of 90 µg of retinol. This can be achieved by including liver, fish liver oils, egg yolk, milk and green leafy vegetables in the diet.

B Vitamins

As calorie and protein requirements are increased during lactation, B vitamin requirements are also increased. Additional B vitamins are required for the amounts that are present in human milk.

Thiamine: The thiamine in breast milk secreted by Indian poor women is below 15 µg per 100 ml. The maximum concentration of thiamine in milk can be achieved by supplementing 20 µg /100 ml. At this concentration with an output of 700 ml of milk 0.14 mg of thiamine would be lost by the mother. Thiamine content of mother's milk depends on mother's diet. Dietary allowances for thiamine for lactating mothers is 0.5 mg/1000 kcal and their daily requirement is computed on the basis of their energy allowance. The daily allowance recommended by ICMR (2020) on the basis of additional calorie allowance is 2.1 mg during lactation.

Riboflavin: The riboflavin content of breast milk of low income Indian mothers is less than 30 µg per 100 ml. With supplements, the concentration can be raised to 30 µg per 100 ml. The amount of riboflavin lost through milk is 0.23 mg per day. Daily allowance of riboflavin corresponding to the increased energy allowance is 3 mg. RDA for riboflavin during lactation is computed on the basis of 0.6 mg per 1000 kcal. If the diet meets the requirement of protein and calcium, the requirement of riboflavin would be definitely met. Milk is not only a good source of calcium but also a good source of riboflavin.

Niacin: The nicotinic acid content of breast milk of Indian women ranges between 100 and 150 µg per 100 ml. The amount lost in milk is between 0.9 and 1.2 mg per day. The dietary allowances for niacin is 6.6 mg niacin equivalents per 1000 kcals. Additional 5 mg is prescribed by ICMR 2020.

Folic acid: The folic acid content of breast milk secreted by Indian women is 1.6 μg per 100 ml. At the higher level, the amount of folate lost by the mother would be about 25 μg a day. An additional allowance of 100–110 μg of folate should be provided during lactation.

Vitamin B_{12}: Amount of vitamin B_{12} present in 700 ml of mother's milk is 0.4 μg/d. And the requirement during lactation adjusted for 50 per cent absorption is 0.8 μg/day. Hence, ICMR suggested 2.2 + 1.0 μg/day for a lactating mother.

Vitamin C

The normal adult woman RDA for vitamin C is 65 mg. The additional needs during lactation are calculated on the basis of vitamin C secreted in milk. Assuming a daily milk secretion of 700 ml milk with an ascorbic acid content of 3 mg/100ml by well nourished women, the additional requirement during lactation is 20 mg. Taking into consideration of the losses (50%) the Expert Committee (2020) recommends an additional intake of 65 + 50 mg per day during lactation. Hence lactating mother requires 115 mg of vitamin C per day.

Fluid

An increased intake of fluids is necessary for adequate milk production, since milk is a fluid tissue. Water and beverages such as juices, soups, butter milk, and milk all add to the fluid necessary to produce milk. A lactating mother should take 2–3 litres of fluid per day.

Nutritional Risk

The lactating woman is likely to be at nutritional risk if

- she is under 17 years of age.
- she is economically deprived.
- her usual diet is nutritionally restrictive or includes unsound nutrition practices.
- she is on a modified diet for chronic systemic disease.
- her weight is less than 85 per cent of ideal weight.
- she has multiple gestation.
- she has had poor weight gain during pregnancy.
- she has had rapid weight loss while breast feeding.
- she is pregnant while breast feeding.
- she has a history of eating disorder.

FOOD REQUIREMENTS

Dietary Guidelines

- Nutritional requirements are maximum during lactation compared to any other age group in a woman's life hence the diet should be balanced and meet the requirement. Number of meals and quantity of each meal can also be increased.
- Like in any balanced diet the food should consist of whole grains, complex carbohydrates and good fats. It should also include plenty of green and coloured vegetables and fruits.

- The lactating mother should be encouraged to take different beverages to meet fluid requirement.
- To prevent osteoporosis, mother should take at least one litre of milk every day.
- To meet additional nutritional requirements, the quantity of food should be increased.
- Variety in the diet helps mother to consume required amounts.
- No food need be withheld from the mother unless it causes distress to the infant. Occasionally, tomatoes, onions, members of cabbage family, chocolate, spices and condiments may cause gastric distress or lose stools in the infant.
- Vitamin and mineral supplements particularly vitamin C, folic acid, vitamin B12, calcium and irons can be taken as the requirements are very high.
- If the mother is under 17 years of age or she has multiple gestation, she needs to take additional care in meeting the nutritional requirement.
- Too much weight gain, should be avoided. When the baby is weaned, the mother must reduce her food intake in order to avoid overweight.
- To increase mono unsaturated fatty acids and polyunsaturated fatty acids, antioxidant vitamin MUFA and PUFA, antioxidant vitamin and minerals, lactating mother should consume whole nuts within the allowance of fat and energy.
- If the mother loses rapid weight loss while breast-feeding, her calorie intake is to be increased.
- Galactogogue or lactogogue act by increasing the prolactin secretion which in turn increases milk production. They also work psychologically and have a marginal effect on milk production. Sucking is the best lactogogue. The diet can include lactogogues which stimulate the production of milk. Garlic, milk, almonds and garden cress seeds are considered to increase the milk production. Some also believe foods of animal origin like goat's meat, fish and mutton increase the secretions of breast milk. Special foods like sonth laddu and gond laddu are given during lactation. This practice can be encouraged as they are nutrient dense.

Early postpartum is a critical period that may initiate consumption of an unhealthy diet which can lead to obesity and adverse lipid profiles. Postpartum is a time of psychological and biological transitions that may affect dietary behaviour.

Consumption of unhealthful diets during this critical period may occur due to demands of infant care, depression, fatigue and weight related distress.

Weight management

Breast feeding for at least 5 – 6 months mobilises fat from the lower body. This may enhance postpartum weight loss. Undesirable weight loss occurs when lactating mother does too much work/exercise.

Low calorie diets are not recommended for obese during lactation due to the possible effects on decreasing breast milk production. Obese women can control their calories by excluding high calorie, low nutrient-dense foods. Nutrient-dense foods should be encouraged within the individual's calorie requirements. Gradual weight loss and adoption of life long healthy eating patterns should be encouraged.

Caffeine

Caffeine is absorbed in human milk and can inhibit the let down reflex. The metabolism of caffeine in the infant takes longer than in the adult. Irritability of the infant can result. Therefore, it is recommended that caffeine-containing beverages be limited to 2 cups per day for the lactating woman. Chocolate, though it contains small amounts of caffeine, does contain theobromide, a stimulant similar to caffeine. Theobromide can cause the infant to become irritable and should be limited in mother's diet.

Allergenic Foods

Sometimes the infant may be sensitive and may react to a food eaten by the mother. Common allergenic foods are cow's milk products, fish, eggs, peanuts or wheat in the maternal diet.

Contaminants

Spices and strong flavoured foods such as garlic, onion and cumin can alter the flavour of the breast milk. Drugs, pesticides, herbicides and other contaminants are transferred to mother's milk. When DDT was used more, mother's milk also contained high amount of DDT. Oral contraceptives lead to lowered milk production and sedatives lead to a decrease in the strength of infant's sucking reflex. Almost all drugs taken by the mother appear to some extent in her milk and hence drugs are to be avoided during lactation.

Medications to the Lactating Mother

All drugs taken by the mother will be excreted in breast milk in low concentrations up to less than 1 per cent. Some drugs are not compatible as given in Table 9.3.

Table 9.3 Effect of medicines taken during lactation on infant

Medicine	*Effect*
• Anti cancer drug	• Immuno suppression in infant
• Anti thyroid drugs and radioactive iodine	• Damage to thyroid gland of the infant
• Ergot therapy	• Ergotism in the baby that manifests as vomiting, diarrhoea, collapse and convultion.
• Oral pill, thiazides, pyridoxine, nicotine	• Suppression of lactation
• Laxatives	• Diarrhoea in the infant
• Antibiotics	• GI disorders like diarrhoea.

Expressed Milk

Breast milk need to be expressed when the infant is not able suck or mother starts working outside the house. Mother should wash her hands before handling the milk, pump or bottles. Milk should be frozen in plastic storage bags, specially designed for it. Freezing milk in 60–120 ml quantities reduce waste and allows for thawing more quickly than larger volumes.

Lactation Failure

It is the inability to produce enough milk to sustain growth of normal newborn for the first 4 months of life. True biological insufficiency of milk is extremely rare. Lactation failure can be due to failure to synthesise milk or movement of milk or failure of both.

Factors Responsible for Lactation Failure

- Maternal malnutrition.
- Acute maternal illness—fever or dehydration.
- Stress, anxiety, negative influence of environment.
- Engorged breast.
- Sore nipples.
- Lack of confidence.
- Occupation and socioeconomic condition.
- Incomplete emptying—weak suckling by the baby, low birth weight babies, pre-term, sick depressed babies and babies with congenital malformation.
- Infrequent feeding, unscheduled feeding.
- Short duration of feeds.
- Prelacteal feeds, hospital practice of separating baby and mother.

Human Milk Bank

In the last few years, awareness of benefits of breast milk has increased. And correspondingly demand for donor breast milk has also been increased.

Human milk banks are established in many Indian hospitals.

Milk from human milk bank is primarily used by preterm or premature babies who are not able to suck the breasts. These infants are fed human milk from their mothers or from other mothers' milk through tube feeding.

Some mothers who may not be able to secrete milk temporarily can take advantage of human milk bank.

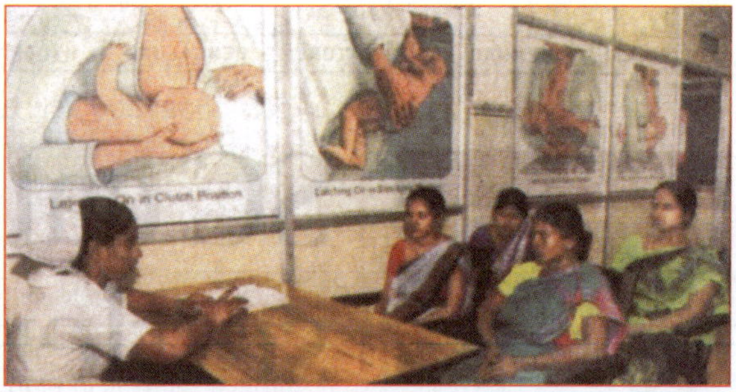

Fig. 9.4 Counselling has proved a key factor in the rise of number of donors of human milk.
Source: Institute of Child Health, Chennai.

Mothers who donate milk are those whose infants are dead or are undergoing treatment and cannot be breast fed. Some mothers may produce excess milk, beyond the requirement of their infants donate milk to the bank.

Donor breast milk has several advantages over formula or supplement. A major benefit is that it brought down the risk of necrotizing enterocolitis, a potentially life-threatening condition in which the baby’s intestine is damaged. Donor breast milk also helps avoid intolerance to formula.

Awareness is key factor both for donors and recipients.

Exercise

The breast feeding mother can do exercise a few weeks after postpartum, when lactation is well established. She can do aerobic exercise at 60–70 per cent of maximal heart rate without any adverse effect on lactation. Exercise improves mother's cardiovascular fitness. However, strenuous exercise is not recommended.

INDIAN NURSING MOTHERS

In poor Indian communities the nursing mother takes only rice supplemented with little pulse and vegetables. Milk is used in tea or coffee. In India it is the custom to breast feed infants for prolonged periods ranging from six months up to even three years, without giving sufficient weaning foods.

Studies conducted by NIN have indicated that women from low income groups do not have adequate weight gain during pregnancy with probably low fat mass accrual start lactation without adequate energy reserves. They breast feed their infants for a period of 18 – 24 months postpartum and have short pregnancy intervals. Energy stress during lactation leads to maternal tissues depletion.

It is fortunate that despite a faulty and insufficient maternal diet the quality of breast milk does not suffer. On the other hand, it compares well with that of nursing mother consuming excellent diets in other parts of the world. Perhaps the Indian nursing mother keeps up the quality by withdrawing nutrients from her own bone, blood and muscle for the formation of milk, since her inadequate diet is incapable of providing the nutrients required for satisfactory milk production. Continuous withdrawal of nutrients from the maternal body may lead to osteomalacia. In order that a mother may breast feed her infant without any undue strain on her own body, she must continue to eat an adequate and balanced diet to meet the requirements of lactation.

Under ICDS programme lactating mothers are given 160 g per day of sathumavu (health mix) in packets of 15 days quota. A lactating mother gets about 600 kcal and 18–20 g of protein by supplementary food.

Suggested recipes for a lactating mother

Recipe	*Reasons*
Badam kheer, groundnut kheer, carrot halwa, caramel custard	Nuts and milk may increase milk production. Concentrated foods help in meeting the increased requirement.
Garlic and onion chutney	May help in increasing the production of milk.
Soups and rasam	Appetisers help in digestion
Fried snacks like vada, bajji etc., parathas, paneer parathas	Help in meeting increased calorie and protein requirements
Goond laddu Gardencress seeds laddu	Rich in lactogogues and nutrient dense foods.

SUGGESTED READINGS

- Calcium rich food supplementation to lactating women from low socio-economic group. Effect on bone density, Annual report 2010–2011, NIN, Hyderabad.
- Kulkarni Bharti *et al*., Regional body composition changes during lactation in Indian women Nutrition News, 2011, NIN, Hyderabad.

QUESTIONS

1. Give ICMR RDA for a lactating mother who delivered the child eight months ago.
2. Explain the reasons for increased nutrient requirement in lactation.
3. Find out the dietary pattern of lactating mothers in your locality and reason out scientifically.
4. Write a note on lactogogues.
5. Explain the role of hormones in milk production.
6. What is expressed milk?
7. Explain the factors affecting the quantity and quality of milk.
8. Inspite of breast feeding, the infant does not thrive. Explain.

TOPICS FOR ACTIVITY

- Plan and prepare a diet for a nursing mother who is a school teacher.
- Survey and find out the locally available lactogogues.
- Make a survey and find out the dietary superstitious beliefs during lactation period.

10

Nutritional Recommendations and Food Requirements of Elderly

Successful ageing is defined not by longevity alone but also by sufficient well being in multiple domains—socially, physically and mentally. The three components for successful ageing are avoiding disease, engagement with life and maintaining high physical and cognitive function.

Old age is best defined as the age of retirement that is, 60 years and above. Improvement in health care technology has resulted in increased life expectancy. The number of persons in old age has increased. Average Indian woman's menopause age is 46.3 years. Life expectancy in 2018 is 70 years.

Poor health is not an unavoidable consequence of ageing. Studies show that healthful eating, physical activity, mental stimulation, active social engagement, moderate use of alcohol maintaining safe environment, social support, regular health care, not using tobacco are important in maintaining good health and independence.

PROCESS OF AGEING

Ageing is not a disease but a biological process. It is a normal process begins at conception and ends only with death. Individuals are known to age at different rates. The changes associated with ageing are partly influenced by genetics, race and gender. Heredity and good nutrition may slow the ageing process so that the individual enjoys physical and mental vigour in his eighties. Goal of nutritional care should be to help the aged achieve a healthy, purposeful and independent living.

One prominent theory of ageing—the free radical theory—involves the continuous formation of free radicals as a result of exposure to oxygen and harmful exposure to environmental factors. These highly reactive substances lead to damage and alterations in the structure of proteins, lipids, carbohydrates and chromosomal material in cells which probably leads to changes associated with ageing.

Tissue damage by free radicals and pro-oxidant radicals like superoxide, peroxide and hydroxyl radicals is the basis for inflammatory and degenerative changes. Endogenous antioxidants are superoxide dismutase (SOD), catalase (CAT), glutathione peroxidase (GPX) which act together with glutathione (GSH) and NADPH. With age and in diseases these antioxidant defenses are lowered and the vitamins A, C and E get excessively utilised and a deficiency state occurs.

The process of ageing brings about physiological, psychological and immunological changes which influences the nutritional status. In the ageing process free radicals are thought to cause degenerative changes, perhaps leading to cancer, cataract formation, atherosclerotic plagues, arthritis and Parkinson's disease.

Inability to prepare food, decreased purchasing capacity and psychosocial problems adversely affect the health and nutritional status of the elderly. Decreased physical activity and dental problems could lead to overall decrease in food intake and poor absorption of nutrients. As part of ageing process the functioning of the organ may change which may influence nutrient status as given in Table 10.1.

Table 10.1 Changes in organ function with ageing that may influence nutrient requirements

Organ function	*Changes*	*Effect on nutrition*
Taste and smell	• Decreased taste buds and papillae on tongue. • Decrease in taste and olfactory nerve endings.	• Loss of ability to detect salt and sweet. • Decreased palatability causing poor food intake. • Decreased sensory stimulation that may impair metabolic processes.
Salivary glands	• Decrease in salivary secretion causes feeling of dry mouth, xerostomia.	• Difficulty in chewing and swallowing make them avoid certain foods particularly crunchy, dry and sticky foods.
Teeth	• Loss of teeth and wearing dentures.	• Decreased consumption of meats and fresh fruits and vegetables particularly which are hard (carrot) and have lot of seeds (guava). In turn this can result in inadequate intake of energy, iron and vitamins particularly vitamin C, folate and β carotene.
Gastric function and emptying	• Decreased secretion of hydrochloric acid, intrinsic factor and pepsin. • Above 60 years of age rapid rate of emptying of liquids.	• Decreased bioavailability of minerals, vitamins and proteins. • Decreased absorption of protein bound vitamin B_{12} and folate.
Small intestine	• Increased proximal small bowel pH and bacterial overgrowth in bowel • Decreased calcium absorption • Decreased secretion of lactase • Constipation—prolonged rectosigmoid transit	• Increase in bacterial folate synthesis to counteract malabsorption. • Poor vitamin D nutriture • Can be a risk factor for developing osteoporosis
Liver and biliary function	• Decreased size and blood flow • Minor structural and biochemical changes • Gall bladder becomes sluggish in releasing bile • Activity of drug metabolising enzymes reduced.	• Rate of albumin synthesis may be decreased • Susceptible to gallstones • Drug dosages may need to be lowered.

Table 10.1 (*Contd.*)

Organ function	*Changes*	*Effect on nutrition*
Metabolic function	• Impaired glucose tolerance	• Requires dietary modifications, exercise and oral pharmacologic agents.
	• Decreased metabolic rate due to changes in body composition and reduction in physical activity.	• Requirement of energy decreases
	• Body protein level decreases	• Activity decreases
Neurologic function	• Confusional states	• Decreased synthesis of serotonin; Carnitine derived from the amino-acids lysine and methionine may be effective in slowing the mental deterioration in Alzheimer's disease. • Carotenoids seem to play a protective role related to ageing and cognitive function.
Immuno competence	• Declines with age	• Supplementation with vitamin E, zinc and polyunsaturated fatty acid can be increased.
Opthalmic function	• Opacity of eye lens	• Increased requirement of antioxidant.
Psychological factors	• Depression	• Can affect appetite, digestion, energy level, weight and well being.
Cardiovascular function	• Blood vessels become less elastic and total peripheral resistance increases.	• Prevalence of hypertension, modification of diet accordingly.
Renal function	• Glomerular filtration rate can diminish as much as 60 per cent; changes in fluid and acid base balance.	• Protein, sodium and potassium nutrition may be affected.

Fatigue, alteration in appetite, alteration in weight, shortness of breath and giddiness and joint pains are the common complaints during old age. Fatigue may be due to co-existing diseases like diabetes or ischemic heart diseases or due to pulmonary tuberculosis. Blunting of taste sensation may be due to degenerative changes in the parietal lobe of brain in old age. Loss of weight during old age may be due to consumption of less calories. Hypertension, diabetes and anaemia may be the cause of giddiness.

Nutritional Screening

It is difficult to get accurate weights and heights due to inability to stand erect, kyphosis, bedridden or wheel chair bound. Alternate methods of determining height should be considered. Total arm span, half arm span, Luft ruler or knee height can be measured.

Luft ruler, an instrument with a retractable rod that extends from a bar at the tip of the head to a bar at the base of the feet, measure the height of patient in the supine position. The Luft ruler has only minor mean variation from the gold standard of stadiometer measurement. Mini nutritional assessment is good.

The stress response can create additional loss of lean body mass. The stress response can occur due to catabolic illness such as wounds, trauma, surgery and infection. It is essentially a normal response to stress that increases energy needs, causes the body to break down protein and lean body mass and can lead to protein calorie malnutrition. Loss of just 10 percent of lean body mass decreases immune response and increases the risk of infection. A loss of 15 per cent or more reduces the rate of wound healing and increases weakness. A loss of 40 per cent results in death often due to pneumonia.

NUTRITIONAL RECOMMENDATIONS

These are based on the physiological changes that take place during old age.

The percentage of muscle tissue decreases and fat tissue increases as the age increases. Resting metabolic rate decreases approximately 15–20 per cent over the life span, primarily due to changes in body composition and reduction in physical activity.

Sarcopenia, an age related loss in skeletal muscle is the result of a decline in muscle strength. Sarcopenia contributes to changes in gait and balance and loss of physical function. Lean body mass declines approximately 2 to 3 per cent per decade. Body protein level in the healthy elderly is 30–40 per cent less than that in young adults. The average body fat percentage in males increases from about 15 per cent when young to 25 per cent.

The average body fat percentage in males increases from about 15 per cent when young to 25 per cent at the age of 60 years. This change in body fat is attributable to less intense physical activity and to an alteration in testosterone and growth hormone production that affects anabolism and lean tissue growth. Lean body mass is also affected by wounds trauma, surgery and infection. It is due to hormonal response to stress that increases energy needs, causes the body to break down protein and lean body mass. Figure 10.1 shows percentage changes in body composition with age.

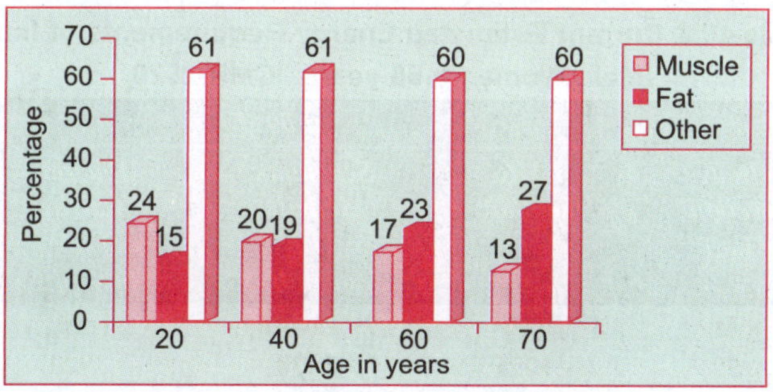

Fig. 10.1 Percentage changes in body composition with age. Change in body composition affects the nutritional needs.

Source: Guthrie A.H., 1989, Introductory Nutrition, Times Mirror/Mosby College Publishing, St. Louis.

Energy

After the age of 30 the basal metabolic rate decreases due to reduced muscle mass and other metabolically active tissue mass. Also there is reduction in physical activity which affects the energy needs.

There is reduction in resting energy expenditure (REE) and with declining PAL ultimately leads to decrease in BMR and energy requirements.

Energy requirement decreases with age beyond 30 years. The adjustment factor given earlier by FAO/WHO/UNU is adopted for Indians are used for computing the energy requirements of different age periods. ICMR has given energy requirements of the elderly above 60 years as shown in Table 10.2.

Table 10.2 Daily Nutrient Recommendations for the Elderly. ICMR-2020

Nutrients	*Men* ≥ *60 years*	*Women* ≥ *60 years*
Energy kcal	1700	1500
Protein g	54	46
Dietary fibre g	30	25
Calcium mg	1200	1200
Magnesium mg	440	370
Iron mg	19	19
Iodine µg	140	140
Zinc mg	17	13.2
Vitamin A µg	1000	840
Vitamin D IU	800	800
Thiamine mg	1.4	1.4
Riboflavin mg	2.0	1.9
Niacin mg	14	11
Pyridoxine mg	1.9	1.9
Dietary folate mg	300	200
Vitamin B_{12} µg	2.2	2.2
Vitamin C mg	80	65

Although the energy requirements decrease, the requirements for protein, vitamins and minerals do not diminish. Hence the elderly are encouraged to consume nutrient-dense foods such as nuts, oil seeds, fruits and vegetables to meet the requirement of all nutrients.

Table 10.3 Current Estimated Energy Requirements of Indian Men, Women > 60 years. ICMR-2020.

Gender	*> 60 y*				
	Body weight (kg)	*BMR (kcal/d)*[a]	*Sedentary Activity TEE (kcal/d)*[b]	*Moderate Activity TEE (kcal/d)*[b]	*Heavy Activity TEE (kcal/d)*[b]
Males	45	1003	1404	1805	2306
	50	1055	1478	1900	2427
	55	1108	1551	1995	2549
	60	1161	1625	2089	2670
	65	1213	1699	2184	2791
	70	1266	1772	2279	2912
	75	1319	1846	2374	3033
Females	40	930	1303	1675	2140
	45	972	1361	1749	2235
	50	1013	1419	1824	2331
	55	1055	1477	1898	2426
	60	1096	1535	1973	2521
	65	1138	1593	2048	2616
	70	1179	1650	2122	2711

[a]BMR calculated using FAO/WHO/UNV, 2004 equation and adjusted to 10% and 9% lower value for males and females, respectively

[b]PAL values. Sedentary-1.40; Moderate- 1.80; Heavy 2.30.

Carbohydrate

An impaired glucose tolerance in the elderly can lead to hypoglycaemia, hyperglycaemia and type 2 diabetes mellitus. Insulin sensitivity can be enhanced by balanced energy intake, weight management and regular physical activity. Emphasis is placed on increasing the consumption of complex carbohydrates and controlling the intake of simple sugars. Whole grain cereals and pulses should be included in the diet.

It is necessary that at least 55–60 per cent of calories are derived from carbohydrates.

Since caloric requirements are reduced, carbohydrates intake is also reduced.

Protein

As people age there is a decrease in muscle mass and skeletal tissue mass. This results in decrease in store of protein provided by skeletal muscle and may be inadequate to meet the needs for protein synthesis. Hence the dietary protein intake is more important to meet essential needs.

A protein intake of 1.0 g per kilogram, the normal adult requirement, is safe during old age. Since calorie requirements are decreased without the corresponding decrease in protein, the food should be protein rich compared to normal adult food. To meet this adequate quantities of protein foods such as milk, eggs and pulses can be included.

Due to decreased appetite and poor digestion, old people are likely to consume less protein. Intake and bioavailability of dietary protein appear to decrease with age. The serum albumin level is the most reliable indicator of protein nutriture. Deficiency of protein results in oedema, anaemia and lowered resistance to infection. Infection, altered gastrointestinal function and metabolic changes caused by chronic disease can reduce the efficiency of dietary nitrogen utilisation and increase nitrogen excretion.

Of the total caloric intake 11–12 per cent should be from protein.

Lipids

Dietary fat should meet 30–40 per cent of total energy intake and saturated fat should be maximum 10 per cent. Epidemiological studies show that dementia and cardiovascular disease may share risk factors including high intakes of dietary total fat, high saturated fat, high ω-6 : ω-3 fatty acid ratio and low fish intake.

Emphasis should be placed on reducing the intake of saturated fat and *trans* fat and choosing monounsaturated or polyunsaturated fat sources. Elders who take sufficient ω-3 fatty acids, have better visual acuity. ω-3 fatty acids may help in conditions such as hair loss, impairment of vision, improper digestion and gas, poor kidney function, tissue inflammation, osteoarthritis, painful joints and muscles and mental depression. ω-3 fatty acids may help to protect the heart and brain.

Minerals

Calcium needs during old age increases. Women over 50 years of age who are not receiving estrogens require more calcium as there is increased losses resulting in demineralisation of bone and osteoporosis. For women over fifty, 800 mg/day is recommended for the following reasons:

(*a*) Calcium is available only from a limited number of foods.

(*b*) To compensate age-related bone loss and to improve calcium balance.

(*c*) To decrease the prevalence of fractures and dental decay.

The physiology of calcium homeostasis in ageing men over 65 is similar to that of women with respect to the rate of bone loss. Calcium absorption efficiency decreases, vitamin D levels decline and hence men also require more calcium.

Milk is an important source of calcium for elderly as it is in the diet of the young. Wise provisions for calcium throughout life may go far in assuring an above average measure of health, an increase in vitality and perhaps in the lengthened prime of life. As caloric requirement decreases, total food consumption decreases, hence calcium supplements are essential.

The iron deficiency seen in the elderly is due to inadequate iron intake, blood loss due to chronic disease and/or reduced non-heame iron absorption secondary to achlorhydria of atrophic gastritis. Iron absorption per se does not appear to decline significantly with age. Vitamin C deficiency may also impair iron absorption.

Mild anaemia affects the health of old people due to less efficient circulation of blood. Iron intake should be adequate to prevent anaemia. Iron requirement can be same as adult man, 30 mg. If there is anaemia, supplemental iron can be given. Consumption of liver once or twice a week is effective in combating such a tendency. Particular emphasis may be placed upon the inclusion of those green leafy vegetables which are good source of iron like amaranth, gogu, curry leaves and mint and whole grain or enriched breads and to certain iron rich dry fruits, and use of iron fortified salt.

Experimental evidence suggests that magnesium deficiency may trigger an increased production of reactive oxygen species and promote a proinflammatory stage contributing to poor muscle strength. Magnesium supplementation may retard the age-related loss of muscle function and performance.

There is no evidence that moderate sodium restriction will delay or prevent the onset of cardiovascular disease. It is believed that great restriction of sodium should not be attempted except under the advice of a physician in the treatment of specific disease condition. Infact, moderate amounts of salt help to improve the palatability and thus the acceptability of the diet.

The status of zinc is especially important in the elderly because immune function decreases with age and even a mild zinc deficiency in humans can impair cell-mediated immunity, increasing susceptibility to infections in the elderly. Chronic malnutrition, history of ethanol abuse and adherence to a vegetarian diet can all result in low dietary intake of zinc. Immunological abnormalities are reversible with zinc supplementation. Zinc has been identified as a factor in the development of age-related macular degeneration, may be due to oxidative damage to the retinal epithelium.

Some features of old age such as delayed wound healing, decreased taste sensitivity and anorexia are also findings associated with zinc deficiency. However, healthy elderly subjects have been shown to be in zinc balance despite an apparent low dietary intake. Older people who avoid flesh foods may be at increased risk of poor zinc status.

Vitamins

Vitamin D: With ageing vitamin D status declines as a result of less efficient skin synthesis of vitamin D, impaired ability of the kidneys to convert the inactive form of vitamin D to the active form, reduced sun exposure and low dietary intake of vitamin D. Elderly lose ability to store vitamin D. Vitamin D insufficiency is now considered a wide spread global epidemic particularly the elderly based on serum levels defined as < 50 m mol/L.

Vitamin D insufficiency is associated with reduced calcium absorption, low blood levels of ionized calcium, increased circulating parathyroid levels and increased bone resorption.

Vitamin D is traditionally linked to healthy teeth and bones. Now it is linked to immune status and to muscle strength and prevention of falls as well as being a factor in insulin production, anti-inflammatory properties and maintenance of vascular integrity.

Adequate supplies of both vitamin D and calcium are needed to prevent nonvertebral fractures, especially hip fractures in the elderly.

Prudent dietary supplementation with calcium and vitamin D improves bone density and may prevent fractures in a healthy elderly population. Recent studies have indicated that people with Parkinson's disease are likely to have low vitamin D levels.

Vitamin D insufficiency is now considered a widespread global epidemic particularly in the elderly, based on serum levels defined as < 50 mmol/L. The capacity to synthesis vitamin D in the skin when exposed to UV radiation is reduced in older adults. In addition, older adults are more likely to stay indoors.

Hypovitaminosis D increases the risk for a number of medical conditions, including osteoporosis, heart disease, hypertension, immunologic conditions, persistent musculoskeletal pain and alterations in glucose and lipid metabolism. Studies have shown that supplementation reduces mortality.

Vitamin D deficiency can be managed through pharmacologic vitamin D_3 doses 50,000 IU once a week for 8 weeks followed by supplementation with D_2 twice a month.

Vitamin E: Vitamin E has also been found to be a potent nutrient for reducing the decline in cellular immunity that occur in the elderly. Changes in immune system can be overcome by taking 200 mg of vitamin E. Protection from DNA damage enhances the body's self defence mechanisms.

Vitamin K: A recent study found that patients with early stage Alzheimer's disease consumed less vitamin K. Consumption of green leafy vegetables may supply enough vitamin K during old age.

B Vitamins: Requirements for the vitamin B_6 are increased in many elderly persons owing to atrophic gastritis which interferes with absorption. Alcoholic and liver dysfunction are additional risk factors for a deficiency of vitamin B_6. It has a significant role in immune function. Alcoholism is a risk factor for folate deficiency. Severe deficiency of folic acid in the elderly may result in anaemias and elevated serum homocysteine levels a risk factor for cardiac disease. Diets are often lacking in folate, so consumption of folate rich foods should be encouraged.

The usual causes of vitamin B_{12} deficiency are atrophic gastritis and bacterial overgrowth, which decrease absorption and can lead to pernicious anaemia. The ageing process reduces the body's ability to cleave the vitamin from its protein carrier, thereby resulting in less bioavailability of the vitamin. Synthetic vitamin B_{12} added to fortified foods and dietary supplements are easily absorbed and may be the best source of B_{12} during old age. B_{12} status should be evaluated in people using medications such as histamine blocker proton-pump inhibitors and antibiotics.

Recent research has shown that increased serum levels of vitamins $B_{6,}$ B_{12} and folate confer protection against elevated serum homocysteine, an independent risk factor for cardiovascular disease, depression and certain neurologic deficits.

Vitamin C: Stress, smoking and some medications can increase vitamin C requirement. The antioxidant vitamins, such as vitamin E, carotenoids and vitamin C have been promoted as agents that enhance the health of the elderly. Vitamin C may be protective against cataract at an intake level of between 150 and 250 mg per day which is possible to achieve from dietary sources alone.

Supplementation with vitamins, carotenoids and polyunsaturated fatty acids provide protection against ultraviolet light. An increase in delayed type hypersensitivity skin responses after supplementation with nutrients has proven beneficial in elderly people. Supplementation of micronutrients may boost cell-mediated immunity.

All vitamin requirements remain the same as the adult requirement.

Water

It is essential for the older person as it is for the younger individual. The kidney can function more adequately when there is sufficient fluid (1.5 litres) to eliminate the waste solids. Water stimulates peristalsis and thus aids in combating constipation. Water can be consumed as such or in the form of butter milk, fruit juices, porridge and soups.

Some elderly individuals may have a fading sense of thirst and may go for long periods without fluid. Others avoid liquid for fear of incontinence. Dehydration can result in mental confusion, headache and instability. Elderly should be advised to consume some fluid at regular intervals even if they are not thirsty.

To maintain normal saliva flow rate, bowel movements, gastric functioning and emptying, metabolic renal, cardiovascular functions and cognition, greater volume of fluid are recommended.

Table 10.4 Water requirement for elderly persons - ICMR-2020

Group	*Body weight kg*	*Energy Requirement kcal*	*Total Water Requirement* ml*	*Water from Food* ml*	*Water from Beverages ml*
Man					
Sedentary	65	1883	2800	850	1950
Moderate	65	2216	3300	1000	2300
Woman					
Sedentary	55	1706	2550	750	1800
Moderate	55	2007	3000	900	2100

* Values are rounded off to the nearest 50.

Fibre

ICMR-2020 suggested requirement of fibre for elderly 30 g/d and 18 g/1000 kcal.

Fibre stimulates peristalsis. There is great enthusiasm to encourage the consumption of fibre containing food but any increase should be gradual otherwise bowel discomfort, distension and flatulence will result. While rough fibre, bran and mature vegetables are not advised for the aged, the fibre of tender vegetables, fruits will make easier the passage of the food pass down the intestinal tract.

Fibre also helps in reducing cholesterol which may reduce the incidence c ··aerosclerosis. Excess of fibre may reduce the absorption of iron and certain trace element

Antioxidants

Research has shown that the decreasing ability to remove free radicals within the body contributes to the ageing process and certain diseases. Several non-nutrient phytochemicals play a key role in reducing oxidative stress. Carotenoids including lycopene, lutein and zeaxanthin that do not have vitamin A activity but have health promoting properties should be included in the diet. Fruits and vegetables which are yellow orange in colour should be taken during old age.

Berries and legumes are especially rich in antioxidants that help bone cells and defend against damage caused by free radicals.

Red wine consumed in moderation may be beneficial in reducing LDL, preventing blood clots and protecting the heart. The flavonoids, procyanidins, present in wine are cardioprotective.

Vitamins like vitamin C, E, B_{12} and folic acid supplementation have a significant role in lowering the risk of dementia. A well preserved memory is the cornerstone of a good life. Catract progression can be reduced by antioxidant rich diet. Good nutrition and a healthy life style would help to achieve this.

Antioxidants-Vitamin E, C and β-carotene along with vitamins B_6 and B_{12} folate and iron have a role in cognitive function, memory performance, immune response, reducing the cancer risk, cardiovascular health, vision and general health.

Saturated fats and high serum cholesterol is associated with increased risk of Alzheimer's disease. Consumption of long chain polyunsaturated ω-3 fatty acids (particularly DHA) and antioxidants such as vitamin E appear to lower risk.

Consumption of foods rich in antioxidants should be preferred to supplemental antioxidants. Diseases like diabetes, atherosclerosis, hypertension, cataract formation, Parkinson's disease and cancer and disability disorders like bone fractures, arthritis and strokes may affect nutrient requirements, intake, digestion, absorption, metabolism and excretion.

FOOD REQUIREMENTS

In nearly 60–65 years of one's life habits, especially those pertaining to diet usually get moulded by factors like heredity, health, family, education, occupation and numerous other socioeconomic and cultural factors. They are set in their ways and they cannot totally modify their whole pattern of eating.

The elderly prefer well cooked food in soft form or semisolid form. This may be due to the fact that elderly suffer from loss of teeth or wear dentures. Due to dental problems if the elderly are not able to eat common raw vegetables they can be used as grated vegetables or chutneys made with green leafy vegetables. Porridge can be prepared with unrefined cereals. If there is difficulty in chewing, whole wheat rava upma can be given instead of chapathis.

Cereal fibre consumption late in life is associated with lower risk of CVD. Hence elderly individual should increase consumption of dietary cereal fibre.

If mastication and deglutition are problems, modification of food and beverage consistency may be indicated. The danger in dysphagia is that the person may choke on foods or beverages that are swallowed too rapidly. Aspiration pneumonia is the greatest risk in such cases.

For many elderly persons, swallowing difficulty occurs as a result of poor dentition, stroke, Alzheimer's disease or other dementias. Thin liquids (other than pure water taken alone in small sips) may need to be avoided. Thickening agents in food can be used.

Alteration in appetite may be due to ageing process affecting the centre in the brain for appetite. Physical, social and emotional problems may interfere with appetite.

There is a considerable difference in taste preference among the elderly which may be attributed to decline in taste perception as age advances. Elders usually do not prefer sweets, salty foods or fried foods.

Plant-based estrogens or phytoestrogens are used as adjunctive therapy for alleviating the symptoms of menopause. Phytoestrogens are nonsteroidal estrogens of dietary origin. Phytoestrogens in soya (isoflavones) may reduce the incidence of hot flushes, one of the symptoms of menopause.

Table 10.5 Modification of diet during old age

Dietary modification	*Reason*
Foods must be soft, easily chewable.	Problems of dentition, fallen teeth or dentures.
Foods should be easily digestible.	Decreased production of digestive enzymes.
Restricted fat in the diet, inclusion of PUFA.	Susceptible to heart disease.
Foods rich in fibre should be given.	To prevent constipation and reduce cholesterol level. Also to prevent colon cancer.
Coffee, tea and cola beverages should be restricted.	May result in insomnia due to over stimulation.
Foods rich in calcium like milk and curd should be given.	To compensate the bone loss and reduce the incidence of osteoporosis. Curd can aid in balance of intestinal flora.
Cereal fibre	Reduces the risk of CVD.
Green leafy vegetables can be given liberally.	Source of nutrients like carotene, calcium, iron, riboflavin, folic acid and vitamin C, besides supplying fibre. Rich in antioxidants.
Foods of the elderly should consist of familiar foods. New foods are difficult to accept.	Unfamiliar or changes in the food pattern may lead to psychological problems like depression.
Clear soup at the beginning of meal.	Aids digestion.
Small and frequent meals instead of three heavy ones.	Favour more complete digestion and free from distress.
A glass of warm milk just before going to bed.	Calcium along with magnesium deactivates adrenaline and promotes sleep. The warmth of milk acts as a relaxant.
Heavy meal at noon and light in the night meal.	Sleep is less likely to be disturbed.
Too many sweets with lot of fats and sugar should be avoided.	Too much of sugar may cause fermentation, discomfort due to indigestion and cause tooth ache and may increase cholesterol level. May lead to obesity and fractures
Plenty of fluid.	To prevent constipation and dehydration.
Consumption of flax seed (40 g/d).	Decreases hot flushes in post menopausal women.
Inclusion of greens and beet root	Prevents age related macular degeneration.

Certain whole pulses may produce flatulence in the elderly. Hence such pulses should be avoided in the diet. Sulphur containing vegetables are avoided if they produce gas and discomfort in the elderly.

The general principles for planning a nutritious diet for the elderly are similar to those for younger adults. The most important guideline is to provide meals and snacks that are nutrient dense, visually appealing, tasteful and of the appropriate consistency. Four or five smaller meals are often more acceptable than three substantial ones.

A summary of the dietary modifications required during old age and the reasons of it are given in Table 10.5.

Dietary Guidelines

- Empty calorie foods should be taken in minimum quantity.
- Foods rich in protein, vitamin and mineral should be included.
- Vegetables and fruits are good sources of antioxidants. A minimum of five servings should be taken.
- Fat promotes weight gain. Fat particularly saturated fat should be limited. Saturated fats is associated with an increased risk of Alzheimer's in addition to CVD.
- Gas forming foods like sulphur containing vegetables and certain type of pulses have to be avoided.
- Soft well cooked foods are preferred.
- Food should be less salty and spicy.
- Fried and concentrated foods should be avoided.
- Caffeine containing beverages should be limited, otherwise they may suffer from insomnia.
- High fibre diet including greens and whole grains are to be included in the diet.
- Easily digestible steamed foods like idlis or idiappam can be part of the diet.
- Plenty of fluids and semisolid foods should be taken.
- Two to three servings of low fat milk should be included in the diet.
- Consumption of ω-3 fatty acids may help in reducing hair loss, impairment of vision, improper digestion and tissue inflammation.
- The elderly persons if needed supplements of vitamin. B_{12} and vitamin D can be taken.
- Tobacco chewing, smoking and betel leaves chewing are the habits which may affect consumption of food in the elderly, hence should be avoided.

Long life of Japanese

According to WHO Japan's average life expectancy at birth is 83.7 years. Global average is 71.4. Longevity of Japanese-diet policy, exercise, cultural factors and genetics making it difficult to single out one cause. Rice, vegetables, fish and meat are staples of the Japanese diet. Fish cosumption is higher than other nations. Pickled, fermented and smoked foods are also common. Fermented foods support healthy digestive system. Soya beans is key part of meal. Low in calories and saturated fat are significant factors in reducing the cardiovascular disease.

NUTRITION RELATED PROBLEMS OF OLD AGE

The elderly are at a risk of poor nutrition due to economic pressures, poor dentition, reduced mobility, depression, loneliness, ageing tissues and inadequate food consumption.

Table 10.6 List of factors that increase nutrition risk in older adults

Presence of chronic disease	Renal dysfunction
Polypharmacy	Reduced vision
Poor oral health	Malabsorption
Dysgeusia	Diminished olfactory senses
Dysphagia	Financial constraints
Ill fitting dentures	Depression
Gingivitis	Lack of transportation
Xerostomia (dry mouth)	Functional limitations
Anorexia of ageing	Recent bereavement
Prescribed therapeutic diets	Feeding dependency
Gastric dysmotility	Lack of socialization
Achlorhydria	Isolation/living alone

Source: Marian Mary and Gordon Sacks, Micronutrients and older adults - Nutrition in clinical practice 2009, **24.**

Sarcopenia

It is an age related multifactorial syndrome resulting in loss of skeletal mass and strength. Adverve outcomes of sarcopenia include functional decline, physical disability, fraility, falls, fractures, poor quality of life and death. Sarcopenia may be caused in part by nutritional inadequacies such as inadequate protein intake.

Osteoporosis

WHO identified osteoporosis as second only to cardiovascular disease as a leading health care problem.

Osteoporosis is a condition where there is loss of bone mineral density due to increase in osteoclast bone resorption activity and a concomitant decrease in osteoblast mediated bone formation. There is a generalized bone disease characterized by low bone density and micro architectural deterioration of bone tissue. It is primarily found in middle age and elderly women who had early menopause and had sedentary life. The early manifestations are an increased incidence of bone pains and of back pain in women. Its major symptom is an increased vulnerability to bone fractures. Post-menopausal women who consume around 800 mg of calcium with life time milk consumption can postpone the incidence of osteoporosis.

The age at which peak bone mass of population is 25–30 (NIN, 2006–2007). In young people in good health, the rate of calcium resorption equals that of bone formation. As people age, resorption begins to predominate over the bone formation, eventually resulting in osteoporosis.

In osteoporosis the total amount of bone is reduced, but the remaining bone is of normal composition and quality.

Signs and Symptoms

Due to the reduction in number of cells, there is a decrease in thickness of the cortex, a thinning of the trabeculae and increased porosity of bone. As a result fractures occur with greater frequency. Common fracture sites include the vertebrae, femur and radius and often these occur in spite of little or no trauma. The rate of femoral fractures alone doubles for each decade after the age of 50.

The cause of osteoporosis may be age related changes such as decreased estrogen production associated with menopause. The decline in circulating 17-β–estradiol is the predominant factor in the accelerated bone loss that begins after the menopause and continues for 6 to 8 years. Decreased intestinal absorption of calcium and production of vitamin D, reduced physical activity and increased parathyroid hormone secretion may also cause osteoporosis. Inadequate protein intake may contribute to osteoporosis in the elderly. Men also suffer from osteoporosis.

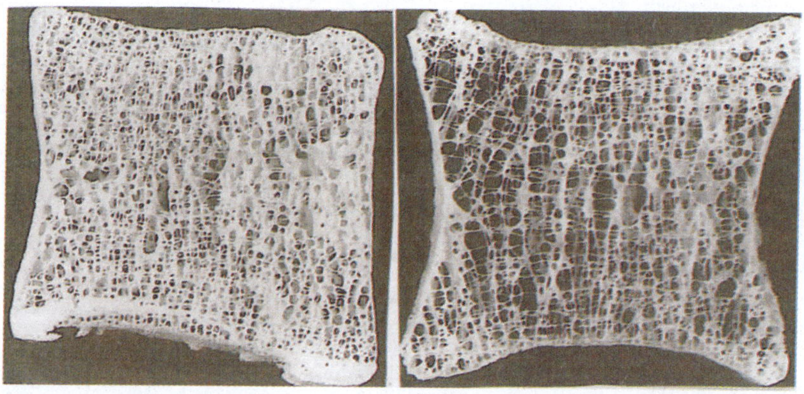

Section of a vertebral body from a normal individual showing the pattern of trabeculae

Section of a vertebral body from a patient with osteoporosis showing the thinning and loss of trabeculae compromising the mechanical strength of the bone

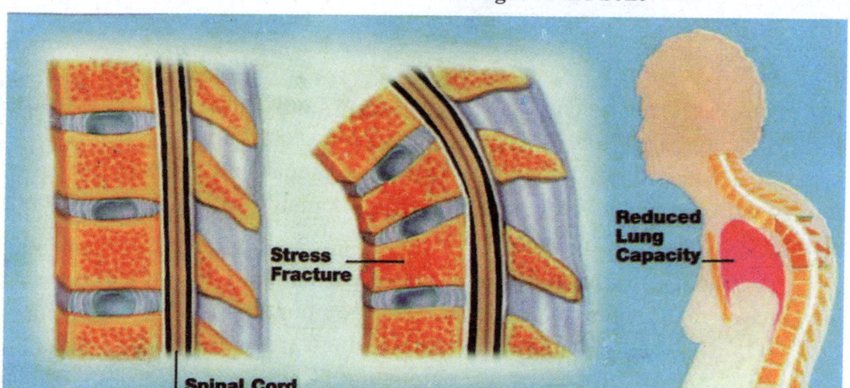

Fig. 10.2 Changes in osteoporosis. Stress fracture and reduced lung capacity and decreased height are characteristics of osteoporosis. About 6" height is decreased after 30 years of menopause

CHAPTER 10

Figure 10.2 shows height loss in post-menopausal woman with osteoporosis. The compact bone mass in the vertebrae is responsible for humped backs characteristic of many elderly people. Dissolution of the jaw bone is another frequent symptom of osteoporosis. It is a major contributing factor in periodontal disease, resulting in premature loss of teeth.

Risk factors and protective factors

Risk factors and protective factors of osteoporosis are given in Table 10.7.

Table 10.7 Risk and protective factors that correlate with osteoporosis

Risk factors	*Protective factors*
High correlation	
• Advanced age • Alcoholism • Chronic steroid use • Female gender • Rheumatoid arthritis • Surgical removal of ovaries or testes • Thin body structure • White race and Asian women	• Black race • Oestrogen long term use.
Moderate correlation	
• Vitamin D deficiency • Chronic thyroid hormone use • Diabetes Type I • Early menopause • Excessive antacid use • Family history of osteoporosis • Low calcium diet • Sedentary life style	• Having given birth • High body weight • High calcium diet • Regular physical activity
Probably important but not yet proved	
• Coffee intake • High fibre diet • Lactose intolerance	• Adequate vitamin K intake • Low sodium diet (later year)

Diagnosis

Dual energy X-ray Absorptiometer, DEXA, is used to know bone mineral density. BMD is correlated with fractures therefore it is used as marker for osteoporosis.

The *T*-score is a standard deviation any site measurement that compares the patient's bone mineral density with the mean value in a reference population of young healthy adults. It is calculated using the following formula

$$T\text{-score} = \frac{\left(\begin{array}{l}\text{Bone mineral density of participant} - \text{mean bone}\\ \text{mineral density of reference population}\end{array}\right)}{\begin{array}{l}\text{Standard deviation of bone mineral density}\\ \text{of reference population}\end{array}}$$

T-Score up to

– 1 = Normal ;

– 1.1 to – 2.5 = Osteopenia

– 2.5 = Osteoporosis

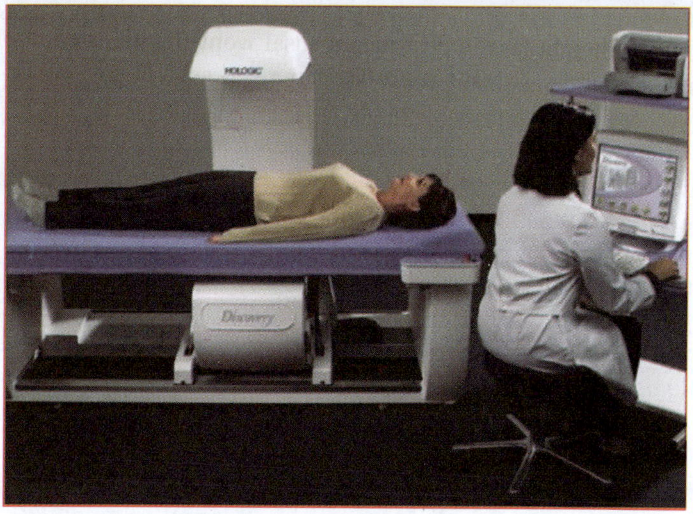

Fig. 10.3 Bone mineral density being estimated using DEXA. BMD test is preferred at the lumbar spine and hip.

Although ageing is one universal and unavoidable factor that brings a risk of osteoporosis many avoidable risk factors like sedentary life-style, emotional stress, inappropriate diet may contribute for osteoporosis. Low calcium intake and family history of osteoporosis are significant risk factors for low bone mass.

Osteoporosis Self-assessment Tool for Asians-OSTA

A simple index based on age and weight. OSTA = 0.2 [weight (kg) – age (years)]

A score ≤ –1 denotes higher risk and > –1 denotes lower rsik. It is the easiest method to calculate.

Osteoporosis Self Assessment Tool for Women

OST = [weight (kg) – age (years)] divided by 5

- – 20 to – 4 high risk
- – 4 to – 1 moderate risk
- – 1 to 20 low risk

Treatment

Treatment is of two types; one is by reducing fracture risk and the other one is by increasing bone mineral density. Antiresorptive agents slow the rate of bone turnover with a net sparing effect. Examples are calcium, vitamin D, calcitonin, bisphosphonates, selective oestrogen receptor modulators and oestrogen.

Anabolic agents stimulate the formation of bone. Parathyroid hormone and sodium fluoride are anabolic agents that increase bone density. But only parathyroid hormone decrease fracture risk. Strontium ranelate non radio active form of strontium appears to inhibit bone resorption and stimulate bone formation.

Teriparatide, a synthetic form of parathyroid hormone is the newest therapy which actually stimulates new bone formation.

Vitamin D supplementation in older individuals in stable health is associated with a 20 per cent reduction in the risk of falls. Patients who are diagnosed with osteoporosis and who comply with treatment are less likely to have fractures. Alendronate and risedronate are first line agents for the prevention and treatment of osteoporosis. Combination therapy with hormone replacement and alendronates is efficious and well tolerated to improve skeletal integrity. Bisphosphonates slow bone resorption without lowering bone formation, increasing bone density. To be effective vitamin D levels should be adequate.

It is sensible to encourage all old people and especially those with radiological evidence of osteoporosis, to be as physically active as possible. The more they are on their feet, less is the risk of pathological fractures of femur and spine.

Prevention

Prevention of osteoporosis can be achieved by adopting a life style that involves regular exercise and avoiding the avoidable risk factors.

Oestrogen therapy in post-menopausal women has been shown to slow the rate of bone loss although it does not stimulate new bone formation. It is much more effective as a preventive measure begun immediately after menopause than as a treatment of osteoporosis that has already developed. In the longer term, oestrogen treatment, results in increased parathyroid hormone and 1,25 $(OH)_2$ D synthesis, which may explain the observed improvement in the intestinal absorption and renal reabsorption of calcium.

Weight bearing exercise may help increase Bone Mineral Density by imposing stresses through repetitive impact loading. Resistance training (weight lifting, squeezing a tennis ball, streching exercises, sit ups, trunk extensions, aerobic exercise) may help by exposing bone to varying loads and rates of strain. Improved muscle strength may enhance coordination and balance and protect against falls and fractures. Although an exercise regimen that includes both weight-bearing and resistance-training routines has a greater impact on BMD, even a simple weight-bearing programme performed at moderate intensity may be beneficial.

The most effective preventive measures are, ensuring additional calcium intake of about 200 mg/d with a total intake of 1200 mg/d. This is to cover at least 30 mg/d extra obligatory loss of calcium in the urine.

It is logical for old people to take a diet with ample calcium that is to drink 2–3 glasses of milk regularly. Some old people have a markedly reduced capacity to absorb calcium from the gut and in such patients therapeutic doses of calcium salt might be of benefit. Adequate protein along with calcium also helps in the formation of bone tissue. Soya isoflavones may protect women against osteoporosis by the action of genistein, which has an effect similar to estrogen. It stimulates osteoblasts, the bone-forming cells.

Osteogenic or bone protective substances are soya proteins, (genestein, daidzein) calcium, casein, phosphopeptides, fructooligosaccharids and inulin. Studies generally found a higher score which reflects a closer resemblence to the Mediterranean diet was associated with a lower risk of hip fractures.

Exercise combined with adequate calcium and vitamin D intake may have a modest effect on slowing the decrease in bone mineral density in post menopausal women. Milk and sardines are good sources of vitamin D.

With the reduction in energy requirement and the low intake of food along with the impaired absorption and utilisation, deficiency of certain vitamins more likely to occur in elderly.

A variety of factors can have an adverse impact of nutrition status in the elderly, including immobility, confusion, forgetfulness, incontinence, isolation, loss of dexterity and coordination, and fatigue. Polypharmacy, the unnecessary and/or excessive use of prescribed and over-the-counter medications, increases the risk of adverse drug reactions and drug-nutrient interactions, The use of multiple medications is common among older adults.

Poor nutritional status increases health services use and cost of care in the elderly. Nutrition screening and intervention, often an afterthought in the management of chronic disease, are cost-effective yet underused tools in the care of this increasingly vulnerable segment of society. As age advances and chronic diseases and conditions accrue, optimizing nutritional status in the elderly becomes imperative and has the potential to significantly improve health and quality of life and cost-effective.

Secondary Osteoporosis

Secondary osteoporosis is defined as bone loss that results from specific well defined clinical disorders. Many a time it is reversible. Adverse use of drug therapy, endocrine disorders, eating disorders, immobilisation, bone marrow related disorders, disorders of the gastrointestinal or biliary tract, renal disease and cancer.

Glucocorticoids suppress osteoblast function, inhibit intestinal calcium absorption leading to secondary hyperparathyroidism and increased osteoclast-mediated bone resorption. All these cause bone loss. Bone loss is also promoted by direct stimulation of renal excretion of calcium by glucocorticoids. Bone density is reduced and rib and vertebral fractures are the most common. Anyone taking glucocorticoids for more than two months should be considered at risk.

Indian Scenario: The life expectancy of both men and women is increasing in India. However, this increased longevity is associated with increased burden of age-related morbidities including osteoporosis.

Studies conducted by NIN (2007), on low socio-economic group shows that osteoporotic hip fractures occur at least 10–15 years earlier in Indians (57–62 years) compared that to reported from the Western region (75 years). However, populations from the high income group in India do not show this early age of fractures. A few studies from India suggest that osteopenia and osteoporosis may occur at a relatively younger age in the Indian population. However, prevalence of fractures of the spine and forearm goes undetected in India because they are usually treated as out-patient cases. Studies reporting the bone density values of the Indian population involving large sample size are however not available. This is important because Indians from low income group subsist on diets that have inadequate calcium coupled with low calories, proteins and micronutrients. In addition, they have low body weights and women attain menopause at an earlier age than their Western counterparts. It is possible that these women are at a risk of osteoporosis and fractures at an early age.

In the near future, developing countries like India may expect the occurrence of hip fractures in epidemic proportions. Osteoporotic fractures, especially hip fractures are associated with considerable morbidity and mortality and increasing high economic and social costs.

Obesity

Ageing is a faltering process. It is more pronounced and sustained for women than men. Height decreases and weight increases. Some of the elderly are obese because their consumption of calories has not decreased though there is steady decrease in calorie requirement. Decreasing basal metabolic rate and sedentary life style may be contributing factors. Obese are susceptible to degenerative diseases and mortality rate may be higher. Maintaining weight promotes healthier ageing and prolongs life span.

By maintaining weight one can reduce stress on the joints and reduce pain and be able to control osteoarthritis.

Anaemia

Anaemia in old age is an independent risk factor for decline in physical performance. Anaemia, characterised by feelings of fatigue, anxiety, lack of energy and sleeplessness is a common result of inadequate iron. Anaemia also decreases myocardial function and can lead to heart failure. Iron inadequacy can be caused by low dietary intake, impaired absorption possibly resulting from lack of haem iron or vitamin C or blood loss. A majority of the anaemia in old age is due to underlying diseases such as cancer and infectious diseases or due to malnutrition. Treatment may involve using iron supplements together with a diet providing iron sources of high bio availability and vitamin C to enhance absorption.

Pernicious anaemia is seen chiefly in middle ages and elderly persons (women aged between 45–65) Plasma vitamin B_{12} is below 160 ng/l while plasma folate is usually normal. Hydroxy cobalamin should be given in a dosage of 1,000 mcg. The diet should include animal foods like liver, egg yolk, shrimps and curd.

Malnutrition

The important causes of malnutrition during old age are, poverty, inability to move around easily, cumulative effects of chronic diseases necessitating multiple medications, social isolation and lack of knowledge for adequate preparation of meals. The studies conducted by NIN showed that the average daily intake of majority of nutrients such as calcium, iron, vitamin A, thiamine, riboflavin and vitamin C were below the recommended levels as evidenced by the low levels of consumption of protective foods. Malnutrition is common among old people who are institutionalised.

According to the studies conducted by NIN the prevalence of Chronic Energy Deficiency is significantly higher among the elderly than their adult counterpart. With increasing age there is decrease in consumption of food and nutrients. There is a need to develop and implement appropriate programmes to improve the health and nutrition in particular, among the elderly population of India.

Constipation

It is the infrequent passage of stools which are most often attributed to prolonged recto sigmoid transit.

The stools become hard and dry because the stool moves too slowly through the colon. The natural contractions or rhythms of the colon might be disturbed due to loss of tone, stress, medication, illness, resisting the urge to defecate, pain from haemorrhoids or tissues, lack of exercise, a low fibre diet or not drinking enough fluids. It may even be caused by overuse of stimulant laxatives or enemas. In the elderly it may be related to inadequate energy intake, fewer meals per day, depression and sedentary life-style.

Generally, it is uncomfortable and elimination can be difficult and painful. Common symptoms of constipation include bloating, sluggishness, a feeling of "fullness" in the rectum and a general sense of "feeling out of sorts".

Constipation can be prevented by eating regular meals, drinking plenty of fluids and doing exercise daily. One should respond to the urge to move bowels and avoid straining. And by adding fibre to the diet, constipation can be prevented.

Dehydration

The ageing process produces physiological changes that can affect fluid balance in the older adult, increasing the risk for dehydration. Total body water decreases with age, which means a decreased fluid reverse. Dehydration risk increases for older adults because of the kidney's decreased ability to concentrate urine, altered thirst sensation, decreased renin activity and aldosterone secretion. Relative renal resistance to vasopressin changes in functional status, delirium and dementia medication side effects and mobility disorders also result in dehydration.

The frail older adult is more prone to dehydration due to cognitive skill impairment, reduced ability to obtain fluids and self-feed and incontinence or self-imposed fluid restrictions. Elders need at least 2 to 3 litres of fluids daily, except those who have cardiac and kidney ailments.

Fruits and fruit juices, butter milk, lime juice with salt in addition to water are recommended.

Lowered Resistance

Recent studies have shown that the gut microbiota changes in old age with an increased number of bacterial groups represented. This change in species evenness coinsides with parallel changes in immune function. The mechanism by which the gut microflora changes with age could be due to decline in immune response which would allow for more of the harmful bacteria to proliferate; excessive use of antibiotics; digestive physiology, decrease in transit time; dietary changes, low fibre and probiotic intake.

The responsiveness of the human immune system has been shown to decrease with age. The clinical implications of immunosenescence include a poor response to vaccination, progressive loss in the ability to recognise foreign antigens, increased autoantibodies and increased susceptibility to infections and chronic disease.

The deficiency of a number of nutrients have been linked to immune function notably vitaminA, vitamin C and zinc, vitamin B_6, iron, copper and selenium. Lower than recommended intakes of selenium and ω-3 fatty acids and higher than recommended intakes of vitamin A may influence overall immune function in elderly persons. Taking 200 mg of vitamin E may bring out changes in the immune system.

Alcoholism

Studies show that light to moderate alcohol consumption has been linked to lower risk of heart diseases, diabetes and has the benefit of prevention of disabilities. For moderate drinking a person can have 15 drinks per week with a daily maximum of five drinks for men and four for women.

Alcoholic and liver dysfunction are additional risk factors for deficiency of vitamin B_6. Alcoholism is a risk factor for folate deficiency.

DEGENERATIVE DISEASES

Oxidative stress promotes the process of ageing. Lowered red cell activity of glutathione peroxidase was observed in the elderly. Such decrease might be a precursor to oxygen mediated damage to the tissue and incidence of degenerative tissue. Diseases like diabetes, atherosclerosis, hypertension, cataract formation, Parkinson's disease, Alzheimer's disease and cancer that occur during old age may be related to low intake of antioxidants.

Cardiovascular disease

Blood pressure continues to increase in women older than 80 years of age but declines substantially in older men. Serum cholesterol levels in men tend to peak at 60 years of age, but total cholesterol levels as well as the low density lipo protein fraction continue to rise in women until the age of 70 years. Correction of hypertension and hyperlipidaemia have been shown to reduce cardiovascular morbidity and mortality in the elderly.

Free radicals are implicated in the cause of atherosclerosis. Studies have shown that vitamin E retards the development of coronary artery disease.

Renal disease

Renal function and glomerular filtration rate can diminish as much as 60 per cent between the ages of 30 and 80. This may be due to certain chronic conditions which reduce the number of nephrons and reduce blood flow. This makes the elderly person less able to respond to changes in fluid status and to challenges to the acid base balance. Geriatric nephropathy may be result of chronic protein over nutrition.

Diseases of the eye

Cataract is the opacification of the eye lens, which interferes with the transmission of light on the retina. The UV radiation may damage the cells like lens protein by generating reactive oxygen species. Antioxidants prevent susceptibility of lens proteins to UV radiation. Studies have shown that people with low serum carotenoid levels had more chances of developing cataracts than those with normal levels. Cataract can be prevented by making the diet rich in β-carotene, riboflavin and ascorbic acid. Studies have also shown that elders who take sufficient ω-3 fatty acids have better visual acuity.

Age related macular degeneration affect the macula, the centre of the retina's inner lining. This progressive disease gradually comprises sharp vision, making it difficult to see and recognize faces. There is no cure only it can be prevented. Lutein, a phytochemical is found mainly in dark green leafy vegetables can be helpful in preventing disease. Dark green leafy vegetables are also rich in other nutrients. Supplement combination of β-carotene, vitamin C, E, zinc, copper can reduce the risk. Dietary approach is better than pharmacy.

Cancer

The incidence of cancer increases progressively with age. Persons with high antioxidant intake are less likely to develop certain cancers.

Changes in the skin

Damage to the collagen fibrous network underlying the skin by free radicals can result in sagging of the tissue, appearance of fine lines, and wrinkles and discolouration of the pigment. This can be slowed down through nutrition or antioxidants.

Alzheimer's disease and Parkinson's disease

Dietary factors may interact with disease-causing or predisposing genes in molecular cascades that either promote or prevent the degeneration of neurons. Epidemiologic findings suggest that high-calorie diets and folic acid deficiency increase the risk for Alzheimer's disease and Parkinson's disease. High homocysteine levels have been implicated as one of the causes of Alzheimer's disease.

Supplementing with vitamin B_6, vitamin B_{12} and folic acid are helpful. Lipoic acid and coenzyme Q and herbs like ginkgo tea may be useful to the patients. Reducing calorie intake has also been found to be of much help.

Eating a Mediterranean diet which emphasizes fruits, vegetables and olive oil includes little red meat is associated with a lower risk for Alzheimer's disease. Individuals who have higher levels of fatty acid docosahexaenoic acid (DHA) in their blood may have a lower risk of developing dementia and Alzheimer's disease. The dietary modifications may be helpful most with cognitive impairment rather than advanced dementia. Keeping the patient mentally active by encouraging reading, making them to solve puzzles is important. Reciting slokas and singing may also be helpful to the patient.

The elderly are more prone to diseases due to lowered synthesis of antioxidants in the body, reduced food intake, physical activity and resistance to infection. The elderly need more calcium, iron, zinc, vitamin A and antioxidants to prevent age related diseases. Present evidence shows that 600 g/day of antioxidants rich in fruits and vegetables should be taken by elderly persons.

Stress

People who are stressed over long periods tend to look haggered and it is commonly thought that psychological stress leads to premature ageing and the earlier onset of diseases of the ageing. Stress is known to affect physical health, act as a risk factor for heart disease and lead to poorer immunity against infection. Psychological stress is linked to oxidative damage to DNA and other cellular components.

The intake of antioxidants such as some vitamins and micronutrients and certain plant products such as greens, tomatoes, carrot or red wine have been shown to retard age-related biological effects as well. Research shows that eating more ω-3 fatty acids and fewer ω-6 fatty acids may help reduce stress and inflammation in the body.

It is a challenge to prevent physiological ageing getting converted into pathological ageing with chronic disease.

Depression

Symptoms of depression include weight loss or weight gain, boredom, lack of interest in activities, increase or lack of sleep, inability to perform activities of daily living, memory problems. Nutrition risk has been associated with higher depression scores, longer hospitalisation and poor appetite. A deficiency of B-vitamins like folate and B_{12} and increased levels of homocysteine are thought to play a role in the cognitive decline and dementia and depression in older adults.

PHYSICAL ACTIVITY

Studies have proved that those who walk or exercise regularly are less likely to experience the memory loss and other declines in mental function that can come with ageing. Weight bearing activities enhance bone and muscle mass. Aerobic exercise increases lung capacity. Exercise is an integral part of maintaining healthy life. It helps to regulate body weight. The risk of degenerative disease is considerably decreased by regular exercise.

Activities that get seniors outdoors-gardening with children can help raise vitamin D levels and provides natural connection with children. Walking is another key activity for multigenerational groups. People who live in intergenerational households walking helps positive and open communication between generations which is the key to healthful eating.

Walking reduces the risk of type 2 diabetes. Walking is also weight bearing exercise that helps to decrease bone loss and keep muscles and heart healthy. In addition walking burns calories.

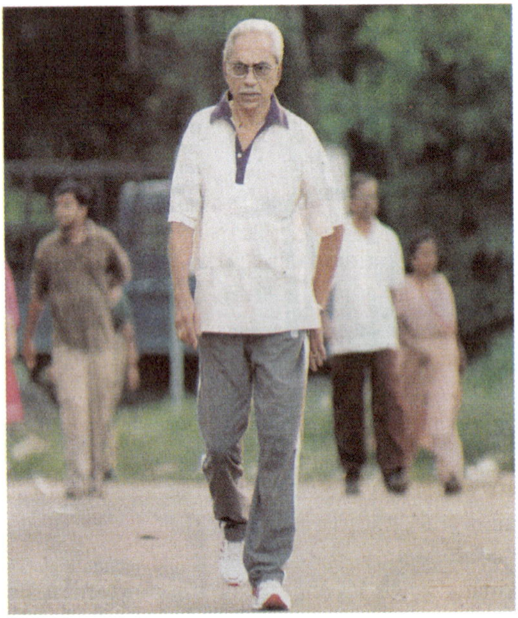

Fig. 10.4 Walkers perform better in tests of mental agility

Points to Remember

- Always warm up and stretch before physical activity. Cold muscles are more prone to injury.
- Try to get atleast 30 mn of moderate physical activity everyday.
- Select proper shoes.
- Listen to the body. As one ages, flexibility may reduce. Injuries can be prevented by modifying the activity.
- Rule of 10 per cent should be used when changing your activity level, increase by 10 per cent per week.
- Develop a balanced fitness programme that incorporates cardiovascular exercise, strength training and flexibility.
- Do new exercise cautiously.

Falls are the leading cause of injuries and deaths. Inactivity contribute to an increase in body fat and a decrease in muscle mass which in turn leads to reduced functional ability.

Life long physical activity is associated with reduced risk of fractures. Regular daily physical activity should be recommended to elderly women with osteopenia.

Beyond the effect on BMD, exercise has many additional benefits in post menopausal women. A number of studies have shown that regular exercise can

- improve psychological health
- increase muscle mass, strength and endurance
- reduce musculoskeletal complaints
- prevent chronic disease
- decrease the risk of falls through improved agility and balance
- promote functional independence

Exercise is an integral part of maintaining healthy life.

DRUGS AND SUPPLEMENTS

The aged constitute only 10 per cent of the total population but they consume about 25 per cent of drugs prescribed because of increased health problems in old age.

At any age there is a risk of harmful drug or drug nutrient interactions, but elderly persons seem to have more than their share. Several things contribute to this increased risk among the elderly.

- They are likely to take more drugs for longer period to control chronic diseases.
- The elderly are at increased risk owing to pathophysiologic changes related to ageing, endocrine dysfunction and the common ingestion of restricted diets.
- Illness, mental confusion or lack of drug information may increase errors in self-care.
- Nutrients can affect drug action by altering the digestion, absorption, distribution metabolism and/or excretion of the drug. Drugs may exhibit their effects on nutritional status through several avenues effects on food intake, alteration of nutrient absorption, and alteration in nutrient excretion.
- Because the rate of drug metabolism and detoxification in the liver is much slower in older people, drugs remain in the body longer to exert their influence on the metabolism of nutrients.

Many older adults regularly take an assortment of dietary supplements for a variety of reasons including to improve health, prevent disease and feel better. Multivitamin-mineral supplements may be needed. Dietary preferences and/or sensitivities and intolerance to particular foods such as dairy products may also necessitate the need for dietary supplements to obtain needed micronutrients. Whey protein prevents negative nitrogen balance.

One of the greatest concerns of older adults, is becoming dependent on others and being unable to live independently. All efforts should focus on offsetting declines in functional status and promoting independence and successful ageing.

Recent research findings suggest that it may be possible to increase 'health span' by reversing the deleterious effects of senescence on cognitive and motor behaviour via nutritional modulation.

Promoting a healthy diet for older adults is the optimal approach for health promoting, disease prevention, risk reduction and maintenance of quality of life. Nutrition as prevention on the mantra for successful ageing. Studies have shown that a sense of purpose and meaning in the lives of older individuals can significantly reduce the risk of early mortality.

Suggested recipes during old age

Pongal, idli, idiappam, adai	Cereal pulse combination easily chewable and digested.
Tomato soup, rasam	Good appetiser, low calorific value aid in digestion.
Amaranth dal	Greens good sources of vitamins, minerals and fibre.
Buttermilk, fruit juices	As they are light old people may feel comfortable.
Banana	Prevents constipation.
Skimmed milk powder	High in protein and low in fat. The requirement of protein, remains the same where is calorie intake is reduced.
Warm milk	Induces sleep.
Mixed cereal Kanjee	Easy to consume and nutritious

'World Alzheimer's Day' is on 21st September.

'World Elders Day' is on 1st October.

'World Arthritis Day' is on 12th October.

'World Osteoporosis Day' (WHO) is on 20th October.

SUGGESTED READINGS

- Dorner Becky *et al.*, Position of the academy of nutrition and dietetics: Individualised nutrition Approaches for older adults, J. Acad. Nutr. Diet. 2018; **118.**
- Bolzetta Francesco *et al.*, Are the recommended dietary allowances for vitamins appropriate for the elderly people? J. Acad. Nutr. Diet. 2015; **115**.
- Kim D. Luke *et al.*, Medication management in older adults, Cleveland Clinic journal of medicine, 2018; **85**.
- Fontana Luigi and Samual Klein Aging, Adiposity and colorie restrition JAMA 2007; **297**.
- Fung T. Teresa *et al.*, Association on diet quality scores and rising hip fractures in post menopousal woman and men aged 50 years and older J Acad Nutr Diet., 2018; **118**.
- NIH Osteoporosis and Related Bone Disease National Resource Centre. www/niams.nih.gov/Health_Info/Bone/Osteoporosis.

QUESTIONS

1. Give RDA for 64-year-old man.
2. What alteration would you suggest in the diet plan for an old man?
3. Discuss the modifications of calorie requirement during old age.
4. Describe the nutritional problems during old age.
5. What are the reasons for malnutrition during old age?
6. Suggest five recipes for an old man, giving reasons.
7. Bring out the importance of calcium and fibre during old age.
8. Explain the differences in body composition of an adult and old man.
9. Why is osteoporosis common during old age? What are the risk factors? Explain the preventive methods.
10. How can degenerative diseases be prevented during old age?
11. Bring out the importance of antioxidants during old age.
12. What is OSAT?

TOPICS FOR ACTIVITY

- Plan and prepare a diet for 65 year old man who is moderately active. Give the RDA.
- Plan and prepare a diet for a 70 year old woman who is suffering from depression.

11

Introduction to Diet Therapy

Diet therapy is concerned with the modification of the normal diet to meet the requirements of the sick individual. Its purposes are:

- To maintain good nutritional status.
- The energy requirements of patients with disease are similar to or less than or more than those of healthy subjects. Basal hypermetabolism of disease often offset by decreased physical activity.
- To correct deficiencies.
- To afford rest to the whole body or the part that is affected.
- To maintain body's ability to metabolise the nutrients.
- To bring about changes in body weight whenever necessary.

Diet therapy in most instances is not a remedy in itself but is a measure which supplements or makes the medical or surgical treatment more effective.

Diet is used as therapeutic purpose not only because of the presence of nutrients but also contains chemical substances which act as antioxidants, detoxifying agents or blocking or suppressing agents or help in excreting toxic substances or maintain proper intestinal flora or to improve the immunity. In planning diets these factors also should be kept in mind. While planning therapeutic diets, understanding drug-nutrient relationship is essential.

GLYCAEMIC INDEX

All foods are not digested or absorbed at the same rate and hence their glycaemic index levels are different. In planning diets one need to consider glycaemic index of food.

The glycaemic index is a ranking of foods based on the postprandial blood glucose response compared with a reference food (Jenkings, 1981).

The ability of the food item to raise the blood sugar is measured in terms of glycaemic index. The area above the fasting glucose concentration is calculated and is expressed as a percentage of the area obtained after the ingestion of 50 g glucose or 50 g carbohydrate from white bread. The higher the area under the curve the higher the glycaemic index.

$$\text{Glycaemic index} = \frac{\text{Incremental area under the 2 hours plasma glucose curve after eating 50 g of CHO from test food}}{\text{Incremental area under the 2 hours plasma glucose curve after taking 50 g CHO from white bread}} \times 100$$

The index integrates multiple influences on glucose availability and is proposed as a means for prescribing diets in different diseases.

Foods low in GI may reduce the insulin demand, improve blood glucose control, reduce lipid concentrations and body weight and thereby could help prevent diabetes.

Factors Affecting the Glycaemic Response to Food

The rate of digestion of the food is an important determinant of glycaemic response. Intrinsic and extrinsic factors that alter the rate of gastrointestinal motility, digestion and absorption and the nature of the starch, cooking method, particle size and the presence of fibre fat and proteins are all found to result in differences in the glycaemic index.

Glycaemic index is not significant in low energy foods in which the ratio of other desirable factors—minerals, vitamins and fibre to available carbohydrate is like carrots.

Factors affecting glycaemic response to food

- Rate of ingestion
- Food components
  - Protein and Fat content
  - Complex carbohydrates
  - Acidity
- Methods of cooking and processing food
- Physiologic effects
  - Pregastric hydrolysis
  - Gastric hydrolysis
  - Intestinal response
  - Intestinal hydrolysis and absorption
  - Pancreatic and gut hormone responses
  - Colonic effects

Rate of ingestion

Sipping 50 g of glucose slowly over a several hour period produces a much smaller increase in blood glucose than rapid intake of the same amount. Eating three apples takes more than 15 minutes whereas their juice can be consumed in 1.5 minutes. As the rate of ingestion increases the glycaemic index also increases.

Food components

Protein and Fat content: Foods rich in fat and protein like ice creams, groundnut and milk have low glycaemic index. But they are not recommended for diabetics because they have high calorific value. Pulses which have high protein are low in glycaemic index compared to cereals.

Complex carbohydrates: Starches have low glycaemic index compared to sugar. As the fruits ripen starch gets converted to glucose and glycaemic index increases.

The glycaemic index of starch is affected by the proportion of amylose to amylopectin in the grains. The higher the proportion of amylopectin, the higher the glycaemic index because amylopectin, which is made up of branched-starch molecules is more easily hydrolysed in the gut than is the single strand amylose. Some starches are more slowly digested not only because of amylose content but also because they are protected in structure for the enzymes to act.

Complex carbohydrates like fibre which is not disrupted adequately, take longer time to pass through the stomach and small intestine. Soluble fibre with the viscosity increasing property slow down passage and delay gastric emptying. Foods with soluble fibre such as beans have a low glycaemic index.

Most varieties of rice have high GI. Rice with higher amylose content is low in GI. Rice bran which is rich in fibre and oil is low in GI. Brown rice and red rice have low GI due to the presence of fibre.

Acidity: An increase in the acidity of a meal can greatly lower its GI. Increasing the amount of vinegar in a meal, for instance, affect the glucose response. The addition of sour dough bread to a meal can result in different GIs, depending on its content of organic acids. These foods apparently affect the glucose response at least partially by slowing gastric emptying.

Phytic acid, usually contained in cereals and pulses may have a more dominant role in decreasing the blood sugar rise than fibre.

Food processing

GI is dependent on the history of processing, storing, ripening, cutting and cooking of the food. The more processed a food is, the higher the glycaemic response. New methods such as extrusion cooking, explosion puffing and instantisation appear to make the starch in these foods more readily digested. Conditions which are known to increase the digestibility of starches are those which produce obvious hydration of the granules (gelatinisation), distinct changes in chemical nature or disruption of the organised granule structure. Such conditions increase the availability of the starch to amylose and are more likely to occur during factory processing because of the higher temperatures and pressures involved. Cornflakes produced from maize grits which are thoroughly cooked at elevated pressure, rolled and then toasted. In contrast, conventional cooking methods such as boiling involve less physical disruption and only moderate heat and are therefore less likely to cause starch damage or complete gelatinisation. The heat and the amount of water utilized and the time of cooking affect GI.

White rice has higher glycaemic response compared to brown rice. Polishing the rice increases glycaemic index. Rice varieties belonging to sona masuri, ponni and surti kolam have high GI, according to the studies conducted at International Diabetes Federation Centre of Education, Chennai. Wheat which is normally eaten as rotis probably has lower GI compared to refined cereals. Higher amount of protein and fibre and the mode of eating makes wheat preferable cereal. Multi-grain atta has better GI values. Presence of acarbose in wheat may also influence GI.

Parboiled rice has lower GI compared to non parboiled rice. During parboiling retrogradation of starch and formation of resistant starch formation occur. When starch undergoes retrogradation it becomes insoluble and not available to hydrolysis in the small intestine. Starch also forms insoluble complexes with proteins such as browning- Maillard-reaction, making it unavailable to digestion and absorption. Pasta products have different GIs depending on its type. The GIs of macaroni, star pasta and spaghetti are 68, 54 and 45.

Physiological effects

Digestion of dietary carbohydrate in the upper gastrointestinal tract provides glucose, fructose and galactose for intestinal absorption. The presence of nonabsorbable oligosaccharides and viscous dietary fibres such as pectins, β-glucans and gums in fruits, vegetables and cereals reduce the efficiency of enzyme hydrolysis and slow the rate at which glucose enters the blood stream.

Starch encased in its seed coat or coarsely ground is not efficiently hydrolysed to glucose because digestive enzymes are prevented from reaching the starch.

Starch granules subjected to moist heat and subsequent cooling become dense and less available to enzyme action. Thus the physical form as well as food processing and cooking methods influence the energy availability of dietary carbohydrate.

Acarbose, present in wheat, is a competitive inhibitor of sucrose and pancreatic amylase. It lowers post prandial blood glucose rise.

Classification of glycaemic foods

Foods are classified according to the GI.

High glycaemic foods 65-75 GI—Sugars, refined cereals processed breakfast cereals, sticky and waxy rice, banana, root vegetables, white bread

Intermediate glycaemic foods 45-55 GI—Fruits, unrefined cereals

Low glycaemic foods 30-40 GI—legumes, nuts.

According to the studies conducted at Dr. Mohan's diabetes specialities centre and Madras diabetes research foundation. GI values of rotis can be reduced when whole wheat flour is mixed with roasted bengal gram flour, psyllium husk powder and debittered fenugreek powder.

Table 11.1 Glycaemic Index of Different Foods

Foodstuff	*Glycaemic index*	*Foodstuff*	*Glycaemic index*
White wheat bread	75 ± 2	Mango (raw)	51 ± 5
Whole wheat bread	74 ± 2	Watermelon	76 ± 4
Wheat roti	62 ± 3	Potato (boiled)	78 ± 4
Chapatti	52 ± 4	French fries (potato)	63 ± 5
White boiled rice	73 ± 4	Carrots (boiled)	39 ± 4
Brown boiled rice	68 ± 4	Milk (Full fat)	39 ± 3
Barley	28 ± 2	Milk (skim)	37 ± 4
Instant oat porridge	79 ± 3	Ice cream	51 ± 3
Rice porridge/congee	78 ± 9	Chick peas	28 ± 9
Millet porridge	67 ± 5	Soya beans	16 ± 1
Sweet corn	52 ± 5	Lentils	32 ± 5
Cornflakes	81 ± 6	Chocolate	40 ± 3
Apple (raw)	36 ± 2	Popcorn	65 ± 5
Orange	43 ± 3	Soft drinks/soda	59 ± 3
Banana	51 ± 3	Honey	61 ± 3
Pineapple	59 ± 8	Glucose	103 ± 3

Cited from: Dietary guidelines for Indians - A manual, 2011, National Institute of Nutrition, Hyderabad.

Glycaemic load

Glycaemic index ignores how much of that food a person eats. Walter Willet of Harvard University pioneered the concept of glycaemic load. The glycaemic load is the product of the dietary glycaemic index and total dietary carbohydrate.

$$\text{Glycaemic load} = \frac{\text{Glycaemic index}}{\text{Carbohydrate}} \times 100$$

Glycaemic load assesses the total glycaemic effect of the diet and has proved to be very useful in epidemiologic studies. The emphasis should be on low glycaemic loads as steady blood glucose also helps keep the appetite in check. One need to choose good carbohydrate to be healthy.

A glycaemic load of 10 or less is considered low, 11 to 19 is medium and 20 or more is high. Consistently eating low glycaemic load foods evens out blood sugar peaks and valleys. According to Willet this helps to keep appetite and weight under control. Good carbohydrate means that the food should be rich in fibre and low in GL.

Glycaemic Index has been endorsed by the FAO/WHO and numerous other international health related organisations.

DIETARY SUPPLEMENTS

Dietary supplements are a group of products intended to supplement the diet. It contains atleast one ingredient that is a vitamin, mineral, amino acid, herb or other botanical or a combination thereof.

Dietary supplements are consumed by apparently normal or diseased individuals with or without prescription by a physician or a dietitian to improve the general well being.

Dietary supplements may contain predigested and easily absorbable nutrients in concentrated form. They may have foods which have nutraceutical properties. Some may be amylase rich foods and some may contain mushrooms, soyabean or milk protein as main ingredient. Some may contain herbs or substances traditionally used for well being but scientifically might not have been proved. Multivitamin and multimineral dietary supplements are the most popular dietary supplements.

A study was conducted by NIN on supplementation of nutritional beverage, additional micro-nutrients in younger school children. The study revealed nutritional supplementation improved physical and mental development of children.

Dietary supplements are required by:

- people who are not taking enough food and have nutrient deficiencies,
- pregnant and lactating women (foliate, iron),
- new born (vitamin K),
- those addicted to alcohol,
- those recovering from surgery, burns, injury or illness,
- vegans,
- people taking medications that interfere with the body's use of nutrient,
- those who have lactose intolerance (calcium),
- chronic drug consumers,
- habitual dieters,
- elderly people,
- patients suffering from infections like AIDS and other wasting diseases.
- to compensate for suboptimal diet
- for medical conditions
- to prevent chronic disease incidence or progression.

Dietary supplements are used more often by non smokers. People who exercise regularly. Those with higher education and incomes and those who report better over all health Adults take supplements for heart health, lower cholesterol and bone health, most common organ specific reasons.

Type of Supplements

Herbal supplements: Garlic, wheat grass, alfalfa, ginseng, aloevera, spirulina, turmeric.

Body building products: Amino acids, anabolic/muscle building.

Laxative supplements: Psyllium, wheat bran, weight loss products, lecithin.

Other biologic and nutrient supplements: Antioxidants, fish oils, bioflavonoids, combination of cereals, pulses, nuts and milk products, amylase rich foods.

Dietary Supplements which are proven claim are given in Table 11.2.

Table 11.2 Dietary supplements proven claims

Dietary supplement	*Claim*
Arginine	Beneficial in CVD, cancer and for wound healing
Bovine	Colostrum Immuene booster for sports persons
Calcium	Prevents osteoporosis
	Reduces blood pressure
Chromium	Helps control diabetes
Coenzyme Q_{10}	Cardio protective
Creatine	Increase in muscular strength
Fish oil	Candio protective
Folic acid	Prevents birth defects
Fructo oligosaccharides	Healthy digestive system
Glycerol	Improves hydration status
Green Tea Extract	Strong antioxidant
β-hydroxy β-methyl butyrate	Increases muscle mass and strength
Sodium bicarbonate	Enhances power and strength
Soya protein and isoflavones	Lower cholesterol
Selenium	Anti cancer

To get the most from the supplement of vitamins and minerals, supplements are to be taken with food. An iron supplement should be taken with foods that assist in its absorption such as meats, fish or poultry or foods that contain vitamin C.

Although dietitians should continue to encourage nutrient dense food choices first, dietary supplements may be a useful approach for meeting some micronutrient needs in certain at risk subpopulations.

Most dietary supplements are expensive. For some they may not be required or may not have any impact on health. Supplements need to be taken only on prescription.

DIET AND INFLAMMATION

It appears that one link between stress and disease is altered immune response that causes inflammation. This is evidenced by an increase in the acute phase response c-reactive protein and proinflammatory cytokines, Interleukin factor-1, Interleukin factor-6 and Tumor Necrosis Factor. Chronic inflammation is caused by life style factors such as poor diet and stress which increases cortisol levels, affecting immune system.

All are subject to physical stress like surgery, infection, burns and pain. Examples of environmental stress are air and noise pollution and crowding. Psychological stress can be due to death of a spouse, friend or loved one. Subclinical conditions such as back aches, head aches, chest pains and fatigue that do not require medical treatment are often stress related.

Increase in cortisol leads to blood sugar imbalance and diabetes, weight gain and obesity, immune system suppression, gastro intestinal problems, increased blood pressure, heart attack, fertility problems. Long term stress and elevated cortisol may be linked to insomnia, chronic fatigue syndrome, thyroid disorders dementia and depression.

Obesity creates a low-grade systemic inflammatory response syndrome. This process involves up-regulation of systemic immunity and is characterized clinically by insulin resistance and the metabolic syndrome.

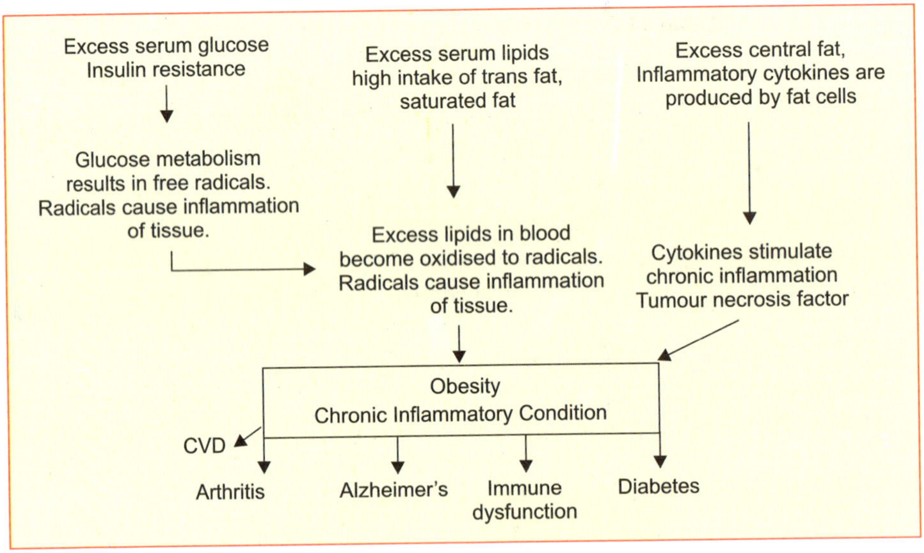

Fig. 11.1 Effect of chronic inflammation

The organs most affected by stress

The adrenal glands produce hormones that regulate many bodily functions. The thymus gland-master gland of immune system. GI tract alter how foods are digested and absorbed and may alter immune function.

Hyperglycemia appears to be a cytokine-mediated indicator of active inflammatory response. Acute onset of hyperglycemia is often a harbinger of brewing infection or other inflammatory events. It is possible that insulin therapy is actually an anti-inflammatory intervention.

Inflammation plays a role in neurodegeneration diseases. Oxidative stress has been implicated in diseases like Alzheimers and Parkinsons diseases. Consumption of diets rich in antioxidant and anti-inflammatory agents may lower the risk of developing these age-related neurodegenerative diseases.

Chronic use of Home Parenteral Nutrition may be associated with low level inflammatory state. The contributory facts for inflammation may include chronic medical conditions, subclinical infections, associated hepatic dysfunction and poor glycemic control. Parenteral nutrition should be replaced be enteral nutrition at the earliest to reduce inflammation.

In acute and chronic protein-calorie malnutrition, at least partially there is a manifestation of inflammatory response that results in an altered metabolic state. Clinical nutrition in SAM involves more than protein and calories.

Anti-inflammatory diet has following characteristics:

- rich in a variety of foods to provide a rainbow of nutrients and anti-inflammatory compounds;
- low in processed, refined, low-nutrient foods;
- packed with fruits and vegetables to provide antioxidant and anti-inflammatory compounds;
- balanced in calories to promote optimal weight;
- contains healthful carbohydrates that are less refined, are high in fiber, and have a low glycemic index;
- moderately low in animal proteins (except for fish);
- focuses on plant proteins such as legumes, soy foods, and nuts;
- includes healthful fats such as extra-virgin olive oil, nuts and avocados and minimizes saturated and *trans* fats;
- includes ω-3 fatty acids from fish and plant sources such as walnuts and flax;
- contains generously flavoured antioxidant spices and herbs such as garlic, green herbs, ginger and turmeric;
- encourages frequent tea consumption;
- promotes moderate consumption of red wine (if alcohol is consumed); and
- allows small amounts of antioxidant-rich dark chocolate (at least 70% cocoa) as a treat.

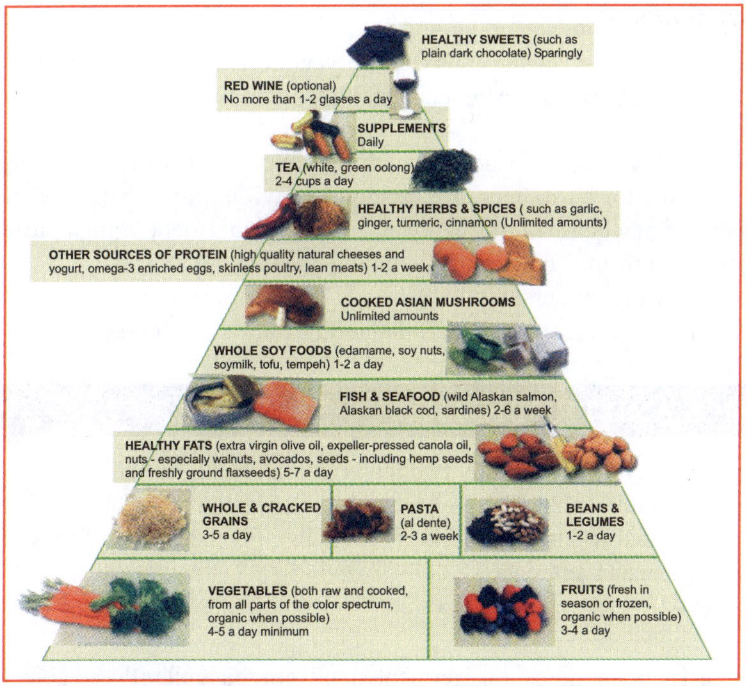

Fig. 11.2 Anti-Inflammatory food pyramid

Andrew Weil, created an Anti-inflammatory Food Pyramid to help people make optimal food choices every day.

Source: Palmer Sharon, Inflammation, today's dietitian, 2011.

CHAPTER 11

According to Andrew Weil all diseases of ageing have a common root: inappropriate inflammation. Inflammatory process promotes diseases like coronary heart disease and Alzheimer's disease. There is also a link to cancer; anything that up regulates inflammation increases the pressure for cells to divide rapidly.

Anti-inflammatory foods

There is inverse association between fibre intake and HS-CRP, High sensitive C-reactive protein, independent of weight but associated with reduction in fasting glucose with higher consumption of dietary fibre.

Linolenic acid, EPA, DHA, GLA (Gamma Linolenic Acid) are anti-inflammatory substances.

Flavonoid compounds, quercetin, kaempferol, malvidin, peonidin, daidzein and genistein each has inverse association with serum HS-CRP concentration. Anti-inflammatory effects of flavonoids may be due to enzyme inhibition. Carotenoids from food is associated with decreased levels of inflammatory markers in serum. A modest increase in beta cryptoxanthin intake, equivalent to 200 ml of freshly squeezed orange juice per day is associated with a reduced risk of developing inflammatory arthritis.

Whole grain is the main contributor to dietary magnesium, followed by green leafy vegetables, nuts and legumes. Green leafy vegetables and nuts consumption is inversely related to high sensitive c-reactive protein. Inverse relationship between dietary magnesium and inflammation is very strong.

HS-CRP is inversely associated with high intake of olive oil, vegetables, legumes, fruits and fish. Mediterranean diet reduces inflammation.

Inflammatory foods

Diets with relatively high glycemic index and glycemic load are inflammatory. *Trans* fatty acids and saturated fatty acids are associated with interleukin factor-6 and high sensitive a-reactive protein.

High ω-6/ω-3 PUFA are also associated with increased levels of inflammation.

Systemic inflammatory diseases are associated with more than one organ system. Atherosclerosis is a major cause of morbidity and mortality in patients with lupus erythematosus as well as other inflammatory conditions including rheumatoid arthritis.

Inflammation is at the cornerstone of the body's healing process it is so powerful yet so destructive. If it is chronic, it creates the foundation of age-related diseases.

PREBIOTICS AND PROBIOTICS

Healthy microflora can be supported by two interventions prebiotics and probiotics. Prebiotics include foods that contain substrated that nourish beneficial gut microbiota. These substrates include dietary fibre and fructooligosaccharides (FOS). Food sources of these FOSs include honey, beer, onion, banana and oats.

Prebiotics

Prebiotics are resistant to digestion, fermented by colonic microflora, able to selectively stimulate growth of beneficial bacteria and beneficial to the host's health.

Nondigestible oligosaccharides inulin, lactulose, galacto oligosaccharides are prebiotics.

Inulin and oligofructose are present in varying amounts in more than 36,000 plant foods as plant storage carbohydrates. Excellent food sources are chicory root and Jerusalem artichokes. Others include wheat, barley, rye, flax, and oatmeal. Other whole grains, onions, garlic, leeks, legumes, greens, berries, bananas and honey.

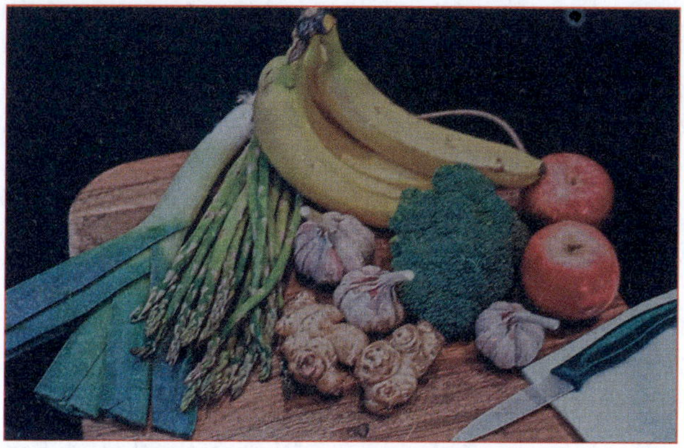

Fig. 11.3 Some foods rich in prebioties

Resistant Starches

It is found in whole grains, fruits and some processed foods, differs from other starches in that it resists digestion in the small intestine. Probiotics ferment it in the colon. Resistant starch is similar to inulin and oligofructose but unlike fructans, resistant starch is fermented slowly resulting in less flatulence. Resistance starch is well tolerated in larger amounts compared with the fructans.

Health benefit of dietary intake of resistance starch is improvement in insulin sensitivity Resistant starch is a low-glycaemic ingredient. It is a functional food.

Prebiotics arrive intact in the colon, where they are digested through bacterial activity. They are selectively fermented by probiotics, specifically *bifidobacteria*, which possess beta-fructofuranosidase, an enzyme that allows preferred utilisation of fructoligosaccharides over sucrose. Fermentation an anearobic process results in the release of short chain fatty acids, organic acids and short-chain carboxyl acids.

Short chain fatty acids have a variety of positive physological effects and health benefits. They decrease the pH level in the colon, which enchances mineral absorption, especially calcium. An acidic environment is favorable for probiotics but detrimental to the survival of pathogenic bacteria.

Short chain fatty acids are also the preferred energy source for colonic epithelial cells and they increase bacterial growth and cell mass resulting in increased faecal bulk and weight. An increase in stool bulk has a laxative effect, increases the excretion of nitrogen and energy and aids in diluting genotoxic substances in the colon.

Propionic acid *in vitro* decreases serum LDL cholesterol levels by inhibiting hepatic fatty acid synthesis. Acetate is a strong acid that effectively lowers the pH level. *In vitro* studies-indicate that butyrate is the preferred fuel for colon cells and may prevent colon carcinogenesis by suppressing cancer cell growth.

Inulin and oligofructose have many fibre like properties. They are water soluble and thus increase the colonic water volume. They increase fecal bulk and weight. There is inverse relationship between stool weight and risk of colon cancer.

Health benefits include inhibiting pathogenic bacteria growth, producing a laxative effect, inhibiting diarrhoea preventing colon carcinogenesis, enhancing mineral absorption, decreasing serum triglycerides and decreasing postprandial glucose and insulin levels.

Probiotics are defined by the World Health Organisation as live microorganisms that when taken in a sufficient amounts, have a beneficial effect on the overall health of the host. The term was originally created in contrast with antibiotic.

To qualify as a beneficial probiotic, a microorganism should meet the following criteria.

- Viability after culture, manipulation and storage
- Ability to survive gastric, biliary and pancreatic digestion
- Existence of sufficient bacteria to affect change
- Ability to provide functional benefits to the host
- Capability to induce a host response once in the intestinal microflora
- High resistance against antibiotics
- No permanent colonisation of colonic mucosa

Probiotics benefit the host animal by improving intestinal microbial balance and promoting health benefits. *Lactobacilli* and *bifidobacteria* are the two most common bacteria used. However not all strains are alike. The effects of any probiotic depend on the particular strain used. Use of each probiotic strain results in a unique profile of cytokines secreted by lymphocytes, enterocytes or dendritic cells interacting with a particular bacterium.

Saccharomyces, *enterococcus* and *streptococcus* are also known to have health benefits.

Probiotics give immunological benefit by activating local macrophages to increase antigen presentation to B lymphocytes. They increase secretory immunoglobulin A production. They modulate cytokine profiles.

Probiotics also give non-immunological benefits. They help to digest food and compete with pathogens for nutrients. They alter local pH to create an unfavourable environment for growth of pathogens. They produce bacteriocins to inhibit pathogens. They scavenge superoxide radicals. They stimulate epithelial mucin production and enhance intestinal barrier function.

Some probiotics have the capacity to activate receptors in the enteric nervous system. These could be used to promote pain relief in the setting of visceral hyperalgesia. Eating food rich in probiotics can influence brain behaviour and help alleviate stress, anxiety and depression.

Probiotics have a significant positive effect on gastrointestinal diseases – pouchitis, infectious diarrhoea, irritable bowel syndrome, IBS, helicobacter pylori, bacteria infection, clostridium difficile infection, antibiotic associated diarrhoea, traveller's diarrhoea and necrotising enterocolitis in infants.

Probiotics can be prescribed for both preventive and therapeutic purposes. Probiotics like *lactobacillus casei* strain *shirota* (LcS) can reduce the risk of diarrhoea.

> **FSSAI - 2018**
>
> According to the food safety standards authority of India, all probiotic foods should specify the complete name on the labels of the products of the probiotic bacteria (genus, species, strain) shelf life, health benefits and storage conditions on the products.

Synbiotics

Synbiotics are foods or dietary supplements that contain a mixture of probiotics and prebiotics. The premise behind developing synbiotcs is that a combination of probiots and prebiotics may improve the survival of organisms as they pass through the stomach and small intestine, thus enhancing their effects in the colon, It is suggested that to improve a probiotic's viability and vitality, as well as its survival chances in the digestive tract and its subsequent attachment and growth rate, a prebiotic ingredient should be included. Currently, the best synbiotic combinations are *bifidobacteria* and Fructo Oligo Saccharides FOS, *Lactobacillus GG* and inulins, and *bifidobacteria* and *lactobacilli* with FOS or inulin. Fermented milks, yogurt, kefir and some cheeses are the most popular synbiotic foods. However, not all fermented milks contain prebiotics.

Table 11.3 Potential uses of probiotics for disease prevention

Table 11.3 Potential uses of probiotics for disease prevention

Disorder	*Rationale*
Cardiovascular disease	May lower cholesterol
Infantile colic	Affect GI motility
Musculoskeletal disorders	Impact on mineral absorption, metabolism, bone composition, and architecture
Fatigue in athletes	Better recovery from fatigue and immune enhancement
Hepatic diseases	Alteration of intestinal microflora
Malnutrition in lactose intolerance	Improving nutrient absorption
Aging processes	Inhibiting immunosenescence and lowering chronic inflammation
Restless leg syndrome	Inhibiting small bowel bacterial overgrowth, which may be a common denominator in chronic pain syndromes
Obesity	Intestinal flora vary in ability for nutrient extraction, and probiotics alter the "obese microbiodata" to "lean"
Maniac depressive disorder	Altered intestinal microflora to affect proinflammatory cytokines, oxidative stress, and improved nutrition
Attention-deficit hyperactivity disorder (ADHD)	ADHD may be an allergic disorder, and probiotics may prevent allergy.

Source: Minocha Anil Probiotics for preventive health, Nutrition in clinical practice 2009; **24**.

Studies conducted at NIN (2013-14) showed that indigenously prepared probiotic curd with combination of *Cactobacillus bulgaricus* and *Streplococus Thermophilus* showed significant changes in the lipid profile parameters upon supplementation in obese subjects. Cholesterol levels and triglyceride levels decreased and HDL levels increased significantly.

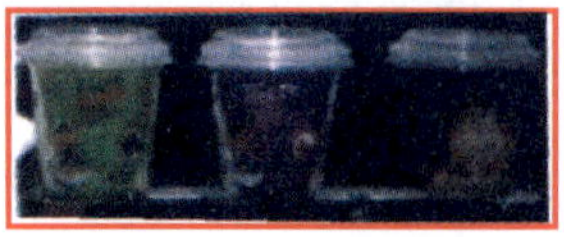

Probiotic ice cream from Amul

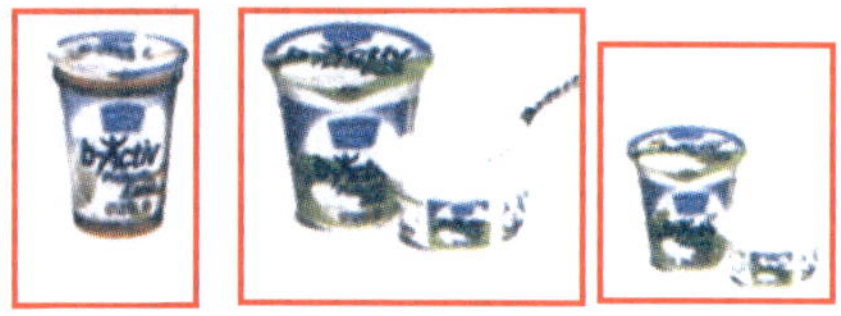

b-Active yogurt and Lassi and b-Active plus fiber rich dahi from Mother Dairy

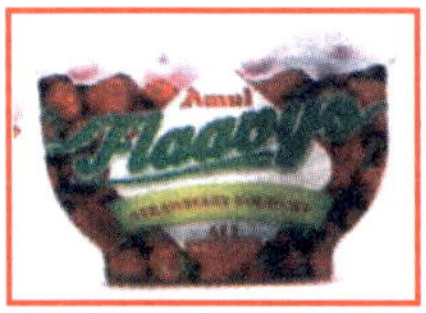

Flaavyo—probiotic fruit yogurt by Amul - Vitamin fortified

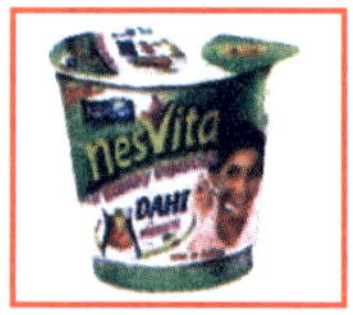

Lactobacillus acidophilus dahi by Nestle

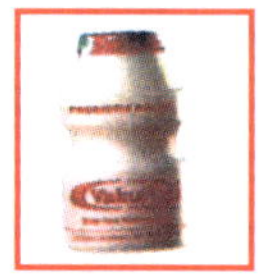

Yakult contains *lactobacillus casei*

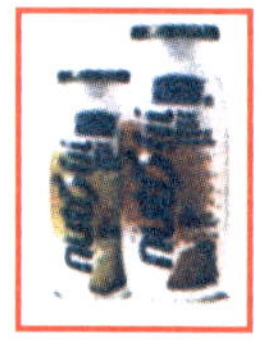

Probiotic drink Nutrifit LA5 Strawberry and mango flavor Kesar elaichi

Fig. 11.4 Probiotic dairy supplements commercially available in the Indian market.

Source: Grover Sunita *et al.*, 2012 Probiotic formulations and delivery in dairy foods: Establishing *in vivo* functionality, Health impact of probiotics, Elsevier, India.

ARTIFICIAL SWEETENERS

An ideal sweetener is as sweet as or sweeter than sucrose, has a pleasant taste with no after taste. It is colourless, odorless, readily soluble, stable, functional and economically feasible. It is non-toxic, does not promote dental cavities and is either metabolised normally or excreted from the body unchanged without contributing to any metabolic abnormalities.

When multiple sweeteners are used together they have a synergistic effect. They reduce the cost and improve the product taste and stability, since the combination often overcomes the limitations of the individual sweeteners. Ideal is multiple sweetener approach.

Low-Calorie Sweeteners

Polyols: Polyols though occur in nature, they are synthesised on industrial scale from easily accessible carbohydrates such as starch, sucrose, glucose, invert sugar, xylose and lactose. Sugar alcohols (xylitol, sorbitol, mannitol, maltitol, lactitol, isomalt) known as polyols are white crytalline, slightly hygroscopic, water soluble powders.

They are less sweet and 50 per cent of energy of polyols is available to human body. Average caloric value is 2.4 kcal/g. Polyols are suitable for diabetics because rapid glycaemic response is avoided. For the same reason sorbitol and xylitol are often included in parenteral nutrition to provide more controllable carbohydrate energy source to glucose or fructose. Due to induced digestibility of polyols, their intake should be restricted to 40-50 g/day for adults and 30 g/day for children in order to avoid gastrointestinal discomfort.

Polyols do not promote and may retard or prevent the formation of dental caries due to the fact that cavity causing oral bacteria cannot readily convert polyols into decay causing acids. Their sweet flavour stimulates the production of saliva reducing plaque formation and increasing mineralisation of tooth surfaces.

Polyols may assist in reducing the diet's overall glycaemic load. Polyols are suitable for diabetics, as they do not increase blood sugar rapidly. For the same reason sorbitol and xylitol are often included in parenteral nutrition to provide more controllable carbohydrate energy.

Carbohydrate counting can be easily done by diabetics when counting carbohydrate.

Polyols are commonly used for weight loss and maintenance as they give half the calories per unit without affecting the sweetness.

Polyols are generally incompletely absorbed and the absorbed portions are either metabolised generally by insulin independent mechanism or excreted via urine. A significant amount of the unabsorbed portion is metabolised to short fatty acids and gases by bacteria in the large intestine.

The epithelial cells in the gastrointestinal tract utilize the short-chain fatty acids for energy and the acids contribute to the formation of an acidic environment, which promotes the growth of beneficial bacteria such as *bifidobacteria* and *lactobacilli*. Thus, many polyols are considered prebiotic due to their ability to promote the growth of beneficial colonic bacteria.

Non-Calorie Sweeteners

Acelsulfame-K: It is a synthetic derivative of acetoacetic acid. It is not metabolised in the body and is excreted unchanged. It has little undesirable after taste. At very high concentrations it exhibits lingering bitter and metallic flavour attributes. Acelsulfame-K, the potassium salt of acelsulfame is up to 200 times sweeter than a 3 per cent sucrose solution.

In mixtures of acelsulfame-K and aspartame (1 : 1 by weight) there is a strong synergistic enhancement of sweetness. Blends are 300 times sweeter than sucrose solutions while individually they are only 100 times sweeter.

Acelsulfame-K is heat stable hence can be used in cooked and baked products. In preparations like baked custard, half the amount of sugar can be substituted with acelsulfame-K without changing the acceptability.

Aspartame: It is made by combining two amino acids—aspartic acid and phenylalanine—and adding methyl alcohol to form a methyl ester. Aspartame is a white, odourless, crystalline powder that has a sugar-like taste and sweetness potency is 180 to 200 times that of sucrose without any bitter aftertaste. Since it cannot be utilised by the body the caloric value is insignificant.

Saccharin: It is sodium ortho benzene sulphonamide of the calcium salt. It is 300 times sweeter than sucrose. It is stable in a wide variety of products under extreme processing conditions. It can be synthesised with relatively few impurities and is inexpensive. It gives bitter after taste at higher concentration. But when used in combination with aspartame or cyclamate, sweetness is enhanced and bitterness is decreased.

Sucrolose: It is a white crystalline solid produced by the selective addition of chlorine atoms to sucrose. It is 600 times sweeter than sugar and has no bitter aftertaste. It is very soluble in water and stable at high temperatures and therefore can be used in baked goods. Sucralose does not interact with any other food components.

Stevia: Stevia, botanically known as *stevia rebandiana* is a sweet herb. Stevia is a calorie free bio-sweetener. This sweet-honey leaf herb finds its use as a natural sweetener, replacing the chemical sweeteners and even table sugar. The sweetness in leaf is due to the presence of an intensive sweetening agent called stevioside and the leaf by itself is about 20 to 30 times sweeter than sugar. Stevioside is 300 times sweeter than sucrose.

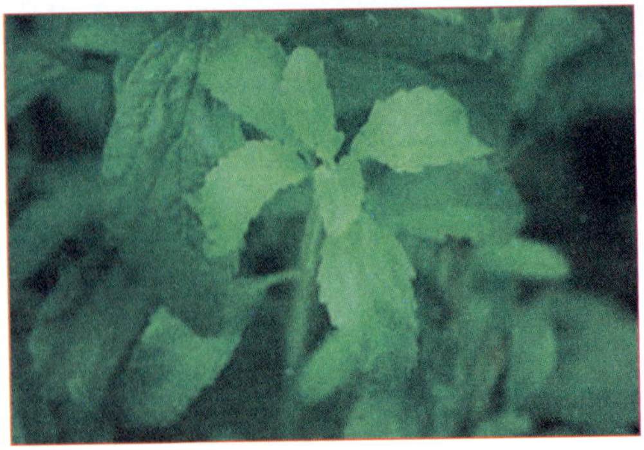

Fig. 11.5 Stevia leaf contains stevioside which is a natural sweet compound. 50 g of stevia powder = 1000 g of cane sugar.

Use of sweeteners by patients is not encouraged as it does not help the patient to wean away from sweet foods.

GUT MICROBIOME

The gut microbiome plays an important role in metabolism, immune defence and behaviour. It changes with age, environment, stress, diet, health status as well as medication exposure.

The typical healthy person is inhabited with trillions of microbes. Two healthy people may have different microbiomes.

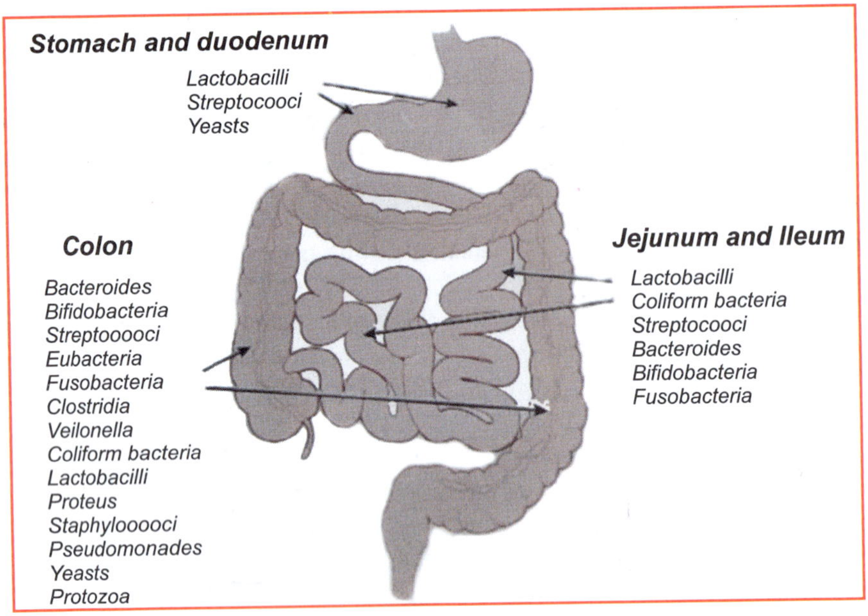

Fig. 11.6 Gut microbiome

The human gut microbiome has a huge number of beneficial bacteria, collectively called commensals, living in it. Key among these are the bacteria of the *bifidobacterium genus*, *bifidobacterium* adolescentis and *B. longum* are found in adult human gut whereas *B. bifidum* are found in infant gut.

The gut is second brain, both are connected through neurons, hormones and chemicals that provide feed back to each other.

Gut microbiome changes with age

When an infant's diet comprises breast milk and formula, microbiome has minimal diversity. When there is introduction of solid foods takes place, the microbiome also changes. When the child is around 3 years of age, the bacterial composition resembles that of an adult and remains stable until old age. The *bifidobacterium* dominated micro biodata of the infant changes over time into the bacteroidetes. This remains fairly stable throughout adulthood in the absence of long term dietary changes or repeated antibiotic usage.

Alterations in gut microbiome are associated with health concerns pertaining to elderly people such as frailty.

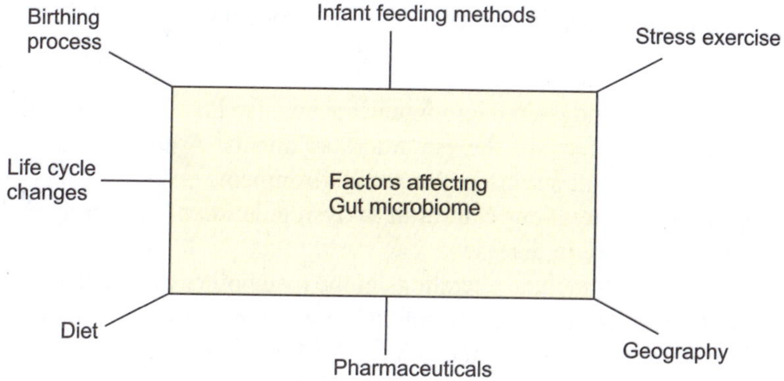

Fig. 11.7 Factors affecting Gut Microbiome.

Gut microbiome changes with geography

Geographical location and ethnicity have been shown to be determinants of the diversity and overall composition of micro biodata. Using the type of micro biodata, functional markers might be used for diagnostic and perhaps even prognostic tools for numerous human disorders. For instance, colorectal cancer and obesity linked comorbidities such as metabolic syndrome, diabetes and cardiovascular disease.

Changes in gut microbiome due to food supply

Diet has emerged as one of the most relevant factors in influencing gut microbiome. Significant and meaningful changes in the gut micro biodata have been associated with dietary alterations, primarily consumption of dietary fibres from foods, vegetables and other plants. A diet that is varied and complex is associated with more diversified microbiome. Diversity of gut microbiome may be future biomarker of long term consumption of a healthy vs unhealthy diet which may be linked to potential disease development.

Stress and microbiome

Stress is defined as an organism's total response to environmental demands or pressures. There are different types of stressors such as or chronic. Stress contributes to susceptibility to disease and disability. The GI tract or the gut micro biodata are sensitive to stress and stress mediators. Enteric bacteria respond to the release of stress related neurochemical mediators by the host which can influence the response to a bacterial infection.

Microbiome and exercise

High intensity exercise is physiological stressor that can lead to GI distress. High intensity training has been associated with the reduced GI bloodflow, tissue hyperthermia, and hypoxia leading to possible alterations of micro biodata and gut barrier. Contrary to the benefits of regular exercise, prolonged excessive exercise can negatively affect the intestinal function.

Microbiome and critical illness

Critically ill, gut has an important role in promoting infectious complications and multiple organ dysfunction syndrome. This is due to deteriorated intestinal epithelium, altered gut immune system, and dysfunctional metabolic activities of commensal bacteria.

Antibiotics

Antibiotics not only affect pathogenic microorganisms but also host associated microorganisms leaving a lasting negative effect on the gut microorganisms. Antibiotics also promote the expansion of antibiotic resistant strains in the gut environment.

Gut microbial immunity alterations can result in dysregulation of host immune homeostasis and an increased susceptibility to disease.

Antibiotic induced changes include alterations in the metabolites produced by the microbiota such as short chain fatty acids which are beneficial to gut health. SCFAs are beneficial for gut health because they serve as a primary fuel source for the colonocyte.

Changes in gut immunity increases host susceptibility to infection by pathogens.

Gut microbial populations contribute to inflammation, altered glucose metabolism and insulin sensitivity and immune response leading to diabetes and obesity.

FOOD, NUTRITION AND DRUG INTERACTION

Food and nutrition affect drug action by altering the digestion, absorption, distribution, metabolism and/or excretion of the drug. Drugs may exhibit their effects on nutritional status through effects on food intake, absorption, alteration of nutrient metabolism.

Diet Effects on Drug Disposition

Food can decrease or increase a drug's rate of absorption. The amount of water, the temperature of food, the osmotic power of a meal, the nature of food (particularly lipids) and the acidity or basicity of food alter the dissolution of drugs and the rate of gastric emptying. Some drugs are to be taken after a meal and some should be taken on empty stomach.

The coumarin anticoagulants (warfarin, coumadin, dicumarol) act through antagonism of vitamin K. Consumption of vitamin K enriched foods or supplements may couteract the effects of the anticoagulants.

A major way in which a food item may affect the action of medicines is by hampering their absorption into the blood stream.

The effect of meals on the absorption of drugs may differ strikingly from one formulations to another and one needs to examine the literature before taking the drugs.

Studies have shown that in the case of aspirin, not only its bioavailability was reduced when taken with food but also the time to reach the peak plasma level was significantly delayed, especially after high carbohydrate meal.

Beverages, fibre, type of meal, milk and milk products or vegetables can affect the absorption of different drugs. For example, absorption of iron tablets is enhanced if they are taken with fruit juice but the tannic acid in tea tends to interfere with iron absorption.

Food may play a role of drug carrier from gastrointestinal tract to systemic blood. Water soluble substances which are absorbed by an active transport mechanism are better absorbed with a concomitant high carbohydrate meal for example, riboflavin, a water soluble vitamin.

Table 11.4 shows the impact of food on the absorption of drugs.

Table 11.4 Effect of food on the absorption of drugs

Decreased absorption	***Increased absorption***	***Delayed absorption***
Avoid taking these drugs with food. Take them at least one hour before or 2 hours after meals	*Foods alter the amount of the drugs absorbed, therefore the drug should be taken at the same time.*	*Foods delay the absorption of these drugs. Take them at least one hour before or two hours after meals.*
Ampicillin	Albenazole	Acetaminophen
Atenolol	Diazepan	Aspirin
Bisphosphonates	Fenofibrate	Digoxin
Cholestyramine	Griseofulvin	Hydrochorthiazide
Erythromycin stearate	Metoprolol	Hydrocortisone
Furosemide	Metronidazole	Indomethacin
Glipizide	Phenytoin	Pentobarbital
Isoniazid	Spironolactone	Pentoxyfyline
Levodopa	Sulfadiazine	Sulfisoxazole
Proton pump inhibitors	Theophylline	Tocainide
Methotrexate	Warfarin	
Tetracycline		

Heimburger C. Douglas and Jamy D. Rrd. 2006, Handbook of Clinical Nutrition Elsevier, New Delhi.

Fat soluble vitamins have their absorption enhanced by fat ingestion. The biliary flow which is increased by a high fat meal enhances micelle formation and thus fat soluble compound absorption.

Phenothiazine may be precipitated as a highly insoluble compound if coffee or more especially tea is taken close to drug administration. Caffeine also decreases the effectiveness of antiepileptic drugs.

When digoxin is taken with food its peak blood levels are lower but persist for longer time. Very high peak levels which might precipitate arrhythmia are avoided.

Plenty of water should be taken with uricosurics to prevent renal precipitation and with cholestyramine and bulk-formers like methyl cellulose.

When milk is consumed with tetracycline, calcium present in milk forms an insoluble complex in the gut and there is no effect of tetracycline.

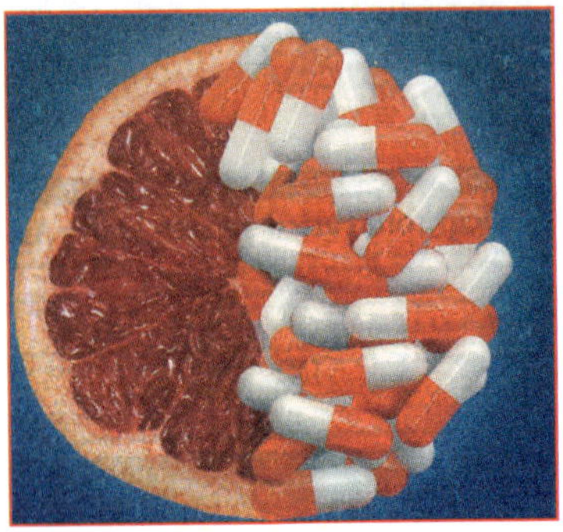

Fig. 11.8 Grapefruit juice-statins is one example of a potentially dangerous pairing.

Grape fruit affects absorption of cholesterol lowering statins. Statins are metabolized (broken down) in the intestines by an enzyme called cyp 3A which normally reduces the amount of drug that enters the blood stream. Grape fruit juice contains compounds called furanocoumarines that stop cyp 3A from doing its job. As a result more of the drug is absorbed making it more powerful that even making it toxic in some cases.

Table 11.5 shows effect of various foods and beverages on drug action.

Table 11.5 Effects of various foods and beverages on drug action

Food or beverage	*Drug*	*Effect*
Beverages		
Coffee, tea, and other caffeine-containing beverages	Theophylline	Increased intake may enhance drug side effects (nervousness, insomnia).
	Neuroleptic agents (fluphenazine, haloperidol)	Increased intake may result in wide variations in plasma concentrations of drug and may reduce its clinical effectiveness.
Citrus juices	Quinidine	Excessive intake may increase blood levels of drug (alkalinization of urine).
Fibre		
Bran	Digoxin	May reduce drug absorption.
Pectin	Acetaminophen	May depress rate of drug absorption.
Beverages		
Food in general	Aspirin	May decrease drug absorption and absorptive rate
	Antimicrobial agents (celphalexin, penicillin G, erythromycin stearate, penicillin V, tetracycline)	May reduce drug absorption
High-protein diet	Levodopa, methyldopa	Amino acids from dietary protein inhibit absorption of drugs
High-fat meal	Griseofulvin	Increases drug absorption
Milk and milk products	Tetracycline	Calcium inhibits drug absorption.
Vegetables		
Broccoli, greens, lettuce, cabbage.	Warfarin	Vegetables rich in vitamin K may inhibit hypoprothrombinemic response to oral anticoagulants.
Soyabeans, cabbage, turnips	Levothyroxine	Decrease the absorption of medication. Should be taken separately

Drug Effects on Nutrients

Drugs affect nutrient intake, functions, absorption, requirements and nutritional status.

Methotrexate inhibits folacin absorption. Phenytoin, non steroidal antiflammatory drugs cholesyramine, sulfasalazine, metformin and triainterene are associated with antifolate. Secondary malabsorption also occurs when phenytoin inhibits absorption of vitamin D which in turn inhibits calcium absorption.

Drugs may induce mineral depletion e.g., diuretics deplete potassium, penicillin causes zinc and calcium depletion and aspirin and salicylates may induce iron deficiency anaemia.

Drugs bind with food itself, for example, interactions between milk and cheese and certain antibiotics (tetracycline, penicillin and erythromycin) the calcium ions contained in these dairy products form insoluble complexes with these drugs.

Drugs induce anaemia due to under production of haemoglobin. Aplastic anaemia can occur when chloramphenical, gold or atabrine is taken. Iron deficiency can occur due to aspirin or corticosteroids. Folate deficiency can occur due to birth control pills or pyrimethamine. Pyridoxine deficiency can occur due to the consumption of isoniazid, a drug taken for the treatment of tuberculosis.

Table 11.6 Examples of drug-nutrient interactions

Drug	*Increased requirement*	*Potential mechanism*	*Deficiency symptoms*
Antacids (aluminum and magnesium hydroxides)	Phosphate	Formation of insoluble salts	Malaise, paresthesia, anorexia
Anticonvulsants (phenobarbital, phenytoin)	Vitamin D	Induction of hepatic microsomal enzymes resulting in inactive vitamin D metabolites	Rickets, osteomalacia
Oral contraceptives (norethindrone/ mestranol)	Folic acid	Inhibition of polyglutamic folate absorption	Megaloblastic anaemia
Antituberculous drugs (isoniazid, cycloserine)	Vitamin B_6	Excretion of pyridoxal hydrazone complex	Peripheral neuropathy
Anticoagulants (coumarin, warfarin)	Vitamin K	Inhibition of vitamin K recycling	Hypoprothrombinemia
Diuretics (benzothiadiazides)	Potassium	Enhancement of renal excretion	Hypokalemia

Interactions of Drugs and Nutrients

- Metabolic link with certain nutrients
  - —penicillium, sulphonamides, chloramphenical combine with serum albumin and may block normal carrier function of proteins.
  - —tetracycline may have chelating effects and bind bone calcium. Isoniazid inactivates vitamin B_6.
  - —chloramphenical may decrease protein synthesis.

- Sulphonamides may decrease intestinal bacterial synthesis of folic acid and vitamin K.
- Neomycin may decrease the absorption of carotene, vitamin B_{12}, glucose, cholesterol, vitamin B_1.
- In undernourished subjects like PEM, hypoalbuminemia reduces the binding capacity of drugs.
- Anatacids may affect the absorption of thiamine.
- Corticosteroids decrease glucose tolerance, decrease muscle protein and increase liver fat.
- Barbiturates and anticonvulsants may cause folic acid deficiency.
- Diuretics deplete potassium levels.
- Oral contraceptives lower folic acid and B_6.
- Anticonvulsant drug, dilatin, causes deficiency of vitamin D and folic acid.

By increasing stomach pH, antacids decrease the bioavailability of vitamin A, folate and thiamine. Sodium overload with development of congestive heart failure can result from intake of antacids containing sodium bicarbonate. Dietary phosphate combines with aluminium and magnesium hydroxide to form insoluble aluminium and magnesium phosphates which are excreted through the gastrointestinal tract. Effects of phosphate depletion include muscle weakness, malaise, parasthesia in the limbs, anorexia, hemolytic anaemia and convulsions.

The milk-alkali syndrome occurs as a complication of excessive ingestion of soluble, absorbable alkali and milk. It is characterised by hypercalcaemia, precipitation of calcium in the kidney and progressive renal insufficiency.

Certain drugs chelate minerals and render both the drug and mineral unavailable for absorption. The best known example of this effect is the chelation of divalent and trivalent cations by tetracyclines. This should not be taken within 2 hours of consuming foods containing calcium, magnesium, iron and zinc. The other drugs that interact with iron include the dopa drugs (methyl dopa, levodopa, carbidopa) ciprofloxin and penicillamine.

Foods containing tyramine and other phenylethylamines should be avoided by persons taking first-generation monoamine oxidase inhibitors. These include not only the antidepressants such as phenelzine, tranylcypromine and pargyline but also the cancer chemotherapeutic drug procabazine.

Dietary phenylethylamines, including tyramine are normally oxidatively deaminated via monoamine oxidase MAO in the gastrointestinal tract and in the liver. When a person is taking MAO inhibitors the phenyl-ethylamines are not deaminated by the gut and liver, so they are absorbed systemically and taken up in the brain. There they displace norepinephrine from storage vesicles. The resulting flood of norepinephrine released into synapses leads to severe acute hypertension with the potential for stroke or myocardial infarction. Attacks of hypertension of short duration are associated with headaches, palpitations, nausea and vomiting.

Fermented foods and protein-rich foods that have begun to spoil contain large amounts of phenylethyl amines. Those at greatest risk of a hypertensive crisis due to phenylethylamines are vegetarians having poor appetites and/or on weight reduction diet, because the phenylethylamines consumed are not diluted by other foods. Iron deficiency and consumption of yeast supplements may present increased risk. Liver, chicken, red wine and aged cheese contain tyramine.

Effect of Drugs on Food Intake and Absorption

Drugs can alter food intake by causing either a perversion or loss of appetite or an increase in appetite. Appetite suppression can be from development of food aversions because of nausea or food avoidance associated with a sore mouth or slow gastric emptying. Impaired oral function, dysgeusia or ageusia, gastric irritation and changes in gastric intestinal tract function (cytotoxic antineoplastic drugs) can affect the appetite.

Dextroamphetamine, which has been used to treat attention deficit hyperactivity disorder in children, causes growth retardation, partly due to appetite suppression.

Virtually every drug can cause nausea and vomiting, either centrally through activation of chemoreceptor trigger zone in the brain (cisplatin) or more commonly peripherally through irritation of the gastrointestinal tract. Digitalis preparations can cause severe wasting because nausea diminishes the desire for food.

Table 11.7 shows the effect of drugs on food intake and absorption.

Table 11.7 Effect of drugs on food intake and absorption

Drug	*Its effect*
I. Increased appetite	
• Antihistamines-Cypropheptadine hydrochloride	Increased in appetite and subsequent weight gain.
• Psychotropic drugs-Chloridiazepoxide hydrochloride, diaxepam, Chloropro-mazine hydrochloride	Hyperphagia (Tranquilisers may cause hypophagia in geriatric patients)
• Steroids	Nitrogen retention, increased lean body mass and weight gain.
• Anticonvulsants-Carbamazepine valproic acid	Increased appetite and subsequent weight gain
II. Decreased appetite	
• Amphetamines	Depress the appetite and loss of weight
• Insulin	Insulin induced hypoglycaemia may cause nausea, weakness and aversion to foods.
• Alcohol	Anorexia, reduced food intake and malnutrition.
• Methylphenidate: Calming effect	Decreases appetite
III. Taste sensitivity	
Chelating agent D-penicillamine used in heavy metal poisoning, rheumatoid arthritis or cystinuria.	Loss of taste (dysgeusia) caused by zinc deficiency
Diuretics; anticancer agents such as methotrexate and agents used to treat Parkinson's disease; antibiotics—ampicillin, griseofulvin, streptomycin; anticoagulant; antihistamine; antihypertensive agents; antiinfectious agent (metronidazole); cholesterol lowering agent (clofibrate); hypoglycaemic agent; sodium lauryl sulphate of tooth paste.	Loss of taste, smell can lead to overeating or may stop from eating.

IV. Nausea	
Cardiac glycosides digitalis; drugs used in cancer chemotherapy.	Nausea and vomiting Malnutrition and weight loss.
Bulking effects-Methyl cellulose	Decreased intake of food may interfere with absorption of nutrients.
Increased absorption-Cimetidine	Reduces gastric acid and volume output; improves absorption of protein and carbohydrate.
Decreased absorption-Colchicine (used in the treatment of gout)	Causes B_{12} deficiency
Alcohol abuse	Malabsorption of thiamin and folic acid.
Laxatives	Osteomalacia
V. Absorption of nutrients	
Cathartic agents and laxatives	Reduce transit time, cause steatorrhoea, loss of calcium and potassium
Cimetidine (for ulcer)	Inhibits gastric acid secretion Impairs absorption of vitamin B_{12} Reduces intrinsic factor
Cholestyramine (hypocholesterolmic agent)	Inhibit fat digestion and absorption, sequester bile acids.

Food aversions develop in more than half of all patients who undergo cancer chemotherapy. The aversions are usually transient, however, lasting several weeks to several months after cessation of therapy.

Drugs that cause a dry or sore mouth and make eating difficult or painful lead to avoidance of food intake. Patients may develop sore mouths, stomatitis (antineoplastics) gum inflammation and hyperplasia because of drugs. Dry mouth may be caused by drugs that decrease salivary flow including atropine and amantadine opioids.

Bezoars. Bezoars, balls of unabsorbed material residing in the stomach, may form from undissolved portions of drugs and from masses of food matter in particular plant fibre. Bezoars tend to form in patients with achlorhydria, in whom tablets may not dissolve and in those with poor gastric emptying. Drugs found in bezoars include sucralfate, cholestyramine, aluminium hydroxide gel and iron and antacid tablets. All of these preparations either form precipitates with foods or require stomach acid for dissolution or both. Bezoars may cause feelings of gastric fullness, pain, nausea, vomiting and gastric obstruction.

Physical interactions between drugs and enteral formulas in feeding tubes lead to sometimes subtle changes in the appearance of the formula with clouding, curdling, flocculation, phase separations and changes in formula's viscosity. Mixing the drug and formula are to be avoided.

The nutritional-pharmacological interactions may have considerable importance in vast segments of the population who undertake weight reducing regimens; in large numbers of post operative patients who receive glucose intravenously as a sole form of nourishment and in large numbers of patients whose disease processes (diabetes, atherosclerosis) require significant nutritional restrictions. Drug dosage may have to be changed to prevent toxic or non-therapeutic blood levels of the drug.

PERSONALISED NUTRITION

The concept of personalised medicine is now being extended to the field of nutrition.

Nutritional genomics is an umbrella term that encompasses two disciplines; nutrigenomics and nutrigenetics which play an important role in establishing personalised nutrition. Nutrigenomics focuses on how bioactive dietary components like macronutrients, micronutrients and antinutrients alter molecular processes such as DNA structure, gene expression and metabolism. These in turn may alter disease-initiation, development or progression.

Food/nutrient affects genome evolution and genome mutation hence susceptibility to a particular disease. A healthy diet provides ligands (special molecule) that 'turn on' disease fighting genes and 'turn off' those that cause disease. Personalised diet or nutrition should be suggested so that the disease causing genes will not 'turn on'.

Nutrigenetics investigates the mechanisms by which genetic variables affects the interaction between the bioactive dietary components and health and disease potential of individual persons.

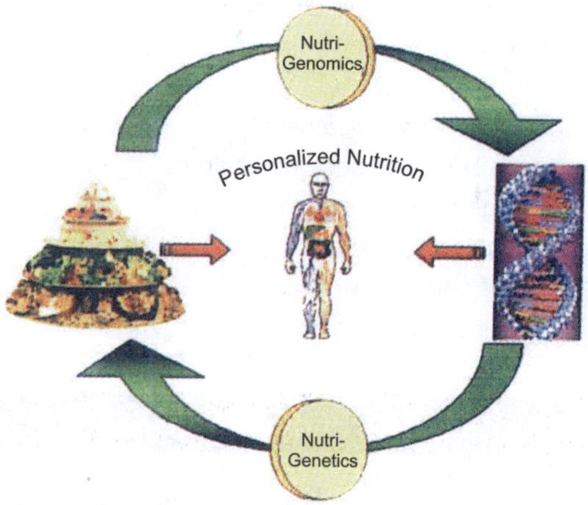

Fig. 11.9 Nutrigenomics and nutrigenetics are two sides of the coin. For the target goal of personalized nutrition to be realized, the effects of diet on whole-body metabolism (*i.e.*, genes, proteins, and metabolites) and the influence of genotype on nutritionally related disease must be considered.

Source: Mutch David M. *et al.*, Nutrigenomics and nutrigenetics: the emerging faces of Nutrition FASEB Journal, 19, 2005.

Genes affect nutrient absorption nutrient utilisation and nutrient requirement. Variants in genes determine how nutrients are metabolized and utilised. This field is the study known as nutrigenetics. Personalised nutrition is required as genetic variation determines the nutrient requirement.

Individual genetic variation can influence how nutrients are assimilated, metabolised, stored and excreted by the body. The same tools and methods used in pharmacogenomics (SNP - single nucleotide polymer prism analysis, gene expression profiling, proteomics, metabolomics and bioinformatics) are being used to examine an individual's response to his or her nutritional environment.

In the near future, quick low cost point-of-care tests will be available to assist patients and physicians to achieve, manage and prolong health through dietary invention. The desired outcome of nutrigenomics is the use of personalised diets to delay the onset of disease and optimise and maintain human health.

SUGGESTED READINGS

- Galland Leo, Diet and inflammation, Nutrition in clinical practice, 2010, **25.**
- Ramakrishna S. 2014 Probiotics in prevention of lifestyle disorders. Elsevier India.
- Shobana S., *et al.*, "Glycaemic Index of Three Indian Rice Varieties." International Journal of Sciences and Nutrition 2011.
- Koshria G. Hemant and B. Sesikeran 2014, The regulatory scene: standardising probiotics in India, Phobiotics in prevention of lifestyle disorders, Elesevier, India.

QUESTIONS

1. Define glycaemic index and glycaemic load. Discuss the factors affecting glycaemic index.
2. Explain the role of dietary supplements in the health of an individual.
3. Bring the importance of prebiotics and probiotics.
4. Explain the relationship between inflammation and diet.
5. What are symbiotics?
6. How is stevia is superior to other sweetness?
7. Explain the effect of food on the absorption of drugs.
8. Discuss the effect of drugs on nutrients.
9. Explain the effect of drugs on appetite.
10. Explain the importance of personalised nutrition.
11. Explain the factors affecting gut microbiome.

TOPIC FOR DISCUSSION

- Dietary supplements – bane or boon?

12

Therapeutic Diets

A therapeutic diet is quantitative/qualitative modified version of a basic nutritious diet which has been tailored to suit the changing nutritional needs of a patient/disease condition. Therapeutic nutrition begins with the normal diet. Advantages of using normal diet as the basis for therapeutic diets are:

- It emphasises the similarity of psychologic and social needs of those who are ill.
- Food preparation is simplified when the modified diet is based upon the normal diet of the family.
- It is useful in finding out the effects of addition or omission of certain foods, for example, if vegetables are restricted, vitamin A and C deficiency can occur.

The normal diet may be modified to provide change in consistency as in fluid and soft diets; to increase or decrease the energy value, to include greater or lesser amounts of one or more nutrients, for example, high protein, low sodium, etc.; to increase or decrease bulk-high and low fibre diets and to provide foods bland in flavour.

While planning meals for a patient, his economic status, his food preference, his occupation and time of meals, the possible duration of the disease and the patient's tolerance should also be considered.

It requires a recognition of the need for dietary supplements such as vitamin and mineral concentrates when the nature of diet itself imposes severe restrictions, the patient's appetite is poor, or absorption and utilization are impaired so that the diet cannot meet the needs of optimum nutrition.

Recommended Dietary Allowances is not applicable to undernourished or malnourished individuals or for those suffering from diseases or infective morbidity.

Diet history should serve as the basis for planning each diet. The dietary history will reveal the patient's past habits of eating with respect to dietary adequacy, likes and dislikes, meal hours, where meals are eaten, budgetary problems, ability to obtain and prepare foods. The likes and dislikes of patients are respected because food habits are deep-seated and it is not possible to change them overnight. It requires considerable encouragement and understanding on the part of the doctor-nurse-dietitian team to bring about important changes in the diet.

IMMUNO NUTRITION

Immune function is depressed in seriously ill patients and they are susceptible to infections particularly nosocomial infections.

The three major factors responsible are

- Severe underlying disease, multiple illnesses, malnutrition, extremes of age and immuno suppressing drugs.
- Invasive medical devices *e.g.*, urinary tract catheters.
- Infected crowded patients.

The potential to modulate the activity of the immune system by interventions with specific nutrients is termed immuno nutrition.

The benefits of nutrition support in general include improved wound healing, a decreased catabolic response to injury, enhanced immune system function and improved clinical out comes including a reduction in complication rates and length of stay in hospital.

The main goals of nutrition support of severely ill patients are to protect lean body mass and to preserve immune function.

Immuno nutrition refers to the addition of specific nutrients in greater than normal concentrations to modulate immune function, and thus improve clinical function. The immuno nutrients comprise of the following:

Arginine: This conditionally essential amino acid plays a pivotal role in maintaining body homeostasis and is prescribed when stress occurs. Arginine also contributes to immunity by increasing macrophage phagocytic activity, neutrophil production by reactive oxygen species and involvement in cell mediated immunity. Arginine is a source of nitrogen in nitric oxide. It stimulates secretion of anabolic hormones and enhances wound healing and cellular immunity but not with severe sepsis. Arginine supplementation may increase production of nitric oxide that may in turn promote vasodilation and hypotension. Arginine supplementation may be beneficial in patients with mild sepsis.

Benefits of arginine supplementation include, decreased production of inflammatory mediators at the site of infection, increased albumin and liver protein synthesis.

Since arginine is a component of immune enhancing enteral products, the evidence-based guidelines address the use of these products rather than arginine alone.

Purine nucleotides: These are precursors for RNA and DNA. Deficiency of purine nucleotides is associated with immune suppression and supplementation improves cell-mediated immunity.

Glutamine: It is a nonessential amino acid present in the body. This becomes conditionally essential in the presence of severe stress and multiple organ failure. It is a major oxidative substrate and enhances the immune function essential in stressed states.

During sepsis, glutamine is released at an accelerated rate from skeletal muscle for use by cells, resulting in low muscle and plasma concentrations. Mortality rate is inversely correlated with glutamine concentrations. Glutamine supplementation may reduce mortality in septic patients by preventing multiple organ dysfunction syndrome and reduce mortality. Consequently glutamine may preserve organ and cellular metabolic functions and modulate inflammation.

It is a substrate for glutathione synthesis. Glutamine supplementation can prevent or ameliorate the gastrointestinal mucosal atrophy seen in prolonged states of parenteral nutrition.

Glutamine also helps the gastrointestinal mucosa heal more promptly after damage by either radiotherapy or chemotherapy.

Clinical trials of glutamine supplementation in critical illness, surgical stress and cancer have shown benefit with regard to mortality, length of stay in hospital and infectious morbidity.

American Society for Parenteral and Enteral Nutrition, ASPEN and Society of Critical Care Medicine, SCCM recommend use of enteral glutamine for critically ill, burn and trauma patients.

Whey proteins has been shown to stimulate cell mediated and humoral immunity to improve the body's nutritional status in stressed individuals. Whey proteins have an antioxidant role by increasing tissue glutathione and inhibits the growth of several types of tumours.

Commercial formulations containing immuno nutrition are now available.

ROUTINE HOSPITAL DIETS

Clear-fluid Diet

Whenever an acute illness or surgery produces a marked intolerance for food as may be evident by nausea, vomiting, anorexia, distention and diarrhoea, it is advisable to restrict the intake of food.

Clear fluid diet is suggested in the following conditions:

- In acute infections before diagnosis.
- In acute inflammatory conditions of the intestinal tract.
- Following operations upon the colon or rectum when it is desirable to prevent evacuation from the bowel.
- To relieve thirst.
- To supply the tissues with water.
- To add in the removal of gas.

This diet is made up of clear liquids that leave no residue, and it is non-gas forming, non-irritating and non-stimulating to peristalitic action. Milk is not suggested in clear fluid diet. This diet is entirely inadequate from a nutritional standpoint since it is deficient in protein, minerals, vitamins, and calories. It should not be continued for more than 24 to 48 hours. The amount of fluid is usually restricted to 30 to 60 ml per hour at first, with gradually increasing amounts being given as the patient's tolerance improves. This diet gives 300 kcal and no protein.

This diet can meet the requirement of fluids and some minerals. It can be given in 1 to 2 hour intervals.

Full-fluid Diet

This diet bridges the gap between the clear fluid and soft diet. It is used following operations, in acute gastritis, acute infections and in diarrhoea. This diet is also suggested when milk is permitted and for patients not requiring special diet but too ill to eat solid or semisolid foods.

In this diet, foods which are liquid or which readily become liquid on reaching the stomach are given. This diet may be made entirely adequate and may be used over an extended time without fear of developing deficiencies, provided it is carefully planned. This diet is given at 2-4 hour intervals. This diet gives 1200 kcal and 35 g of protein.

Soft Diet

This diet is one of the most frequently used routine diets; many hospital patients are placed on this until a diagnosis is made. It bridges the gap between acute illness and convalescence. It may be used in acute infections, following surgery, and for patients who are unable to chew. The soft diet is made up of simple, easily digested food and contains no harsh fibre, low in fat and no rich highly seasoned food. It is nutritionally adequate when planned on the basis of normal diet. Patients with dental problems are given mechanically soft diet. It is often modified further for certain pathologic conditions as bland and low residue diets. In this diet, three meals with intermediate feedings should be given. This diet gives 1500 kcal and 35-40 g of protein. Light diet is given before regular diet.

Regular Normal Diet

It is most frequently used in all hospitals. It is used for ambulatory and bed patients whose conditions does not necessitate a special diet of one of the routine diets. Many special diets progress ultimately to a regular diet.

Table 12.1 gives contents allowed in clear fluid, full-fluid and soft diets.

Table 12.1 Contents of clear fluid, full fluid and soft diets

Types of food	*Foods allowed*		
	Clear-fluid	*Full-fluid*	*Soft diet*
Cereals	Barley water	Gruels, porridges kanji, ragi malt	Refined, finely ground whole grain
Pulses	Dal water	Dal soups, dal payasam	All dals
Vegetables and Fruits	Clear strained fruit juice	Strained juices, cooked and pureed fruits	Juices, pureed, cooked and mashed, baked, ripe banana
Milk	Whey water	Milk and milk beverages, milk shakes, lassi	Milk and milk products, cheese, fine cream
Fats and oils	—	Butter, oil and cream	Butter, oil, cream, margarine
Meat and fish	—	—	All except pork, minced fish poultry
Eggs	Egg white well beaten in fruit juices	Only in beverages	All except fried
Sugar and jaggery	Sugar or glucose	Sugar, jaggery and glucose	All
Nuts and oil seeds	None	None	None
Beverages	Tea, coffee (without milk) non-carbonated beverages, coconut water,	Tea, coffee, egg, non-carbonated beverages	All
Soups	Fat free broth,	Strained	All
Desserts	Plain gelatin	Custards, ice cream plain gelatin	Custards, kheer, puddings

The regular hospital diet is simple in character and preparation. This diet is easily digested. It gives maximum nourishment with minimum effort to the body. The diet is well balanced, adequate in nutritional value and attractively served to stimulate a possible poor appetite. This diet gives 1800–2000 kcal and 42–45 g of protein.

NUTRITION SUPPORT SERVICE

Nutrition support does not mean merely giving protein, calories and minerals but providing substrates for the biological process of healing. It involves screening all patients on arrival—barring those with simple problems—for malnutrition underlying their disease, planning therapy and monitoring progress, using standard guidelines.

Nutritional support needed in the following conditions

- A previously well nourished patient with current or anticipated complications of multi organ dysfunction, infection, trauma or cancer.
- One who has not consumed sufficient nutrition for 5–7 days prior to admission.
- A patient found to be malnourished by standard nutritional assessment on admission.

The ideal team for providing nutrition support service is headed by a physician, who has a special interest in nutrition. The co-director of the team is always a dietitian with a clinical dietitian and a food service dietitian as assistants. The role of clinical dietitian is to take charge of nutritional assessment, enteral and parenteral feeding, cholesterol control, and diabetes education. The food services dietitian oversees the food services manager and others who deliver the diet. Other members of the team are a part-time nurse, who maintains peripheral and central vein catheters and feeding tubes and a pharmacist, especially at centres where total parenteral nutrition solutions are prepared.

SPECIAL FEEDING METHODS

Enteral Nutrition

Enteral nutrition can be provided either orally or by tube feeding. By definition enteral means 'within or by the way of the gastrointestinal tract'. Enteral nutrition is given to an individual who has functioning gut and is unable or unwilling to achieve adequate oral intake. If the gut is functioning, it should be used. Enteral feeding retains epithelial structure and function of GI tract. It also increases mucosal immunity. In practice enteral nutrition is generally considered as tube feeding.

Enteral infusion of nutrients prevents adverse structural and functional alterations of the gut barrier induced by injury, increases epithelial proliferation, maintains mucosal integrity, decreases gut permeability improves gut blood flow and improves local and systemic immune responsiveness. There is an increase in immunoglobulin A secretion, maintenance of the gut associated lymphoid tissue, improved mucous secretion, decreased bacterial translocation increased tropic hormone secretion and decreased infection. Apoptosis occurs in many clinical conditions that include ischaemia reperfusion injury caused by free radicals. Early enteral feeding may also decrease apoptosis in the gut.

Providing even small amounts of enteral nutrition as much as the patients can tolerate decreases the gut mucosal atrophy. "If the gut works, use it".

Oral feeding is the best for the nourishment of a patient. But in the following conditions it is not possible to give the feeding orally and tube feeding or partenteral feeding is resorted.

- Those who cannot swallow due to paralysis of the muscles of swallowing (diptheria, poliomyelitis) or cancer of the oral cavity or larynx.
- Those who cannot be persuaded to eat.
- Those with persistent anorexia requiring forced feeding.
- Semiconscious or unconscious patients.
- Severe malabsorption requiring administration of unpalatable formula.
- Short bowel syndrome.
- Those who are undernourished or at risk of becoming so.
- Those who cannot digest and absorb.
- Post surgery.
- Patients with neurological and renal disorders and those with fevers or diabetes.
- Babies with very low birth weight.
- Severe diarrhoea.

Oral Supplements

Commercially available supplementary sip feeds are used in patients who can drink but in whom appetite is impaired. These feeds typically provide 200 kcal and 2 g of nitrogen in each 200 ml carton. There is some evidence to suggest that sip feeds taken in the pre-operative period may enhance post-operative recovery and reduce hospital stay.

Tube Feeding

Figure 12.1 shows enteral tube placement.

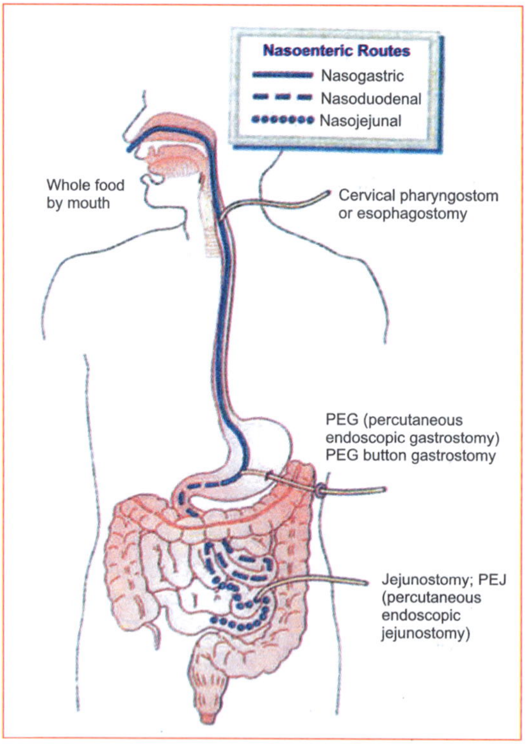

Fig. 12.1 Enteral tube placement

Source: Mahan L. Kathleen and Sylvia Escotl-stump, 2000, Krause's Food, Nutrition & Diet therapy, W.B. Saunders Company, Philadelphia.

Tube feeding is done by passing a tube into the stomach or duodenum through the nose which is called nasogastric feeding or directly by surgical operation known as gastrostomy and jejunostomy feeding. Short term (3-4 weeks) feedings usually are administered via nasogastric, nasoduodenal or nasojejunal tubes. For long term feedings, a gastrostomy or jejunostomy is usually indicated.

In order to minimise the risks of aspiration, tubes should not be placed in the stomach unless there is normal gastric emptying and an intact gag reflex and if possible, nasoenteric rather than nasogastric feeding tubes should be employed. This may be especially valuable in post operative and critically ill patients in whom gastric motility is impaired.

A satisfactory tube feeding must be

- nutritionally adequate
- well tolerated by patient so that vomiting is not induced
- easily digested with no unfavourable reactions such as distension, diarrhoea or constipation
- easily prepared and
- inexpensive.

Nutrient guidelines are the same for enteral and parenteral nutrition.

Proteins: Maintenance dose 1g/kg/d
In stress 2g/kg/d
Increasing protein in ICU decreases mortality.

Non protein calories: To start with 20–25 kcal/kg/d with gradual increase to 30–35 kcal/kg/d. Upto 50 per cent caloric intake may be given as fat. Less emphasis on calories more on proteins.

Electrolytes: Standard requirements plus replacement for losses.

Types of Food

Many enteral formulas contain fructooligo saccharides. FOS are rapidly fermented by intestinal bacteria that produce short chain fatty acids which stimulate water and electrolyte absorption and may help treat diarrhoea. FOS are preferred like substrate for *bifido* bacteria but not used by potentially pathogenic *clostridia* bacteria. Thus FOS help to maintain and restore the balance of healthful gutflora.

Tube fed patients with constipation or diarrhoea who are known to have otherwise healthful gastrointestinal tract can be given fibre containing enteral formula, especially for long term enteral feeding.

Natural liquid foods: Foods like whole or skim milk, eggs and some form of carbohydrate such as cooked strained cereals, sugar or molasses can be given. Vegetable oil or cream and non fat dry milk are also incorporated to increase the calorie and protein levels respectively. Supplements can be added to different foods to increase the nutritive value. Many convalescent patients who are often depressed and have little appetite benefit from appetising foods of high nutrient density.

Blenderised feeding: In this the food items are cooked and blended to make thin liquid which can pass through nasogastric tube.

- Water added to make the volume to 1500 ml.
- Gives 1500 calories.
- Each ml provides one calorie.
- Gives 50 g protein.
- Cost is no more than an average meal in hospital.
- Contains probiotics and prebiotics.

Blenderised feeding can also be prepared by using starch, milk, skim milk powder, egg, soya flour, refined oil, salt and curd. Blenderised tube feedings are well tolerated and are only infrequently associated with diarrhoea. They are less expensive than commercial formulas.

Kitchen prepared blenderized feedings are to be given through large bore feeding tubes. Access to a hospital kitchen at all times is difficult and there is a high risk of bacterial contamination when food is stored. Calculation of calorie and protein intake may not be accurate.

Blenderised tube feeding is used for adults in home enternal nutrition patients.

Elemental diets: Normal foods may be replaced by preparation of protein or amino acids, fats and carbohydrates in easily assimilable forms. Such preparations are known as elemental diets. For tube feeding commercially supplied polymeric mixtures can also be used.

Semi-elemental diets are peptide based formulas also contain free amino acids. Carbohydrates are usually hydrolysed. The fat content is very low. Some formulas contain medium chain triglycerides and short chain fatty acids. These together with small peptides allow for ease of absorption. A small peptide based diet may be beneficial in patients with short bowel syndrome. Semielemental diet is less expensive than TPN. Peptide based enteral diets are associated with better hepatic protein response and cause less diarrhoea compared to intact proteins.

Commercial preparations possess the advantage of convenience, constant composition, presterilisation, minimal preparation time and ease of administration. The disadvantages are high cost and unpleasant taste and sometime high osmolarity. Elemental diets though can be given orally, palatability may be a problem and tube feeding can be resorted. Though elemental diets are better tolerated the human gut is capable of absorbing complex moieties as well. Patients with pancreatic insufficiency, malabsorption or massive bowel resection may require an elemental formula. Newer feeding formulations include glutamine and fibre to optimise intestinal nutrition. Some may contain immuno stimulatory mixture of amino acids such as arginine and fish oils.

Special hepatic formulas are high in branch chain amino acids and low in aromatic amino acids. Renal failure formulas are calorie dense 2 kcal/ml and low in K, P, and Mg.

Commercial preparations are available in liquid or powder form. Generally feedings provide 1 kcal/ml.

Feeding Requirements

A concentration of about 1 kcal per millilitre is satisfactory. Lesser concentration increases the volume which must be given to meet the nutrient and energy needs. A concentration of 1.5 kcal/ml is given for patients with increased caloric needs or patients with fluid restrictions. Greater concentration is more likely to produce diarrhoea and may be too thick to pass through the nasogastric tube.

There are four different infusion techniques:

1. Continuous method is to feed via an infusion pump or gravity flow 50 ml/hr.
2. Cyclic method has off and on periods in 24 hrs e.g., 8 hrs on and 16 hrs off.

3. Interrupted method is a regular period of interruption in 24 hrs e.g., 4 hrs on and 4 hrs off.
4. Bolus method where large volumes are given in a short time e.g., 200cc in a minimum of 10 min. time.

Careful monitoring is needed to see that the patient is in fluid balance.

Table 12.2 Feeding requirements in tube feeding

Nutrient	*Amount*
Fluids	30 ml/kg
Energy	25–45 kcal/kg
Protein	1–2.5g/kg
Non Protein calories	
Carbohydrate: fat (in critical illness)	50 : 50
Carbohydrate: fat (in noncritical illness)	60 : 40

Vitamins and minerals supplementation should be given.

Parenteral Nutrition

In parenteral nutrition, a sterile nutrient dense solution is infused intravenously by a peripheral or a central venous access, entirely bypassing the digestive tract. Parenteral nutrition is for those patients who are not capable of digesting and absorbing nutrients and who are severely malnourished and for catabolic patients. Parenteral nutrition reduces mortality.

Parenteral nutrition is a life saving modality in critically ill patients. Undernourished patients scheduled for high risk surgeries can benefit from parenteral nutrition with lower complication rates and shorter hospital stays. Reducing the intake of total calories to a moderate level may improve outcome in mechanically ventilated ICU patients. Providing high protein hypo caloric parenteral nutrition can minimize the risk of overfeeding in obese critically ill patients and facilitate good glucose control in patients with diabetes.

Peripheral Parenteral Nutrition is a means of nutrition support in which the parenteral solution is administered directly into the peripheral vein. PPN is indicated for anticipated short-term use (less than 10 days) because PPN usually does not meet all the nutritional needs of the patient (1000–1500 kcal/day). Central venous access is used when higher concentration solutions to be administered for longer period.

Total Parenteral Nutrition

Total Parenteral Nutrition is defined as provision of all nutrients essential for normal homeostasis and growth in the required amounts through parenteral route, that is, directly into a vein. The same process is called hyperalimentation when at least 150 per cent of daily requirements are provided to produce a positive nitrogen balance for weight gain.

Partial parenteral nutrition provides 30–50 per cent of daily nutrients while the rest is provided through enteral route.

Table 12.3 **Parenteral nutrition support order**

Type of Line	*Rate*	*Total Volume*	*Administration*
☐ CVC ☐ PICC ☐ Peripheral	___ mL/hour	___ mL/day	☐ Continuous ☐ Cyclic over__________ hours

Custom Formulas

☐ *Central Standard 2-in-1 Formula*	☐ *Central Standard 3-in-1 Formula*	☐ *Central High Nitrogen 3-in-1 Formula*	☐ *Central Non-standard Formula Dose Range Guidelines*	☐ *Peripheral 3-in-1 Formula*
50g Amino Acids	50g Amino Acids	75 g Amino Acids	Amino Acids ___g (1.2–1.5 g/kg)	50g Amino Acids
250g Dextrose	210g Dextrose	210g Dextrose	Dextrose___g (4–7 g/kg)	50g Dextrose
	40g IV fat emulsion	40g IV fat emulation	IV fat emulsion ___ g (1g / kg)	60g IV fat emulsion
1050 Kcals	1300 Kcals	1400 Kcals	Sterile water to make total volume	970 kcals
Per 1000 mL	Per 1000 mL	Per 1000 mL		Per 1000 mL

Source: Baylor Healthcare System US.

Cancer patients comprise the largest percentage of patients receiving long-term TPN. It is recommended for cancers which associates malnutrition. Preoperative and postoperative parenteral nutrition is recommended for severely malnourished patients. It is given in short-bowel syndrome, hepatic disease and pancreatitis. This nutrition support should be initiated in patients who are not expected to resume oral feeding for 7 days, for example during renal failure, acquired immuno deficiency syndrome and respiratory failure.

TPN includes

- glucose—a minimum of 100 g per day is given to prevent protein catabolism.
- emulsified fat—provide essential fatty acids and calories.
- crystalline amino acids—commercial amino acids are available in concentrations 3.5, 5.5, 7.5, 8.5, 10, 11 and 15%.
- vitamins including B_{12}, folic acid and vitamin K.
- electrolytes: sodium, chlorine, phosphorus, potassium, calcium and magnesium.
- trace elements: zinc, copper, chromium, manganese and iodine.
- water.

Polyols have low glycaemic response. They give 2.4 kcal/g. For this reason sorbitol and xylitol are often applied in parenteral nutrition to provide more controllable carbohydrate energy source compared to glucose. Due to reduced digestibility of polyols, the intake should be restricted to 40–50 g/day for adults and 30 g/day for children. Adequate non-protein calories 150 NPC/g of nitrogen are provided in the programme so that aminoacids are used for protein synthesis. TPN is indicated for (greater than 7–10 days) anticipated long-term use. TPN is also used as a vehicle for drug delivery.

The selection of parenteral nutrition solution should be determined by patient's tolerance to glucose (diabetes), amino acids (renal and hepatic disease) and fat (critical illness or sepsis).

Total Parenteral Nutrition for Children

Table 12.4 Energy requirements of children

Age	*Dietary reference intake (DRI)(kcal/kg)*	*Basal Energy, Expenditure (BEE) kcal/kg*
0–3 months	102	54
4–6 months	82	54
7–12 months	80	51
13–35 months	82	56
3 years	85	57
4 years	70	47
5–6 years	65	47
7–8 years	60	47

Table 12.5 Protein requirements of children

Age	*Dietary reference intake DRI (g/kg/day)*	*Paediatric ICU (g/kg/day)*
0–6 months	1.52	2–3
7–12 months	1.2	2–3
13–23 months	1.05	2–3
2–3 years	1.05	1.5–2
4–13 years	0.95	1.5–2
14–18 years	0.85	1.5

Fluid Requirements: Holliday segar formula;

- 0–10 kg = 100 ml/kg/day
- 10–20 kg = 1000 ml + 50 ml for each kg > 10 kg.
- >20 kg = 1500 ml + 20 ml for each kg > 20.

Table 12.6 Glucose infusion rate (GIR) / dextrose guidelines

Age	*Initiate*	*Advance*	*Maximum*
Below one year	6–9 mg/kg/mins	1–2 mg/kg/mins	Goal 10–12 mg/kg/mins 14 mg/kg/mins
1–10 years	1–2 mg/kg/mins	1–2mg/kg/mins	8–10 mg/kg/mins
>10 years	1–2 mg/kg/mins	1–2 mg/kg/mins	5–6 mg/kg/mins

Table 12.7 Parenteral amino acid guidelines

Age	*Initiate*	*Advance*	*Maximum*
< year	1–2 g/kg/day	1 g/kg/day	4 g/kg/day
1–10 years	1–2 g/kg/day	1 g/kg/day	1.5–3 g/kg/day
> 10 years	1–2 g/kg/day	1 g/kg/day	0.8–2.5 g/kg/day

Parenteral Lipids:

- Below one year = 3 g/kg/day
- 1–10 years = 2–3 g/kg/day
- > 10 years = 1–2.5 g/kg/day

Table 12.8 PN–electrolyte dosing guidelines

Electrolyte	*Preterm neonates*	*Infants/Children*	*Adolescents/ Children 0.50 kg*
Na^+	2–5 mEq/kg	2–5 mEq/kg	1–2 mEq/kg
K^+	2–4 mEq/kg	2–4 mEq/kg	1–2 mEq/kg
Ca^{2+}	2–4 mEq/kg	0.5–4 mEq/kg	10–20 mEq/day
Phos	1–2 mmol/kg	0.5–2 mmol/kg	10–40 mmol/day
Mg^{2+}	0.3–0.5 mEq/kg	0.3–0.5 mEq/kg	10–30 mEq/day

Source: Tables 12.4 to 12.8 cited from Krishnamurthy, P. Parenteral Nutrition Calculation in PICU, Nutrition Management in Surgery, An Inter-Professional Approach, Seminar. Madras Medical Mission, Chennai 2017.

Total Parenteral Nutrition for Adults

TPN solution is given 100 ml per hour. For 24 hours, 2400 ml is given.

Calories from carbohydrates

TPN solution contains 30% dextrose	
That is, 100 ml contains 30 g	
800 ml contains	240 g
1 g of dextrose in monohydrate form gives	3.4 × 240
∴ 240 g of dextrose gives	= 816 kcal

Calories from Protein

TPN solution contains 10% amino acids with electrolytes	
That is, 100 ml contains 10 g	
800 ml contains	10 × 8 = 80 g
1 g of amino acid gives	4 kcal
80 g of amino acid gives	= 4 × 80 = 320 kcal

Calories from Fat

Minimum requirement of fat is 50 g	
1 ml of 20% fat emulsion gives	= 2 kcal
400 ml of 20% fat emulsion	2.0 × 400
(to run over 6 hours)	= 800 kcal
Total calories	
Calories from carbohydrate	816
Calories from protein	320
Calories from fat	800
	1936 kcal

Total calories given in TPN solution is 1936 kcal.

Adult requirements of minerals and vitamins are added to TPN solution.

Patient monitoring while on TPN

Daily weight, weekly skinfold thickness and midarm circumference are monitored. Biochemical indices like blood glucose, electrolytes, acid base balance, creatinine, haemoglobin and ammonia are monitored.

Complications of TPN

Enternal nutrition maintains intestinal epithelium, whereas parenteral nutrition causes villous atrophy.

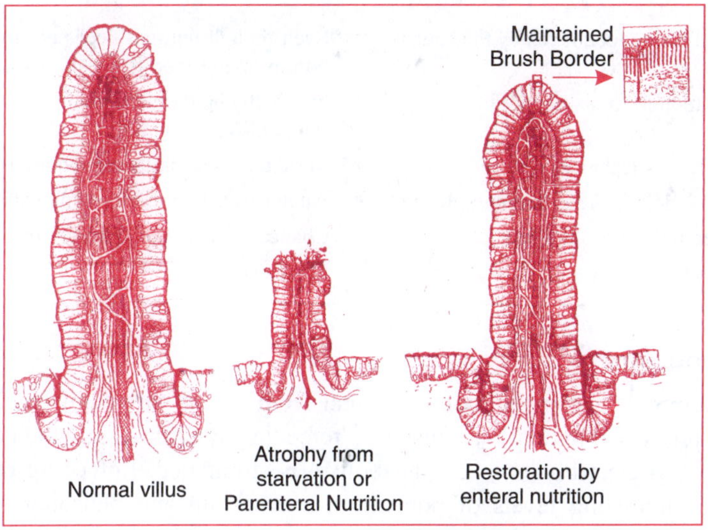

Fig. 12.2 **Enteral nutrition maintains and restores intestinal epithelium, whereas starvation or parenteral nutrition causes villous atrophy. Even short period of starvation diminish the function of mucosa of the ileum and colon making it permeable to toxins and bacteria.**

Source: Bessey Q. Palmer, Third National Conference on critical care and ISPEN annual conference and workshop, 1997.

Catheter related cardiac arrhythmias, air embolus, thrombosis, perforation and sepsis can occur. Metabolic complications like hyperglycaemia, osmotic diuresis, azotaemia (nitrogen in blood), electrolyte disturbance, acid base change and fatty degeneration of liver can also occur. In addition, nutritional complications like loss of lean body weight, bone demineralisation vitamin deficiency, vitamin toxicity, increase in fat and water, essential fatty acid deficiency and trace metal deficiency can also occur.

Derick and Ruberg summarised that **TPN is given to all patients who cannot eat, should not eat, will not eat and cannot eat enough**.

Table 12.9 Differences between enteral and parenteral feeding

Enteral	*Parenteral*
• Oral feeding directly or through nasogastric tube or through gastrostomy or jejunostomy	• Feeding through peripheral or central vein
• If oral feeding is not possible, tube feeding is given	• If enternal feeding is not possible, parenteral feeding is given
• Food is given in modified form	• Nutrients are directly absorbed into the vein
• The normal health of intenstinal mucosa is well maintained	• Atrophy of the intestinal mucosa may take place
• Satisfaction of taking food is felt by the patients	• Even though nutrient needs are fulfilled, satisfaction of taking food is not felt by the patient
• Biochemical monitoring is required	• Frequently biochemical monitoring and maintaining standards are essential
• Comparatively less technical skill required	• More technical skills are required
• Calculation of food intake is less complicated	• All nutrients in prescribed amounts must be present
• Chances of complications are less	• Chances of complications are more
• Less expensive	• More expensive

Refeeding Syndrome

Refeeding syndrome is a complication of enteral feeding and parenteral feeding. Refeeding of severely malnourished patient may result in 'refeeding syndrome' in which there are acute intracellular shift of electrolytes as cell anabolism is stimulated. Refeeding can cause acute decrease in the circulating levels of potassium, magnesium and phosphorus. Hence these electrolytes should be monitored and replaced as needed to maintain normal circulating levels by supplementation.

Clinical symptoms include weakness, convulsions, respiratory failure, cardiac decompensation and death. This may be the result of aggressive nutrition support in a malnourished patient.

Refeeding syndrome complications can be avoided by anticipating the problem and initially feeding only 20–30 kcal/kg, checking initial serum levels of potassium, magnesium and phosphate. Supplementation with vitamins specially thiamine is given. Fluid overload and congestive failure need to be monitored.

Special feeding methods should be avoided for three reasons

- Supplementary, tube and intravenous feeding are each more expensive than normal feeding. So they should not be used when the patient can get adequate nourishment from an appetising diet, well served and with coaxing to eat it.
- Tube and intravenous feeding inevitably cause inconvenience and some discomfort to a patient.
- Although tube feeding is safe, at least in comparison with a prescription for most drugs, parenteral nutrition carries complications.

If there is not enough hemodynamic stability and no reasonably good tissue perfusion the administered nutrients will not be utilized and may result in septic and metabolic complications.

Role of dietician

The dietician should be well versed in the principles of artificial nutritional support, learn how to detect problems in the early stages, modify the enteral and parenteral formulas as needed and be responsible for the overall metabolic needs of the patients.

MALNUTRITION IN HOSPITALISED PATIENTS

Malnutrition in hospitals remains a serious issue. It occurs worldwide and affects patients of all ages.

Malnutrition may result in increased morbidity such as higher infection rates, increased mortality, longer length of hospital stays and increased costs.

Causes

Many patients are already malnourished at the point of admission, while others become malnourished during their hospital stay. Aetiology includes alterations in the intake, digestion absorption and/or metabolism of food. Risks include GI disorders, chronic disease, malignancies, lower socioeconomics status, psychological disorders, alcohol and drug abuse, older age and lower levels of education.

The diseases that prevent oral food intake, such as oral cancer, tumours or strictures in the throat or esophagus, stroke and degenerative neurologic disorders that result in dysphagia. Trauma patients and others who are ventilator dependent rely on the timely initiation of nutrition support. Conditions such as chronic obstructive pulmonary disease, chronic infections and cancer can result in increased metabolic demand and weight loss due to cachexia and poor oral intake.

Patients with GI disorders are among those who are most prone to developing malnutrition. Surgical resections of the GI tract for cancer or Crohn's disease can result in severe maldisgestion and malabsorption of nutrients as can chronic digestive disorders such as cystic fibrosis. Chronic liver disease contribute to poor nutrient digestion, absorption reduced anabolisum and increased catabolism. Patients with pancreatitis often present with malnutrition.

Even for patients who can eat orally, nutritional intake often decreases during hospitalization. Patients are required to undergo many tests and procedures. Delays or the need for several procedures result in prolonged periods without nutrition. Patients' appetite usually decrease during illness due to pain, nausea, weakness and altered mood or mental status and they can become dissatisfied with repetitive menu cycles, dietary restrictions and the food which may not be the type they order.

Those who have been eating poorly are unlikely to start eating better unless the underlying problem has been corrected.

Treatment

Malnutrition is closely associated with poor out comes. Hence the patient must be fed to preserve lean body mass, aid in recovery and healing, protect immune function and maintain strength and energy.

For patients who can eat orally, between meal snacks and liquid nutritional supplements can be helpful. Patients who are either unable or expected to be unable to take sufficient oral nutrition for 7 to 14 days are candidates for nutrition support. Enteral nutrition should be used if the GI tract is functional and parenteral nutrition is necessary in patients with prolonged ileus, complete bowel obstruction, bowel perforation, mesenteric ischaemia, severe GI bleeding or short bowel syndrome with insufficient absorptive capacity.

Enteral nutrition is a nutrition support modality used in certain patients to increase nutrition intake, thereby maintaining or improving nutrition health. Enteral nutrition reduces the negative impact of malnutrition, improves patient outcomes and results in costs savings.

Refeeding risk is the most critical aspect early in the treatment of malnourished patients. It is important that clinicians initiate feedings at low calorie levels while monitoring serum electrolytes. Intracellular shifts of potassium, magnesium and phosphorus can result in dangerously low serum levels; thus clinicians should monitor atleast daily with the onset of feeding and replete electrolytes when necessary. Avoidance of excessive fluid administration is also important, especially in patients who are cachetic. Provision of multivitamin or single nutrient supplements or atleast thiamine repletion is often necessary.

Prompt identification, treatment and monitoring of malnourished patients as well as helping to educate other healthcare professionals will continue to make a positive impact in healthcare.

NUTRITION AND WOUND HEALING

Wound healing is a complex multifactorial process in which nutrition plays an important role.

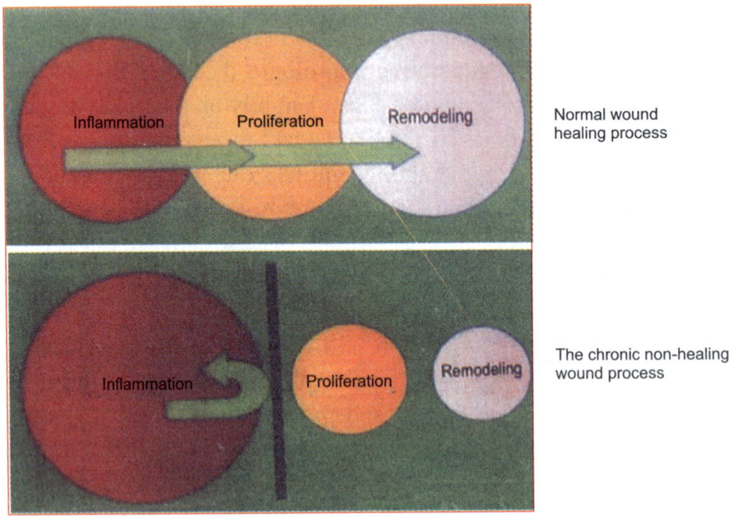

Fig. 12.3 Process of wound healing

Source: Abbott USA

Nutrient deficiencies or malnutrition can have negative effects on wound healing by prolonging the inflammatory phase, decreasing fibroblast proliferation and altering collagen synthesis. Chronic wounds represent a significant cause of morbidity and mortality for many patients.

Malnutrition places the patient at risk for infection by decreasing T-cell function, phagocytic activity and complement and antibody levels and delay clean surgical wounds.

Table 12.10 gives nutritional requirements during wound healing.

Table 12.10 Nutritional requirements during wound healing

Nutrient	*Reasons for increased requirement*
Energy 30–35 kcal/kg/d	Anabolism-nitrogen synthesis collagen formation and wound healing.
Protein 1.25–1.5 g/kg/d	Synthesis of enzymes, collagen formation
Agrinine 17–30 g/d	It is a substrate for protein synthesis, collagen deposition and cellular growth.
Glutamine 0.57 g/kg/d	Involved in immune function, improve nitrogen balance.
Methionine, lysine and proline	Stimulates fibroblast proliferation and collagen synthesis
Linoleic acid, arachidonic acid	Essential for the synthesis of prostaglandin which play a major role in cellular metabolism and inflammation
ω–3 fatty acids	Anti inflammatory, improved immune function, reduced infection rates.
Vitamin A 700 μg/d for females 900 μg/d for males	Stimulates the immune system by increasing the number of macrophages and monocytes in the wound during inflammation, Stimulates epithelialisation.
Vitamin C 100–200 mg/d	Essential for the synthesis of collagen connective tissue protein.

PRE- AND POST-OPERATIVE NUTRITION

Malnutrition affects up to 40 per cent of patients on admission to hospital. About 25 per cent of patients admitted to common medical and surgical specialities have evidence of moderate to severe nutritional depletion.

Inadequate food provision, inability to eat due to anorexia or disease of the oesophagus or pharynx and impaired digestion and absorption are common causes of starvation. The loss of 10 per cent body weight is associated with increased surgical risks. This may be difficult to detect because the anthropometric measurements may remain in the normal range. They may require nutritional support.

Patients who are having BMI less than 19 are considered malnourished. Albumin concentration reflects surgical risk rather than nutritional status.

Patients who require elective intestinal surgery should receive nutritional assessment before their operation. Enteral nutrition is cheaper and safer than parenteral nutrition and may help or preserve the immune function of the intestine. Parenteral nutrition is reserved for patients intolerant of adequate enteral nutrition and those with intestinal failure.

Preoperative Diet

Patients who have lost much weight prior to surgery benefit considerably by ingesting a high protein, high-calorie diet for even a week or two prior to surgery. The diet may be of liquid, soft or regular consistency depending upon the nature of the pathologic condition. Parenteral nutrition or semisynthetic fibre-free diets are sometimes used. In addition, the maintenance of metabolic equilibrium as in diabetes or other diseases must not be overlooked.

Foods which provide a maximum amount of nutrients in a minimum volume are essential. Small feedings at frequent intervals are likely to be better accepted than large meals which cannot be fully consumed.

For additional protein, milk beverages may be fortified with non-fat dry milk or commercial protein supplements. Fruit juices fortified with glucose or high carbohydrate food, increase carbohydrate intake and facilitate storage of glycogen. Butter incorporated into foods and light cream mixed with equal amounts of milk are also useful for increasing the calorie intake. One should remember that the excessive use of sugars and fats may cause nausea.

Food and fluids are generally allowed until midnight just preceding the day of operation, although a light breakfast may be given when the operation is scheduled for afternoon and local anaesthesia is to be used. It is essential that the stomach is kept empty prior to administering the anesthesia so as to reduce the incidence of vomiting and subsequent danger of aspiration of vomitus. When an operation is to be performed on the gastrointestinal tract, a diet very low in residue may be given 2 to 3 days prior to operation. In acute abdominal conditions such as appendicitis and cholecystitis, no food is allowed by mouth until nausea, vomiting, pain and distension have passed in order to prevent the danger of peritonitis.

Preoperative education includes nicotine and alcohol avoidance and nutrition support for malnourished patients. These are effective in reducing complications. Avoidance of overzealous and unnecessary preoperative starvation and preoperative carbohydrate loading are considered useful. Reducing calorie deficit and promoting nitrogen retention and judicious use of immunonutrients, antioxidants, vitamins, minerals and trace elements are to be considered in preoperative diet. Specialized enteral feeds with L-arginine and ω-3 fatty acids are cost effective. TPN is given preoperatively only when absolutely essential.

Postoperative Nutrition

The patient is under catabolic stress after surgery. It is characterised by the presence of an inflammatory response associated with depletion of conditionally essential nutrients. This leads to a dysregulated immune response that increases the risk for postoperative complications especially infections. An optimal nutrition state is an important precondition to provide successful post operative outcomes. In addition to disease, surgical procedure arising complications, metabolic and immune response to injury induces a catabolic state and insulin resistance. The more complex the surgical procedure, the more insulin resistant the patient becomes. Laproscopic techniques render minimal resistance whereas open techniques render in upto 50 per cent fall in sensitivity. Insulin resistance affects protein, fat in addition to carbohydrate metabolism. Insulin resistance is associated with increased morbidity, mortality and length of hospital stay.

Nutritional Requirement

Energy

Without sufficient caloric intake, tissue proteins cannot be synthesised. Excess metabolism of body fat may lead to acidosis, whereas depletion of the liver glucose may increase the likelihood of damage to the liver. With 2500 to 3000 kcal patients make progress.

Obesity delays healing. Whenever possible, it should be corrected. Rapid weight loss results in loss of lean body mass and should be avoided.

Protein

A satisfactory state of protein nutrition ensures:

- rapid wound healing
- increases the resistance to infection
- exerts a protective action upon the liver against the toxic effects of anaesthesia and
- reduces the possibility of oedema at the site of the wound.

When protein is depleted in post-operative condition complications are increased. Protein catabolism is increased for several days immediately following surgery or injury, patients undergo negative nitrogen balance even though the protein intake may be appreciable. The degree of negative balance can be reduced through higher intakes of protein and calories.

Glutamine supplement increases glutathione levels which act as an antioxidant. It has direct anticatabolic effects and hence preserve lean body mass in the post operative patients. Glutamine is available as a dipeptide with alanine for parenteral administration. The dosage should be 0.3–0.5 g/kg/d and should not exceed 30 per cent of the total protein requirement.

The level of protein to be used in pre-operative and post-operative diets depends on the previous state of nutrition, the nature of the operation and the extent of the post-operative losses. Intake of 1.0 to 1.5 g per kilogram or about 100 g of protein are necessary as a rule.

ω-3 fatty acid

ω-6 fatty acid is a proinflammatory agent and checked by anti inflammatory ω-3 fatty acid in the cell membrane of the cells in the body. By increasing the ω-3 fatty acids in the cell membranes of the cells the production of proinflammatory products are checked and finally the immune stimulation is under control in surgical patients.

Fish oil is rich in ω-3 fatty acids and it is a great source for parenteral use. A dose of 0.1–0.2 g/kg/d can be given. It should not exceed 20 per cent of the total fat.

Various studies have proved reduction of the infectious complications, reduced mortality and decreased length of hospital stay in the surgical patients when they receive ω-3 fatty acids in the perioperative period.

Minerals

Phosphorus and potassium are lost in proportion to the breakdown of body tissue. In addition, derangements of sodium and chloride metabolism may occur subsequent to vomiting, diarrhoea, perspiration, drain of fluids, anorexia and dieresis or renal failure.

Iron-deficiency anaemia occurs in association with malabsorption or excessive blood loss. Diet alone is ineffective in correction of anaemia, but a liberal intake of protein and ascorbic acid, together with administration of iron salt is of value in convalescence. Transfusions are usually required to overcome severe reduction in haemoglobin level.

Vitamins

Ascorbic acid is especially important for wound healing and should be provided in increased amounts prior to and following surgery. Vitamin K is of concern to the surgeon since there is evidence of failure to synthesise vitamin K in the small intestine since the inability to absorb and/or the defect in conversion to prothrombin which is likely to result in bleeding. Haemorrhage is especially likely to occur in patients who have diseases of the liver.

Fluids

The fluid balance may be upset prior to and following surgery owing to failure to ingest normal quantities of fluids and to increased losses from vomiting, exudates, haemorrhage, diuresis and fever. A patient should not be operated in a state of dehydration since the subsequent dangers of acidosis are great. When dehydration exists prior to operation, parenteral fluids are administered, if the patient is unable to ingest sufficient liquid by mouth.

Postoperative Dietary Management

In the postoperative patient, starvation leads to increased morbidity in the nutritionally depleted and stressed patient. Nutritional support in depleted patients improves clinical outcome and reduces the length of hospital stay.

Following minor surgery, liquids are often tolerated within a few hours and rapid progression to a normal diet is made. After major surgery, oral intake may be delayed for days. Fruits like papaya and sapota are given postoperatively to initiate bowel movement. Complete nutritional support are provided by conventional intravenous feedings, catheter jejunostomy, total parenteral nutrition, tube feedings or semisynthetic fibre free diets.

Medical and surgical ICU patients are insufficiently fed during their ICU stay when compared with their RDA. Feeding practices differ significantly in medical and surgical ICU patients. Lipid-based sedatives and dextrose containing intravenous fluids are used more frequently in surgical populations. Until the evidence is clear regarding optimal nutrition support of severely ill ICU patients, a thorough review of all energy sources should be routinely monitored and energy delivery to be limited to 80 per cent of the target.

ERAS Enhanced recovery after surgery

It is a fast-track programme to improve the patient's general well-being after surgery.

ERAS protocols involve a curtailed fasting and pre-operative carbohydrate loading. Early post-operative diet initiation is part of this protocol too. These guidelines have been formed to decrease the protein loss, insulin resistance and metabolic stress response to surgery, thereby reducing the harms of conventional post-operative care such as fatigue and decline in nutritional status.

Protocol of Enhanced Recovery After Surgery

A. Postoperative hypoglycaemia of glucose: ERAS affects insulin action and resistance. No risk of causing hypoglycaemia such as avoiding fasting.

B. Fluid balance: Preoperative oral carbohydrate and fluid loading and restrictive intra operative and post operative intravenous fluids.

C. Post operative nausea and vomiting: It is one of the causes of delay in recommencement of oral intake. Early feeding after surgery has been associated with early recovery of bowel function.

D. Early post operative diet and artificial nutrition: Providing sufficient support for wound healing and to avoid excessive loss of lean body mass.

E. Early mobilisation: Post operative exercise should be initiated as soon as possible.

Source: European Society of Parenteral and Enteral nutrition.

NUTRITION SUPPORT IN BURN PATIENTS

The aim is to maintain or attain nutritional status in patients with burn injury by providing nutritional support enterally and/or parenterally. Nutrition support promotes wound healing, prevents infection and prevents loss of more than 10 per cent of the patients preburn weight.

Metabolic changes

- Protein lost depends upon the extent and depth of the burn
- There is an increase in nitrogen excretion due to open wounds.
- The sooner a burn wound is closed the more rapidly positive nitrogen balance is reached. If infection develops, the nitrogen losses are even greater.
- Fluids and electrolytes (K, Na, Cl) are lost through exudation.
- Anemia may be an additional problem.
- First seven days, patient is hypercatabolic and will not retain much of the protein given.
- Six to eight weeks after the burn there is high rate of metabolism.
- Resting energy expenditure increases by 50–125 per cent due to increased per cent release of catecholamines which are directly related to the extent of burn.

First, adequate fluid and electrolytes are provided to maintain circulating volume and to prevent renal failure. Weight gain from fluid is common during this stage and is generally mobilised slowly over the next two weeks. Therefore, preburn weight should be used in estimating kilocalories and protein needs. Serum albumin drops with post burn even if normal on admission due to increased loss of albumin as plasma leaves from micro vasculature to the area of damage.

Patient is given oral supplements. Tube feeding is resorted if the patient is unable to consume enough orally. Parenteral nutrition is the least used route as there is high risk of catheter infection as burn wounds are likely to be colonised with microorganisms.

A. Energy requirements (Major burns)

Adults = 25 × body weight (kg) + 40 × % TBSA burned (With maximum 50% Total Body Surface Area)

Paediatric group

< 1 year = RDA + 15 × % TBSA burned

1–3 years = RDA + 25 × % TBSA burned

4 – 15 years = RDA + 40 × % TBSA burned

B. Protein requirement

Adults

1.3 – 3.0 g/kg ideal body weight

or 20 – 25% of total energy

Children

0–2 years - 2–3 g/kg/d

3–13 years - 1.5–2 g/kg/d

13–18 years - 1.5g/kg/d

C. Non protein energy

Fat = 15–20% of total calories

Carbohydrates = 50–60% of total calories

D. Micronutrients

Multivitamin = 2 × RDA

Vitamin A – 5 × RDA

Vitamin C – 1-2 g

Zinc – 1 × RDA

Studies show that there is a diminished capacity to produce vitamin D among children with severe burns. Hence such children should receive vitamin D supplements. Even skin that is not burned cannot make enough vitamin D in burned children. After being burned, children lose bone mass and during periods of growth there is a heightened risk for fractures. To prevent this, vitamin D supplements should become part of the burned children's therapy during their treatment and after they are discharged from the hospital.

Indian Society for Parenteral and Enteral Nutrition (ISPEN) is an association that is involved in nutrition support service to help reduce morbidity and mortality among patients.

Antioxidant micronutrients in major trauma and burns

The relationship between the amount of Reactive Oxygen Species and natural scavengers of free radicals determines the outcome of local and distant tissues damage in burn injury. If prolonged, this inflammation favours development of organ failure. Lipid peroxidation is particularly intense in burns and caused in part by the direct effect of the burn on lipids contained in the skin and by an increased free radical production which is initiated directly by the burn and indirectly by leukocytes.

In patients with burns > 20% TBSA the inflammatory response spreads rapidly to the whole body, resulting in a general capillary leak syndrome with edema formation.

Endogenous Antioxidant Defences: AOXs are substances that inhibit or delay oxidation. Endogenous AOX defences are both non-enzymatic (uric acid, glutathione, bilirubin, thiols, albumin and nutrition factors including vitamins and phenols) and enzymatic (SODs, the glutathione peroxidases (GSHPx) and catalase).

The trace elements Cu, Se, Mn and Zn have AOX properties as essential compounds of the AOX enzyme system in the cytosol mitochondria or in plasma.

This includes copper-zinc superoxide dismutase and the various types of glutathione peroxidases.

In addition to antioxidants vitamin C and E, selenium is an important AOX micronutrient in the critically ill particularly in burn and trauma patients.

SUGGESTED READINGS

- Clinical Dietetics Manual. Indian Dietetic Association, 2011.
- Stechmiller K. Joyce, Understanding the role of nutrition and wound healing, Nutrition in clinical practice, 2010; **25**.
- Phillips Wendy, The effectiveness of the Braden scale as a tool for identifying nutrition risk, J. Acad. Nutr. Diet 2018; **118**.
- Elless Steenhagen, It's time to change practice. Nutrition in clinical practice 2015; **31**.
- Mayes Theresa *et al.*, Investigation of bone health subsequent to vitamin D supplementation in children following burn injury, Nutrition in Clinical practice, 2005; **30**.
- Disease-related malnutrition and enteral nutrition therapy; A significant problem with a cost effective solution. Advocacy and public policy special report, Nutrition in clinical practice, 2010; **25**.
- Indian society for Parenteral and Enteral Nutrition. www.ispen.org

QUESTIONS

1. Write a short note on soft-diet.
2. Explain the drawbacks of full-fluid diet.
3. Give three recipes for soft-diet, liquid-diet and full-fluid diet.
4. Write a note on tube feeding.
5. What is parenteral feeding? Give a sample of TPN regimen for an adult.

6. Bring out the nutritional importance of pre-operative and post-operative conditions.
7. Discuss the advantages of tube feeding over parenteral feeding.
8. Which conditions necessitate to special feeding methods?
9. Explain the following terms:
   (*a*) Immuno nutrition
   (*b*) Refeeding syndrome
   (*c*) Elemental diet
   (*d*) Peripheral parenteral nutrition.
10. Discuss the different types of tube feeds used.
11. Normal nutritional needs are the basis for diet therapy. Comment.
12. Mention two situations where TPN is given.
13. Give four low residue recipes.
14. Name three foods to be included and three foods to be avoided in low cholesterol diet.
15. Name four conditions in which protein requirement is modified.
16. Name five foods to be avoided in sodium restricted diets.
17. What are the advantages of high fibre diets?
18. In which conditions high protein diet is given? Why?
19. How do you assess the nutritional status of a patients? Give a sample proforma.

TOPIC FOR ACTIVITY

- Collect data on the nutrient composition of enteral and TPN formulae used in hospitals.

13

Nutritional Anaemia in Physiological and Pathological Conditions

Nutritional anaemia may be defined as the condition that results from the inability of the erythropoietic tissue to maintain a normal haemoglobin concentration on account of inadequate supply of one or more nutrients leading to reduction in the total circulating haemoglobin.

Nutritional anaemia is caused by the absence of any dietary essential that is involved in haemoglobin formation or by poor absorption of these dietary essentials. Some anaemias are caused by lack of either dietary iron or high quality protein; by lack of pyridoxine (vitamin B_6) which catalyses the synthesis of the haem portion of the haemoglobin molecule; by lack of vitamin C which influences the rate of iron absorption into the tissues; or by a lack of vitamin E which affects the stability of the red blood cell membrane. Copper is not part of the haemoglobin molecule but aids in its synthesis by influencing the absorption of iron, its release from the liver or its incorporation into haemoglobin molecule.

PREVALENCE

Poor density and bioavailability of dietary iron from staple foods are the major etiological factors for wide spread prevalence of iron deficiency in India.

It is an important public health problem affecting people from all walks of life. Anaemia is very widespread, more among females than males and higher among infants and children than adults. Severe anaemia (with haemoglobin levels < 8 g/dl) is more frequently seen in severely undernourished children who also exhibit signs associated with deficiencies of calories, proteins, vitamins and minerals.

Food insecurity could affect nutritional quality of diet and increased chances of developing anaemia. At all India level 53 percent of women between 15–49 ages are anaemic.

CAUSES

Causes of anaemia in different age groups is given in Table 13.1.

Table 13.1 Causes of anaemia in different age groups

Age	*Causes*
Infancy	• Inadequate iron stores at birth due to low birth weight or due to preterm. • Multiple births • Infant who is breast fed by a mother who is a strict vegetarian (vegan) • Infant who is on milk diet without proper weaning foods • Late weaning • Impaired absorption of folate • Regional enteritis, Crohn's disease, celiac disease
Childhood	• Dietary deficiency • Due to hook worm infestation—occult blood loss • Inflammatory bowel disease • Neglect of female child • Chronic intestinal blood loss induced by exposure to a heat labile protein in whole cow's milk.
Adolescence	• At the time of menarche • Growth spurt with a suboptimal haematopoitic contents • Gender discrimination • Iron depletion occurs in girls who take part in Intensive exercise • Early marriage with pregnancy • Excess blood loss during menstruation
Adults	• Chronic infection—tuberculosis, malignancy • GI surgery • Blunting of the villi are present in advanced iron deficiency anaemia and may cause leakage of blood and decreased absorption of iron • High amounts of tannins and oxalates in the diet • Infestation with tapeworm-*diphyllobothrium latum* • An over growth of intestinal bacteria within diverticula or duplication of the small intestine may cause B_{12} deficiency by consumption of or competition for the vitamin or by splitting of its complex with intrinsic factor. • Drug induced anaemia, methetrexate (an immuno suppressive) interferes folate metabolism.
Pregnancy	• Increased requirements • Increased parity • Hemodilution • Low maternal age • Cultural beliefs, taboos and inappropriate food practices • Infections which may interfere with intake, absorption and assimilation of nutrients • Pregnancy related complications

(*Contd...*)

Table 13.1 (Contd...)

Age	Causes
	• Atrophic gastritis and bacterial over growth (B_{12}) • Gastro intestinal blood loss from malignant disease, peptic ulcer disease • Use of nonsteroidal anti inflammatory drugs • Psychological problems • Loneliness • Poor absorption • Chronic inflammatory disease

High levels of anaemia among women in the child-bearing age is linked to high levels of malnutrition. Due to lack of sanitation and open defecation women and young children are susceptible to worm infestation in turn to anaemia.

TYPES

Hypochromic and Microcytic Anaemia

If there is an insufficiency of iron for the formation of haemoglobin, the red blood corpuscles are pale and small and the anaemia is said to be hypochromic and microcytic.

Megaloblastic Anaemia

Vitamin B_{12} and folic acid are co-enzymes in the DNA synthetic pathway. A deficiency of the vitamins or impairment in their utilisation results in damaged or inadequate synthesis of DNA. The synthesis of RNA and protein is unaffected so there is cytoplasmic enlargement, not matched by DNA synthesis which appears to delay or block mitotic division. Thus there appears to be asynchronism between cytoplasmic maturation and nuclear maturation. If the maturation of the red blood corpuscles in the bone marrow is impaired by lack of folate or vitamin B_{12}, the cells which enter the blood stream are irregular in size and shape, but usually larger than normal, and contain their full complement of haemoglobin. This is also known as orthochromic macrocytic anaemia.

Dimorphic Anaemia

If both iron and either folate or vitamin B_{12} are deficient it gives rise to hypochromic macrocytic or dimorphic anaemia.

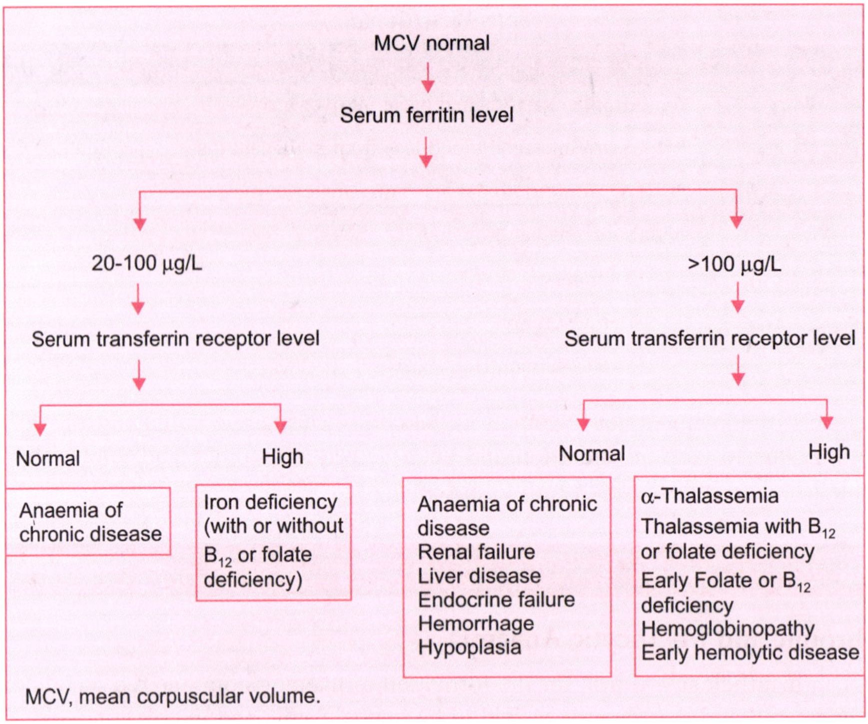

Fig. 13.1 Workup of Normocytic Anaemia

Source: Consultant, 2002.

IRON DEFICIENCY ANAEMIA

Iron is necessary for the formation of haemoglobin. Iron deficiency results in anaemia.

This is the most common form of anaemia throughout the world affecting mainly women in their reproductive years, infants and children. In both rural and urban areas in the tropics, this type of anaemia is extremely common.

Aetiology

Deficiency of iron may occur as a result of the following:

Inadequate iron intake: A few foods like greens and enriched processed foods and raisins dried, black are rich sources of iron. People who do not include these foods in the diet may suffer from anaemia. Availability of iron from plant sources is not as good as haeme iron. Haeme iron present in foods of animal origin which are expensive. The average cereal-legume based diets as consumed in most developing countries would appear adequate in iron content (20–22 mg) for an adult. But the availability of iron from such diets is very poor. Only 3–5 per cent of dietary iron is absorbed in normal apparently healthy individual.

Pregnant anaemic mother gives birth to an infant whose iron stores are inadequate and in turn the infant is susceptible for anaemia.

Infants and children suffer from iron deficiency anaemia due to prolonged breast feeding without the addition of supplementary feeding.

Intergenerational anaemia

It is caused when a severely anaemic mother delivers a premature child with anaemia who suffers throughout childhood and adolescence. Finally, she turns into an anaemic young mother and the cycle continues.

Inadequate utilisation of iron: This can take place secondary to chronic gastrointestinal disturbances, defective release of iron from iron stores into the plasma and defective iron utilisation owing to a chronic inflammation or other chronic disorder.

Blood losses: This can occur in accidental haemorrhage, in chronic diseases such as tuberculosis, ulcers or intestinal disorders, or excessive blood donation or due to hookworm infestation. The mean daily loss of blood from one *Ancylostoma duodenale* is 0.15 ml and *Necator americanus* is 0.03 ml. Figure 13.2 shows cycle of hookworm. Excessive loss of blood during menstruation and childbirth can cause anaemia. Perinatal bleeding may result from obstetric complications such as placental abruption.

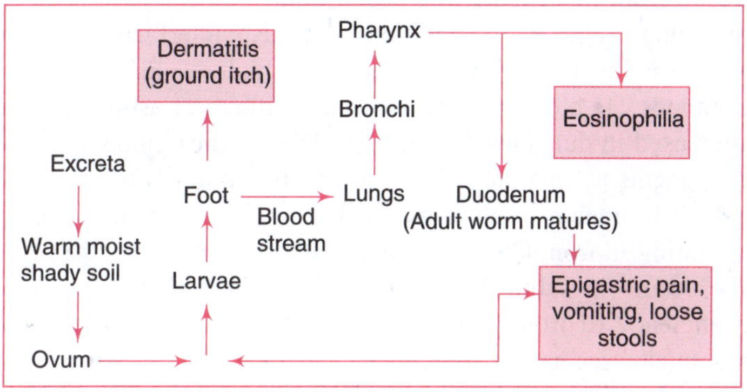

Fig. 13.2 **Hookworm infestation causes anaemia**

In rural areas, post partum haemorrhage on account of poor obstetric spaced pregnancies and prolonged periods of lactation deplete iron stores with each successive pregnancy. This is reflected in the high incidence of anaemia with higher parity. Resurgence of malaria is another important factor resulting in high incidence of anaemia. In women using intrauterine contraceptive device, menorrhagia (increased blood loss) may result in further depletion of already poor stores of iron.

Chronic diarrhea in early childhood may be associated with considerable unrecognized blood loss induced by exposure to a heat labile protein in whole cow's milk. Loss of blood in the stools can be prevented either by reducing the quantity of whole cow's milk or by using heated or evaporated milk.

Increased requirements: During periods of accelerated demand like in infancy (rapidly expanding blood volume), adolescence (rapid growth and onset of menses in girls) and pregnancy and lactation can result in anaemia. Losses of iron may occur due to excessive sweating in tropical climate and due to intense exercise.

Inadequate absorption of iron: This can occur in diarrhoea (sprue and pellagra) or when there is lack of acid secretion by the stomach or in chronic renal diseases when antacid therapy is given. Gastrectomy impairs iron absorption by decreasing hydrochloric acid and transit time through the duodenum. Excessive amounts of phytates and phosphates in the diet and excess consumption of tea can decrease the absorption of iron.

Histologic abnormalities of the mucosa of the GI tract such as the blunting of villi are present in advanced iron deficiency anaemia and may cause leakage of blood and decrease absorption of iron further compounding the problems.

Disease and Drugs can induce anaemia

Medication can alter nutrient metabolism, influence erythropoiesis and blood coagulation and sometimes lead to increased red blood cell destruction.

Anaemia can occur in patients who have chronic infections, inflammatory conditions, autoimmune disorders or cancer. As a result of the inflammatory response macrophages in the liver, spleen and bone marrow sequester iron, making it unavailable for erythropoiesis and hence slowing the rate of production of new blood cells. In addition, RBC are destroyed more rapidly than usual and reduced production of RBC cannot keep pace. Iron absorption is impaired, possibly intestinal cells inhibit release of iron into blood. Eventually, outright iron deficiency may result from inadequate iron absorption.

Several pharmacologic agents or conditions can also interface with iron absorption or transport, leading to iron loss or defective absorption which results in iron deficiency anaemia in adults. These include H_2 blockers, proton pump inhibitors, aspirin or non-steroidal anti-inflammatory drugs used in duodenal and gastric ulcers and carcinoma.

Many cirrhotic patients are malnuorished and key micronutrients are malabsorbed.

In liver disease, it is unable to store as ferritin and cannot synthesise transferrin which transports iron, resulting in iron deficiency anaemia.

Iron deficiency occurs in subtotal gastrectomy and in bariatric surgery. Several factors contribute to a deficiency of iron after the surgical intervention. One reason is merely the reduction in food intake secondary to reduced gastric capacity. Another aspect relates to poor iron absorption due to less food exposed to the stomach's acidic environment, which is responsible for converting ferric iron to be more absorbable ferrous form.

In celiac disease, iron deficiency occurs due to malabsorption or due to occult GI bleeding. Intolerance to the food protein gluten causes villous atrophy in the proximal duodenum, leading to malabsorption of nutrients such as iron.

Chronic inflammation mediates mechanisms that sequester iron from the body pool. Upregulation of ferritin and down regulation of transferrin systhesis are classic host defence mechanism that occur during inflammation leading to functional iron deficiency. Iron is simply unavailable for a delivery to the bone marrow and thus erythropoiesis is compromised producing anaemia.

Inflammation induced anaemia and resistance to erythropoietin are familiar characteristics in patients with chronic kidney disease.

Diagnosis

Progressive stages of iron deficiency can be evaluated by four different measurements.

- The plasma ferritin level provides a measure of iron stores.
- Transferrin saturation can be used as a guage of iron supply to the tissues. It is calculated by dividing serum iron by Total Iron Binding Capacity. Levels less than 16 per cent are considered to be inadequate for erythropoiesis.

- Both haemoglobin and hematocrit measurements can indicate anaemia. Most patients develop symptoms of anaemia when the haemoglobin level is approximately 8–11 g/dl.

Large survelliance system use haemoglobin or haematocrit level for screening. These can only identify anaemia not specifically IDA (Iron Deficiency Anaemia). Without the additional biochemical indication of IDA like transferrin saturation, erythrocytes protoporphyrin level and ferritin level it is impossible to determine iron deficiency as the cause of anaemia.

Table 13.2 Diagnosis of iron deficiency

Indicator	*Interpretary guidelines*
Peripheral smear	Microcytic hypochromic
MCHC pg	< 30
Serum Iron μg/dl	< 60
Total Iron Binding capacity μg/dl	> 300
Transferrin Saturation %	< 15
Erythrocyte protoporphyrin μg/dl	> 100
Protoporphyrin Haeme ratio	> 32
Serum ferritin μg/l	< 12
Bonemarrow iron (by Perl stain)	0 or +

Source: Raman Leela and K.V. Rameshwara Sarma, 2009, *Nutrition and Anaemia*. Textbook of Human nutrition. Edited by Bamji M.S. *et al.* Oxford and IBH Publishing Co. Pvt. Ltd., New Delhi.

Haemoglobin concentration alone is unsuitable as a diagnostic tool in cases of suspected iron deficiency anaemia for three reasons:

- It is affected only late in the disease.
- It cannot distinguish iron deficiency from other anaemias.
- Haemoglobin values in normal individuals vary widely.

Table 13.3 WHO Cut-off points for haemoglobin values for diagnosis of anaemia

Group	*Haemoglobin g/dl*
Adult men	< 12
Adult women	< 12
Pregnant women	< 11
Lactating women	< 12
Children < 6 years	< 11
Other Children	< 12

Stages of iron deficiency

First stage is characterised by decreased storage of iron without any other detectable abnormalities.

An intermediate stage of latent iron deficiency, that is, iron stores are exhausted, but anaemia has not occurred as yet. Its recognition depends upon measurement of serum ferritin levels.

The percentage saturation of transferrin falls from a normal value of 30 per cent to less than 15 per cent. This stage is the most widely prevalent in India.

The third stage is that of overt iron deficiency when there is a decrease in the concentration of circulating haemoglobin due to impaired haemoglobin synthesis.

In case of selecting indicators for detecting iron deficiency anaemia in the community, the filter paper method is the most suitable to carry out haemoglobin estimation in field conditions although haemocue or haemotology counter provide accurate results.

Table 13.4 The spectrum of iron status in relation to the major tests available for clinical application

	Iron Overload	*Normal*	*Depleted iron stores*	*Iron deficiency without anaemia*	*Iron deficiency with anaemia*
Serum ferritin	↓	N	↓	↓	↓↓
Transferrin	↑↑	N	N	↓	↓
Erythrocyte Protoporphyrin	N	N	N	↑	↑↑
MCV	N	N	N	N	↓
Haemoglobin	N	N	N	N	↓

Source: Kleinman E Ronald. 2004, Paediatric Nutrition Handbook, American Academy of Paediatrics.

Clinical Findings

The end result of iron deficiency is nutritional anaemia which is not a disease entity. It is rather a syndrome caused by malnutrition in its widest sense. Besides anaemia, the following clinical findings are observed.

Immunocompetence: Deficiency of iron diminishes the number of T-cells and the production of antibodies. A sign of early iron deficiency is reduced immunocompetence, particularly defects in cell-mediated immunity and the phagocytic activity of neutrophils, which may lead to an increased propensity for infection.

Diminished work performance: Inadequate muscle function is reflected in decreased work performance and exercise tolerance. This has profound economic implications on the individual and on the nation.

Cognitive development: Iron deficient young adolescents have been shown to score relatively lower in tests of academic performance. There is evidence of impaired motor and language development, lack of concentration and behavioural changes in IDA. Such changes may be related to functional changes in iron containing enzymes at cellular levels. Recent observations indicated that IDA at a time of crucial brain growth and development may produce permanent and irreversible abnormalities in those functions.

Behavioural implications: Anaemic children have been found to be more disruptive, irritable and restless in the classroom. Iron deficiency is also sometimes associated with pica especially pagophagia (ice eating). Temper tantrum and breath holding spells are also observed in anaemic children. Mono Amino Oxidase, an iron dependent enzyme, has a crucial role in neuro chemical reaction in the central nervous system. Iron deficiency produces decrease in the activities of enzymes such as catalase and cytochrome. Administration of iron may decrease the frequency of breath holding spells.

Pica is well documented feature of anaemia in children, craving to eat unusual substances such as dirt, clay, ice, laundry starch, salt or cardboard are seen in almost 70–80 per cent of patients and are usually cured by prompt iron therapy.

Structure and function of epithelial tissues: Mostly tongue, nails, mouth and stomach are affected. The skin may appear pale and the inside of the lower eyelid may be light pink instead of red. Finger nails can become thin and flat and eventually koilonychia (spoon shaped nails)

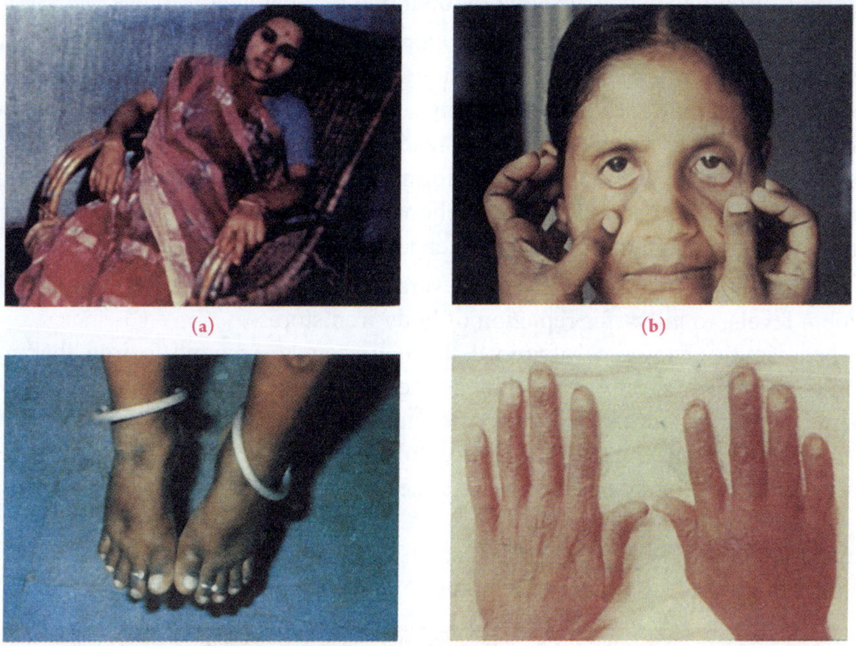

(a) (b) (c) (d)

Fig. 13.3 Symptoms of anaemia. Fatigue, paleness of conjunctiva, oedema and spoon shaped nails

Source: Food and Nutrition Board, Chennai

develop as shown in Figure 13.3. Mouth changes include atrophy of the lingual papillae, a completely smooth waxy and glistening appearance to the tongue (glossitis). Angular stomatitis and dysphagia may occur. Gastritis occurs frequently and may result in achlorhydria. Progressive, untreated anaemia results in cardiovascular and respiratory changes that can eventually lead to cardiac failure as the fall of haemoglobin is gradual. The onset of symptoms is insidious. Initially, pallor, anorexia and irritability may be noticed. Later hyper dynamic circulation leads to palpitations, shortness of breath, fatigue, reduced exercise tolerance and congestive heart failure.

Chronic long-term iron deficiency symptoms reflect a malfunction of a variety of body systems. The general symptoms are lassitude, fatigue, breathlessness on exertion, palpitations, dizziness, tinnitus, headache, dimness of vision, insomnia, paraesthesia in fingers and toes and angina. Growth abnormalities are also observed in anaemic children.

The triad dysphagia due to oesophageal webs, koilonychia and splenomegaly in a patient with iron deficiency anemia is known as Plummer Vinson or Patterson Kelly Syndrome.

Treatment

Treatment should focus primarily on the underlying disease or situation leading to anaemia. Oral administration of inorganic iron in the ferrous form—ferrous sulphate 50–200 mg (60 mg elemental iron) 3 times daily for adults and 6 mg/kg for children. Other salts absorbed at about same degree are ferrous forms of lactate, fumarate, sulphate, and gluconate. Ferric hydroxide poly maltose complex has proved to be a suitable effective and safe alternative to oral salts in the treatment of iron deficiency anaemia by both oral and parenteral routes.

Iron is best absorbed when the stomach is empty. However, under these conditions, it tends to cause gastric irritation. Gastrointestinal side effects of nausea, epigastric discomfort and distention, heart burn, diarrhoea or constipation can be minimised by increasing the dose slowly over a few days until the required dosage is reached and by giving the iron in divided doses at least three times per day. Use of chelated form of iron (bound to amino acids) can result in improved absorption and can reduce the likelihood of gastrointestinal distress. Ascorbic acid greatly increases iron absorption through its capacity to maintain iron in the reduced state.

Iron therapy should be continued for several months even after restoration of normal haemoglobin levels, to allow for repletion of body iron stores.

Some behavioural symptoms of iron deficiency seem to respond to iron therapy before the anaemia is cured, suggesting they may be the result of tissue depletion of iron-containing enzymes rather than of a decreased level of haemoglobin.

In iron deficiency anaemia when dietary folate is also low, treatment with iron alone precipitates folate deficiency because more is needed for production of erythrocytes and the supply of folate becomes insufficient.

Treatment improves work performance and productivity in adults. In children there is improvement in intellechal and psycho motor development.

MEGALOBLASTIC ANAEMIA

Haemopoietic tissue is one of a number of rapidly proliferating tissues in which DNA synthesis is intense. Both vitamin B_{12} and folate are essential for DNA synthesis and deficiency of either or both causes disordered cell proliferation. Haemopoiesis is particularly susceptible and division of cells is delayed and eventually halted. Morphological changes appear in the marrow cells. In the erythrocyte series these changes are described as megaloblastic because the cells appear abnormally large. They are nucleated red cell precursors. Megaloblasts appear in bone marrow as well as in peripheral blood.

VITAMIN B_{12} DEFICIENCY

Vitamin B_{12} must be bound to intrinsic factor, produced by the parietal cells of the stomach, before it is absorbed in the terminal ileum. Inability to produce intrinsic factor results in pernicious anaemia. The red cell count is often less than 2.5 million and a large proportion of the cells are macrocytic. The anaemia occurs chiefly in middle aged and elderly persons and may be a genetic defect. Antibodies against gastric mucosa can probably be responsible for destroying the mechanism of producing intrinsic factor. The disease thus arises as an autoimmune disorder.

Nutritional vitamin B_{12} deficiency is not very common, even in populations where intake of the vitamin B_{12} is far below the daily requirement of 0.5 µg–1 µg. Vitamin B_{12} deficiency takes at least 3 years to appear as vitamin B_{12} is stored in the liver.

Prevalence

The majority of patients with vitamin B_{12} deficiency have Addisonian pernicious anaemia. This appears to be relatively uncommon in tropical countries. Addisonian pernicious anaemia is due to a failure of secretion of intrinsic factor by the stomach. The disease is rare before the age of 30, occurs mainly between 45 and 65 years and affects females more frequently than males.

Causes of Pernicious Anaemia

Inadequate ingestion: A poor diet lacking in microorganisms and animal foods can lead to vitamin B_{12} deficiency. Vegans are susceptible for B_{12} deficiency. Chronic alcoholism, poverty, religious taboos and dietary fads can also cause B_{12} deficiency. Infants solely breastfed for long period of time develop anaemia due to dietary vitamin B_{12} deficiency.

Inadequate absorption and utilisation: Inadequate or absence of secretion of intrinsic factor due to heredity or congenital production of defective intrinsic factor can lead to B_{12} deficiency. Gastric atrophy, endocrine disorders associated with gastric damage or gastrectomy can reduce the production of intrinsic factor leading to vitamin B_{12} deficiency. Bacterial proliferation in stagnant loops and in tropical sprue there is malabsorption of B_{12}. In these cases, haematologic response may follow appropriate antibiotic therapy. Parasitic infestation such as fish tapeworm (*diphyllobothrium*) may remove vitamin B_{12} from the gut.

Inadequate utilisation: This is due to the presence of vitamin B_{12} antagonists.

Increased requirements: Hypothyroidism increases haematopoiesis. During infancy and pregnancy there is increased requirement of vitamin B_{12} as it is essential for nucleic acid synthesis.

Clinical Features

Patients with pernicious anaemia have a lemon yellow or pale skin. Anorexia, glossitis, achlorhydria, abdominal discomfort, frequent diarrhoea, weight loss and general weakness can also occur. The surface of the tongue is usually smooth and atrophic but sometimes it is red and inflammed. Gastric secretions are devoid of pepsin, acid and intrinsic factor. Numbness of limbs, coldness of extremities and difficulty in walking are manifestations of neurologic changes. The haemoglobin content may be as low as 8 per cent. Demyelination of white fibers of spinal cord occurs in severe cases. Psychiatric symptoms may occur associated with low levels of vitamin B_{12} in the plasma, but in the absence of other signs of neuropathy. Pernicious anaemia is associated with an increased risk of gastric cancer. Clinical manifestations are mental apathy, pigmentation, growth retardation and megaloblastic bone marrow. In young females there may be infertility.

Diagnosis

The differential diagnosis of pernicious anaemia from other forms of megaloblastic anaemia depends upon the age of the patient (common among females aged between 45 and 65), the finding of histamine-fast or pentagastrin-fast achlorhydria, upon the absence of pregnancy and the lack of evidence of malnutrition, malabsorption of structural change in the small intestine. Plasma vitamin B_{12} is below 160 ng/l while plasma folate is usually normal. The schilling test shows subnormal absorption which is corrected if intrinsic factor is given at the same time.

Treatment

If the haemoglobin level is under 4 g/dl blood transfusion should always be given. Physical activity should be at a minimum until the haemoglobin is above 7 g/dl.

Hydroxocobalamin should be given in a dosage of 1,000 mcg intramuscularly twice during the first week, then 250 mcg weekly until the blood count is normal. Then 1000 mcg every six weeks is given. Folic acid should never be used alone in the treatment of pernicious anaemia as it does not prevent the development of neurological complications and may precipitate them.

Within 48 hours of the first injection of a cobalamin the bone marrow shows a striking change from a megaloblastic to normoblastic state. Within two or three days the reticulocyte count begins to rise, reaching a maximum about the 4th or 7th day.

To cope up with regeneration of blood, ferrous sulphate 200 mg thrice daily is given.

Vitamin B_{12} levels in maternal milk and serum are low in pernicious anaemia. The clinical picture gets corrected by administering a single dose of 50 µg of vitamin B_{12} to the mother or to the infant.

Dietary Consideration

Poor appetite and gastrointestinal discomfort seriously interfere with an adequate food intake so that the patients often present a picture of general nutritional deficiency. A high protein diet of 100 to 150 g of protein with high calorie diet is recommended. Supplementation of liver extracts would be effective in the treatment of pernicious anaemia.

Achlorhydria retards digestion, hence fat in diet should be kept to moderate levels, restricting especially fried foods that may further delay gastric emptying.

A soft or clear liquid diet is preferable until glossitis completely disappears. Spicy food should be avoided. A soft diet is recommended since there is anorexia and irritation of gastrointestinal tract.

Supplementation with ascorbic acid is essential if citrus fruits and other rich sources of vitamin C are not ingested. High protein-high calorie beverages, two or three times daily should be given. They may be prepared from milk, non fat dry milk, protein concentrates and fruits.

FOLATE DEFICIENCY

In tropical countries, most cases of megaloblastic anaemia are due to folate deficiency associated with malnutrition, infection and pregnancy. It is common in the age group 20–30 years.

Aetiology

Poor dietary intake: Megaloblastic anaemia is common among poor vegetarians. This is due to poor intake of milk, fresh fruits and vegetables. As such the Indian diet is a poor source of folic acid and cooking practices commonly encountered tend to destroy the folic acid to a considerable extent.

Low absorption: This anaemia in babies is more frequent in those born to mothers who also have a folic acid deficiency. Anaemia is present in infants whose diet lacks in vitamin C because folic acid cannot be converted to its active form of folinic acid. Low folic acid absorption can occur in coeliac disease and in tropical sprue. Folate absorption is impaired in pregnancy.

Vitamin B_{12} deficiency can result in folic acid deficiency by causing folate entrapment in the metabolically inactive form of 5 methyl tetrahydrofolate.

Increased requirement: Increased requirements due to growth and pregnancy are believed to be the most frequent causes. In haemolysis, when there is cell proliferation there is folic acid deficiency.

Infestation and infection: Malarial infection may play a part in pathogenesis of megaloblastic anaemia. Chronic infections and parasitic infestation may impair absorption of folic acid.

Drugs: Loss of folic acid occurs in hemodialysis. Oral contraceptives may impair folic acid absorption in some women. Drugs such as sulphasalazine (ulcerative colitis), anticonvulsants inhibit folate absorption causing anaemia. Methetrexate (immuno suppressive), triamterene (diuretic) and pyrimethamine (antimalarial) interfere with folate metabolism.

Alcoholics comprise the only group that generally has all metabolic defects leading to folic acid deficiency. Less utilisation and increased excretion, increased requirement and increased destruction of folic acid results in deficiency state in alcoholics.

Clinical Features

General symptoms of iron deficiency are present in folic acid deficiency, Glossitis is less common than in vitamin B_{12} deficiency. Neurological problems are very rare.

Diagnosis

Haemoglobin levels may be as low as 4 g/dl. Glossitis is often present. Paraesthesia is a common complaint. Demonstration of FIGLU (formimino glutamic acid excretion test) in the urine is a test of folic acid deficiency. Plasma folate is less than 3 ng/ml. There is free hydrochloric acid in the gastric juice. Serum homocysteine level is increased during folate deficiency due to impaired folate dependent conversion of homocysteine to methionine.

Treatment

Folic acid in dose of 5 to 10 mg daily is effective. Patients who have less than 5 g/dl of haemoglobin need blood transfusion. Iron and B_{12} are often required before a full haematological response can occur.

Dietary Considerations

Foods rich in folic acid like pulses, green leafy vegetables like spinach and gogu leaves, fish, liver and eggs should be included in the diet.

HAEMOLYTIC ANAEMIA

Haemolytic anaemia results due to vitamin E deficiency. Red blood cells have an abnormal membrane resulting from deficiency of vitamin E that makes them extra sensitive to haemolysis. This type of anaemia is found in premature infants who are given milk formulas containing PUFA without vitamin E. It is also found in adults with deficiency of vitamin E.

There is increased rate of distruction of red cells resulting in this anaemia. Oedema and some of its consequences like swollen legs, noisy breathing and puffy eye lids can be observed. In severe deficiency encephalo malacia - softening of the brain occurs.

Administration of 25 IU of vitamin E daily in water soluble form is effective. Administration of iron should be avoided as it interferes with the utilization of vitamin E.

Anaemia can also be caused due to the deficiency of nutrients like copper, protein, energy, and vitamin B_6.

DIFFERENTIATING ANAEMIAS

Figure 13.4 shows microscopic differences between iron deficiency anaemia and megalobastic anaemia.

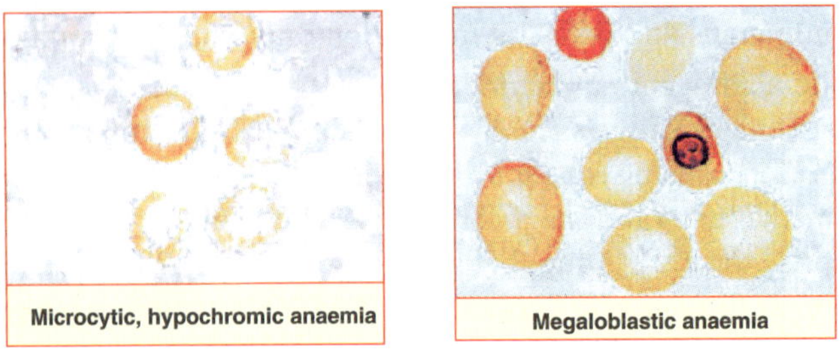

(a) (b)

(a) Microcytic anaemia. This blood smear of a patient with iron deficiency anaemia shows hypochromic, and microcytic red blood cells.

(b) Megaloblastic anaemia-view of red blood cells. This picture shows large, dense, oversized, redblood cells (RBCs) that are seen in megaloblastic anaemia.

Fig. 13.4 Microscopic differentiating characteristics of anaemia

Table 13.5 gives the differences between the different types of anaemia.

Table 13.5 Differentiating characteristics of anaemias

Characteristics	*Iron deficiency*	*B_{12} deficiency*	*Folic acid deficiency*
Type of anaemia	**Hypochromic microcytic**	**Megaloblastic**	
Pathological changes	RBC's are pale and small in size	Variation and irregular shape and size of RBC usually larger than normal, have their full complement of Hb normo-chromic RBC life span reduced to 60 days.	
	MCV < 80	MCV > 100	MCV > 100
Vulnerable groups	Pregnant and lactating women, infants and children	Vegans (no milk, eggs or animal food or fermented food), pregnant women, after gastrectomy	Infants, pregnant women, elderly patients.
Causes	A. Blood loss a. Accidental haemorrhage b. Chronic diseases, cancer ulcer c. Excessive menstrual losses d. Excessive blood donation e. Parasites like hookworm f. Repeated pregnancies B. Deficiency of iron in diet C. Increased demand pregnancy, lactation and infancy	A. Less intrinsic factor. B. Complete vegetarian diet, with no fermented foods. C. After gastrectomy D. Tape worm infestation E. Malabsorption	A. Destruction of folic acid during cooking. B. Increased demand (infancy, pregnancy, alcoholism). C. Malabsorption D. Congenital defects E. Prolonged use of anti-epileptic drugs, oral contraceptives and folate anti-metabolites. F. Loss in haemodialysis.

Table 13.5 (*Contd...*)

Characteristics	*Iron deficiency*	*B_{12} deficiency*	*Folic acid deficiency*
Type of anaemia	**Hypochromic microcytic**	**Megaloblastic**	
	D. Inadequate iron absorption a. Diarrhoea b. Lack of acid secretion by stomach c. Antacid therapy		
Symptoms	General fatigue, breathlessness, giddiness, dimness of vision, headache, anorexia, palpitation, angular stomatitis, koilonychia, glossitis, impaired, language and scholastic achievement, decreased physical activity.	Achlorohydria lemon yellow or pale skin, anorexia, glossitis, diarrhoea, weight loss, coldness of extremities, increased risk of gastric cancer.	Paraesthesia, tropical sprue, fatigue, diarrhoea, glossitis
Diagnosis	Hb level < 12 g/dl in adult < 7.5 g/dl indicates advanced cases.	In Schilling test, 1 μg dose of radioactive B_{12} is given, 30% recovered in faeces of healthy one, 70% in pernicious anaemia patients.	A. Folic acid content of serum. B. Absorption least with tritium labelled folic acid C. FIGLU excretion test
Treatment	A. Oral iron preparation (280 mg of $FeSO_4$) has 60 mg of elemental iron B. For infants the dose is about 6 mg/kg ($FeSO_4$ mixture)	1000 μg of hydroxocobalamin given by intramuscular injection twice weekly until Hb is normal. Intramuscularly 100 mg every six weeks is given. If Hb level is 4g/dl blood transfusion is given.	Folic acid dose of 5–10 mg daily. Hb level is 5 g/dl blood transfusion given; for anticonvulsant therapy-FA is 10–15 mg daily 1000 μg vitamin B_{12} weekly.

Mean Corpuscular volume, mean corpuscular haemoglobin can be used to detect type of anaemia.

PREVENTION

Anaemia can be prevented by diet, supplementation, education and fortification.

Diet

Balanced diet rich in protein, vitamins and minerals should be consumed. Anaemia can be prevented by taking proper diet. Once anaemia is developed there is need for supplementation. Sometimes like in pregnancy some amount of supplementation with blood forming nutrients may be required.

Supplementation

To prevent anaemia under National Nutritional Anaemia Prophylaxis Programme distribution of iron and folate tablets to pregnant women during last trimester and for pre-school children is in operation as part of MCH services. Expectant and nursing mothers are given 60 mg of elemental iron and 0.5 mg of folic acid. Children in the age group 1–5 years are given 20 mg of elemental iron and 0.1 mg of folic acid.

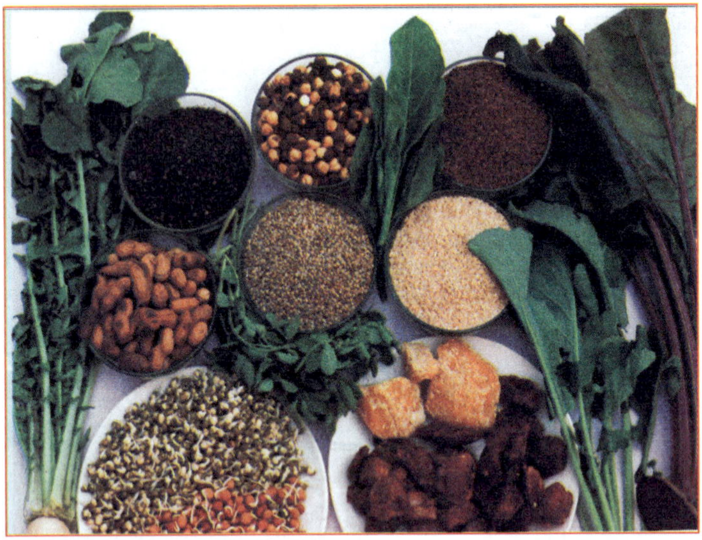

Fig. 13.5 By regular consumption of green leafy vegetables, cereals such as wheat, ragi, jowar and bajra, pulses, jaggery and foods of animal origin anaemia can be prevented. Fruits rich in vitamin C help in the absorption of erythropoietic nutrients.

Source: Food and Nutrition Board.

Table 13.6 Dietary sources of nutrients that prevent anaemia (per 100 g)

Iron mg		*Vitamin B_{12} µg*		*Total folates µg (B9)*	
Coriander seeds	17	Sheep liver	91	Bombay duck	2784
Gingelly seeds	15	Goat Liver	90	Crab	2304
Mustard seeds	13	Shrimp	9	Sardine	2266
Gogu leaves red	9	Egg yolk	4	Rohu	1263
Tamarind pulp	9	Goat meat	2	Moth bean	349
Horse gram	8	Mutton	2	Rajmah	330
Curry leaves	8	Hen egg	1	Soyabean	297
Quinoa	7	Skim milk powder	1	Sheep Liver	206
Sheep liver	6			Spinach	142
Egg yolk	3			Egg	49

Source: Longvah, T, *et. al.,* 2017, Indian Food composition tables, National Institute of Nutrition, Hyderabad.

Education

Emphasis should be laid on educating both the health functionaries as well as the general population about anaemia. All medical, health and social workers, horticulture department and voluntary oganisations have roles to play in promoting the consumption of iron-rich foods. Extensive efforts by community level workers and effective use of modern media are recommended for achieving success in this strategy. Following points need to be considered for promotion of the strategy:

- Promotion of consumption of pulses, green leafy vegetables, eggs and fish (which are rich in iron and folic acid) and meat products—rich in bioavailable iron, particularly by pregnant and lactating mothers. To get vitamin B_{12} consumption of meat, curds, and eggs need to be encouraged.
- Creation of awareness in mothers attending antenatal clinics, immunisation sessions, anganwadi centres and creches about the prevalence of anaemia, ill effects of anaemia and its preventable nature.
- Addition of iron-rich foods to the weaning foods of infants.
- Regular consumption of foods rich in vitamin C such as oranges, guava or amla need to be promoted.
- Promotion of home gardening to increase the availability of common iron rich food such as green leafy vegetables like mint and gogu leaves.
- Encouraging the use of iron pans and iron ladles.
- Periodical administration of antihelminthic drugs to control parasitic worms. Malaria should be controlled.
- Discouraging the consumption of tea immediately after a meal as tannins affect the iron absorption.
- Encouraging consumption of fortified salt. One gram of salt contains one mg of iron.

Fortification

Fortification of a commonly consumed food item with iron has been considered as one of the practical approaches for the prevention and control of iron deficiency anaemia.

Salt is considered as eminently suitable vehicle for iron fortification in India as it satisfies all the criteria for an ideal vehicle. Salt is consumed in India by all segments of population, rich as well as poor perhaps more by the poor. Salt consumption lies within a narrow range of 12–20 g/day with an average intake of 15 g/day/person. Of the estimated annual production of 7 million tons of salt about 4.5 million tons are estimated to be available for human consumption, most of which is produced in about 120 manufacturing centres principally in two States of India—Gujarat and Tamil Nadu.

Now-a-days salt fortified with iron, iodine, folic acid, vitamin B_{12}, vitamin A and zinc is available in the market. Iron fortification of wheat flour and bread is currently employed in the developed countries for the prevention of iron deficiency. Fortification with iron has been successfully adopted for rice, sugar, milk, fish sauce and curry powder.

Policies for combating micronutrient malnutrition must be firmly rooted in food based rather than drug based approaches. One should look to farms and not pharmacies for the solution of nutritional problems.

SUGGESTED READINGS

- Meta analysis approach on micronutrients food fortification and its effect on health, social and economic factors. Annual report, 2013-14, NIN, Hyderabad.
- Clark F. Susan, Iron deficiency anaemia, Nutrition in clinical practice 2008; **23**.

QUESTIONS

1. Define anaemia. Discuss the causes of anaemia in pre-school children.
2. What are the different types of anaemias? How do you distinguish them?
3. Explain the role of different nutrients in erythropoiesis.
4. Discuss iron deficiency anaemia under the following:
   Aetiology, Diagnosis, Clinical findings.
5. Why is it that folic acid deficiency common during pregnancy?
6. What is pernicious anaemia?
7. Vitamin B_{12} is present only in animal sources. How do vegetarians meet its requirement?
8. What is the diagnostic test for folic acid deficiency?
9. Give the list of foods to be included in the diet of a patient suffering from megaloblastic anaemia.
10. List any five foods rich in iron and vitamin C. What is the special advantage of this combination?
11. Iron deficiency occurs in some pathological conditions. Name any two and explain.
12. Why is it gastric resection leads to iron deficiency anaemia?
13. Explain the interrelationship between drugs and iron deficiency anaemia.

TOPIC FOR ACTIVITY

- Check the haemoglobin levels of classmates or a community.

14

Diet in Infections and Fevers

Infection is invasion of the body by harmful organisms such as bacteria, fungi, protozoa, rickettsiae or viruses. The infective agent may be transmitted by a patient or carrier in airborne droplets expelled during coughing and sneezing or by direct contact.

Fevers are usually caused by bacterial or viral infections and can accompany any infectious illness. Fever can also result due to antigen-antibody reaction, malignancy or due to graft rejection.

A catabolic response occurs with all infections even when they are subclinical and not accompanied by fever. Infection stimulates interleukin 1 release from leukocytes which is followed by endocrine changes and mobilisation of amino acids from the skeletal muscle resulting in depletion of body proteins from muscles. The amino acids are used for gluconeogenesis in the liver and the nitrogen released in excreted in urine.

In severely undernourished children there is protein depletion and deficiency of vitamin A, ascorbic acid, pyridoxine, folic acid, thiamine and riboflavin reducing the activity of phagocytes.

Dietary inadequancies decrease resistance of the tissues to infection by causing pathological changes in epithelial and other cells. Vitamin A and B complex deficiencies affect the health of the epithelial cells.

Changes in the normal intestinal flora induced by diet can influence susceptibility to some intestinal pathogens. Intestinal organisms which are non-pathogenic in normal human subjects may become pathogenic in acute diarrhoeal diseases in malnourished children. Lysozymes activity is reduced in human subjects suffering from vitamin A deficiency.

The effect of infection on nutritional status

Impaired Appetite: At central level a transient reduction in plasma levels of micronutrient like zinc or increase in circulating interleukins during acute infection could possibly impair appetite.

In some infections such as gastroenteritis, vomitting and abdominal pain are obvious causes for impaired appetite.

In HIV infection poor appetite is primarily due to mouth ulcers and throat sores.

Depression and mental state also contribute to poor appetite.

Impaired absorption: There is poor absorption of fats, proteins and carbohydrates and certain fat soluble vitamins like vitamins E and A during infections. Fat and protein metabolism is altered and faecal fat and protein loss may be 20–40 per cent with infections. Loss of nutrients may occur with vomiting and diarrhoea.

Increased requirements: The caloric requirement is increased as much as 50 per cent if the temeperature is high and tissue destruction is great.

Drug Nutrient Interactions: The primary task in caring for the infected person is to identify and eliminate the invading organism. Often physicians prescribe anti-infective agents. These drugs may alter nutrient status; nutrients may also interfere with drug effectiveness.

Increased Blood Loss: Hook worm infection causes blood loss leading to anaemia. Malaria causes hemolysis of RBC leading to anaemia.

Development of fever due to exogenous agents is shown in Fig. 14.1.

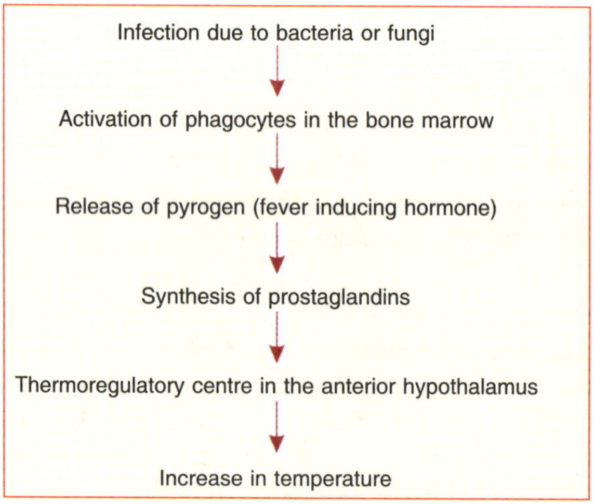

Fig. 14.1 Development of fever due to exogenous agent

There are three types of fevers:

- Short duration: Cold, tonsillitis, influenza and typhoid
- Chronic: Tuberculosis and AIDS
- Intermittent: Malaria

Drugs like aspirin are effective in reducing fever because they inhibit prostaglandin synthesis, though they do not affect the cause of the disease.

Metabolic changes in fever

- An increase in the metabolic rate amounting to 13 per cent for every degree celsius rise in body temperature (7 per cent for each degree Fahrenheit); an increase is also due to restlessness and hence a greatly increased caloric need.
- Decreased glycogen stores and decreased stores of adipose tissue.
- Increased catabolism of protein places an additional burden upon the kidneys.

- Accelerated loss of body water owing to increased perspiration and excretion of body wastes.
- Increased excretion of sodium and potassium.

GENERAL DIETARY CONSIDERATIONS

Energy: Basal metabolic rate increases during infection and fever and calorie requirement increases. Restlessness also increases the calorie requirement. Initially, the patient may be able to ingest only 600 to 1,200 kcal daily, but this should be increased as rapidly as possible.

Protein: About 100 g protein or more is prescribed for an adult when fever is prolonged. This will be most efficiently utilised when the calorie intake is liberal. High protein beverages may be used as supplements to the regular meals.

Carbohydrates: Glycogen stores are replenished by a liberal intake of carbohydrates. Glucose which is less sweet and readily absorbed into the blood stream is preferred.

Fats: The energy intake may be rapidly increased through the judicious use of fats but fried foods and rich pastries may retard digestion unduly.

Minerals: A sufficient intake of sodium chloride is accomplished by the use of salty broth and soups and by liberal sprinklings of salt on food. Fruit juices and milk are relatively good sources of this element.

At the onset of an infection, blood iron rapidly declines as iron moves into the liver for storage. This shift helps fight the infection by depriving the infecting microorganigms of the body's iron which they require for their metabolism. Infact, providing large doses of oral or intravenous iron can worsen the infection. Without medical intervention, the liver will return iron to the blood as the infection resolves.

Vitamins: Fever apparently increases the requirement for vitamin A and ascorbic acid just as the B-complex vitamins are needed at increased levels proportionate to the increase in calories. Oral therapy with antibiotics and drugs interfere with synthesis of some B-complex vitamins by intestinal bacteria, thus necessitating a prescription for vitamin supplements for a short time.

Fluid: The fluid intake must be liberal to compensate for the losses from the sweat and to permit adequate volume of urine for excreting the wastes. Daily 2500-5000 ml is necessary, including beverages, soups, fruit juices and water.

Dehydration is usually not a problem unless a person has diarrhoea, vomiting or excessive sweating. When these losses do occur, fluid needs may be as high as 3 to 4 litres per day. It is also possible that the infected person will retain fluids due to the hormonal changes that accompany fever. Giving fluids in these cases can cause fluid overload.

Ease of digestion: Bland, readily digested food should be used to facilitate digestion and rapid absorption. The food may be soft or of regular consistency. Fluid diets can be used initially. If it is continued there are disadvantages:

- Most fluid diets occupy bulk, out of proportion to their calorie and nutrient values, so that reinforcement with solids is essential.

- A liquid diet sometimes increases abdominal distension to the point of acute discomfort, whereas solid foods may be better tolerated.
- Many patients experience less anorexia, nausea and vomiting when they are taking solid foods.

Intervals of feeding: Small quantities of food at intervals of 2 to 3 hours will permit adequate nutrition without overtaxing the digestive system at any time. With improvement, many patients consume more food if given three meals and bedtime feeding.

The duration of many fevers has been shortened by antibiotic and drug therapy and nutritional needs are usually met without difficulty. During an acute fever the patient's appetite is often very poor and small feedings of soft or liquid foods as desired should be offered at frequent intervals. Sufficient intake of fluids and salt is essential. If the illness persists for more than a few days, high-protein, high calorie foods need to be emphasised.

TYPHOID

Typhoid is an infectious disease with an acute fever of short duration and occurs only in humans. *Salmonella typhi* causes typhoid and *salmonella schottmulleri* causes paratyphoid B. Faeces and urine of the patients or carriers of the disease are the source of infection. Drinking water or milk and food contaminated by intestinal contents of the patients or 'carriers' or by flies which often transmit the disease.

Typhoid bacilli do not multiply in water but some may survive for about 7 days. They may survive for over a month in ice and ice-cream. Typhoid bacilli grow rapidly in milk without altering its taste or appearance in anyway. Vegetables grown in sewage farms or washed in contaminated water are a positive health hazard.

Incubation period is usually 10–14 days. But it may be as short as three days or as long as three weeks depending upon the dose of bacilli ingested.

The disease begins in the small intestine, where the bacteria attach to the epithelium of intestinal wall, penetrate this layer, multiply in the mesenteric lymphnodes and eventually reach the blood stream. Here lysis of the bacteria by the action of antibodies and complement results in the liberation of endotoxin which causes generalised symptoms such as fever. Some bacteria pass from the liver to the gall bladder and bile ducts and are secreted into the intestine where they establish a secondary infection and may cause diarrhoea. Bacterial excretion may occur for weeks and some persons may become chronic carriers.

Symptoms and Signs

The disease is characterised by a continued, high inflammation of the intestine, formation of intestinal ulcers, haemorrhage and enlargement of spleen can occur, Peyer's patches or flat patches of lymphatic tissue situated in the small intestine but mainly in the ileum are the seat of infection in typhoid fever. The patient may complain of diarrhoea or constipation and severe stomach ache. Intestinal absorption of nutrients is decreased and the patient may feel headache and anorexia.

Principles of Diet

A high calorie, high protein, high carbohydrate, low fat, high fluid, low fibre and bland diet is suggested for typhoid patients.

Dietary Suggestions

The general principles of dietary treatment of fever is followed for typhoid also.

At first clear fluid diet is given, followed by full fluid and soft diet. On liquid diets the patient may not meet high calorie and high protein requirements. As the patient is improving soft diet can be given. The febrile period may upset water balance and liquid diets are helpful in meeting water and electrolyte requirements.

Foods to be included	*Foods to be avoided*
Fruit juices with glucose, coconut water, barley water, milk, milk shakes if there is no diarrhoea, custards, thin dal, eggs, baked fish, curds, cottage cheese, cereals, gruels, steamed vegetable juices, milk puddings, vegetable puree	Butter, ghee, vegetable oil, no irritating fibres foods, chillies and other spices, rich pastries, fried foods, puddings and cream soups

Due to intestinal inflammation, great care must be exercised to eliminate all irritating fibres and spices in the diet. Refined cereals, bread, eggs, boiled potato simple desserts like custards, porridges can be given.

Adequate nutrition reduces convalescence period.

INFLUENZA

Influenza is an acute infection of short duration. It spreads from person to person by contact inhalation of virus. A sneeze or cough from an infected individual produces many droplets containing virus and these may be inhaled by those nearby.

Symptoms

The incubation period is about 2 days with a range of 1–7 days. Onset is usually sudden and consists of headache, lassitude, myalgia, shivering and fever. The patient usually has dry cough but there is frequently sneezing or sore throat. The illness is associated with pyrexia and lasts for about 5 days. The patient may complain of lassitude and depression for one or two weeks. A secondary but small rise in temperature may occur but if temperature remains elevated after the fifth day then one of the pulmonary complications is likely. Bronchitis and pneumonia are the most important and frequent complications of influenza.

Principles of Diet

General principles of dietary treatment is followed for influenza patient.

MALARIA

Four species of the genus plasmodium are responsible for human malaria. *P. vivax*, *P. malariae*, *P. ovale* and *P. falciparum*.

Malaria is transmitted from human to human by the bite of infected female anopheles mosquitoes. Induced malaria occurs due to congenital transmission or transmission by blood transfusion.

Symptoms and Signs

Typical malarial attacks show sequentially over 4–6 hours. Shaking chills (the cold stage) and fever (the hot stage) to 41°C or higher and the sweating stage.

Associated symptoms include fatigue, headache, dizziness, gastrointestinal symptoms (anorexia, nausea, slight diarrhoea, vomiting, abdominal cramps) myalgia, arthralgia, backache and dry cough.

Either from the onset or with progression of the disease, the attacks may show an every-other-day periodicity in vivax, ovale or falciparum malaria or an every-third-day (quartan) periodicity in malariae malaria. Splenomegaly usually appears when acute symptoms have continued for 4 or more days.

Principles of Diet

Dietary management is same as for fever.

TUBERCULOSIS

Tuberculosis is one of the leading causes of morbidity and mortality among the adult population of India. Everyday 1,200 Indians die of tuberculosis (2018). TB creates poverty. Poverty creates TB. Mumbai has the highest incidence due to overcrowding in houses and trains; migrant labourers, alcoholism, HIV and missing cases of diabetes. Incidence is common in the age group 25–35.

The sources of infection by *mycobacterium* tuberculosis are inhalation of street dust or house dust and coughing adult. It can also enter through alimentary tract by ingestion-infected milk, edibles and utensils. It is also spread through the inoculation through sputum.

Tuberculosis is an infectious disease caused by the bacillus *mycobacterium tuberculosis*. It affects the lungs most often but may also be localised in other organs such as the lymphnodes, intestine, meninges, bones and joints, skin or it may be generalised. Infection is life long, with bacilli lying dormant in the body. This phase is latent tuberculosis and 40–70 per cent of the population are living with latent tuberculosis. A few progress to TB even after 20 years if the immunity becomes low.

Progression occurs when bacilli become active, multiply and cause disease.

Clinical Features

Pulmonary tuberculosis is accompanied by wasting of tissues, exhaustion, cough, expectoration (cough with respiratory secretions) and fever. The acute phase resembles pneumonia, with high fever. The chronic phase is accompanied by low-grade fever and though the metabolic rate is high, it is lower than in acute fever. Due to protracted illness, wasting may be considerable.

As the disease progresses the patient begins to exhibit loss of appetite, pain in chest, fatigue, weight loss, night sweats and a persistent worsening cough. If a blood vessel is eroded in the lungs, the sputum coughed up by the patient may become streaked with blood, also the tubercle bacilli may gain access to the blood and be transported to various parts of the body, establishing numerous secondary foci of infection. Death ultimately results when sufficient damage has occurred in the lungs or other vital organs. Lymphnodes and kidneys can also be affected. There is increased catabolism of tissue proteins and increased loss of water from body due to perspiration, increased loss of sodium chloride and potassium salt from body.

Treatment

Rifampicin, isoniazid, pyrazinamide and ethambutol are drugs used in combinations for treating tuberculosis. These drugs are supplied free to the patients through government hospitals and health centres. The progress is monitored under the Revised National TB Control Programme based on the Directly Observed Treatment Short Course (DOTS). The treatment lasts for a minimum period of nine months.

Modification of Nutrients

Energy: Since the metabolic rate is not as high as in other fevers, satisfactory weight can be maintained with 2500 to 3000 calories. 45–50 kcal/kg body weight for adults and 90 kcal/kg body weight for children are suggested. It is not desirable to gain more than 10 per cent above the ideal weight for the body frame. High calorie diet is prescribed.

Protein: A protein intake somewhat in excess of normal requirements is necessary in tuberculosis, since the serum albumin value especially in advanced tuberculosis and in cases of long standing, may be low. The daily requirement may be from 80 to 120 g. 1.5–2 g/kg body weight for adults and 3–3.5 g/kg for children are suggested.

Minerals: The drug isoniazid interferes with vitamin D metabolism. This in turn can decrease absorption of calcium and phosphorus. Calcium, especially should be provided liberally since it is also essential for healing tuberculosis lesions. Atleast one litre of milk should be taken daily. The iron needs may also be increased if there has been haemorrhage. Calcium, iron and phosphorus help in regeneration of cells, blood and fluids.

Vitamins: The metabolism of vitamin A is adversely affected in tuberculosis. Carotene appears to be poorly converted to vitamin A so that the diet should be planned to provide vitamin A as such. The inclusion of eggs, liver and dietary supplementation with vitamin A is essential.

If ascorbic acid deficiency is present, increased amounts of orange juice is prescribed. Vitamin C is essential for many regenerative purposes. To get antioxidants, 5 servings of different types of fruits and vegetables should be given.

Isoniazid used as a chemotherapeutic agent for tuberculosis is an antimetabolite to pyridoxine, preventing the formation of pyridoxal phosphate. Pyridoxal phosphate functions as a coenzyme for transaminases that are required for the conversion of amino acids like glutamic acid. Glutamic acid being the only amino acid that the brain can metabolise, lack of pyridoxal phosphate depresses utilisation of glutamic acid and leads to the onset of neuritis. Treatment with large doses, 50 to 100 mg of pyridoxine daily prevents this effect.

Isoniazid also interferes with vitamin D metabolism. This in turn can decrease absorption of calcium and phosphorus. Hence supplementation of vitamins and minerals is required.

Principles of Diet

A high calorie, high protein, high vitamin and minerals and high fluid soft diet is recommended.

Dietary Management

- Patients have poor appetite initially hence food must be appetising and patient's likes and dislikes must be considered.
- During the acute stage a high-calorie fluid and soft diet are prescribed.

- Initially small quantities of fluid diet should be given once in three hours. When the fever comes down, the interval can be increased to every 4 hours.
- With medication patient improves. There will be no fever and cough but due to catabolic process the patient is emaciated. Hence, high calorie and high protein diet should be given. One litre of milk and 3 to 4 eggs per day are given.
- Two to three servings of different type of fruits are suggested to meet micronutrient and antioxidant requirement.
- As the patient progresses, normal, attractive and palatable food should be given. The patient should come back to ideal weight. Rest, fresh air and good nutrition are the key elements for recovery from tuberculosis.

Prevention

By 2025 India aims to eradicate TB. BCG vaccine is effective for children against TB, but not for adults. Improving malnutrition and having diagnostic centre in every district can help in eradicating tuberculosis.

To outsmart tuberculosis bacilli, we must intercent infection, progression and transmission. All these steps can be overcome with well nourishment which develops immunity in an individual.

ACQUIRED IMMUNODEFICIENCY SYNDROME (AIDS)

Primary infection with Human Immunodeficiency Virus, 'HIV' is the underlying cause of AIDS. HIV invades the genetic core of the CD4 + or T-helper lymphocyte cells. HIV infection causes a progressive depletion of CD4 + cells which eventually leads to immunodeficiency, constitutional disease, neurologic complications, opportunistic infections and neoplasms.

The virus can be transmitted via any one of five body fluids: blood, semen, preseminal fluid, vaginal fluid and breast milk. Saliva, tears and urine do not contain enough virus. The most common way of HIV is transmitted via blood and semen. Transmission can also occur by sharing contaminated needles, blood products as well as by across the placenta from an infected mother to her baby.

The virus is not transmitted by casual contact, touching, hugging or kissing or through using the same plates or drinking glasses. All persons should use universal precautions to protect both themselves and others when working with body fluids.

Perinatal HIV transmission can happen three ways; in utero, during birth while through the birth canal or during breast feeding.

Manifestations

Four stages of HIV disease have been characterised:

Acute HIV Infection: It is 4 to 7 weeks period immediately after primary infection when there is rapid viral replication. The infected person develops an acute syndrome characterized by fever, malaise, lymphadenopathy syndrome, pharyngitis, headache, myalgia and sometimes rash which may last for a week to a month.

Asypmtomatic HIV: It is the stage where few if any, noticeable symptoms occur. This stage could last an average of 10 years. Decrease in lean body mass without apparent total body weight change, vitamin B_{12} deficiency and increased susceptibility to food and water borne pathogens.

Symptomatic HIV: In this stage, symptoms like fever, sweats, skin problems and fatigue can be seen. A decline in nutrient status or body composition may also occur.

AIDS: A small proportion of persons infected with the virus develop AIDS and die within months following primary infection. Some HIV infected individuals exhibit no signs of disease progression. A lowered viral load set point, lesser virulence of the virus and protective genetic mutations appear to contribute to this state.

Nutritional Problems in HIV Patients

Causes of nutritional deficiencies

- Decreased nutrient intake
  - Primary anorexia
  - Peptic disease
  - Opportunistic infections of upper GI tract
  - Idiopathic aphthous ulcers
  - Dysgeusia (Zinc deficiency)
  - Pancreatic/hepatobiliary disease
  - Encephalopathy
- Gastrointestinal malabsorption
  - Mucosal disease
  - Infections
  - Inflammatory
  - Disasccharidase deficiency
  - Protein-losing enteropathy
  - Fat malabsorption
  - Hepatobiliary
    - Cholangitis
    - Chronic pancreatitis
- Increased nutritional requirements
  - Protein wasting
  - Hyper metabolism
- Psycho social factors
  - Poverty,
  - Illness in biological family members
  - Limited access to health care

Micronutrient deficiencies

During HIV infection, nutrient requirements are increased to sustain immune cell turnover. In particular, deficiencies of vitamin A, zinc, and iron adversely affect immune function through different mechanisms, and their correction can restore immune function, though they do not compensate for T lymphocyte depletion, which occurs in HIV infection. Iron is a key component of cytochromes that mediate cellular energy metabolism, as well as of important enzymes, potentially influencing immune cell turnover. Zinc is important in the activity of many enzymes, DNA-binding proteins, and the thymic hormone, thymulin, and its deficiency impairs lymphocyte function. The active metabolite of vitamin A, retinoic acid, affects the thymic hormone production of immunologically significant cytokines such as gamma interferon and interleukin-4, and influences the ability of cells to respond to these cytokines.

In addition, low levels of 1, 25-dihydroxyvitamin D and vitamin E have been reported in various HIV-infected populations. Deficiencies in B-vitamins can also compromise immune function by virtue of their roles as cofactors in many enzymes, including those involved in nucleic acid synthesis. Vitamin B_{12} deficiency is very prevalent in the pre-HAART (Highly Active Antiretroviral Therapy) era and was related to absent intrinsic factor secretion and to abnormal ileal B_{12} absorption. Serum levels of other water-soluble vitamins also have been reported to be low, despite apparent normal intake, whereas fat-soluble vitamin deficiencies occur in subjects with diarrhoea and malabsorption.

Depletion of antioxidant nutrients (e.g., vitamins E and C, and selenium) and of various regulatory molecules, such as reduced glutathione and nitric oxide, impairs immune responsiveness and allows greater oxidative damage to immune and other cell types. Selenium deficiency has been associated epidemiologically with increased mortality risk, while autopsy studies have shown low myocardial concentrations of selenium in HIV-infected subjects. Antioxidant requirements are increased in HIV patients.

Macronutrient deficiencies

In asymptomatic patients, mild weight loss may be noted. Early studies documented disproportionate depletion of body cell mass in AIDS patients with clinical complications. Body cell mass depletion is associated with variable amounts of fat depletion, and with expansion of the extracellular space. Patients with malabsorptive illnesses demonstrated depletion of total body water. Weight loss and body cell mass depletion in HIV infection are associated with shortened survival and diminished quality of life.

Malnutrition is an important and complicated consequence of HIV infection. Protein Energy Malnutrition is a frequent complication of AIDS. Weight loss, body cell mass depletion, decreased skinfold thickness and midarm circumference, decreased iron-binding capacity and hypoalbuminemia are frequently reported.

Weight loss and wasting are due to lack of adequate intake, malabsorption, metabolic irregularities, uncontrolled opportunistic infection and lack of physical activity.

Nutrient deficiencies may play an important role in the pathogenesis of HIV disease. Medical nutrition therapy and counselling are critical aspects of treatment.

Components of Medical Nutrition Therapy

Nutritional Screening

Ideally, all persons with HIV infection should be screened for nutritional problems and concerns at the time of their first contact with a health care professional. Routine monitoring should be performed and action should be taken accordingly.

Nutrition Referral

Referral information should include the following:

- Current diagnosis and medical history.
- Referring health care provider's nutrition prescription or desired outcome.
- Clinical symptoms and feeding route.

- Weight history and body composition.
- Recent biochemical data.
- Current medications including drugs, vitamins and minerals and dietary supplements.
- Life style.

Nutritional Assessment

The diet should be evaluated for nutrient adequacy especially of nutrients involved with immune function.

Psychosocial conditions should also be assessed. Fear, anxiety, depression and social isolation all affect appetite and nutrient intake. Illness or ostracism often leads to a lack of employment and subsequent loss of social contact as well as income and medical care.

Height, weight, hip-to-waist ratio, neck circumference and measurements of either lean body mass (using triceps skinfold and midarm muscle circumference) calculations should be compared to each other, rather than to published reference.

Serum albumin, prealbumin, retinol binding protein, transferrin and total iron binding capacity can be used to monitor changes in visceral protein status.

Nutritional Requirements

The goals for nutrition therapy should be to educate these individuals about the importance of consuming a well-balanced diet, to provide adequate nutrition for maintenance or improvement in nutritional status and to prevent severe acute malnutrition.

Energy: Energy and protein needs vary depending on the health status of the individual at the time of HIV infection, the progression of the disease and the development of complications that impair nutrient intake and utilisation. The Harris Benedict equation can be used to determine basal energy expenditure which can be multiplied by a stress factor (1.3) to allow for maintenance and anabolism (1.5). An adjustment must also be made in the presence of fever. Activity can also affect energy requirements. Generally a patient may require 30–45 kcal/kg body weight at different stages of the disease.

Protein: High protein diets promote positive nitrogen balance and lean body mass repletion. Protein requirements may be estimated at 1.0 and 1.4 g/kg for maintenance and 1.5 and 2.0 g/kg for repletion.

Fat: In individuals with malabsorption or diarrhoea, use of a low-fat diet may aid in management. Medium chain triglyceride oil should be given for decreasing stool fat and stool nitrogen content and in reducing the number of bowel movements and abdominal symptoms. MCT is more readily absorbed than long-chain triglycerides.

Fish oil (ω-3 fatty acids) when given with MCT oil may improve immune function because this combination is less inflammation-promoting than the usual ω-6 fatty acids.

Fluids and Electrolytes: Fluid needs in HIV-infected individuals are similar to those of normal individuals and are calculated to be 30–35 ml/kg. Additional amounts are required to compensate for losses from diarrhoea, nausea and vomiting, night sweats and prolonged fever. Replacement of electrolyte losses (sodium, potassium and chloride) in the presence of vomiting and diarrhoea is also recommended.

Vitamins and Minerals: Studies have indicated that there is increased need of β-carotene, vitamin E, ascorbic acid, vitamin B_{12} vitamin B_6 and folic acid. Selenium is a biological anti-oxidant. Supplementation of selenium with 70 mg/day would benefit the patient. Excessive zinc is deleterious. Immuno nutrients and antioxidants can also be supplemented. Probiotics improve immunity. Those who are taking inadequate diet, vitamin-mineral supplementation should be taken. Use of doxorubin hydrochloride requires adequate riboflavin to reduce drug toxicity. Excellent nutritional status enhances the ability to fight subsequent infections.

Food Modifications

- **Mouth pain or sores:** It is difficult to eat is there is mouth pain or sores or problems in swallowing. Cool, smooth and mildly favoured foods make eating more enjoyable.
    - Food should be served at moderate temperature as very hot and very cold foods may be irritating.
    - Mild foods and drinks like apple juice can be given. Acidic foods like oranges, grape fruit and pineapple may cause a burning feeling in the mouth.
    - Species like chillie powder and masala powders and salt foods should be limited in the diet.
    - Hard foods like chapattis or toast should be made soft with milk or soup.
    - Easy to swallow foods like egg puddings noodles should be given.
    - Sherbets which numb the pain can be given.
- **Difficulty in swallowing**
    - Foods that irritate the throat should not be taken.
    - Coarse particle foods like nuts, corn not mash rice may get stuck in the throat.
    - Sticky dry foods like peanut butter, should be avoided.
    - Straw can be used for drinking beverages.

Oral Supplements

An elemental diet containing medium-chain triglycerides (MCT) and hydrolyzed whey protein produce improvements in fat and nitrogen balance, accompanied by weight maintenance and decreased diarrhoea. The use of high-protein/high-calorie supplements in AIDS patients is associated with weight gain, provided there are no active opportunistic infections. Enteral formulas that contain peptides, MCT, ω-3 fatty acids, β carotene, vitamins and minerals, and soluble fiber as given to HIV-positive patients. This reduces hospitalisation rate without affecting weight or immune function.

Neuropsychological abnormalities associated with low serum vitamin B_{12} concentrations improved after specific supplementation. High doses of vitamin A are shown to stabilize CD4+ cells in an inner-city intravenous drug use population. In vitro, addition of antioxidant vitamins to experimental systems block this activation and inhibits HIV replication. Supplementation with vitamins C and E produced a significant decrease in oxidative stress indices and a trend toward reduced HIV viral load.

When supplements fail to control wasting, enteral or total parenteral nutrition can be given to the patient.

Drugs and Nutritional Complications

Antiretroviral drugs are given to AIDS patients. The disease and the drugs may affect the nutritional status. Nutritional management of common ARV side effects is given in Table 14.1.

Table 14.1 Nutritional management of common ARV side effects

Side effect	*Recommended nutritional management*	*Avoid*
Anorexia	• Eat small and frequent meals. • Eat favourite foods. • Select foods that are rich in energy. • Take multivitamins.	• Avoid strong smelling foods.
Nausea or vomiting	• Eat small quantities of food at frequent intervals. • Drink after meals and limit intake of fluids with meals. • Limit salt intake and eat dry foods to calm the stomach. • Sip oral rehydration solution (ORS) if vomiting. • Rest between meals.	• Avoid having an empty stomach for too long. • Avoid lying down after eating.
Change or loss of taste	• Use flavour enhancers such as salt, spices or lemon. • Chew food well and move around in mouth to stimulate receptors. • Select foods that smell good to help improve the desire to eat.	
Constipation	• Eat foods high in fiber content. • Drink plenty of fluids. • Exercise regularly according to capacity.	• Avoid processed or refined foods.
Diarrhoea	• Drink plenty of fluids (clean boiled water). • Continue eating during and after illness. • Prepare and drink ORS regularly. • Eat banana or potatoes to replace potassium and sodium. • Take soluble fibre foods (like oranges, mangoes, oats, and legumes). • If diarrhoea is severe check for lactose intolerance. Decrease intake of dairy products and see if diarrhoea improves. Lactose intolerance is often temporary. • Seek medical care if there is blood in the diarrhoea.	• Avoid fried foods. • Avoid alcohol. • Reduce the amount of dietary fat.
Fever	• Drink plenty of fluids. • Eat energy and nutrient dense foods. • Eat small, frequent meals.	

Wasting and diarrhoea occur sooner or later during the course of AIDS. In many persons death appears to be determined more by nutritional status than any particular opportunistic infection. Other common nutrition related complications are anorexia, fatigue, fever, dehydration, nausea and fat and metabolic abnormalities. Successful lowering of viral load, especially through the use of potent protease inhibitors, helps to maintain nutritional status.

Since there is immune suppression food and water safety should be the main concern.

COVID -19

There was an outbreak of corona virus disease in 2019. This was caused by a novel corona virus, severe acute respiratory syndrome coronavirus 2 (SARS-COV2). And this has become a global catastrophe.

Data from the early months of 2020 suggests that most people with COVID-19 have comorbidities, the most prevalent of which are diabetes, cardiovascular disease and hypertension. A significant association with worse outcomes is seen in people with these comorbidities. Studies have also shown that COVID-19 is associated with hyperglycemia particularly in the elderly with type-2 diabetes. Depending on the global region, 20-50 per cent of patients with COVID-19 pandemic had diabetes. A risk of fatal outcome from COVID-19 is upto 50 per cent higher in patients with diabetes than in those who do not have diabetes.

In general, people with all forms of diabetes are at increased risk of infection because defects in innate immunity affecting phagocytosis, neutrophill chemotaxis and cell-mediated immunity.

Symptoms

The most commonly reported symptoms are fatigue, cough, shortness of breath, chest pain, difficulty in concentrating, arthralgia, low grade fever and headache.

Other reported symptoms include cognitive impairment, olfactory and gustatory dysfunction, sleep difficulty, depression, gastrointestinal upset, alopecia and rashes.

Sometimes symptoms continue for 6 months after acute COVID-19 diagnosis.

COVID-19 is primarily considered a respiratory illness but the kidney may be one of the target of SARS-COV2 infection. The virus enters cells through the angiotensin-converting enzyme 2 receptor which is found in abundance in the kidney.

Mechanism

There are at least two specific mechanism that might play a vital role in COVID-19 infection. First, to gain entry to its target cells, the SARS-COV-2 virus hijacks an endocrine pathway that plays a crucial role in blood pressure regulation, metabolism and inflammation. Angiotensin-converting-enzyme 2(ACE2) has been identified as the receptor for the coronavirus spike protein. ACE2 has protective effects primarily regarding inflammation. COVID-19 infection reduces ACE2 expression inducing cellular damage, hyper inflammation and respiratory failure. Acute hyperglycemia has been shown to upregulate ACE2 expression on cells which might facilitate viral cell entry. However, chronic hyperglycaemia is known to downregulate ACE2 expression making the cells vulnerable to the inflammatory and damaging effect of the virus.

Furthermore, the expression of ACE-2 on pancreatic β cells can lead to a direct effect on β cell function. Although these findings have not been verified in humans, they suggest that diabetes might not only be a risk factor for a severe forms of COVID-19 disease but also that infection could induce new onset diabetes.

Nutritional Implications

Protein energy malnutrition from inadequate dietary intake can increase risk of an infectious disease. Reciprocally any exposure including infectious disease that impairs immune functions and causes malabsorption, increased catabolism or decreased nutrients intake can increase risk of malnutrition.

Individuals infected with COVID-19 may have baseline nutrient deficiencies or increased nutrient needs due to COVID-19 pathology.

Suspected efficiency of providing additional micronutrients to patients to reduce disease severity is based on known mechanisms of micronutrients including optimising the immune system and reducing inflammation as well as results from trial with human infected with other viruses and in animal models of coronavirus. Providing micronutrients, particularly ascorbic acid and cholecalciferol may treat underlying insufficiencies or deficiencies to benefit immune function prior to and after contracting COVID-19 infection.

Nutritional support is in high demand for critically ill patients being treated in Intensive care units during the pandemic. Conditional amino acids become essential in the context of critical care.

Socio-economic factors such as gaps in access to health care no doubt play a role in the incidence of COVID-19. But another possible factor has been largely overlooked which is Vitamin D deficiency that weakens the immune system. Researchers found that the nations with the highest mortality rate are Italy, Spain and France and also had the lowest average Vitamin D levels among countries affected by the pandemic. Supplements may promote immunity especially in people with a darker skin.

Viral infection is a cause of acute pancreatitis. Novel coronavirus has a potential risk of triggering acute pancreatitis. The association of COVID-19 with acute pancreatitis is important in the context of nutritional therapy as it has immulogic effect, prevention of bacterial overgrowth and decreased bacterial translocation and intestinal permeability. COVID-19 infection and acute pancreatitis are considered highly catabolic disease processors and have nutritional risk.

March 24th is World Tuberculosis Day

December 1st is World AIDS Day

SUGGESTED READINGS

- Mahendri N.V., 2011, "HIV." Clinical Dietetics Manual. Indian Dietetic Association.
- "Micronutrient Status in HIV Infected Population in India." Annual Report National Institute of Nutrition Hyderabad.
- Park K., 2010, Park's Textbook of Preventive and Social Medicine. Jabalpur: Bhanarasidas Bhanot Publishers.
- Rozga Mary et al., Effects of Micronutrients and Conditional Amino acids on COVID-19 related out comes, J Acad Nutr Diet, 2021; 121.
- ADA Nutrition fact sheet: HIV/AIDS. www.eatright.org/nfs42.html.
- CDC National Centre for Infectious Diseases, www.cdc.gov/ncidod/diseases/foodborn/foodinfections.htm.

QUESTIONS

1. State the basic principles to be observed in planning diets for patients recovering from typhoid fever.
2. What is fever? What are the causes of fever? List the types of fever. Explain the metabolic changes in fever.
3. Give a diet plan for a patient recovering from tuberculosis.
4. Describe the contributing factors in the development of tuberculosis. What are the common signs and symptoms in this condition? State the mode of treatment and the dietary modifications prescribed.
5. State the principles involved in the dietary management for (a) typhoid (b) tuberculosis. Plan a diet for a male adult admitted in hospital for treatment of tuberculosis.
6. What dietary principles are recommended in planning diets for fever of short duration?
7. Suggest protein concentrates and nutrition supplements available in the market for a patient recovering from tuberculosis.
8. Explain the components of medical nutrition therapy.
9. Describe the nutritional problems in HIV patients.
10. Give the nutritional requirements for HIV patients.
11. Bring out the importance of oral supplements for HIV patients.
12. Explain COVID-19 under the following headings.
    (*i*) Symptoms (*ii*) Nutritional implications

TOPIC FOR DISCUSSION

- Discuss how COVID-19 was controlled in India and the implications of those methods.

15

Diet in Obesity and Underweight

OBESITY

Obesity is a chronic disease that can begin in childhood adolescence or adulthood.

Obesity is due to positive energy balance, the intake of calories is more than the expenditure of energy. The underlying influences of this energy imbalance are multi dimensional and complex comprising an intricate interaction between biological, behavioural and environmental factors. Obesity is a state in which there is a generalised accumulation of excess adipose tissue in the body leading to more than 20 per cent of the desirable weight. Over weight is a condition where the body weight is 10–20 per cent greater than the mean standard weight for age, height and sex. Obesity invites disability, disease and premature death. Obesity is a chronic disease. Excess body weight is a hindrance, leading to breathlessness on moderate exertion and predisposes a person to diseases like atherosclerosis, high blood pressure, stroke, diabetes, gall bladder diseases and osteoarthritis of weight bearing joints and varicose veins.

In children and adolescents overweight is defined by the percentile rank of BMI within the population distribution. BMI between the 85th and 95th percentile indicates increased risk for overweight, whereas BMI > 95th percentile is used to define obesity.

AETIOLOGY

Obesity is a complex multi factorial chronic disease developing from interactive influences of numerous factors—social, behavioural, psychological, metabolic, cellular and molecular (genetic).

The desire and drive to eat food, satiety choice of food, digestibility of the food eaten and its absorption in the body, metabolism of nutrients and the metabolic rate, drive and ability to exercise are the factors that determine body weight.

Genetic factors: Genetic inheritance probably influences 50–70 per cent a person's chance of becoming fat more than any other factor. A genetic base regulates species differences in body fat and sexual differences within a species. Within families the chance is 80 per cent if both parents are obese and 50 per cent if one parent is obese. A mutation in the human gene for the B3 receptor in adipose tissue, involved in lipolysis and thermogenesis markedly increase the risk of obesity.

Many genes play a role in energy homeostasis (UCP1, UCP2, UCP3), food intake regulation (MC3R, MC4R; CCKAR), appetite (NPYRS), and ultimately obesity (ASIP, CPE, LEP, LEPR, TUB, POMC), in mammals.

In addition, there are reports about ethnic differences in metabolic rate, increasing the tendency to gain weight in races with lower metabolic rate compared to other races of similar size.

Age and sex: It can occur at any age in either sex as long as the person is under positive energy balance. Studies conducted at Nutrition Foundation of India have shown more females than males are found to be over weight among all age groups. Hormonal predisposition put women at higher risk of obesity when compared to men.

Eating habits: Certain type of eating habits may lead to obesity.

- Nibbling between meals is common among housewives and is a potential cause for obesity.
- Some may eat faster taking less time for chewing, therefore they tend to consume more food. Eating in the absence of hunger also leads to over weight.
- Neurotransmitters or chemicals in the brain that respond to outside stimuli such as sight, taste, smell and temperature transmit signals to other areas of brain and body. Obese respond to external cues to eat rather than internal hunger signals. They eat when it is mealtime or when they are surrounded by tasty foods instead when they are hungry.
- Housewives who are fond of cooking variety of foods or persons who are working in the kitchens may become obese.
- Business executives who frequently attend business lunches have more chance of becoming obese.
- Housewives who do not want leftover foods to be thrown out may consume forcibly and put on weight.
- People who eat outside home more frequently are prone to obesity. Large portions of food served outside the home promote high calorie consumption.
- People who eat more junk food (high fat, high carbohydrate, high salt) or fried food snacks may become obese.
- Certain cultural practices like making and distributing sweets on festive occasions contribute to increased calorie consumption.
- Non-inclusion of fruits and vegetables and non-vegetarian diet with high fat favour weight gain.
- People who like to eat processed, concentrated and high fat food are susceptible to obesity.
- Some may eat more food when they are unhappy or bored as a compensation mechanism.
- There is an abundance of palatable, calorifically dense food available in the market. Aggressive and sophisticated marketing in the mass media, super markets and restaurants tempt the people to eat more.
- Sugar added beverages when frequently consumed may contribute to weight gain.
- Personnel who work in different shifts, whose body clock is disturbed, may over eat.
- There is a potential link between low water consumption and obesity.

- People may have extra feeding during night may be due to sleep disorder.
- Type of food consumed-high carbohydrate food increases insulin levels and interfere in the leptin signaling and increase appetite and increase fat storage.

Physical activity: Obesity is found in persons who lead sedentary lives and pay less importance to physical activity. Though obesity can occur at any age, this is more common during middle age when physical activity decreases without corresponding decrease in food consumption. Obesity can also be seen among school children who spend too much time on studies, who do not do physical exercise, who do not participate in school games and who use vehicles for commuting to schools.

Stress: Food is one of the many stimulants of endorphin, 'feel good' neurotransmitter. Self gratification, self punishment, depression, anxiety and stress may lead to excess caloric intake. Recent studies have shown that school children tend to take more fatty foods as their lives grow stressful. Chronic sleep deprivation may increase appetite in some.

Endocrine factor: Obesity is found in hypothyroidism, hypogonodism and cushing's syndrome. Obesity is common at puberty, pregnancy and menopause, suggesting endocrine may be a factor in obesity.

Trauma: Obesity may follow due to damage to hypothalamus after head injury because it is not able to regulate appetite or satiety.

Prosperity and civilisation: Obesity is common in prosperous countries like UK, USSR and USA and among people from higher socioeconomic status of developing countries, since they have the purchasing power and availability of surplus food. Obesity is rare in primitive societies and in wild animals. Civilisation has brought plentiful supply of appetising foods, concentrated foods and variety of foods in the market.

Drugs: Some drugs promote weight gain. Psychiatric drugs like antidepressants, steroid hormones, contraceptives, diabetic drugs and antihistamines may increase weight in an individual.

THEORIES

Fat cell theory: Number of fat cells is determined early in life to provide space to store fat. Once they have been formed, fat cells have a tendency to remain full of fat. Total number of fat cells was set early in life, supporting the notion that juvenile onset obesity was caused by an increase in the number of fat cells while adult-onset was caused by an increase in the size of fat cells.

The number of fat cells can increase in adult life and that the number of fat cells can also actually diminish as a result of sustained weight loss. People with a large number of fat cells have more difficulty in maintaining body weight than those with fewer fat cells. Research has shown that risk for medical problems is related to the size of fat cells present more than the number of fat cells or the person's weight.

Set point theory: Each person has an ideal biological weight or set point. Once body weight reaches this point, a whole set of signals is produced that influences the person's food intake to maintain this weight.

ROLE OF HORMONES

Obesity gene is expressed in the fat cells and codes for the protein leptin. It acts as a hormone in the hypothalamus. It promotes negative energy balance by suppressing appetite and increasing the energy expenditure. People with genetic defect of leptin show signs of poor appetite control, constant hunger and eat more and may gain weight. In obesity there is sufficient leptin production but there is insensitivity or resistance of the adipose tissues to leptin. The concentration of leptin in blood is usually proportional to the amount of stored fat. Leptin plays an important role in the long term regulation of energy balance. During starvation and weight loss, leptin production from adipose tissue decreases.

Leptin is regarded as a body weight regulatory hormone. It binds to a specific receptor in the brain and functions as a lipostat. When the fat stores in adipose tissue are adequate, leptin levels are high. This signals to restrict the feeding behaviour and limit fat deposition. Leptin stimulates lipolysis and inhibits lipogenesis. Any genetic defect in leptin or its receptor will lead to obesity.

Insulin and leptin are hormones that act as medium to long term regulators of body weight through their actions to decrease food intake and increase energy expenditure (metabolic rate), ensuring that energy intake and energy expenditure is closely matched.

People who do not produce leptin due to genetic deficiency or who have defects in the leptin receptor have dramatically increased appetites and over eat to the point of becoming massively obese. The effects of leptin deficiency are ameliorated by the administration of recombinant leptin.

Insulin, in addition to its effects in the central nervous system to inhibit food intake acts in the periphery to ensure the efficient storage of incoming nutrients. Insulin also has an indirect role in body weight regulation through the stimulation of leptin. Both insulin and leptin are transported into the central nervous system, where they may interact with a number of hypothalamic neuro peptides known to affect food intake and body weight.

Insulin and leptin are released and circulate in the blood stream at levels that are proportionate to body fat content. Secretion and circulating levels are also influenced by amount and type of foods eaten, with decreased concentrations noted during fasting or energy restricted diets.

The decrease of leptin during a prolonged energy-restricted diet has been shown to be related to increased sensations of hunger suggesting a role for low leptin levels to increase appetite during dieting in humans, and therefore to the predisposition for weight regain, after initially successful dieting.

Increased insulin secretion has been suggested to protect against weight gain in humans. Circulating concentrations of both insulin and leptin, reduce in women who consume high fat meals. Insulin stimulates leptin production, which acts centrally to reduce energy intake and increase energy expenditure. Decreased insulin and leptin production during the consumption of high-fat diets could help contribute to the obesity promoting effects of dietary fat.

There is a direct relationship between leptin, BMI and waist circumference and inverse relationship between total grehlin, BMI and waist circumference regardless of age and sex.

Table 15.1 Hormones and obesity

Hormone	Level in obesity	Effect of weight loss
Insulin	80% of obese patients have hyperinsulinemia. Obesity enhances insulin resistance.	Improves insulin sensitivity. All aspects of glucose uptake are improved.
Thyroid hormones	Serum total and free thyroxine levels are usually normal but obese patients may have reduced number of cellular receptors. Hypothyroidism has minimal effect on long-term body weight.	Decreases concentrations of T_3 combined with reduced fat-free mass may contribute to decreased resting metabolic rate in formerly obese patient.
Growth hormone	Decreased; may be adaptive.	Levels normalise
Leptin	Elevated; leptin resistance common	Reduces plasma leptin levels but level remains higher than those who were never obese.

ASSESSMENT

Visual inspection of a patient can give a subjective but fairly accurate estimate of the degree of obesity.

Body weight: Tables of average weights by height and age and tables of desirable weights for height are used to assess the patient. An adult weighing 10 per cent more than the standard weight is overweight and 20 per cent more is obese.

Table 15.2 Body weight in relation to degree of obesity

% Body weight excess to normal	Degree of obesity
25	mild
50	moderate
75	severe
100	very severe

Body Mass Index: Body mass index is used as an indicator of whether or not a person is overweight or underweight. BMI is accepted as a better estimate of body fatness and health risk than body weight. It is also called Quetlet Index. This index does not require any standard tables.

$$\text{BMI} = \frac{\text{Weight (kg)}}{\text{Height}^2\,\text{(m)}}$$

The following classification scheme is endorsed by the ICMR.

Grading of obesity based on BMI.

Obesity	> 25.0
Overweight	– 23–24.9
Normal	– 18.0–22.9
Underweight	< 18

BMI is a good tool for policy makers such as national health organization when they are assessing a large group and BMI correlate with body fat composition.

This index has limitations as it does not distinguish between overweight due to obesity and muscular hypertrophy as it happens in athletes and BMI provides no information about body fat distribution. BMI does not accurately measure the amount and location of body fat or the portion of muscle to fat. BMI may be normal but may have insulin resistance and higher risk of heart disease which may be due to having more body fat and less muscle mass. People with obese BMI may be healthy because they have a lot of muscle.

Nomogram for determining Body Mass Index is given in Appendix.

Figure 15.1 gives relation of weight to height by giving desirable range (0) to grade III obesity as per the definition of BMI.

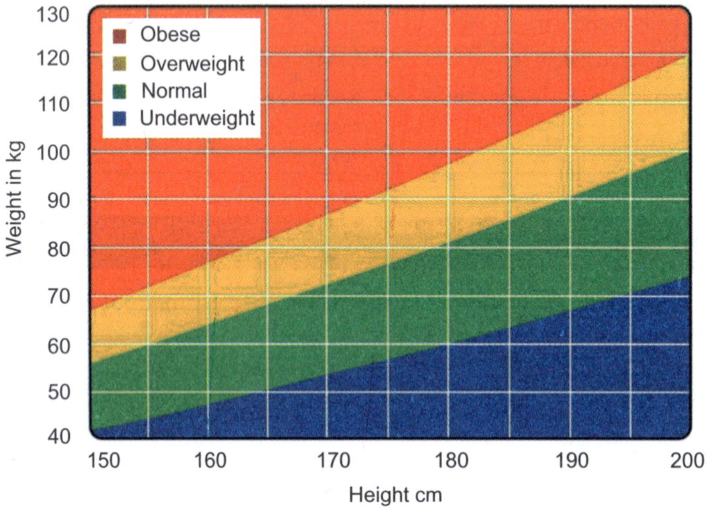

$$BMI = \frac{\text{Weight in pounds}}{\text{Height in inches}^2} \times 703.1$$

$$BMI = \frac{\text{Weight in kg}}{\text{Height in meter}^2}$$

Fig. 15.1 Relation of weight to height giving the desirable range

Waist circumference: It is the most practical tool a clinician can use to evaluate a patient's abdominal fat before and during weight loss treatment.

High risk waist circumference:

Men: > 40 inches (> 102 cm) Women: > 35 inches (> 88 cm)

Waist circumference has been shown to be a better predictor of visceral abdominal fat than BMI, percentage body fat and waist hip ratio.

Measurement of body fat: A more accurate definition of overweight and obesity should be based on the total amount of body fat. The upper limit of body fat for defining obesity have been set as 25 per cent for males and 30 per cent for females. Duel Energy X-ray Absorptometry is one of the most widely accepted methods of measuring body composition. It is safe, convenient and noninvasive method. It can measure per cent fat with great precision and it correlates well with other methods of measuring body composition. A simple instrument called body fat analyser gives the percentage of body fat. Asian Indians have a characteristic phenotype, consisting of excess body fat, abdominal adipocity, and less lean tissue. The study conducted at

National Institute of Nutrition (2004-2005) confirms that Indian women have high levels of body fat per cent at comparatively lower BMI levels than the values reported for the other ethnic groups.

Table 15.3 Criteria for obesity in terms of percentage body fat

Category	*Males*	*Females*
Normal	12–20%	20–30%
Borderline	21–25%	31–33%
Obesity	> 25%	> 33%

Subcutaneous fat is less likely to cause insulin resistance. Sumo wrestlers never suffer from insulin resistance though they have excessive subcutaneous fat and very negligible visceral fat.

Ponderal Index: The ponderal index is the ratio of height to the cube root of weight. This index is given by the formula

$$PI = \frac{\text{Height (inches)}}{3\sqrt{\text{weight (lbs)}}}$$

An index less than 13 is associated with obesity.

Waist to Hip ratio: The predominant distribution of fat in an obese person, whether in the upper part or the lower part of the body, may determine the disease pattern.

$$\text{The normal ratio } \frac{\text{waist}}{\text{hip}} = 0.7$$

but with upper body obesity the ratio is 0.85 in women and greater than 1.0 in males. Abdominal obesity does not always go hand in hand with overweight or obesity.

Broka's index: The formula for Broka's index is

$$\text{Height (cm)} - 100 = \text{ideal weight (kg)}$$

This measurement is easy to calculate and accurate.

GRADES

Grade I obesity: These people have body mass index more than 25 but less than 29.9. Overweight does not affect their health, they lead normal health and life expectancy is above normal. They may reduce on their own.

Grade II obesity: The body mass index is between 30–39.9. These patients should be treated by doctors and dietitians. Although they appear to be in good health, they have reduced tolerance to exercise with shortness of breath on exertion and they are unduly fatigued. This is due to the burden of increased weight they carry always and reduced capacity of the circulatory and respiratory systems that are handicapped by masses of internal fat and fatty infiltration of muscle. For mechanical and metabolic reasons these patients are at increased risk of diabetes, atherosclerosis, hypertension, fatty liver, gall bladder diseases, osteoarthritis, hernias and varicose veins. Mortality rate also increases.

Grade III obesity: The body mass index is above 40 and these patients are in pathetic condition. Their day to day activities are restricted due to their enormous mass and more susceptible to diseases mentioned in Grade II. They are susceptible to atherosclerosis, prone to accidents and have serious psychological disturbances.

REGIONAL DISTRIBUTION OF ADIPOSE TISSUE

Fat mass is distributed differently in men and women. The android or male pattern is characterised by fat distributed predominantly in the upper body above the waist, whereas as gynecoid, or female pattern shows fat predominantly in the lower body that is lower abdomen, buttocks, hips and thighs. In abdominal obesity the waist : hip ratio is high. Abdominal adipose tissue is influenced by environmental factors and not genetic like female adipose tissue.

Recent findings suggest that waist circumference increases less with high fruit and high red meat intake. Waist circumference increases more with a diet high in fat, unhealthful snack choices and sweatened beverages.

There is conclusive evidence that obesity located in the central abdominal parts of the body is statistically associated with a number of metabolic derangements such as insulin resistance, hyperinsulinemia, non insulin dependent diabetes mellitus, hyperlipidimia and hypertension. The mechanism might be due to the lipolytically sensitive abdominal depots providing excess free fatty acids to a muscle tissue that has a decreased capacity for their oxidation. The excessive exposure of tissues to fatty acids impairs insulin function and increases blood insulin levels. All this ultimately results in reduced insulin sensitivity making a person insulin resistant. This in turn result in hyperinsulinemia which might be the starting point for most of the other metabolic derangements. Majority of Indians suffer from diabetes due to insulin resistance and not due to insufficient insulin secretion.

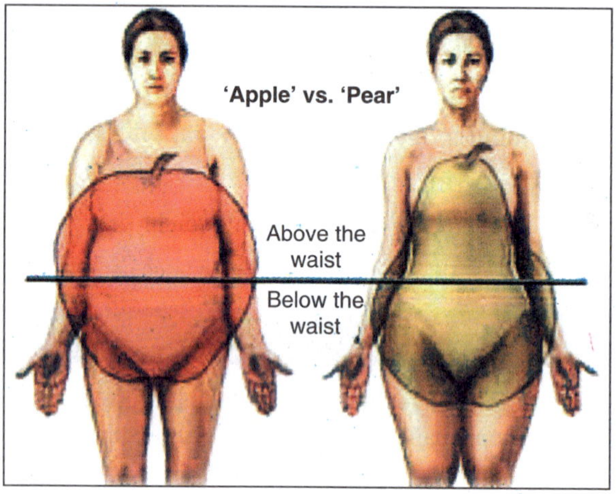

Fig. 15.2 Regional distribution of adipose tissue

Weight gain in the area of and above the waist (apple type) is more harmful than weight gain around the hips and flank area (pear type). Fat cells in the upper body have different qualities than those found in hips and thighs. Indians have significantly greater abdominal fat and visceral fat at Normal Body Mass Index. The relationship between per cent body fat and BMI is ethnic specific.

Source: Medline Plus Medical Encyclopedia: Different types of weight gain. www.nlm.nih.gov/medlineplus/ ency/imagepages/19265/htm.

Trunkal obesity is associated with high blood insulin levels which also increases the activity of lipoprotein lipase and fat storage and may indirectly cause over eating.

Fat cells from the upper body seem to be functionally different from fat cells in the lower body. Primarily by hypertrophy (increase in size of cells) of the existing cells, whereas lower body fat deposition is by hyperplasia (increase in number of cells). Reducing the number of cells in the lower body hyperplastic depot is difficult compared to reduce trunkal obesity where there is increase in size of adipocytes. This may explain the weight loss difficulties of many women with lower body obesity. Central adiposity is often related to menopause.

Percentage of body fat, subcutaneous truncal fat or abdominal fat and visceral fat in the abdominal cavity are the components of body fat that are associated with health risk. According to the studies conducted by National Nutrition Monitoring Bureau (2005–2006) the prevalence of abdominal obesity in terms of waist circumference (> 102 cms) was about 1 per cent among men while it was 7 per cent among women (≥ 88 cms). Heredity plays a role in fat distribution. Android obesity can also occur in women. It is not always associated with general obesity.

Hyperinsulinemia is a cardinal feature of obesity. It may be due to increased insulin secretion, decreased clearance by the liver or both. Hyperinsulinemia may lead to decreased insulin sensitivity by down regulation of insulin receptors.

The low capacity of android muscle to remove free fatty acids by oxidation may render the muscle particularly sensitive to the effects of excess free fatty acid. Both adipose tissue and muscle might contribute to the insulin resistance in android obesity. Waist : Hip ratio is a stronger independent risk factor than Body Mass Index for myocardial infarction or premature death both in men and women.

Table 15.4 Differences between android obesity and gynacoid obesity

Type	*Adipose tissue and consequence*	*Muscle and consequence*	*In muscle*	*In glucose homeostasis*
Android obesity	Abdominal adipose tissues enlarged, elevated free fatty acid mobilisation and excess FFA turnover resulting in hypertriglyceridemia.	Few slow twitch fibres, many fast twitch fibres, slow oxidative capacity. Physical exercise increases slow-twitch fibres.	Decreased glucose transport, insulin resistance.	Insulin resistance, decreased glucose tolerance resulting in diabetes mellitus.
Gynacoid obesity	Femoral, gluteal adipose tissues enlarged, low FFA mobilisation, normal FFA turnover.	Many low twitch fibres, few fast twitch fibres, high oxidative capacity.	Normal glucose transport, insulin sensitivity.	Normal glucose tolerance.

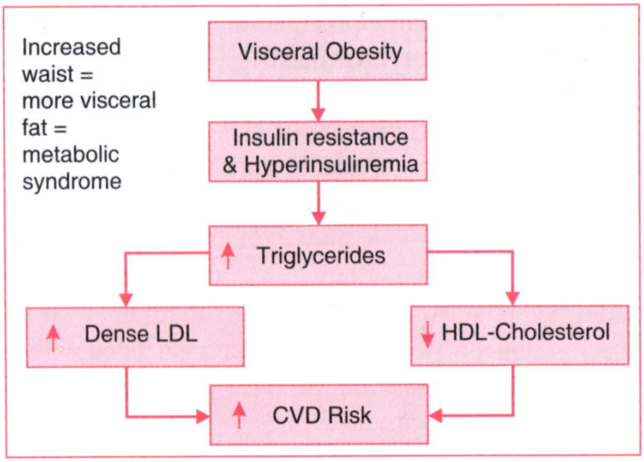

Fig. 15.3 Android obesity leads to metabolic syndrome

Lean men with body fat concentrated abdominally are at the highest risk for myocardial infarction or premature death.

Table 15.5 Diagnosis of metabolic syndrome

Risk factor		*Defining level*
Abdominal obesity		
	Men	> 102 cm
	Women	> 88 cm
Triglyceride		≥ 150 mg/dl
High density lipoprotein cholesterol		
	Men	< 42 mg/dl
	Women	< 50 mg/dl
Blood pressure		≥ 130/≥ 85 mm Hg
Fasting glucose		≥ 110 mg/dl

TYPES

Juvenile Onset Obesity

Juvenile obesity occurs due to hyperplasia and most rapidly in the first few years of life. There is a marked increase in the adipose tissue cells—thus the term hyperplastic obesity is used. Too many calories injected in infancy and early childhood leads to an overproduction of fat cells followed by hypertrophy (enlargement of the fat cells). Fat cells once developed do not disappear nor differentiate. For this reason, fat children are inclined to be fat adults. As many as 80 per cent of obese children will become obese adults.

The repeated offering of a bottle as a method of dealing with a fretful or crying infant may establish a habit that leads the infant to expect or seek food whenever experiencing frustration. Early introduction of high calorie solid foods may lead to rapid weight gain and obesity. Studies suggest that in normal infants, infant autonomy in feeding may be advantageous in appropriate regulation of weight during the first year of life.

The incidence of childhood obesity relates strongly to family variables, including parental obesity, small family size and family patterns of inactivity.

An increased amount of time spent viewing television, playing videogames or 'surfing' the Internet appears to correlate with an increased incidence of childhood obesity and may relate not only to the sedentary nature of the past time but also to subtle effects promoting food consumption through advertisement of food products particularly those of low nutritional value such as snack foods high in sugar, fat and salt. Feeding young children with excess amount of ghee may result in obesity.

Obesity may become evident at any age, but it appears most frequently in the first year of life, at 5-6 years of age and during adolescence. Obesity occurs when thyroid function is affected.

Psychologic disturbances, glucose intolerance, and sleep apnea are increasingly identified in obese children and adolescents. Eating disorders can lead to obesity.

Adult-onset Obesity

In adult-onset obesity (hypertropic obesity) the size of the individual cell is greatly enlarged. A distended adipose cell leads to further physiological, biochemical, anatomic aberrations in individual's organs and organ systems. Hypertropic obese patients have been reported to maintain weight loss better than hyperplasic ones.

TREATMENT

Obesity is a chronic disease that requires long-term treatment. Even a 5-10 per cent loss from initial weight may produce marked improvement in diabetes, dyslipidemia and even sleep apnea. The ease of weight gain and difficulty in losing and maintaining weight all make obesity a challenging illness to treat. The goals set for weight loss should be realistic. Nonreachable targets result in frustration and failure.

Multidisciplinary approach is used in treating obesity.

Table 15.6 Multidisciplinary scope of treatment for obesity

Provider	*Roles in multidisciplinary setting*
Registered dietician	Assess dietary patterns and preferences. Develop and implement nutrition goals with formal monitoring
Behavioural counsellor	Counsel patient and family as needed. Structure a behavioural programme Identify behavioural issues interfering with treatment.
Exercise specialist	Assess musculoskeletal and physical activity Develop and implement rehabilitation and activity plan.
Physician	Coordinate multidisciplinary team

Source: Ross. M. Michael, Multidisciplinary treatment of paediatric obesity. Nutrition evaluation and management, Nutrition in clinical practice, 2010, **25.**

Strategies for weight loss and weight maintenance

Initial goal is to reduce body weight by approximately 10 per cent from base line. Many obesity related conditions significantly improve with this modest weight loss, even when patients remain considerably overweight. If this goal is achieved, further weight loss can be attempted.

Successful weight loss strategies embrace small changes, moderate losses, and reasonable goals. Steady weight loss should be achieved by decreasing calorie intake, choosing nutrient dense foods and engaging in regular physical activity is much more likely to maintain those losses and reap health benefits than if more weight is lost in less time by adopting a radical fad diet.

It is not only loss of weight but body composition should be considered. Fat should be lost without loss of muscle mass.

A reasonable time for a 10 per cent reduction in body weight is six months.

Principles

- Diet therapy
- Physical activity
- Stress management
- Pharmaco therapy
- Behaviour therapy
- Weight loss surgery

Diet Therapy

Very low calorie diet < 800 kcal: Although much weight is initially lost on very low calorie diets, more weight is usually regained. Rapid weight reduction does not teach behaviour changes. Patients on very low calorie diets have increased risk for developing gallstones. Very low calorie diets (400 to 800 kcal/day) can be used safely in extremely obese individuals (greater than 50% overweight) when under the care of a physician and registered dietitian.

Reducing diet: The initial goal of weight loss therapy is to reduce body weight by approximately 10 per cent from baseline. If this goal is achieved, further weight loss can be attempted. A reasonable time line for a 10 per cent reduction in body weight is 6 months of therapy.

The person should be on negative energy balance ideally 500–1000 calories less than RDA. An ideal reduction of 500 g–1 kg/week is approved. Once the target is fixed, progress should be checked once a month. Usually 3 kg are lost in the first month largely due to utilisation of carbohydrate store and water. Reducing diets should provide adequate amounts of protein, vitamins and minerals.

Calorie restriction for weight reduction is the safest and most effective method. One pound of body fat is equivalent to 3500 kcal; therefore, intake must be reduced by 500 kcal daily to produce a loss of one pound of body fat weekly (500 kcal × 7 days = 3500 kcal). A caloric deficit of 1000 kcal/day is required to lose 2 pounds or approximately 1 kg of body fat weekly. This is the maximum weekly weight loss recommended since a more restrictive diet may not be nutritionally adequate.

The caloric recommendation can be determined from actual food intake and not from formulas. A detailed 24-hour food recall and/or 3-day diet history are generally adequate to determine intake.

Energy Deficit Calculation

Step 1: Estimate the recommended individual calorie requirement (kcal/day) by calculating the Resting Energy Expenditure (REE).

REE of adult males = 10 × weight (in kg) + 6.25 × height (in cm) – 5 × age (in years) + 5.

REE of adult females = 10 × weight (in kg) + 6.25 × height (in cm) – 5 × age (in years) – 161

Step 2: Multiply REE by Activity Factor of 1.5 for women and 1.6 for men for light activity to estimate daily caloric need.

REE × AF = estimated total calorie need (kcal/day) to maintain weight

Step 3: From this number, subtract 500 kcal/day to obtain adjusted calorie intake required to achieve weight loss of approximately 500 g/week.

Example

Expected loss of weight—500 g/week

Recommended Dietary Allowance—2320 kcal

1 g of body fat is equivalent to—7.7 kcal

∴ 500 g of body fat is equivalent to—7.7 × 500 = 3850 kcal

Less calories per week = 3850 kcal

Less calories per day $\frac{3850}{7} = 550$ kcal

Prescribed calories to be 2320 – 550 = 1770 kcal

To achieve a loss of 500 g/week, 1800 kcals are prescribed for adult man.

As weight loss progresses, further calorie reduction may be necessary as calorie requirement decreases with body size.

Table 15.7 Loss of weight on low calorie diet

BMI	*Less calories/day*	*Weight loss/week*	*Weight loss in six months*
27.35	300–500	0.5 kg	10% weight loss
> 35	500–1000	0.5–1 kg	10% weight loss

Actual meal plans can be based on food groupings such as the exchange system. Counting calories may be appropriate for some individuals who dislike the regimentation of food groupings.

Reducing excessive food sources of fat and sugar can dramatically reduce calories for many overweight people, and general guidelines to accomplish such a change may be as effective as a specific meal plan. Regardless of the method chosen to produce weight loss, the patient must eventually learn to eat a healthy diet to maintain body weight. This is when behaviour modification techniques and exercise programs are useful.

Calorie level below 1500 kcal/day is inadequate in most nutrients, therefore, should be supplemented with appropriate vitamins and minerals.

The body composition should be maintained throughout and after reducing weight

Total body water L– 26.4 – 32.2

Protein kg – 7.0 – 8.6

Minerals kg – 2.44 – 2.98

Body fat mass kg – 10.3 – 16.6

Nutritional Requirements

Low calorie, normal protein, vitamin and mineral (except sodium), restricted carbohydrate, restricted fat and liberal fluid, high fibre diet are suggested in obesity.

Energy: To lose weight, energy output must exceed energy input. The person has to be in negative energy balance. About 20 kcal per kg ideal body weight is prescribed for a sedentary worker and 25 kcal for moderately active worker.

Proteins: About 0.8–1 g of protein/kg body weight is prescribed for tissue repair and for specific dynamic action.

Carbohydrates: High carbohydrate diet enhances insulin resistance, which causes the body to store excess carbohydrates as fat. To lose weight is to decrease insulin by reducing carbohydrate intake. High carbohydrate content foods like potatoes and rice are restricted. Sugar which gives empty calories should be totally avoided. Fruits rich in carbohydrate like banana should be avoided. Complex carbohydrates which are good carbohydrates have low glycaemic index should be consumed.

Fat: Experiments have shown that when fat content of the diet increases, those without body weight problems are able to regulate their body weight by unknowingly reducing the amount of food eaten and hence, controlling the number of calories eaten. But low fat or no fat diet should be given to reduce the energy value of food. Foods rich in fat substances like nuts and oil seeds should be restricted. Skim milk should be the choice. Saturated fat and *trans* fats are avoided.

Vitamins: With prolonged restriction of fats, there is likely to be a restriction of fat soluble vitamins A and D which need to be supplemented.

Minerals: Restriction of sodium as common salt is helpful in weight reducing diet as excess sodium predisposes to retention of fluid. Research suggests that a calcium rich diet especially one that includes dairy sources (with limit in total calories) not only helps young women keep weight in check but may reduce overall levels of body fat. Calcium may depress certain hormones which consequently improves the body's ability to breakdown fat in cells and slow fat production.

Fluid: Fluids can be taken liberally as extra fluids are excreted by healthy kidneys. Also a glass of water before meals helps to cut down food intake.

High fibre: High fibre low calorie foods like green leafy vegetables, fruits, vegetable salads, whole grain cereals and pulses can be included in the diet. Inclusion of high fibre foods in diets for obese has many advantages. They are 1. Low in calorie density 2. Foods like greens provide many vitamins and minerals (which are difficult to meet with restricted food) 3. Give satiety 4. Help in regulating bowel movements 5. Reduce blood cholesterol 6. Promote chewing and decreases rate of ingestion. Higher intake of fibre automatically cut down fat and calories. To reduce weight, taking high fibre is considered less expensive and less torturous than medical treatment of obesity.

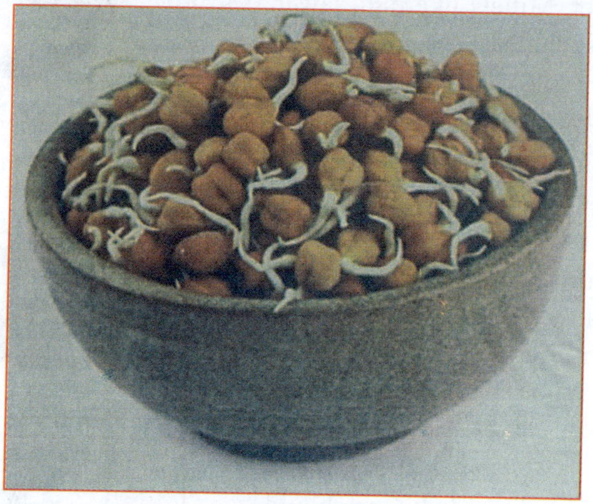

Fig. 15.4 Sprouted pulses are low glycaemic foods

Glycaemic Index: Low GI foods may benefit weight control in two ways

- By promoting satiety
- By promoting fat oxidation at the expense of carbohydrate oxidation.

Mixed meals with low GIs induce greater cholecystokinin secretion and greater satiety. Due to slower rate of digestion and absorption in the small intestine, nutrient receptors in the gastrointestinal tract are stimulated for a longer period of time resulting in prolonged feed back (through signals such as cholecystokinin and glucagon like peptide) to the satiety centre in the brain.

When high GI foods are consumed, rise in glucose and insulin concentrations increase carbohydrate oxidation through rate limiting enzymes. For example, malonyl-CoA, an intermediate of glucose oxidation, strongly inhibits fatty acid transport into mitochondria resulting in decreased fatty acid oxidation which is linked with greater weight gain.

The patient should be convinced that there is no other way of reducing weight except by consuming less calories and by spending more energy.

Maintaining weight is life long process and a permanent change should be brought in dietary habits. Anyone who is fit and looks great is working at it. It does not just happen.

Modification of normal diet is the best way of planning good reducing diet.

The diet should be adequate in all other nutrients except calories. The diet should consist of all five food groups.

Dietary Guidelines

- The diet should consist of variety of whole grains. White rice is to be replaced with brown rice or whole grains. Oats should be included in the diet. Millets like ragi, jawar and bajra are to included. The quantity of cereal should be reduced. Refined cereals such as polished rice and maida are avoided.
- The diet should include whole grams and other legumes. Sprouted grams are nutrient dense. Legumes have low GI and give satiety.
- Skim milk should be used in the diet. Probiotics with low fat can be included. Butter cream and ice cream should be avoided. Cheese can be sparingly used. Low fat cheese or paneer can be used.
- Red meat should be avoided. Fatty portions of chicken should be discarded. One should learn to enjoy preparations using little fat. Fish can be included in the diet. Restricted amount of eggs can be included.
- Plenty of colourful fruits and vegetables should be included in the diet. Green leafy vegetables should be part of every meal. This will ensure to meet the requirement of antioxidants on a low calorie diet. Salads without oils should be part of the diet.
- The diet should be rich in fibre. Meals can be started with salads. Diet should include whole grains, sprouted grams, unprocessed foods and natural foods in raw form. Fruits can be taken as snack item (instead of making juice or pulp). Whole fruits are healthy snacks.
- Diet is low in calories hence carbohydrate intake should be reduced. Measured quantities of rice should be taken. Intake of chapatis should be limited.
- The diet should be low in fat. No saturated and trans fatty acids to be included in the diet. Fried foods should be avoided. Gravy dishes having saturated fats should be avoided. Junk foods like chips and french fries should be strictly avoided. Foods naturally rich in oil like nuts should be taken in restricted amounts.

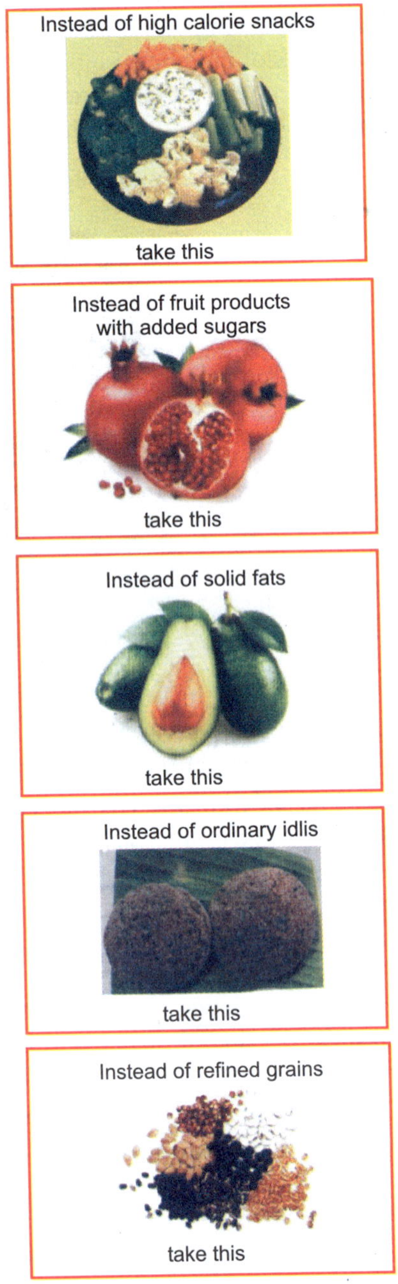

Fig. 15.5 Shifting to healthier food choices.

Source: Modified, Dietary guidelines for Americans 2015-2020.

- The diet should be low in sugar. Sweets, cakes and chocolates should be strictly avoided. Concentrated foods like condensed milk, honey and sugar syrups should be avoided.

Implications of some fat loss methods

High carbohydrate and low fat diets: Low calorie intake favours negative energy balance. Wise food selection can make the diet nutritionally sound. Initial water retention from glycogen storage may be discouraging.

High carbohydrate and high protein diets: Low calorie intake favours negative energy balance.Initial rapid water loss acts as incentive.Increased thermic effect of protein.

Low carbohydrate and high fat diets: Increased ketone excretion removes energy from the body. Fat intake often voluntarily decreased resulting in low calorie intake. Inclusion of rich foods has psychological appeal. Initial rapid water loss acts as incentive. Ketogenic high fat intake is contraindicated for heart and diabetic patients. Diet is nutritionally inadequate.

- Water can be consumed in unlimited quantity. Carbonated and sweetened beverages should be avoided. Fruit juices, coffee and tea can be consumed without sugar. Alcohol should be restricted. Foods giving empty calories should be avoided.
- Method of cooking should be modified. Boiling, poaching steaming, pressure cooking and simmering with no additional fat should be the methods of cooking.
- To reduce the intake of food, serving size can be reduced; small size plates and ladles can be used.
- Food should be consumed regularly in measured amounts. Meals should not be skipped. Snacking fried foods between meals should be avoided.
- Feasting should be avoided. One should learn to select proper foods at the time of festivals and while attending parties. A psychological change can be brought out in them to celebrate festivals without giving much importance to food. Parties can be followed by playing team games like cricket.
- Fasting should be avoided as one tend to eat more food later. Substitute foods during fasting time are generally rich in calories like potatoes, sago and ground nuts. People who eat once a day usually consume concentrated foods.
- Generally food taken outside the home is rich in calories. To reduce the calories, one should choose the foods wisely. Buying fried foods should be avoided. One should be accompaniments which are not charged separately may contribute to calories. Single serving packages are preferred than ala car te. Avoiding outside food is the best.
- Unsweatened beverages and yogurt in which fibre is added can potentiate the satiating property, suppress appetite and control food intake. Yogurt with added sugar should not be taken.
- Even low calorie foods should not be taken in unlimited quantities.
- Home prepared meals that emphasise more variety and include fruits vegetables, whole grains and dairy products may reduce the chances of android obesity.
- Small meals evenly spaced throughout the day should be taken.
- While eating one should focus on food and not get diverted to watching T.V. or working on computer.
- Excess socialization hinders weight reduction programme.
- Meals should be taken at specified time and place.

> **Dietary Education is a Necessary Ingredient for Complying Dietary Restrictions**
>
> Following points need to be educated:
> - Energy value of different foods
> - Composition of foods like fats, carbohydrates, fibre and proteins
> - Invisible fats
> - Reading nutrition labels
> - New habits of purchasing—low calorie high in micro nutrients
> - Food preparation—avoiding high calorie ingredients while cooking like fats, coconut, cashewnuts and sugar
> - Avoiding over consumption of high calorie foods. Maintaining adequate water intake
> - Reducing portion sizes
> - Limiting alcohol consumption

Improved Diet Quality Decreases Inflammation

Chronic inflammation is associated with obesity and its comorbidities including cardiovascular disease and cancer. Low grade, asymptomatic inflammation results in prolonged elevation of inflammatory cytokines leading to cellular damage. Inflammation not only is a consequence of obesity but may contribute to progression of obesity. Dietary components such as marine sources ω-3 fatty acids and plant foods rich in fibre and phytochemicals (whole grains, fruits, vegetables and legumes) have anti-inflammatory properties. Added sugars increase inflammatory markers. Better diet quality is inversely related to inflammation, independent of body weight.

Weight Maintenance

- After six months of weight loss treatment, efforts to maintain weight loss should be put in place. If more weight loss is needed, another attempt at weight reduction can be made. This will require further adjustment of the diet and physical activity prescriptions.
- Adjusting to reduced body weight is difficult. Lost weight usually will be regained unless a weight maintenance programme is followed indefinitely.

Table 15.8 Most common facilitators and barriers in weight control

Facilitators	*Barriers*
• Change in eating behaviour	• No self control
• Increase in physical activity	• Special occasions
• Attitude and motivation	• Not exercising enough
• Monitoring	• Attitude and motivation
food records	• Stress
weighing oneself	• Eating habits
• Social support	• Eat everything on plate
• Awareness of calorie content of food	• Eat fast foods
• Balanced diet	• Eating quickly
	• Having lot of food around
	• Liking for fatty food
	• Liking for sweets

- Maintaining an active life style will help offset some of these metabolic changes.
- For patients unable to achieve significant weight reduction, prevention of weight gain is an important goal.

These diets provide 1500 to 1800 kcal. When the body weights are reduced to optimal level on reducing diets, these diets maintain at this level. Weight maintenance program consisting of dietary therapy, physical activity and behaviour therapy is continued indefinitely.

Quackery in Obesity Treatment

With many wanting to lose weight, it is no surprise that many people have cashed on weight loss products and programmes that do not work. Some may carry significant risk. Unscrupulous businesses count on unproven weight loss schemes. Creams, teas, magnets and numerous food supplements are sold for weight loss.

Fradulent weight loss methods proclaim guarantees of specific amounts or rapid weight loss; a single price for all weight loss participants; weight loss without effort; and promises of long-term or permanent weight loss.

Detox diets promise to help to shed weight in days or weeks with starvation mode, a person loses weight. But as the metabolism slows, the weight eventually creeps back. The body has its own built in detox system.

Bizarre diets claim fast results with minimal effort. Such diets would lead to nutritional deficiencies. The proposed diets are impractical and are abandoned after a few weeks, with subsequent guilt feeling.

Crash diets reduce water and protein and not fat. Loss of muscle leads to weak body and weaken immune system.

Physical Activity

Most obese patients lead sedentary lives. A low calorie diet accompanied by moderate exercise will be effective in causing weight loss. Aerobic exercise directly increases the daily energy expenditure and is particularly useful for long-term weight maintenance. Exercise also preserves lean body mass and partially prevent the decrease in basal energy expenditure seen with semi-starvation. Exercise is extremely beneficial in weight management because it helps to regulate appetite, increases the basal metabolic rate and reduces the fat deposit 'set-point' level. Exercise also helps to reduce stress related eating, since it provides physical outlet for working off the hormonal physiologic events produced by stress in the body.

Tai chi trims belly fat.

The government is encouraging physical exercise. This includes making pedestrian paths in parks in urban design, school and business houses, have provision for physical activity, serve healthy meals and integrate health education into their routines. As a general rule, exercise in the range of 45 mts is recommended. Physical activity in overweight and obese adults increases cardio respiratory fitness independent of weight loss. The best exercise for an obese person is walking. A major reason that many adults do not exercise as a weight loss mechanism is that their level of physical fitness is so low they cannot sustain a moderate level of exercise intensity for very long. However, this will change as one continues to do exercise.

Body-Motion-Sensors

Objective measures of physical activity using body-motion sensors are a promising advance in the field of physical activity. Unlike self-reported questionnaires, these devices can accurately quantify total activity over several days.

A fitness tracker is an objective device and offer continuous wrist based heart rate tracking, all day activity tracking and automatic sleep detection. It also gives information on calorie intake. It helps in controlling the body weight by monitoring energy intake and expenditure. If can also be used by downloading app in smartphones and the results can be viewed on the computer.

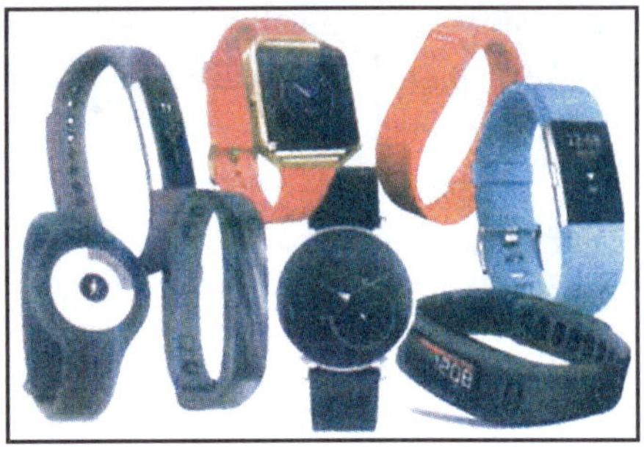

Fig. 15.6 Wrist band fitness activity trackers.

A pedometer is a device, usually portable and electronic or electro mechanical, that counts each step a person takes by detecting the motion of the person.

Obese can use these tracking devices to monitor exactly the calorie intake and energy expenditure which are needed to maintain body weight.

Most objective activity instruments best measure vertical movement activity. Swimming and cycling are not captured by these instruments. Even pedometers do not measure intensity or frequency of activity and cannot capture upper body movement.

Tracking devices are helpful to obese to establish the routine and standardizing energy expenditure and energy intake which ultimately help in maintaining body weight.

Barriers of Physical Activity

- Early years - no time
- Later life - joint pain
- Weather - hot or cold
- Too busy schedule
- Fear of reverting to previous status on stopping exercise.
- Losing motivation with time
- Perceived sense of well being
- Lack of regularity, monotony
- Starting problem
- Lack of energy
- Social influence
- No side walks - walkable neighbourhood
- Recreation - no physical activity
- Use of cars

Activity and Appetite Control

Physical activity regulates appetite. People think that exercising will make them hungry but this is not entirely true. Active people have healthy appetite. Immediately after a good workout most people do not feel like eating. They want to shower and may be thirsty. But they are not hungry. The reason is that the body response to the stress of exercise by mobilizing fuels from storage; Glucose and fatty acids are abundant in blood. At same time the body has suppressed its digestive functions. Hard physical work and eating are not compatible.

Physical activity helps especially to curb the inappropriate appetite that prompts a person to eat when bored, anxious or depressed.

Stress Management

Stress is a major reason for overeating and relapse. Patients can reduce stress-related overeating by learning how to implement methods other than eating to deal with or reduce stress. Some examples include diaphragmatic breathing, deep muscle relaxation, meditation, yoga and physical activity. These techniques provide a distraction to the stressful event and may be helpful in alleviating myriad health-related problems.

Pharmacotherapy

Drug therapy may be used as part of a comprehensive weight loss programme, including diet therapy and physical exercise for patients with a BMI of 30 with no concomitant obesity related risk factors or diseases. Weight loss drugs should never be used without life style modifications. Continual assessment of drug therapy for efficacy and safety is necessary.

The new drugs, sibutramine and orlistat combined with phentermine, provide helpful tools to assist health care professionals manage the weight of patients more successfully.

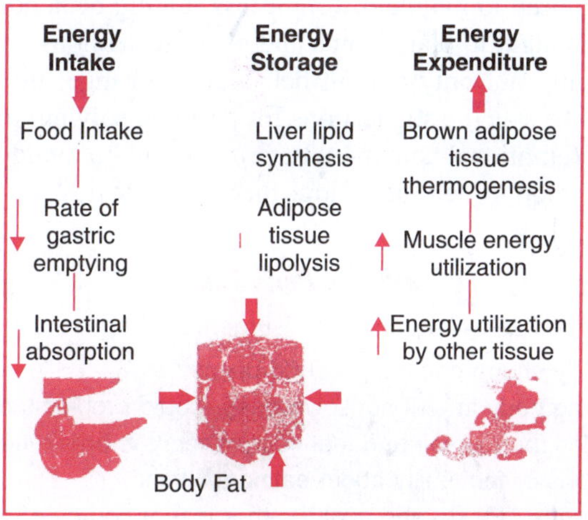

Fig. 15.7 Potential Sites of Pharmacological Intervention in Obesity

Orlistat is a potent and irreversible inhibitor of gastric and pancreatic lipases, inhibiting digestion of dietary fat by 30 per cent. It also reduces absorption of some fat-soluble vitamins and β carotene hence patients should take a multivitamin supplement. Most commonly observed adverse events are faecal urgency, oily evacuation, and increased defecation. Treatment with orlistat + diet for 1–2 years promotes weight loss, lessens weight regain and improves fasting LDL and insulin levels.

Sibutramine is a potent re-uptake inhibitor of serotonin and noradrenaline. It enhances satiety and increase thermogenesis, increasing energy expenditure. It improves lipid profile. Side effects are lethargy, constipation, nausea, tachycardia and insomnia. It should be used in conjunction with a reduced diet.

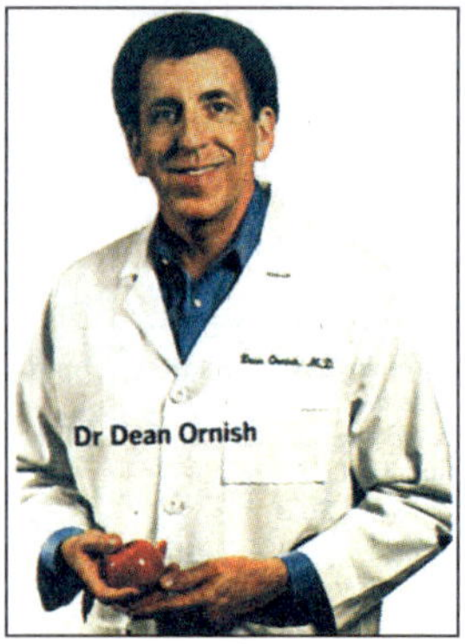

Fig. 15.8 Ornish's diet recommend loss of weight through nutrition, exercise, stress management and love and intimacy.

Behaviour Therapy

Psychological problems involved in overeating need to be understood. Behaviour therapy strategies to promote diet and physical activity should be used routinely. Long term changes in eating behaviour are required to maintain weight loss. Eating behaviour is not instinctive but learned. Patients can be taught to plan menus and exercise sessions and to record their actual behaviour. Record keeping not only aids in behavioural change; the availability of records helps the provider to make specific suggestions for problem solving. Patients can be taught to recognise 'eating cues' (emotional, situational etc.) and how to avoid or control them. Stress management and social support help behaviour therapy strategies.

Improve Body Image

This guide is not intended as a treatment for disordered eating.

- Learn to accept body shape-emphasize good points.
- Realize that reducing body fat will not solve deep rooted problems or an emotional crisis.
- Do not set rigid rules for yourself and feel guilty when you break them.
- Do not ban any foods or feel guilty about eating anything.
- Think of foods in terms of taste and health rather than a source of calories.
- Establish a sensible healthy eating pattern rather than strict diet.
- Listen to your natural appetite cues - learn to eat when you are hungry.
- Enjoy ur exercise or sport for its own ends. Have fun instead of enduring torture to lose body fat.
- Set positive exercise goals not related to losing weight.

Source: Bean Anita 2009, A complete guide to sports nutrition A & C Publishers Ltd.

Surgery

Weight Loss Surgery

For morbidly obese patients bariatric surgery remains the only option. Bariatric surgery is the use of surgical interventions in the treatment of obesity. The most common approach is to reduce the volume of the stomach, producing an early sense of satiation.

Bariatric surgery is advised in patients with a BMI > 40. Persons with a BMI in the 35–40 range having a comorbid factor such as diabetes are also considered candidates for surgery. Gastric bypass surgery is the preferred method for most obesity surgeons. Weight loss is dramatic, compared with medical treatment. The average weight loss at five years is about 65 per cent of excess weight and most complications resolve in about 80 per cent of cases. Surgery produces striking improvement in emotional out look.

Patients who have undergone bariatric surgery need special attention. These patients may be at increased risk for refeeding syndrome because of rapid weight loss that typically follows surgery.

The diet immediately after the operation starts with small volumes of liquid that are gradually advanced to well-chewed foods over several weeks.

Less common but also worth noting are cases of sudden death from protein malnutrition. Fatal ventricular arrhythmia have been reported following very low calorie diet. Deficiency of water soluble vitamin B_1 presents the greatest risk acutely. Marginal status challenged by carbohydrate feeding can result in Wermicke-korsakoff syndrome of central and peripheral neuropathy with rapid progressing weakness of the extremities and numbness.Post surgical complaints are nausea, vomiting anorexia, dehydration., dumping syndrome, constipation, diarrhea, flatulence, lactose intolerance and reactive hypoglycaemia.

There is convincing evidence that bariatric surgery results in dramatic improvement of medical conditions such as sleep apnea and other hypoventilatic syndromes, type 2 diabetes mellitus, obesity related candiomyopathy and hypertension, hyperlipidemia, asthma, osteoarthritis, back pain, female urinary incontinence and infertility.

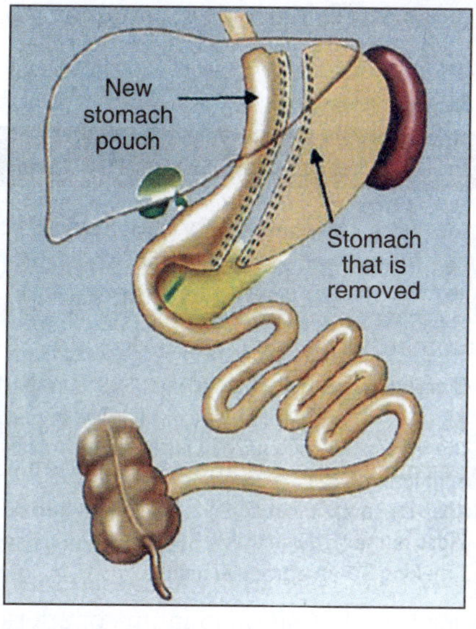

Fig. 15.9 **Sleeve/Vertical gastrectomy where the size of stomach is reduced.**

Ghrelin is the hormone that sends hunger signals to the brain. It is produced by the cells located in the fundus of the stomach. Sleeve gastrectomy removes much of the stomach with its ghrelin-producing cells. After sleeve gastrectomy, people eat less because stomach capacity is smaller and less ghrelin is released.

Source: Lito M. Kathryn, The weight loss surgery, today's dietetian, 2008, **10**.

Micronutrient and vitamin deficiencies follows bariatric surgery are of concern despite oral supplementation. Deficiencies can persist because of restricted intake, food intolerance, poor eating habits and diminished absorptive capacity.The development of iron deficiency has been described as a major cause of anaemia following bariatric surgery.

Plastic surgery removes excess fat from the skin level. This procedure can be done only to certain individuals who have isolated deposition of fat in the abdomen and thigh areas. These surgeries do not tackle the root cause of obesity.

Social support is essential for a successful weight loss programme. Continued close contact with the therapist and involvement of the family and peer group are useful techniques for reinforcing behavioural change and preventing social isolation.

Most successful programmes employ a multidisciplinary approach to weight loss with hypocaloric diets, behaviour modification to change eating behaviour, aerobic exercise, pharmacological therapy and social support. Emphasis must be on maintenance of weight loss.

Similar to iron, the bioavailability of vitamin B_{12} is dependent on HCl of the stomach. HCl facilitates cleavage of vitamin B_{12} bound to food. Just as gastric acid-blocking agents have been shown to result in decreased serum vitamin B_{12} levels, gastric acid production following bariatric surgery is low and protein-bound vitamin B_{12} absorption will decrease. For absorption of B_{12} in the terminal ileum requires the presence of intrinsic factor produced by the parietal cells of the stomach. Lack of intrinsic factor causes pernicious anaemia. Body stores of B_{12} are sufficient to prevent the onset of B_{12} deficiency for many years and bariatric patients respond well to vitamin B_{12} supplementation.

Folate is predominantly absorbed in the upper part of the small intestine but absorption can occur along the entire part of the small intestine when necessary such as after surgical procedures. For maintaining folate status under achlorhydric conditions bacterial folate synthesis is increased in upper small bowel.

COMPLICATIONS

Physical disability: Since the feet have to carry extra load, complications like flat feet, osteoarthritis of knee, hips and lumbar spine are common. The abdominal muscles that support the viscera and leg muscles are infiltered with fat hence their normal mechanical action is impaired with abdominal hernias and varicose veins. Adipose tissues around chest and diaphragm interferes with respiration and predisposes to bronchitis.

Metabolic disorders: Obesity is a chronic inflammatory condition and can lead to CVD, arthritis, Alzeimer's disease, diabetes and immune disfunction. There is a close association between obesity and diabetes. In simple obesity, there is a insulin resistance especially in muscle and there is hyper insulinemia because of impaired insulin uptake by receptors in target tissues. Plasma cholesterol level is generally high therefore prone to develop gall stones. Excess cholesterol in plasma leads to deposition in intima of arteries producing atherosclerosis. Gout is common.

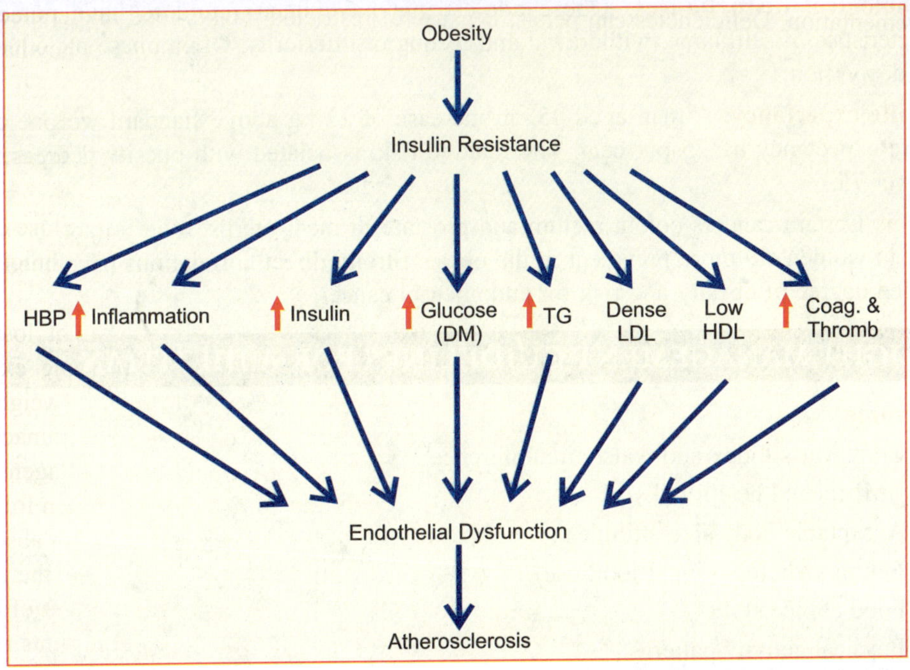

Fig. 15.10 Interrelationship between obesity, insulin resistance, diabetes, and atherosclerosis.

Source: Resident and Staff Physician, 2002; 48.

Cardiovascular disorders: Apart from atherosclerosis, obese people with BMI higher than 30 develop high blood pressure and increased incidence of varicose veins.

Sleep apnea: A transitory cessation of breathing is increasingly identified in obese children and adolescents.

Prone to accidents: Obese people are likely to meet with accidents by falling down on slippery floors and crossing streets.

Gastrointestinal disturbance: Obesity is associated with increased risk for gastro oesophageal reflux disease (GERD) symptoms such as erosive oesophagitis. These include increased incidence of hiatal hernia as well as abdominal wall hernias and gall bladder disease. Obese people have higher out put of cholesterol in bile. So their bile is constantly in danger of forming gall stones.

Osteoarthritis: Degenerative disease of weight-bearing joints is a very common complication of obesity, in the knees of middle-aged women and causes significant disability.

Obsterical risks: Obese women when pregnant have greater obsterical risks because of hypertension, diabetes and postpartum infection. Restriction of weight gain in these individuals may cause complication during pregnancy. There is an increased risk of neural tube defects in children of obese mothers. There is reduced fertility in obese people.

Psychological disturbances: Obese adolescents have been found to have personality characteristics of selfblame, withdrawal and feeling of inferiority. Often obese patients suffer from depression.

Low life expectancy: A man aged 45, an increase of 12 kg above standard weight reduces his life expectancy by 25 per cent. The relative risk associated with obesity decreases with age over 75.

Cancer: Certain cancers colon, rectum and prostate in men; uterus, biliary tract, breast and ovary in women are more prevalent in the obese. Strong direct correlations have been found between degree of obesity and risk for endometrial cancer.

WEIGHT MANAGEMENT GUIDELINES FOR A DIETITIAN

Determine

- Body Mass Index and waist circumference
- BMI-related health risks.
- Acceptable body size attitude
- Eating style (emotional food use)
- Food choice skills
- Physical activity patterns
- Weight management history
- Weight expectations
- Support system.

Decide

- Short term
- Long term.

Apply: Food choice strategies

- Low energy dense foods
- Whole grains
- Fruits and vegetables.

Practice: Internal regulation

- Hunger recognition
- Enjoy physical activity

Monitor: Consistent professional support

- Food records
- Weight expectations
- Quality of life.

Dietitian during interviewing the patient should define realistic, achievable and sustainable initial weight loss goals. The achievement of more healthy weight should be stressed as an important goal rather than the achievement of a 'normal' weight.

Dietitian should have individual prescriptive approach and not general lifestyle advice because most of the younger clients may have eating patterns that may not be structured.

Once a weight goal has been achieved a modest level of calorie restriction may be necessary to maintain weight loss and prevent weight gain.

Advantages of Weight Loss

- Reduction in blood pressure
- Reduction in total cholesterol and LDL cholesterol
- Increase in physical activity improves HDL levels
- Lower blood glucose level.

Weight loss reduces the risk factors for diabetes mellitus, coronary heart disease and cancer.

Thermogenic Foods as Dietary Supplements

Thermogenic foods promote fat breakdown without affecting the lean muscle mass by increasing the basal metabolic rate, they maintain the negative energy balance in the body. Thus decreases the stored body fat. These foods improve the sensitivity of fats to insulin helping in regulation of blood glucose, cholesterol and triglyceride levels.

Today dietary supplements are available incorporating thermogenic ingredients. The effect may not be proven scientifically.

Table 15.9 Thermogenic foods and their mechanisms

Thermogenic ingredients	*Mechanism*
L-Carnitine	It transfers the acyl group across the second mitochondrial membrane, thus facilitates oxidation of fatty acids
Conjugated linoleic acid (CLA)	CLA enhances fat loss and increases lean body mass
L-Tyrosine	It is an appetite suppressant because it is precursor to cholecystokinin which is a satiety hormone
Ephedrine	Ephedra increases the metabolic rate of the fat tissue
Caffeine	Caffeine stimulates nervous system and metabolism by neurotransmitter modulation
Chromium	Glucose metabolism is increased
Choline Bitartarate	It is a lipotropic agent
Inositol	It is also lipotropic agent
L-Methionine	It assists in breakdown of fats
Lecithin	It is a lipotropic factor

Source: Sharma Prateek et al., Thermogenic foods and supplements, Food Pack, 2004.

PREVENTION

Methods of prevention of obesity and overweight at different ages are given in Table 15.10.

Table 15.10 Prevention of obesity and overweight

Age	*Preventive methods*
Infancy	Breast feeding is to be given.
1–6 years	Too much of processed food should not be given. Forced feeding should not be done.
6–12 years	Physical activity is to be encouraged at school and at home Encouraging eating fruits and vegetables and creating healthful eating habits.
Adolescence	Outside food and skipping meals should be avoided.
	Junk food is to be avoided. Outdoor games are to be encouraged.
	T.V. watching, electronic usage to be limited.
	Mobile phone to be used only when necessary.
Adult	Encouraging ovo vegetarian diet.
	Exercise should be everyday routine.
Expectant mothers	Special foods like gond laddu should be given in limited quantity. Simple exercise like walking should be encouraged.
Lactating mothers	Should breast feed the child at least for six months.
	Encouraging eating fruits and vegetables which are rich in antioxidants. Consumption of sugary sweets should be rarely consumed and not on daily basis.
Old Age	BMR is decreased. Intake of food should be decreased. Simple exercise like walking should be encouraged.

The role of physical activity, games and sports are to be emphasized in the schools by teachers and managements. The focus should be given on promotion of healthy food and lifestyle practices and regulated T.V. viewing and working with computers. Schools should make participation in sports and games mandatory and they should be part of the school curriculum. Health and nutrition education should be imparted regularly.

Suggested recipes

Reason	*Foods*
Vegetable salads	Low calorie and high fibre.
Chapathis using multigrain atta	More protein and high fibre give satiety.
Dals, steamed foods like idlis	Limit calories, increase protein content.
Thin soups	Provide fluids, low calorie value, give fullness.
Cut fruits	Give satiety and rich in antioxidants.
Poached fish	Low in calories, high in protein of good quality.
Boiled chowli/sundal	Rich in protein and B vitamins.
Greens Porial	High in fibre, vitamins, minerals and antioxidants.
Coffee, tea without sugar	Low calorie beverages
Boiled eggs	Gives good quality protein
Brown/Red rice/Millets	Glycaemic index is low

Future obesity treatment places greater emphasis on broader definitions of treatment success rather than focussing on weight loss as the primary treatment outcome. Improvements in metabolic profiles, physical activity, self esteem, body image, self efficacy, quality of life and functional capacity are to be considered. Moderate weight losses (5–10 per cent) provide significant health benefits. Realistic expectations of success must be established since achieving ideal weight is not realistic. A stepwise decrease in weight should be aimed.

Type 2 diabetes, cardiovascular disease and hypertension are comorbidities associated with obesity. Treatment and prevention strategies for these comorbidities of obesity are often assumed to be - weight loss. Medical nutrition therapy for obese persons with comorbidities should be refocused from weight loss to attaining and maintaining metabolic parameters - normal blood glucose levels, optimal lipid levels and blood pressure levels within normal limits should be physically fit.

Restricted energy diet even without weight loss. spacing of meals through out the day and fat intake modifications have been shown to improve glycaemia. Dyslipidaemia can be improved by reducing or changing the fat content of the diet. Blood pressure levels can be reduced by a diet high in fruits and vegetables and low in fat.

Not only weight loss but also lifestyle strategies should be directed toward the improvement of metabolic parameters associated with the comorbidity.

UNDERWEIGHT

Half the Indian rural population is underweight with up to three-quarters being so classified in deprived communities.

A very large proportion of rural Indian households have inadequate food supplies. Chronic energy deficiency is due to chronic food deficiency.

Classification

Children who are subjected to socioeconomic and dietary constraints during the critical years of growth and development end up with small body size. Such adult may be apparently healthy but there is evidence that their productivity and earning capacity may be impaired. Recent survey in the rural India revealed 55 per cent of preschool children are underweight.

All those whose BMI is less than 18.5 are considered as underweight. If BMI is 17–18.49. They are classified as mild underweight. Moderate underweight people have BMI 16–16.99. Severely underweight have BMI less than 16.

Limitation of Underweight

- Adults with BMI < 18.5 have reduced VO_2 max, reduced capacity for sustained heavy work and a lower productivity.
- Underweight pregnant women have increased risk of getting underweight baby.
- Progressively greater proportions of time are spent off work or in bed ill when BMI levels are below 17 in men and women.

- There is a progressive curvilinear increase in mortality in group of men with BMIs ranging from 18.5 to below 16.0.
- Immunological deficits are seen particularly in men with low BMIs and concomitant micronutrient deficiencies are present.
- Undernourished children have lower heights and weights.
- The age of menarche is delayed in undernourished girls by about 1–2 years.

Figure 15.11 shows signs and symptoms of underweight.

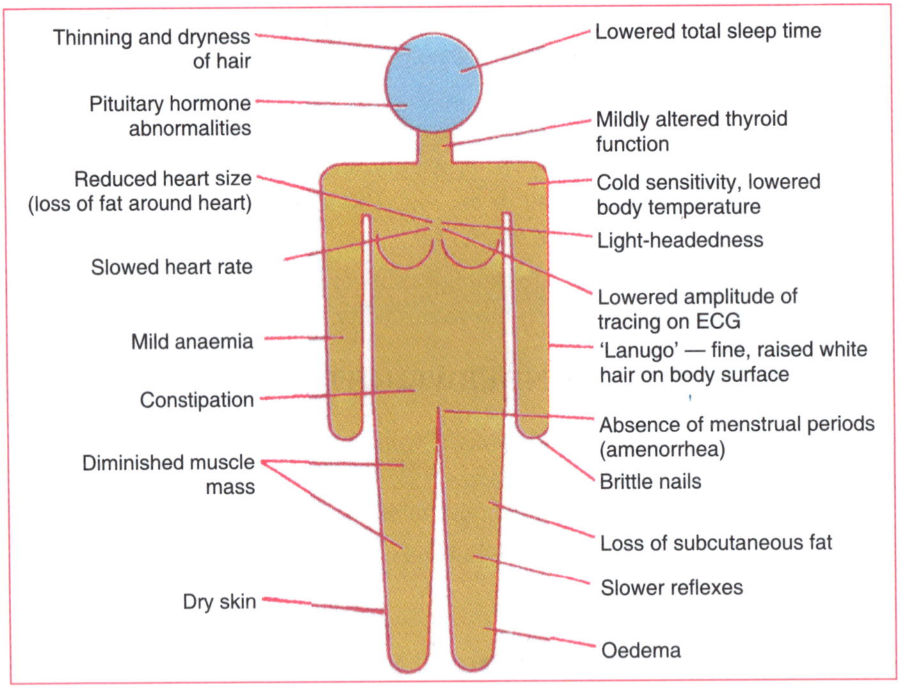

Fig. 15.11 Signs and symptoms of underweight

AETIOLOGY

Some of the causes of underweight are:

- Starvation occurs either due to famine conditions or an inadequate diet in proteins or an attempt at reducing weight. During starvation fatty tissue is lost and the skeletal, heart muscles and small intestine are atrophied losing its absorptive function. This results in low blood pressure, marked emaciation, loss of hair and inelastic skin. Since the feeding programme should be gradual, initially glucose water, fruit juice and skimmed milk powder may be given.
- Underweight also results from debilitating diseases like tuberculosis, diabetes, malabsorption syndrome or cancer. Infections are common among them. In these cases tonics are not useful as they only help to improve the appetite but they do not increase weight. It is wise and necessary to spend money on nourishing high calorie foods.

- Psychological factors may contribute to eating very little food (anorexia nervosa). Some mental patients reject food leading to severe weight loss. Anorexia nervosa is seen in girls between the age of 15 and 25 years. Usually it arises from a desire to lose weight. If untreated this condition may prove fatal due to progressive starvation. Electrolytes are lost in vomiting at the sight of food, or during eating. Transient stoppage of menstruation may occur which becomes normal with dietary treatment. In such cases, patients must be admitted to a hospital and should be given specific directions to have high calorie intake of bread, wheat and milk products.
- Underweight occurs in people who are active, tense, nervous and who never take rest. When it reaches a severe state, psychological efficiency as a whole is reduced and their power for concentration, decision making and withstanding calamities are very poor. Working efficiency is poor and the productivity is less. He cannot work continuously for a long period.
- It occurs in pathological conditions such as fevers, gastrointestinal disturbances, where the digestion and absorption capacities are decreased and in hyperthyroidism.

NUTRITIONAL AND FOOD REQUIREMENTS

A high calorie, high protein, high fat diet with liberal vitamin intake is recommended. But before going into the diet the first step is to determine and eliminate the cause for undereating. Then a balanced diet should be planned based on the requirements.

Energy: The calorie requirements vary depending upon the activities. For increasing weight the total calorie intake should be in excess of the energy requirement. An additional 500 kcals per day is recommended. The increase should be gradual over one or two weeks otherwise digestive disturbances may occur.

Proteins: Instead of 1 g of protein, over 1.2 g per kg is recommended for tissue building. Good quality protein is completely utilised by the body and as far as possible best protein sources must be liberally included at the initial stage.

Fats: Even though fat content is increased, easily digestible fats are to be included. Fried and fatty foods are not recommended as they may cause diarrhoea. Fatty food should not be taken at the beginning of a meal as they reduce appetite. High calorie fatty foods such as cream, butter, margarine and oils help to increase the weight.

Carbohydrates: High carbohydrate sources must form the basis of the diet. Leafy vegetables should be restricted and preference to be given to potato and yam. Dried fruits, sweets, nuts, desserts, jam, jelly, cereals, cereal products and nonvegetarian foods are rich sources of energy and can be liberally included in the diet. The number of meals should be increased. Two feeds incorporating soups, juices or sweets in between major meals improve the nutritive value of the diet. Easily digestible foods should be given. Porridge, cutlets, desserts, potato chips, high protein drinks like milk, malted milk, and badam kheer can be included. Thick soups are easily digestible and highly nutritious items.

Vitamins and minerals: With a liberal diet there is no need for extra vitamin and mineral supplement.

Fluids: Fluids should not be taken before or with a meal but only after a meal so that food intake is not reduced. Enough fluids must be taken so as to avoid constipation.

Dietary Guidelines

- Underweight person has to be on positive energy balance. Calorie intake should be more than the energy expended.
- Energy dense foods hold key to weight gain.
- Under weight person should have regular meals. He should make meals a priority and take the time to plan, prepare and eat each meal.
- They should at least eat three major meals a day and snacks in between.
- Underweight person should learn to eat more food at each meal. Serving size can be increased, for example, drinking milk from a larger glass.
- Dietary supplements can be given.
- Food should be appetising.
- Diet can be varied and new foods and recipes can be tried.
- Eating can be made in different locations and ambience and with friends and family members.
- A walk before taking meals can make an individual more hungry.

Exercise and Bowels

Regular outdoor exercise helps to stimulate appetite. Exercise with high kilocalorie intake ensure that lean body mass is built up and not just fat. Emotional well-being is essential to have a good appetite. Constipation may reduce the appetite so the bowel movements should be regulated with adequate fluids, exercise and fruits. Synthetic drinks, soft drinks, alcohol, aerated drinks, too much of tea and coffee reduce appetite and should be avoided.

Antiobesity Day is on 26th November.

SUGGESTED READINGS

- Jasper W. Phillip *et al.*, Effects of bite count feedback from a wearable device and goal setting on consumption in young adults, J. Acad. Nutr. Diet 2016: **116**.
- Puzziferri Nancy, Sleeve gastrectomy for weight loss, JAMA, 2018; **319**.
- Obesity Foundation India. www.ofi.co.in

QUESTIONS

1. How do you assess an obese and underweight individual?
2. What are the parameters used in the diagnosis of obesity?
3. Explain grades of obesity.
4. Write the principles of dietary management in obesity.
5. State the reasons for the dietary restrictions recommended for an obese individual.
6. Explain the treatment for obesity.
7. Explain the etiology of obesity. Plan a 1200 kcal diet for an adult businessman who is obese.
8. What are the important causes of underweight?
9. Describe the symptoms of underweight and explain the dietary modifications in underweight.
10. What are the complications of obesity?
11. Bring out the role of android obesity in the complications of obesity.
12. Explain the role of hormones in obesity.
13. Explain how stress can lead to obesity and underweight.

TOPICS FOR ACTIVITY

- Find out the BMI of classmates and classify.
- Plan and prepare a low calorie diet for an obese middle aged executive. Suggest in detail lifestyle modifications.
- Plan and prepare a diet for an adolescent girl who is underweight. Suggest other treatments she has to undergo in addition to diet.

16

Diet in Cardiovascular Diseases

Cardiovascular disease (CVD) is a general term describing diseases of the heart and blood vessels. Coronary Heart Disease (CHD) is the most common form of CVD and is caused by atherosclerosis in the large and medium sized arteries that supply the heart muscle with oxygen and nutrients. Atherosclerosis is a man made disease.

PREVALENCE

Cardiovascular disease remains the leading cause of death in many countries. CHD is highly predictable, preventable and treatable. In India the onset of CVD is at an early age; it is more severe and the progression is rapid and aggressive.

Those in the higher socioeconomic group are the first ones to adopt to an adverse life style such as high saturated fatty acid diet, sedentary life style and cigarette smoking. They are also the first to revert to a healthier life style. Thus the poor in the developed countries and the rich in the developing countries consume the highest amount of high saturated fatty acid.

CLINICAL EFFECTS

The clinical effects of atherosclerosis are manifested principally in medium sized arteries including the coronary, carotid, cerebral arteries as well as several arteries supplying the lower limbs particularly the iliac and femoral arteries. The coronary arteries generally demonstrate the most intense involvement.

The principal clinical results of atherosclerotic lesions are due to partial or total occlusion of the arterial lumen. The cracks and fissures developed in the lesions leads to thrombosis which is the principal cause of angina pectoris (pain in the chest provoked by exercise), myocardial infarction (death of heart muscle tissue) and sudden ischaemic death (deficient blood supply).

Plaques usually develop slowly and insidiously over many years beginning from childhood. They may progress from a fatty streak to a fibrous plaque and then to a complicated plaque that is likely to lead to clinical effects.

Impairment of the heart is manifested by dyspnoea on exertion, weakness and pain in the chest. In severe failure there is marked dilation of the heart. The circulation to the tissues through the kidney is so impaired that sodium and water are held in tissue spaces. Oedema fluid collects first in the extremities and with increasing failure in the abdominal and chest cavities. This is referred to as congestive heart failure.

Desirable Cholesterol Levels and Risk Prediction

CHD risk prediction can be based on serum lipid levels.
Table 16.1 gives the desirable cholesterol levels.

Table 16.1 Desirable cholesterol levels

Cholesterol	*Desirable*	*Normal risk*	*High risk*
Total cholesterol mg/d	< 160	200–240	> 240
HDL cholesterol mg/d	> 55	35–55	< 35
Triglycerides mg/d	< 50–150	200–400	> 400
LDL cholesterol mg/d	< 130	130–160	> 160

Total CHL/HDL Ratio : 4.0 to 5.7
LDL/HDL Ratio : 5 : 1 in men
4.5 : 1 in women

Desirable cut off level for cholesterol is found to be 160 mg/dl for Indians. The risk of CHD increases slowly as serum cholesterol values rises from 150 to 200 mg/dl but there is steep rise (2 to 4 fold) beyond 200 mg up to 300 mg/dl. Hyper cholesteraemia occurs when the cholesterol level exceeds 240 mg/dl.

The normal serum triglyceride level is 50–150 mg/dl.

Viseral/abdominal obesity is a major risk factor for CVD. Waist hip ratio correlates well with abdominal obesity.

RISK FACTORS

Various risk factors have been classified into four categories

Category I	*Category II*	*Category III*	*Category IV*
Risk factors for which interventions have been proven to lower CVD risk.	Risk factors for which interventions are likely to lower CVD risk.	Risk factors associated-with increased CVD risk, that if modified, might lower risk,	Risk factors associated-with increased CVD risk-which cannot be modified
• Cigarette smoking • LDL cholesterol • High fat/cholesterol diet • Hypertension • Left ventricular hypertrophy • Thrombogenic factors	• Diabetes mellitus • Physical inactivity • HDL cholesterol • Triglycerides, small dense LDL • Obesity • Postmenopausal status	• Psychological factors • Lipoprotein (*a*) • Homocysteine • Oxidative stress • No alcohol consumption	• Age • Male gender • Family history of early-onset CVD

Source: (Modified) Davidson H. Michael 1998 Cardiovascular risk factors. Cardiovascular nutrition. The American Dietetic Association.

Category I: Risk factors for which interventions have been proven to lower CVD risk

Cigarette smoking: Cigarette smoking enhances endothelial damage, increases heart rate and blood pressure, lowers high-density lipo protein cholesterol, increases LDL, constricts blood vessels and promotes thrombus formation. There is reduction of cardiovascular risk of those who quit smoking after a myocardial infarction compared with those who continue to smoke.

High-saturated fat, high-cholesterol diet: High intake of saturated fatty acid increases plasma cholesterol and so promotes formation of atheroma. Raised levels of both factor VII and blood cholesterol may be a parallel consequence of an increased intake of total and saturated fatty acids. Saturated fats appear to accelerate thrombosis formation. One possible mechanism may be via the inhibition of antiaggregatory prostacyclin. Saturated fats reduce the formation of LDL receptors or VLDL receptors. Animal fat like egg yolk, butter, meat fat have not only high amount of saturated fatty acids, but also contain high amount of cholesterol. Margarine, ghee, hydrogenated fat and coconut oil also contain high amount of saturated fat.

Elevated low-density lipoprotein cholesterol: Extensive epidemiologic, laboratory and clinical trial data have shown that LDL-C is associated with the development of atherosclerosis.

Hypertension: Hypertension is an independent risk factor for both CHD and stroke. High blood pressure leads to enhanced endothelial cell damage and target organ involvement including retinopathy and renal insufficiency. In addition hypertension is often associated with other risk factors, such as obesity, blood lipid abnormalities, insulin resistance and glucose intolerance. Reducing blood pressure has been unequivocally shown to lower the incidence of stroke, CHD and heart failure.

Thrombogenic factors: The final event precipitating a myocardial infarction is usually the development of an intracoronary thrombosis. High circulating fibrinogen concentrations appear to increase CHD risk in a graded fashion. Plasminogen activator inhibitor-1, platelet aggregability and factor VII, among others, are also linked to increased risk.

Category II: Risk factors for which interventions are likely to lower cardiovascular disease risk

Diabetes mellitus: Patients with diabetes mellitus have at least a threefold greater risk of CHD than does the general population. Diabetes eliminates the protection against CHD afforded by female gender. People with diabetes have metabolic alterations like insulin resistance, blood lipid abnormalities, hypertension and central obesity.

Metabolic syndrome is a biological risk factor for type 2 diabetes mellitus and coronary artery disease and enhances the risk of coronary heart disease at any given low density lipo protein cholesterol levels.

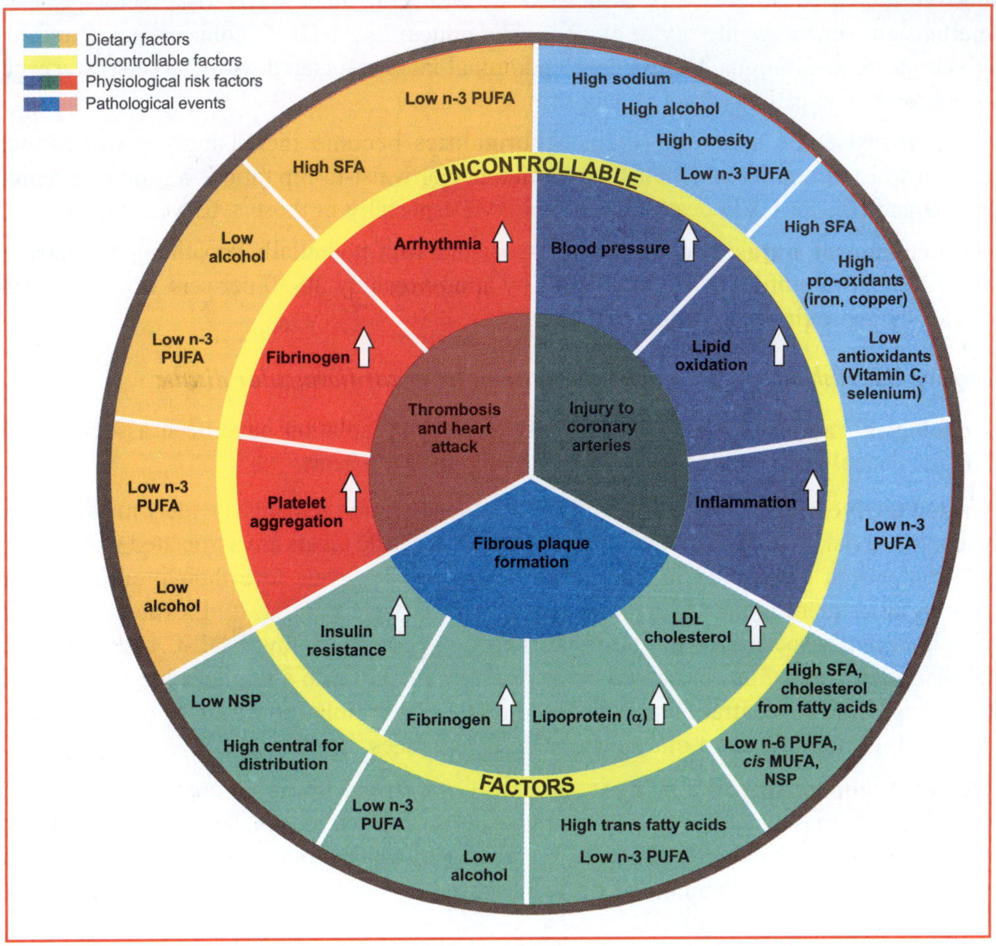

Fig. 16.1 Factors involved in the development of coronary heart disease. Note the dietary factors involved in thrombosis, injury to coronary arteries and in fibrous plaque formation.

Source: Dwight Jeremy, Coronary bypass or angioplasty, The Practitioners, 1994, 238

Physical inactivity: A sedentary life style and low cardio respiratory fitness are each associated with a two fold or more increase in CHD risk. Regular aerobic exercise reduces blood pressure, lowers triglyceride concentration, increases HDL-C, aids in weight control and improves insulin sensitivity. Other potential benefits of exercise include increase in myocardial electrical stability and decreases in platelet aggregation and fibrinogen levels.

Low high-density lipoprotein cholesterol: There is a strong inverse relationship between HDL-C concentration and coronary events. Cigarette smoking, obesity and post-menopausal status are associated with lower HDL-C concentrations, whereas moderate alcohol consumption and aerobic exercise raise HDL-C concentrations. HDL-C concentrations are also strongly influenced by family history.

Obesity: Increased adiposity is associated with several other CHD risk factors, such as hypertension, sedentary life style, glucose intolerance, low HDL-C concentrations and high triglyceride concentrations. Excess deep abdominal fat is associated with marked disturbances in lipoprotein and carbohydrate metabolism.

Insulin resistance and lipoprotein abnormalities become increasingly prevalent with elevated waist circumference. Waist circumference or waist-to-hip ratio is a primary predictor of CHD and risk for CVD death rather than BMI especially in those ≤ 65 year of age.

Post-menopausal status: Menopause is associated with potentially proatherogenic changes in the blood lipid profile. LDL-C increases by approximately 20-30 per cent whereas HDL-C declines by approximately 10 per cent.

Category III: Risk factors for which interventions lower cardiovascular disease

Psychological factors: Depression, hostility and social isolation have been associated with CHD incidence. Poor relationships might literally hurt the heart.

Elevated triglycerides: Circulating triglyceride concentration remains a widely misunderstood and controversial coronary risk factor. Increased triglyceride levels are associated with elevated CHD risk, when considered in isolation but triglyceride levels lose their predictive power when an adjustment is made for other risk factors especially HDL-C. Elevated triglyceride levels are often associated with obesity, diabetes, hypertension, low HDL-C and small dense LDL particles. Apart from increased energy intake, alcohol also stimulates hepatic synthesis. Thus triglyceride concentration may not be directly responsible for increased risk, but may be a marker for the presence of other metabolic disturbances.

Elevated Lipoprotein (*a*): Lp (*a*) is an LDL-C particle with apolipoprotein (*a*) attached. Apolipoprotein(*a*) is a large protein structurally similar to plasminogen, an important contributor to clot lysis. Lp(*a*) by interfering with the action of plasminogen may impair fibrinolysis, perhaps favouring the formation of occlusive thrombi. An Lp(*a*) concentration greater than 30 mg/dl doubles the risk of CHD.

Elevated Homocysteine: Hyperhomocysteinemia is atherogenic by causing oxidative damage to LDL. It modifies apolipoproteins and impairs uptake by LDL receptors. Hyperhomocysteinemia causes loss of vasodilation. It inhibits anticoagulants like prostacyclin and activates procoagulants. An increase in plasma homocysteine of 5 μ mol/l could increase coronary risk similar to an increase of 20 mg/dl in serum cholesterol. Heterozygosity for the enzyme disorder cystathiomine synthase deficiency or inadequate intake of vitamins B_6, B_{12} or folate causes elevated blood homocysteine concentrations in adults. Homocysteine is a possible marker for the development of vascular disease.

Individuals with rheumatoid arthritis have increased risk of CVD. The requirement of B_6 increased when methotrexate is taken. Pyridoxal phosphate decreases and homocystein levels increase. Supplementation decreases homocysteine levels.

Homocyteine may have direct effect on vessel walls by promoting vascular smooth muscles proliferation. Homocysteine may increase platelet adhesion, interfere with clotting and enhances oxidation of LDL cholesterol.

Oxidation and antioxidants: Blood concentration of antioxidants affect the susceptibility of LDL and lipoprotein (*a*) to oxidation, because it is the oxidised LDL that attracts circulating monocytes which then adhere to the arterial wall forming atherosclerotic plaques. Decreased levels of these substances that protect against oxidation increases atherosclerotic risk. Studies show that a dietary intake of antioxidants including flavanoids (polyphenolic antioxidants) naturally present in coloured vegetables and fruits, tea and wine and vitamin E is associated with a decline in coronary heart disease event. Low levels of β-carotene are seen in patients of myocardial infarction especially among smokers. Studies with vitamin C supplementation in CAD patients have been controversial. In patients with CAD, who have undergone previous coronary bypass surgery, progression of the disease was less in subjects with a supplementary vitamin E intake of 100 I.U. per day or more compared with lower intake.

Alcoholic beverage consumption: Individuals who consume moderate amounts of alcohol (one to three drinks per day) have 40 to 50 per cent lower rate of CHD than those who abstain. People who abstain should not be advised to begin consuming alcohol to prevent CHD due to associated risks.

Category IV: Risk factors that are not generally amenable to modification

Age: The incidence of the disease increases with age having peak at middle age around 50 to 55 years.

Sex: Coronary Artery Disease morbidity is twice as high in men as in women. After menopause the incidence is increased in women, by the age of 70 there is no difference between the sexes. Relative immunity of women during their reproductive life is due to secretion of ovarian hormones. If ovaries are removed before the age of 35 there would be a rise in cholesterol level. There is increased risk of CHD with oral contraceptives. The incidence of the disease among males and females is in the proportion of 9 : 1.

Family history: In some families there is early onset of cardiovascular disease. Some families are susceptible for hyperlipidemia. There are 30 genes involved in the disease process with many variants. The gene for apolipoprotein E, a fatty protein molecule that helps remove cholesterol from blood has three variations. It appears that people with one form of gene are more prone to fatty streaks and plaques than people with the other two.

If there is history of heart attack before 55 in father and before 65 in mother, the offsprings are likely to get a heart attack at an earlier age.

In recent years, high levels of factor VII have been found to be associated with increased risk of heart attack. Some people may not have inherited a natural ability to contain the level of a blood protein implicated in clot formation.

People with a combination of risk factors have the greatest risk of developing CHD.

In India smoking is prevalent in poorer households and urban locations face risks from high body mass index, high blood glucose and high systolic blood pressure.

ROLE OF FAT IN THE DEVELOPMENT OF ATHEROSCLEROSIS

Cholesterol and triglycerides are the main forms of fat carried in the blood stream. These fats or lipids come partly from food, and partly from the body's own production in the liver. Fats are not water soluble and hence cannot travel through the blood easily. With the help of lipoprotein, digested fat from the liver is carried to various parts of the body by the blood vessels. The cholesterol returns to liver and repeats its job.

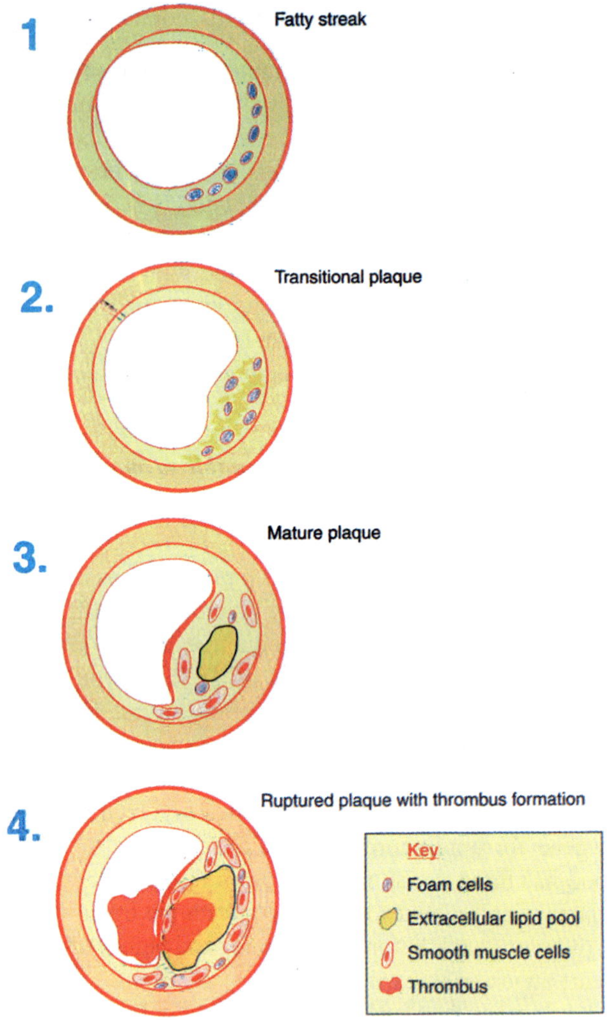

Fig. 16.2 Development of vascular atherosclerosis

Source: Edwards, CRW, *et al*, 1995. Davidson's principles and practice of medicine, ELBS with Chunchill Livingstone.

The smaller the LDL particle size, the higher the number particles resulting in increased surface area for oxidation and thus promoting inflammation and the atheroscerotic process. Once oxidized an LDL particle is no longer recognized by its receptors but rather by scavenger receptors on macrophages which can lead to foam cell formation and fatty streaks and damage the vessel wall. The plaque that is most likely to rupture known as vulnerable plaque has several common characteristics. Its core contains lipids and scavenger cells called macrophages that damage the vessel wall. The plaque has a large amount of the chemical that stimulates the formation of blood clots.

The liver places cholesterol into packages called lipoproteins, made from lipids and protein. There are mainly four kinds of lipoprotein packages namely chylomicrons, VLDL (very low density lipoprotein), LDL (low density lipoprotein) and HDL (high density lipoprotein). High density lipoprotein has more protein content.

Chylomicrons, carry triglycerides whose fatty acids contain more than 10 to 12 carbon atoms, monoglycerides, glycerol and small amounts of cholesterol and phospholipids.

VLDL also transport triglycerides but mainly endogenous triglycerides formed in the liver. The VLDL travels through the blood vessels to unload fat throughout the body. The 'empty' VLDL becomes LDL. VLDL has 85–92 per cent triglycerides.

LDL is the main carrier of cholesterol. Some LDL pieces get stuck to the blood vessel walls, narrowing the same. High LDL decreases Endothelium Derived Relaxing Factor and blood vessel becomes narrow and cannot dilate. LDL is called 'bad' cholesterol because it causes atherosclerosis. LDL has 50 per cent cholesterol.

HDL plays a role in the reverse transport of cholesterol from tissues throughout the body back to the liver for conversion to bile acids or excretion as biliary cholesterol. HDL is called good cholesterol. HDL has 15–20 per cent cholesterol.

Experimental studies have shown beneficial functions of HDL-cholesterol including endothelial, antiapoptotic, antithrombotic, antioxidant and antiinflammatory effects all of which may contribute to its antitherosclerotic properties.

The second potential anti-atherogenic activity of HDL relates to its role as an antiaggregant in the vessel wall.

If too much of fat is consumed, the liver makes extra VLDL to carry the fat. More LDL pieces get stuck if there is not enough HDL to rescue them all. The blood vessel may become blocked. If this happens to a blood vessel in the heart, a heart attack may result.

Hyperlipidaemia and excess of modified lipoprotein fractions/peroxides/free radicals

↓

Endothelial injury or dysfunction

↓

In the intima oxidised LDL is formed and sticks to the blood vessel

↓

Monocytes turn into macrophages
Promote contraction of the vessel

↓

Formation of foam cells

↓

Development of lipid pool

↓

Smooth muscle cell proliferation
Wall becomes thickened, hardened narrowing the lumen

↓

Fatty streak

↓

Transitional plaque

↓

Mature plaque

↓

Ruptured plaque with thrombus formation

Fig. 16.3 Development of atheroma

All the three layers—intima, media and adventia of the arteries are damaged in atherosclerosis.

Genetically, Indians have a low level of HDL and high triglyceride levels.

Coronary heart disease is a process, not a single event. The sequence of development of atheroma is given in the schematic Fig. 16.3.

Cholesterol

Dietary cholesterol can increase LDL cholesterol levels although to a lesser extent than saturated fat. Most foods high in saturated fat are also sources of dietary cholesterol. Hence reduced intake of such foods provides the additional benefit of limiting cholesterol intake. Cholesterol rich foods that are relatively low in saturated fatty acid content (egg yolk and to a lesser extent shell fish) have smaller effects on LDL cholesterol levels.

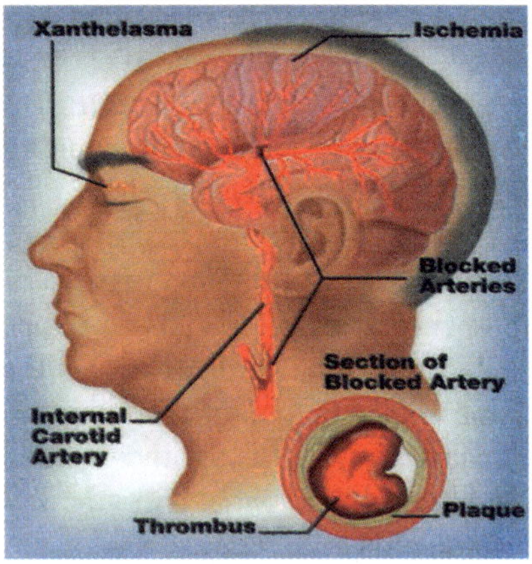

Fig. 16.4 Ischemic storke

Source: Applegate, W (ed.), 1995, Patient Education Center Target Media, Inc. Cincinnati, Ohio.

Saturated Fatty Acids

Saturated fatty acids raise the level of LDL and total blood cholesterol level. Both of these effects increase the risk of CHD. The activity of LDL receptor—its ability to mediate the entry of LDL—appears to be suppressed by saturated fatty acids. When LDL receptor activity decreases, LDL catabolism decreases and blood levels of LDL increase.

A study of Indian adolescents and young adults found that dietary saturated fatty acids are the single most important one contributing to increase in serum high sensitivity C-Reactive protein levels, which is an inflammatory marker.

Individual saturated fatty acids differ in their ability to change blood LDL-cholesterol levels. Palmitic, myristic and to a lesser degree lauric acids increase the LDL-cholesterol level. In contrast stearic acid and medium to short-chain saturated fatty acids do not.

Trans Fatty Acids

Trans fatty acids have proinflammatory effects and increase Tumour Necrosis Factor-α and Interleukin factor. Interleukin factor-6 and C-Reactive proteins are associated with markers of vascular endothelial dysfunction and are most striking when compared with the effects of *cis* unsaturated fatty acids.

Trans fatty acids raise LDL cholesterol to the same extent as myristic acid and in addition lower HDL cholesterol. Thus *trans* fatty acids turning out

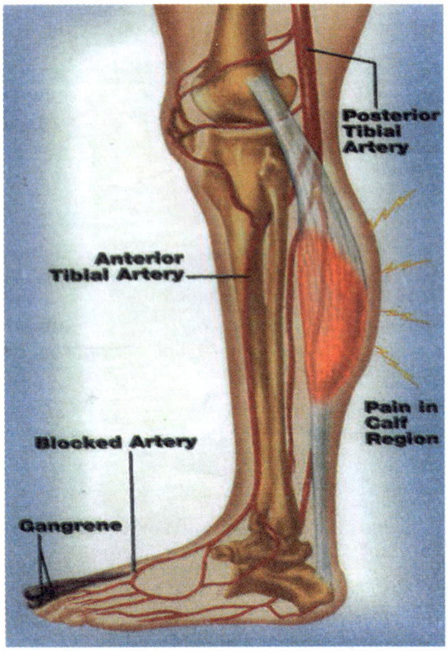

Fig. 16.5 Peripheral vascular disease

Source: Applegate, W (ed.), 1995, Patient Education Center Target Media, Inc. Cincinnati, Ohio.

to be even more atherogenic than myristic acid. Further *trans* fatty acids have been found to raise lipoprotein (*a*) levels, thus raising the risk of CHD.

Trans fatty acids in the diet come from two main sources.

- Bacterial fermentation: In the gut of ruminants *trans* fatty acids are produced. Meat and dairy products contain *trans* fatty acids.
- Hydrogenated fats: Hydrogenation of vegetable oils alter the geometric structure of the polyunsaturated fatty acids from natural '*cis*' to '*trans*' forms. Only *cis* forms can serve as essential fatty acids which are to be incorporated in cell structure. Depending on the degree of hydrogenation, *trans*-fats in food products contain anywhere from 5 per cent to as high as 40 percent. Most bakery products contain *trans* fat.

Triglycerides

Plasma triglycerides and VLDL cholesterol levels may also contribute to increased risk for coronary artery disease. Triglyceride levels are increased when there is excess body weight, reduced physical activity and increased intake of sugar and refined carbohydrates particularly in the setting of insulin resistance and glucose intolerance. Increased alcohol intake can aggravate hypertriglyceridaemia. Individuals with the combination of low HDL cholesterol and elevated triglycerides should make an effort to reduce weight, increase physical activity and reduce carbohydrate and fat intake and increase ω-3 fatty acids.

Summary of Fat as the Cause of Atherosclerosis

- High intake of saturated fatty acid can lead to
  - (*a*) ↑ Plasma cholesterol →↑ Atheroma formation.
  - (*b*) ↓ LDL receptors →↑ LDL cholesterol.
  - (*c*) Arrhythmia → Thrombosis.
  - (*d*) ↑ Lipid oxidation → Injury to coronary arteries.
  - (*e*) ↑ Factor VII level → Thrombosis.
  - (*f*) ↓ Antiaggregatory prostacyclin.
  - (*g*) ↓ HDL cholesterol.
  - (*h*) ↑ Plasma triglycerides.
- High cholesterol intake can lead to
  - (*a*) ↑ Plasma cholesterol
  - (*b*) ↑ LDL synthesis
  - (*c*) ↓ LDL catabolism by cells.
- Low ω-3 Fatty acids intake
  - (*a*) Arrhythmia → Thrombosis
  - (*b*) ↑ Fibrinogen → Thrombosis
→↑ Fibrous plaque.
  - (*c*) ↑ Platelet aggregation → Thrombosis.

(*d*) ↑ Lipoprotein (*a*) →↑ Fibrous plaque

(*e*) ↑ Inflammation → Injury to coronary arteries.

(*f*) ↑ B.P. → Injury to coronary arteries.

Figure 16.6 summarises fat as the cause of atherosclerosis.

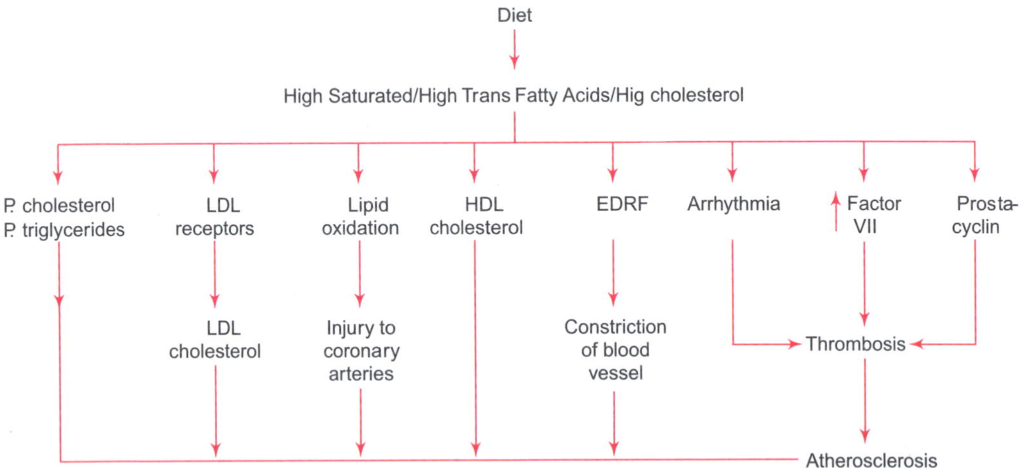

Fig. 16.6 Fat as the cause of atherosclerosis

TREATMENT

Principles

Principles of treatment are the following:

- Dietary management
- Drugs
- Physical activity
- Smoking cessation
- Stress management

DIETARY MANAGEMENT

Principles of Diet

Diet therapy remains the first line of treatment for patients with high blood cholesterol levels. Low calorie, low fat particularly low saturated fat, low trans fat, low cholesterol, high in PUFA with ω-6 to ω-3 ratio 4–10 : 1, low carbohydrate and normal protein, minerals and vitamins are suggested. High fibre diet with increased amount of antioxidants is also recommended.

Total Energy

Those patients whose weight is at a desirable level are permitted a maintenance level of calories during convalescence and their return to activity. The total calories should be restricted so as to reduce the weight to the expected normal for the height, age and sex.

Mild degree of weight loss for the cardiac patient of normal weight is recommended. Usually a 1000 to 1200 calorie diet is suitable for an obese patient in bed.

Loss of weight by the obese leads to a considerable reduction in the work of the heart because the basal metabolism is at a lower level. There is a slowing of the heart rate, a drop in blood pressure and thereby improved cardiac efficiency.

A brief period of undernutrition during the first few days after the attack is advisable as increased cardiac output is needed with high intake of food.

Fat

The first step involves restriction of fats to no more than 20 per cent of the total calories consumed. Levels as low as 20 per cent are tolerated without side effects. It is not desirable to restrict all forms of fat as severe restrictions result in mental depression. According to ICMR the proportion of polyunsaturated fat to saturated fat should be 0.8 : 1.0.

Poly Unsaturated Fatty Acids: The important n-3 polyunsaturated fatty acids are α-linolenic acid, eicosapentaenoic acid and docosahexaenoic acid. The n-6 polyunsaturated fatty acids are linoleic acid and arachidonic acid. n-6 and n-3 fatty acids are also known as ω-6 and ω-3 fatty acids.

PUFA promote esterification of cholesterol and make into easily utilisable form. PUFA, especially arachidonic acid are precursors of prostacyclins, thromboxanes and leukotrienes. Thromboxanes are vasoconstrictors while prostacyclins are vasodilators and hence help in the prevention of thrombus formation. These substances also decrease the stickiness of platelets (PUFA contain antiplatelet aggregate factor) and prevent their aggregation decreasing the tendency of blood platelet clot. ω-3 fatty acids raise endothelial derived relaxing factors. Hence PUFA reduce thrombosis. Linoleic acid prevents accumulation of cholesterol in blood serum and walls of blood vessels and therefore plays a key role in the transport of cholesterol. PUFA decrease the synthesis of the precursor of VLDL which are associated with an increased incidence of CHD. PUFA decrease the production of LDL and triglycerides. They also help in the clearance of LDL. High levels of linoleic acid lower HDL-cholesterol levels. α-linolenic acid do not lower HDL-cholesterol levels.

Foods rich in ω-3 polyunsaturated fatty acids, specially eicosapentaenoic acid and docosahexaenoic acid, confer cardioprotective effects. Apart from improving blood lipoprotein profiles, they reduce the incidence of sudden death, decrease risk of arrhythmia, lower plasma triglyceride levels and reduce blood clotting tendency. α-linolenic acid, reduces risk of myocardial infarction and fatal ischaemic heart disease among women. ω.3 fatty acids also reduce platelet aggregation.

Fish oil increases HDL levels and reduce plasma triglyceride levels by decreasing the synthesis in liver.

Fish consumption improves endothelial function and reduce resting heart rate.

Inflammation is a major contributor to atherosclerosis. EPA and DHA reduce tumour necrosis factor. Immune-modulatory effects of n-3 fatty acids may suggest prevention of atherosclerosis due to beneficial effects on platelet activities.

Both EPA and DHA are readily incorporated into cell membranes and may result in increasing membrane fluidity in cardiac cells, there by preventing atrial fibrillation and reducing the binding of inflammatory cytokines to their receptors and cardioprotective.

Those Eskimos living in Greenland and the fishing community in Japan, who have a daily consumption of fish is 200–400 g, enjoy complete freedom from cardiovascular diseases. The beneficial effect of dietary fish is attributed to the fatty acid composition of the fish.

Fish are good source of ω-3 fatty acids especially fatty fish such as salmon. Consumption of 100–200 g of fish two to three times a week helps to prevent heart disease (National Institute of Nutrition, Hyderabad). Vegetable substances such as mustard oil, flax seed oil, canola oil,

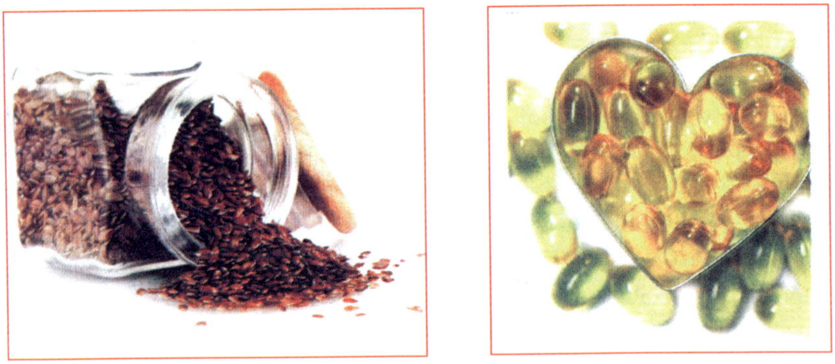

Fig. 16.7 **Flax seeds and fish oils are good sources of ω-3 fatty acids.**

Table 16.2 **Approximate fatty acid composition of dietary fats and oils consumed in India (% of total fatty acids)**

Fats/oil	*SFAs*	*MUFAs*	*LA*	*ALA*
High (medium chain) SFAs				
Coconut	92	6	2	—
Palm kernel	83	15	2	—
Butter/Ghee	68	29	2	1
High SFAs & MUFAs				
Palmolein	39	46	11	< 0.5
High MUFAs & Moderate LA				
Groundnut	19	41	32	< 0.5
Rice bran	17	43	38	1
Sesame	16	41	42	< 0.5
High LA				
Cotton seed	24	29	4	1
Corn	12	35	50	1
Safflower	9	13	75	—
Sunflower	12	22	62	—
LA & ALA				
Soyabean	14	24	53	7
Canola	6	60	22	10
Mustard/rape seed	4	65	15	14
Flax seed	10	21	16	53
High TFAs				
Vanasapti	46	49	4	—

Source: Nutrient requirements and recommended dietary allowances for Indians, 2010, ICMR.

soyabean oil and walnuts are good sources of ω-3 fatty acids. Moderate levels of linolenic acid are present in groundnut and rice bran oil. The daily consumption of 10–15 g of fish oil extract, representing 3–5 g ω-3 fatty acid is probably adequate to control moderate hypertriglyceridemia.

HDL levels for regular fish eaters (who do not eat meat) have been shown to be significantly higher than vegetarians, vegans and regular meat eaters.

FAO and WHO recommend ω-6 to ω-3 fatty acid ratio to be between 4 : 1 and 10 : 1. Among vegetarians excessive intake of linoleic acid is avoided.

Monounsaturated Fatty Acids: The monounsaturated fatty acids are oleic acid and erucic acid. Monounsaturated fats are present in vegetable sources such as olive oil, canola, almond oil and groundnut oil. They lower LDL without lowering HDL cholesterol and do not raise triglyceride levels. Larger proportion of MUFA in diet may be conducive to thrombolysis and may be anti-inflammatory. Uncontrolled peroxidation of PUFA in cell membrane may lead to cellular damage while maintenance of a balance with MUFA is conducive to maintain cell function.

Table 16.3 Fatty acid composition and cholesterol content of animal foods* (g/100 g)

Item	*Fat g/100 g*	*Saturated fatty acids g/100 g*	*Cholesterol mg/100 g*
Butter	80	50	250
Ghee	100	65	300
Milk (cow)	4	2	14
Milk (buffalo)	8	4	16
Milk (skimmed)	0.1	—	2
Milk (condensed)	10	6	40
Cream	13	8	40
Cheese	25	15	100
Egg (whole)	11	4	400
Egg yolk	30	9	1120
Chicken without skin	4	1	60
Chicken with skin	18	6	100
Beef	16	8	70
Mutton	13	7	65
Pork	35	13	90
Organ meats			
Brain	6	2	2000
Heart	5	2	150
Kidney	2	1	370
Liver	9	3	300
Fresh water and sea food			
Prawns/shrimps	2	0.3	150
Fish (lean)	1.5	0.4	45
Fish (fatty)	6	2.5	45

* Values vary depending on the feed of the animals.
* One whole egg or yolk of one egg contains 210 mg. cholesterol.
* Consumption of excess fat, saturated fat and cholesterol can lead to atherosclerosis.

Source: Ghafoorumissa and Kamala Krishnaswamy, 1998, Diet and heart disease, NIN, Hyderabad.

Studies provide evidence that both low fat diets and diets higher in monounsaturated fatty acids decrease LDL-oxidative susceptibility and thereby contribute to a decreased risk of coronary heart disease.

MUFA lower the level of LDL cholesterol by decreasing the input of very low-density lipoproteins, the precursor of LDL, by reducing the cholesterol content of LDL particles and by increasing the activity of LDL receptors.

The mediterranean style diet that focuses on fruit, vegetables, MUFA, legumes and grains and includes only small portion of meat products has beneficial effects.

The trans isomers of oleic acid (present in margarine) raise LDL to the same extent as SFA.

Saturated fatty acids: Saturated fatty acid content of meat fat is 46 per cent, which is double that of fish oils while it is intermediate in chicken, 35 per cent. The only dubious advantage of coconut oil and butter is that these are richer in lauric (C_{12}) and myristic (C_{14}) acids. Myristic acids raise HDL alongwith LDL. Yet both are atherogenic and thrombogenic. Palmitic acid, the chief constituent of palm oil, raises serum cholesterol to a much lower extent than myristic acid of coconut and dairy fat.

Saturated fatty acids are avoided; polyunsaturated fatty acids should be taken in limited quantity; and monounsaturated fatty acids are preferred to protect cardiac health.

Cholesterol: The contribution of dietary cholesterol to plasma value is small (10 mg/d). Intake of cholesterol may contribute modestly to plasma cholesterol only when intake of saturated fatty acid is high. Cholesterol level in the diet should not exceed 300 mg. If cholesterol levels are above 260 mg/dl, it is almost impossible to bring about a drop, by diet alone. No vegetable substance contains cholesterol. Table 16.3 gives fatty acid composition and cholesterol content of animal foods.

The advantages of a vegetarian diet are that it is low in calories, fat and cholesterol and that it has a high p/s ratio and it has adequate fibre which helps in binding cholesterol and increase the excretion of cholesterol. Vegetable oils diminish the plasma cholesterol not only due to polyunsaturated fatty acids but also because the plant sterol inhibits cholesterol absorption.

Table 16.4 Effect of fatty acids on atherosclerosis

	SFA	*Oleic*	*n-6*	*n-3*
Blood cholesterol	↑	↓	↓	↓
HDL cholesterol	↓	no change	↓	no change
Triglycerides	↑	no change	no change	↓
Platelet aggregation	↑	no change	↓	↓↓↓

Source: Ghafoorunissa, 1989, *Nutrition aspects of fats in Indian diets*, 35, Proceedings of the Nutrition Society of India.

Blended Oils: Mustard oil and soyabean oil are rich in (n-3) α linolenic acid. Safflower oil and corn oil are rich in (n-6) linoleic acid. Blended oils help in getting correct proportion of n-6 and n-3 fatty acids and prevent atherosclerosis.

Use of more than one source of oil gives an additional advantage of providing greater variety of minor components present in oils which may enhance their antioxidant properties. The various combinations that have been recommended give the consumer an option to select oils according to their pattern of purchase and culinary habits. Government of India has permitted admixture of any two edible vegetable oils. Blended oils that could ensure optimal balance of fatty acids are available in the market.

Table 16.5 Recommended combinations of oils for optimal health benefits

Oils containing ↑ ALNA (n-3)				Oils containing ↑ LA (n-6)		
GNO	: MO	3 : 1		SAF	: POL	1 : 2
GNO	: CAN	2 : 1	–	SUN	: POL	1 : 1
GNO	: SBO	2 : 1		SES	: POL	1 : 1
POL	: SBO	1 : 1		SAF	: GNO (RBO)	1 : 3
SAF	: PO : MO	1 : 1 : 1		SUN	: GNO (RBO)	1 : 3
SUN	: PO : MO	2 : 1 : 1		SES	: GNO	1 : 3

GNO — Groundnut Oil	MO — Mustard Oil	CAN — Canola Oil
SBO — Soyabean Oil	POL — Palmolein Oil	SAF — Safflower Oil
SUN — Sunflower Oil	SES — Sesame Oil	RBO — Rice bran Oil

Source: Gafoorunnissa 1999, Antiatherogenic potential of oils in Indian subjects consuming cereal based diets, 1999, Proceedings Nutrition Society of India, *46*.

Diet therapy remains the first line of treatment for patients with high blood cholesterol levels.

Recommendations of NCEP of USA for the amount and type of fat to be consumed is given in Table 16.6. In step III there are recommendations for fibre.

Table 16.6 Composition of National Cholesterol Education Programme (NCEP) diet

Fat	*NCEP Step I diet*	*NCEP Step II diet*	*NCEP Step III*
• Per cent of calories from fat	≤ 30	≤ 30	25–35
• Per cent of calories from saturated fat	≤ 10	≤ 7	< 7
• Daily dietary cholesterol mg	≤ 300	< 200	< 200
• Fibre g	–	–	20–30

Polyunsaturated fatty acids (10%) monounsaturated fatty acids (Remaining total fat energy), carbohydrates (55%), protein (15-20%) is same both in step I and step II diet.

Patient should maintain desirable body weight.

Carbohydrate

Only complex carbohydrates should be included in the diet. Simple sugars reduce HDL levels. Since total calories are restricted, carbohydrates intake would be reduced. High carbohydrate intake can increase fasting triglyceride levels. By restricting carbohydrate intake, serum triglyceride levels can be controlled. Carbohydrate intake should be limited to 60 per cent of total energy in patients with metabolic syndrome.

Soluble fibres like oat products, psyllum, pectin, guargum reduce LDL particularly in hypercholesterolmic patients.

Low Glycaemic Foods: Burkilt and Trowell (1977) suggested that foods that are more slowly absorbed may have metabolic benefit in relation to the reduction of CHD.

Studies showed a negative relation between glycaemic index and HDL cholesterol suggesting that low glycaemic index diets may preserve HDL cholesterol and thus have a potentially positive effect in reducing CHD risk.

Low glycaemic foods lower post prandial fatty acid concentration which may be associated with increased glucose uptake by muscle, reduced VLDL synthesis and inturn reduce LDL and increase HDL. Low GI diets may reduce plasma fatty acids and may suppress production of release of signaling hormones from adipose tissue in turn tending to reverse dyslipidaemia and insulin resistance. The foods that are more slowly absorbed may have metabolic benefits to the decrease of CHD risk. Reduced LDL concentration with low glycaemic index diets preserve HDL cholesterol. Low glycaemic index food is beneficial for those with greater degree of insulin resistance (BMI > 23).

Protein, Vitamins and Minerals

Normal allowances are recommended. Animal proteins are not suggested for an atherosclerotic patient.

Since total fat, animal fat, organ meats, eggs and sea food are restricted, vitamin A deficiency may occur. Therefore supplement of vitamin A is essential.

Mega doses of niacin has been known to be an effective treatment of dyslipidemia. Niacin increases high density lipoprotein cholesterol levels while lowering the levels of low-density lipoprotein cholesterol, triglycerides and lipoprotein (*a*). Combining niacin with statins or bile acid sequestrant therapy is safe and effective for improving lipid levels and decreasing coronary risk.

Vitamins B_6, B_{12} and folic acid supplementation decreases the risk of cardiovascular disease related to homocysteine risk factor.

Vitamin C is known to be involved in regulating cholesterol metabolism and in maintaining the structure of blood vessels and the antioxidant effects of the vitamin might prevent the tissue damage that leads to CHD. Vitamin C activates the adrenals and reduce cholesterol. Cholesterol is converted to cholic acid by ascorbic acid. 200–300 mg of vitamin C reduces cholesterol.

There is some evidence to suggest that patients with coronary heart disease and stroke have lowered serum and leucocyte vitamin C levels.

Epidemiologic studies have shown an inverse relation between blood selenium concentrations and coronary heart disease. Selenium is a constituent of glutathione peroxidase an enzyme that inactivates the toxic hydrogen peroxide and hydroperoxides. In lactovegetarian diet, the legumes namely red gram, black gram, wheat, parboiled rice and milk provide selenium. Selenium intake in urban South Indian is low especially among vegetarians and could contribute to the development of CHD. In CHD red cell selenium is lowered and is in the range of 27–131 ng/g. Selenium can be increased in the diet by increased consumption of parboiled rice, wheat and finger millet.

Sodium is restricted when there is hypertension. Usually a restriction of sodium of 1600 to 2300 mg is satisfactory among patients with CHD. When sodium is restricted other sources of iodine should be prescribed. A severe restriction of sodium also reduces the intake of vitamin A because egg and green leafy vegetables that are high in sodium, are restricted. Sodium content of different foods is given in Table 16.7. Sodium restriction should not be a standing order but should be ordered individually as the condition of the patient requires.

Intake of salt 3 g/d is probably both safe and adequate for healthy adults. In tropical countries like India, where sodium loss can occur through sweat the requirements are probably not more than 7g/d, (NIN).

Potassium helps to maintain cell fluid balance and plays a role in muscle contraction. Low levels of this mineral have been associated with high blood pressure. Magnesium helps muscles relax, affects the muscle tone of blood vessels and keep heart rhythm steady. Magnesium intake has also been associated with a decreased incidence of CHD and low magnesium levels have been correlated with high blood pressure and angina.

Salt and Sodium conversions

Milligrams of sodium × 2.5 = milligrams of salt

Milligrams of salt × 0.40 = milligrams f sodium

$$\frac{\text{Milligrams of sodium}}{23\,(\text{atomic weight of sodium})} \times 1\,(\text{valence}) = \text{milliequivalents of sodium}$$

Milliequivalents of sodium × 23 = milligrams of sodium

Milliequivalents of sodium × 58.5 = milligrams of table salt (NaCl)

Table 16.7 Sodium content of foods per 100 g

< 25 mg	*25–50 mg*	*50–100 mg*	*> 100 mg*
Bitter Gourd, Bottlegourd, Brinjal, Cabbage, Colocasia, Cow pea, Cucumber, Beans French, Grapes, Guava, Honey, Horse Gram, Ladies finger, Maida, Oil, Onion, Orange, Papaya, Peas, Plantain, Potato, Pumpkin, Ragi, Sapota, Semolina, Sugar, Sweet Potato, Tomato ripe, Vermicelli, Wheat, Yam, Water melon, Banana, Broad bean, Green gram dhal, Lentil, Mango, Pine-apple, Radish, Tomato, Green, Red gram dhal.	Bengal gram (whole) Black gram dhal, Carrots, Cream, Spinach, Mutton, Raisins, Milk Buffalo, Bengal gram dhal, Cauli-flower, knofkhol.	Beetroot, Chicken, Coriander leaves, Field bean, Liver, Prawn.	Bacon, Egg, Lobster, Beef.

Source: Longvah, T. *et al.*, Indian Food Composition Tables 2017, National Institute of Nutrition, Hyderabad.

Water

Some scientific evidence suggests that heart diseases are more common in areas with soft water than where the water is hard. Minerals such as calcium and magnesium and trace metals like chromium and vanadium present in hard water appear to be protective.

Restriction of fluid is not required as long as sodium is not restricted.

Table 16.8 Therapeutic Lifestyle changes diet to reduce risk of coronary heart disease.

Nutrient	*Amount*
Saturated fat	< 7% of total calories
PUFA	upto 10% of total calories
MUFA	upto 20% of total calories
Total fat	25-35% of total calories
Carbohydrate	50-60% of total calories
Fibre	20-30 g/d
Protein	15% of total calories
Cholesterol	< 200 mg/d
Calories	Balance energy intake and exercise to maintain healthy weight and prevent weight gain.
For at least 30-60 minutes of physical activity at least 5 days per week.	

Dietary Modification Immediately after Myocardial Infarction

In the initial phase the basic clinical objective is cardiac rest.

After myocardial infarction, metabolism of the heart switches from utilisation of free fatty acids for the primary source of energy to the preferential oxidation of glucose. Since glucose is so critical in the metabolism of the failing ischaemic heart, it is important to monitor a patient's daily caloric intake and look for ways of increasing energy intake no matter what the consistency of food served. A typical clear fluid diet provides only 500–600 kcal/day.

Small frequent feeding permits provision of calories and nutrients without taxing the need for splanchnic (intestinal) circulation. A brief period of undernutrition during the first few days after the attack is advisable. The caloric level recommended for this period is 800 to 1200 kcal. The caloric level may be gradually increased, depending on the patient's progress and such factors as nearness to ideal weight, presence of diabetes and hyperlipoproteinaemia.

Soft food with small and frequent feedings and moderate food restriction per meal, would also prevent distension of the stomach and stimulation of reflexes which may produce arrhythmias.

During this stage the patient must not even be permitted to feed himself. When the patient's condition improves, he may be given foods which do not cause strain but easy to chew and digest.

Liquids are used for 2 to 3 days. All liquids are served at room temperature. Extremes of temperature such as very hot or iced beverages are contraindicated because they may induce arrhythmias. Beverages containing caffeine are omitted because of their stimulating effect on heart rate.

Constipation must be avoided. This can be relieved through judicious use of fruits and vegetables. The choice of foods must be restricted to those which are non-distending. There is variation in individual tolerance in this regard.

As the patient improves eggs can be included in the diet in restricted amounts. It is also 'safe' to include shrimp, crab and other edible crustaceans to a low cholesterol diet. Skim milk can be given as it has cholesterol lowering effect.

Low sodium diet consisting of 2 g is usually prescribed. During recovery of acute phase calories are limited to 1000 to 1200 calories. Cholesterol and saturated fats are restricted.

In the rehabilitative stage, calories are adjusted as necessary to bring about weight change if needed. All the other principles maintained earlier should be followed.

Three or four smaller meals are suggested instead of two big meals. Evening meals must be two hours before retiring to bed.

Smoking and drinking of alcohol should be stopped.

Functional foods for CHD

A functional food is any food that has a positive effect on a person's health, physical performance or state of mind. It reduces the risk of chronic diseases and has physiological benefits when eaten on a regular basis in adequate amounts. Foods rich in antioxidants, hypocholesterolemic agents and phytochemicals protect from CHD. Antioxidants including vitamins C, E and β-carotene have potential health benefits of reducing CVD.

Vitamin E: It maintains the integrity of all membranes by preventing the oxidation of polyunsaturated fatty acids. Besides reducing LDL oxidation as a result of its potent antioxidant properties, vitamin E reduces platelet aggregation and thrombus formation. Patients with high levels of Lp (*a*) and familial hypercholesterolaemia may benefit from vitamin E supplementation. Food sources of vitamin E include vegetable oils, dark green leafy vegetables, nuts and whole grain cereals. Studies conducted at AIIMS showed that almonds decrease cholesterol concentration and improve platelet function. Intake of vitamin E from foods protect against nonfatal coronary heart disease. Vitamin E is the most concentrated antioxidant.

Carotenoids and β-carotene: β-carotene is an antioxidant and quenches singlet oxygen and reacts directly with free radicals generated during lipid peroxidation. Green leafy vegetables and yellow orange coloured vegetables are good sources of carotenoids.

Vitamin C: It is an antioxidant found in the blood and cytosol of cells, reduces the damage caused by free radicals during oxidation process.

Vitamin C, beta-carotene and vitamin E may work synergistically in preventing cellular oxidation. Fruits and vegetables are good sources of vitamin C.

Fruits and vegetables are good sources of anthocyanins, vitamin C, β-carotene and dietary fibre which are all cardio protective. Guavas, red grapes and pomegranate have the maximum antioxidant properties and pineapple, sapota and banana have the least. Green leafy and cruciferous vegetables contain nutrients and phytochemicals that protect the heart. Five servings of fruits and vegetables are recommended to fulfil antioxidant requirements.

Selenium: Selenium is essential for the production of glutathione peroxidase, the enzyme that catalyses the breakdown of hyperoxides. Seafood, kidney and liver are good sources of selenium.

Selenium intake in urban South Indians is low, especially among vegetarians and could contribute to the development of coronary heart disease. In CHD, selenium content of red cell is lowered and is in the range of 27–131 ng/g. Selenium in South Indian Vegetarian diet can be enhanced by substituting polished rice with parboiled rice, wheat and finger millet.

Soya protein: Soya protein reduces the plasma total cholesterol concentration in hypercholesterolemic subjects. The isoflavones, genistein and daidzein occur in high concentrations in soyabeans. *In vitro* genistein blocks the action of platelet-derived growth factor and other growth factors, thereby inhibiting the proliferation and migration of arterial smooth muscle cells and halting the transition of fatty streaks to advanced lesions. Genistein may also reduce overall thrombosis associated with atherosclerosis by interfering with the activation of platelets. Daidzein is a potent antioxidant and may also slow the development or progression of atherosclerosis. High intake of soya protein can reduce LDL cholesterol when it is replaced by animal protein. Soya protein sources include soya bean and its products like isolated and textured soya protein supplements. The current recommendations to consume 25 g/day soya proteins as a means of reducing cardiovascular disease risk is not feasible.

Beans: The components of beans that decrease cardiovascular disease are soluble fibre, phytosterols, magnesium, potassium, copper and folate. Greater consumption of legumes was linked to a lower incidence of hypertension. Soluble fibre lowers blood cholesterol by binding bile acids and preventing cholesterol reabsorption. Pinto bean reduces total and LDL blood cholesterol. The chemical structure of flavonoids enables these compounds to scavenge free radical and thus have antioxidant effects.

Table 16.9 Bioactive constituents that reduce CHD biomarkers

Anti inflammatory	*Reduce Oxidation*	*Improve Endothelial function*
Antioxidants	Antioxidants	L. arginine
Tocopherols	Tocopherals	α linolenic acid
Phenolic compounds	Phenolic compounds	Antioxidants
α-linolenic acid	Phytosterols	Tocopherals
Magnesium	Selenium	Phenolic compounds
	Monounsaturated fatty acids	Folic acid
		Magnesium

Source: Coleman Ellen, Chocolate and nut lovers take heart, today's dietician 2011, **13.**

Fruits and Vegetables: Flavonols, powerful health giving chemicals which can protect against heart disease are found in wines, fruits and vegetables. Small cherry tomatoes contain more flavonols than larger ones. Red onions are full of flavonols whereas white onions have practically none.

Unlike many vitamins flavonols are not easily destroyed by cooking. Although flavonols are mostly present in fresh foods, high levels remain after food has been fried and to a lesser extent boiled.

Fish/Fish Oil: Fish reduces the risk of dying from heart attack. It also lowers the risk of stroke Fish oils are richest source of ω-3 fatty acids and cardio protective. It steadies heart rhythm, lowers artery clogging triglycerides, reduces chronic inflammation in the arteries and produces modest drop in blood pressure. Supplements of fish oil are as effective as fish. Fish high in ω-3 fatty acids are bass (striped), herring, mackerel, oysters, sable fish, salmon, trout and tuna.

Garlic: Garlic consumption for extended period of time is followed by a modest reduction in cholesterol, LDL cholesterol and triglyceride concentration in severe hypercholesterolemic patients. One half or one clove of garlic per day is sufficient to reduce cholesterol level. Sulphur compounds within garlic such as allicin, diallyl disulphide and allyl mercaptan are all effective in blocking cholesterol biosynthesis. Allyl sulphur compounds found in garlic can alter cellular thiols. More than one mechanism may occur because nicotinic acid, adenosine and other compounds found in garlic are also recognised to depress HMG-CoA reductase activity. Garlic extracts and several of its constituents possess significant antithrombolic properties. Allicin and ajoene are likely to contribute to antiplatelet effects. Garlic is also valuable for hypertensive patients. Deodourised garlic preparations are also effective.

Nuts: A growing body of scientific evidence suggests potential beneficial effects from the ingestion of tree nuts such as pecans, walnuts and almonds. They contain high amount of monounsaturated fat in the form of oleic acid. Magnesium and copper present in nuts may protect against CHD. Since they are rich in calories and fat, one should consume in small quantities.

Nuts can be included in and even used to design cholesterol lowering diets that have desirable fat contents and fatty acid profiles. Due to the distinguishing macronutrient and fatty acid characteristic of nuts it can be used to reduce the SFA content of the diet by replacing SFA energy with energy from unsaturated fatty acids while maintaining the amount of dietary fat. This is an effective strategy for achieving reductions in total and LDL cholesterol concentrations. Low fat and high carbohydrate diets lower HDL cholesterol and increase triglyceride levels.

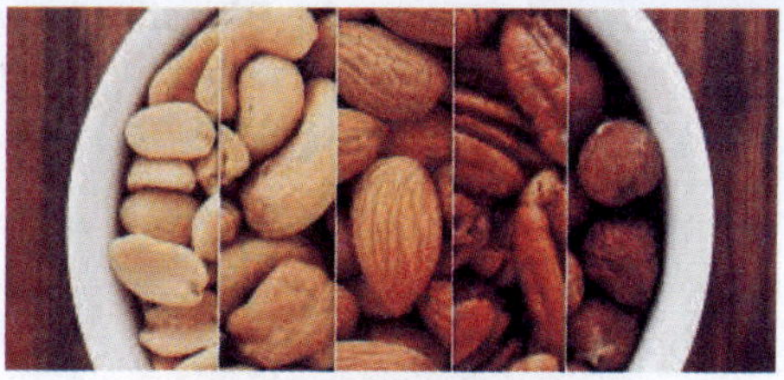

Fig. 16.8 Nuts are rich in unsaturated fatty acids. They are sensitive to light, oxygen and heat. If the fats in the nuts become rancid or denatured from roasting they lose their benefit and become inflammatory. It is best to choose raw nuts over roasted.

Almonds are the best source of the α-tocopherol form of vitamin E and among the best whole food sources. Seventy per cent of fat in almonds is MUFA. This helps to reduce cholesterol. Eating almonds consistently lowers total cholesterol and LDL cholesterol respectively by 4 to 5 per cent. The skin of almond contains fibre and antioxidants. The natural antioxidants are easily absorbable in human system. Walnuts contain high concentration of ω-3 fatty acid, which has cardio protective effect. Walnuts have highest antioxidant activity.

Nuts, in addition to being a rich source of fat and unsaturated fatty acids, they are a unique source of plant protein that is high in arginine, fibre and various micronutrients. Nuts are also sources of phytosterols and other phytochemical compounds with potential serum cholesterol modulating effects. The phytochemicals in nuts include ellagic acid, flavonoids, phenolic compounds, lutein a major antioxidant.

Resveratrol is a phytochemical present in red skin of ground nut, grapes and wine. It is cardio protective.

Consumption of 3/4 to 1 oz of unsalted nuts daily (almonds or walnuts are the nuts researched) is suggested to confer cardiovascular benefits.

CHAPTER 16

Table 16.10 Role of nutrients and food in the prevention of CHD.

Substance	*Chemical involved*	*Prevention of CHD*
Vitamin E	Vitamin E antioxidant	• prevents the oxidation of polyunsaturated fatty acids • Reduces LDL oxidation • Reduces platelet aggregation and thrombus formation
Carotenoids	β-carotene antioxidant	• It quenches singlet oxygen and reacts with free radicals generated during lipid peroxidation.
Vitamin C	Vitamin C antioxidant	• It reduces the damage caused by free radicals during oxidation process
Selenium	Selenium antioxidant	• Essential for the production of glutathione peroxidase
Soya protein	Isoflavones–genistein and daidzein	• Inhibit the proliferation and migration of arterial smooth muscles • Halts the transition of fatty streaks to advanced lesions • Genistein reduces thrombosis. • Daidzein is a potent antioxidant.

Beans	Soluble fibre, phyto-sterols, magnesium, potassium, copper and folate.	• Reduce hypertension • Soluble fibre lowers blood cholestrol.
Fruits and vegetables	Flavonoids Flavonols	• Flavonoids scavenge free radicals and have antioxidant effects Protect against heart disease
Garlic	Allicin, diallyl, disulphide and allyl mercaptan	• Reduces cholesterol: LDL cholesterol and triglycerides • They block cholesterol biosynthesis
Nuts	Monounsaturated fatty acids, magnesium, copper	• Protect against CHD by reducing LDL cholesterol without affecting HDL. • Walnuts contain ω 3 fatty acids, act as antioxidant. • Skin of almonds contain fibre and antioxidant.
	Resveratrol	• Groundnut skin contains this phytochemical which is an antioxidant.
Yogurt and milk	Hydroxy methyl glutarate	• Reduces cholesterol biosynthesis. • Casein and calcium have hypocholesterolemic effect.
Tea	Polyphenols	• Prevent the oxidation of LDL cholesterol
High fibre	Pectin	• Reduces serum cholesterol • Enhances excretion of faecal steroids.
	Guargum (duster beans)	• Hypocholesterolemic effect • Lower the blood pressure • Reduces serum fibrinogen
	β glucon (oats),	• Have hypocholesterolemic effect • Reduces triglycerides level
	Fenugreek seeds (Saponins, Diosgenin Tigogenin)	• Increases bile acid excretion, deplete cholesterol stores
	Curry leaves	• Anti lipidemic effect
	Turmeric	• Reduces cholesterol and triglyceride levels.

Yogurt and Milk: Synthesis of cholesterol is reduced when yogurt and milk are consumed. The postulated mechanism is that the hydroxy methyl glutarate content of yogurt may inhibit the activity of production of hydroxymethyl glutanyl coenzyme A reductase, the enzyme that catalyses the rate limiting step in cholesterol biosynthesis. Casein and calcium have a hypocholesterolemic effect.

Tea: Polyphenols present in tea prevent the oxidation of low density lipoprotein, LDL cholesterol, thereby inhibiting the formation of artherosclerotic plaques. Green tea contains more polyphenols than black tea.

Green tea may effect the cardiovascular function through mechanisms of action related to LDL-cholesterol oxidation. The oxidation of LDL-cholesterol associated with a risk of atherosclerosis and heart disease is inhibited by green tea due to EC (epicatechin) and EGCG (epigallocatechin-3-gallate) antioxidant activity.

Myocardial infarction was estimated to decrease by 11% with an increase in green tea consumption of three cups per day.

High fibre: High fibre in the diet reduces cholesterol. Pectin (apples, guavas) lowers the level of serum cholesterol and enhances the excretion of faecal steroids. It has no effect on serum triglycerides and HDL cholesterol. Guargum (extracted from seeds of cluster beans) has hypocholesterolemic effect. Legumes, vegetables and fruits can lower the level of serum cholesterol, but the effect is usually small when compared with the well known effect on HDL and serum triglycerides. Psyllium which contains soluble fibre reduces LDL cholesterol.

Studies show that blood pressure can be reduced by using fibre rich diets. Dietary fibre also reduces serum fibrinogen levels, which in turn lower the risk of blood clot formation and myocardial infarction.

Oats contain soluble and insoluble fibre. Oat products, which contain high amount of β–glucan content has hypocholesterolemic effect. One of the postulation was that cholesterol synthesis is inhibited by acetic, propionic and butyric acids, generated by the colon bacteria and concurrent clearance of LDL cholesterol.

Tips for Adding Fibre to the Diet

- Choose fresh fruits rather than canned fruits or juices. Raw foods contain more fibre than processed ones.
- Choose whole-grain cereals and pulses.
- Eat the skins on fruits such as apples, pears, and peaches.
- Eat the skins on vegetables such as potatoes, squash, and carrots.
- Have a salad everyday.
- Use brown rice rather than white rice.
- Choose raw vegetables and fresh fruits for snacks.
- Have a serving of dried beans or peas daily.
- Eat foods in their most naturally occurring state.

Dietary fibre intake is inversely associated with blood pressure, serum triglyceride level, and serum fibrinogen levels.

Fenugreek seeds are rich in fat, protein and fibre. It contains 20 per cent mucilaginous fibre and 50 per cent total fibre. The mechanism of hypercholesterolemic effect of fenugreek seeds is same as that of rice bran oil. Incorporation of fibre in the diet brings about reduction in serum cholesterol by preventing its absorption. Twenty seven per cent of total energy derived from fat, 59 per cent from carbohydrate and 55 g dietary fibre/2500 calories produce most favourable lipid profile.

Saponins of fenugreek are composed of diosgenin and tigogenin in ratio 9 : 1, which have lipid lowering activity. Fenugreek increases the excretion of bile acid and neutral sterols and depletes the cholesterol stores of the liver.

Among the three main food contributors to total fibre intake (vegetable, fruit and cereal) cereal fibre is most strongly associated with a reduced risk of myocardial infarction.

Dietary fibre remains as an acceptable and less expensive alternative to costly medical or surgical intervention to the consumers to manage the potential risk of CHD.

Spices: Curry leaves and turmeric have anti-lipidemic effects. They reduce cholesterol and triglyceride levels.

Table 16.11 Role of food in CHD at a glance

Protect from CHD	*Increase risk of CHD*
• α-linolenic acid (ω-3)—fish	High calorie diet
• Mono unsaturated fatty acids—walnuts and almonds	High amount of fat
• Anthocyanins—red wine	High amount of sugar
• Vitamin C—amla	High amount of dietary cholesterol
• Vitamin E—vegetable oils	High amount of saturated fatty acids
• β-carotene—carrots	High amount of trans fatty acids
• Flavonoids—soyaprotein	Hyperhomocysteinemia
• Dietary fibres—whole grains	High amount of coffee
• Allyl sulphur compounds—garlic	

Dietary Guidelines

- Patient should maintain the body weight slightly lower than the standard weight. Accordingly total calories should be restricted. Calorie intake and physical activity should be balanced to maintain a healthy body weight. For the obese, weight reduction is the key to prevent and treat CHD.
- The patient should know the energy requirement to maintain healthy body weight. He should know the energy content of foods he consumes.
- The patient should eat variety of foods which are low in fat, saturated fat and cholesterol. *Trans* fat should be avoided. Intake of bakery products should be limited. Soft margarines have less trans fatty acids than stick margarines.
- Vegetable oils rich in poly unsaturated fatty acids like safflower and sunflower oil should be included in the suggested combinations as given in Table 16.5. Solid fats should be avoided. Olive oil rich in monounsaturated fatty acid can be included.
- Small quantities of almonds and walnuts can be consumed to bring down the cholesterol levels. High amounts of nuts and oil seeds increase the calories and fat content in the diet.
- Coconut should be restricted in the diet as it contains high amount of saturated fatty acids and it is a concentrated source of energy.
- Egg yolk contains cholesterol. Hence eggs should be restricted to 2–3 eggs/week. Cholesterol containing foods should be limited in the diet.
- Animal foods like meat and pork which contain high amount of saturated fat should be avoided. Chicken can be taken instead of red meat. Shrimps and crabs have less amount of fat and can be included in the diet. All sea foods are rich in sodium. Hence hypertensive patients should avoid these foods.
- Two servings of fish per week in the diet is beneficial as they contain ω-3 fatty acids People who do not eat fish can take one gram fish oil capsule per day.
- Patient should take skim-milk or low fat milk.
- Olive oil which contains monounsaturated fatty acids and phenolic compounds has favourable effect on blood lipids. It increases HDL and decreases oxidative stress.

- Boiling, steaming, grilling and baking without fat are preferable methods for cooking.
- Five servings of fruit and vegetables should be included in the diet not only to meet the nutritional requirement but also to meet antioxidant and fibre requirements. Fruits and vegetables can be taken as snacks.
- Foods rich in antioxidants, containing carotenoids and vitamin-E, protect from cardiovascular diseases. Whole grain cereals, fruits and vegetables increase the antioxidant content of the diet.
- The diet should be rich in fibre by including foods like raw salads, fruits, green leafy vegetables, whole grains and sprouted grams.
- Constipation should be prevented by including plenty of water and fibre in the diet.
- The patient should avoid taking preserved foods, especially high energy syrups, sauces and gravies.
- Foods giving only empty calories like sweetened beverages, alcohol, sugar and sago are totally avoided.
- Concentrated foods like sweets, chocolates, cakes, pastries, ice creams and fried foods should be restricted or preferably avoided.
- Artificial sweeteners can be included occasionally in the diet.
- Intake of beverages and foods with added sugars to be minimised.
- Coffee and tea can be taken in moderation. Excess amount of caffeine increases the heart rate.

The Mediterranean diet is associated with significant reductions in the risk of recurrent CHD and mortality.

Table 16.12 Substitution food for an atherosclerotic patient

Instead of this	Reach for this
• Palak paneer	Greens dal
• Whole milk	Skim milk
• Fruit juice with milk	Whole raw fruit
• Potato chips	Papad (grilled)
• French toast	Vegetable sandwich
• Lassi	Buttermilk
• Cake	Bread
• Carrot halwa	Raw carrot salad
• Chole	Boiled or seasoned channa
• Rice	Wheat or ragi
• Ghee or vanaspathi, butter,	Oil
• Ice cream	Cut fruits
• Paratha, puri	Phulka
• Dosa	Idli, Idyappam
• Curries with lot of oil and coconut	Curries with little oil and no coconut

Foods to be included	*Foods to be restricted*	*Foods to be avoided*
Fruit juice like tomato, lime juice without sugar Green leafy vegetables, avocado, black grapes, green tea, flax seed, all boiled vegetables except roots and tubers.	Nuts, egg and egg yolk, learn meat chicken without skin, fish cooked without fat, olive oil, unrefined cereals.	All fats like butter, ghee, vanaspati, coconut oil, fried foods, chips, samosa, cakes, pudding, sweets, pickle, mutton, ham, baken, cheese, khoya, cream.

- Foods that have hypocholesterolemic effects like soyabean, fenugreek, garlic, onion, flax, oats and turmeric should be included in the diet.
- If the patient is suffering from hypertension, sodium should be restricted.
- Heavy meals should be avoided. Small and frequent meals are preferred.
- Taking outside meals should be avoided as they are mostly high in fat or calories and low in fibre and micro nutrients.
- Elevated C-reactive protein levels, a marker of systemic inflammation is a risk factor for cardiovascular disease and diabetes. Multivitamin supplementation (α-tocopherol, B_6 and vitamin C) reduce C-reactive protein levels.

These dietary guidelines are not presented as diet plan, per se, but as something that can be thought of as a life style prescription to promote cardiovascular health.

DRUGS

Drugs lower blood LDL and total cholesterol. Statins reduce the amount of lipid deposited in artery walls, reduce heart attacks, unstable angina and stroke. May reduce the fat content of the plaque.

Along with dietary and life modifications, exercise and proper medication can reduce the risk of atherosclerosis though one cannot substitute the other. Lipid lowering agents such as statins, HMG CoA reductase inhibitors, fibrates, niacinamide and fish oils are not substitute for diet and exercise. The patient should stop smoking and reduce the stress as part of the treatment of CHD.

HYPERTENSION

Worldwide about 12.8 per cent of total deaths is due to raised blood pressure. Raised blood pressure is a major risk factor for coronary heart disease and ischaemic as well as haemorrhagic stroke.

Every individual has blood pressure which is necessary to move blood through arteries and to provide oxygen to the tissues of the body. Hypertension is elevated blood pressure. WHO defines hypertension as a condition in which systolic pressure exceeds 140 mm Hg and diastolic pressure exceeds 90 mm Hg. With diastolic pressures of 100 or more therapy should be initiated with drugs as well as diet. High blood pressure is not a disease but only a symptom indicating that some underlying disease is progressing.

According to NNMB survey (2005–2006) the over all prevalence of hypertension $\geq$ 140 mm Hg (SBP) and $\geq$ 90 mm Hg (DBP) was about 25 per cent among men and 24 per cent in women. The prevalence tended to increase with age from 13.6 per cent among 20–30 years group to 54.4 per cent among $\geq$ 80 year age group. The prevalence of hypertension is high among the adults, who are overweight/obese (48 per cent) when compared to normal (26 per cent). There are more hypertensive people in urban areas than in villages.

When genetic predisposition causes hypertension it is called primary hypertension. High BP caused by illness or medication it is called secondary hypertension.

Causes

Cardiovascular diseases, renal diseases like glomerulonephritis, polycystic renal disease, pyelonephritis, tumors of the brain or adrenal glands, hyperthyroidism or diseases of ovaries and pituitary may cause hypertension.

Predisposing factors of hypertension are heredity, stress, obesity, smoking, high viscosity of blood due to too many red blood cells in the circulating blood, narrowing of the main blood vessels due to hormone secretions especially cortisone, aldosterone, adrenaline and noradrenaline.

Apart from ageing, obesity, alcohol consumption, salt sensitivity and a person's dietary choices may influence hypertension risks. Nearly half of all diabetics are hypertensive.

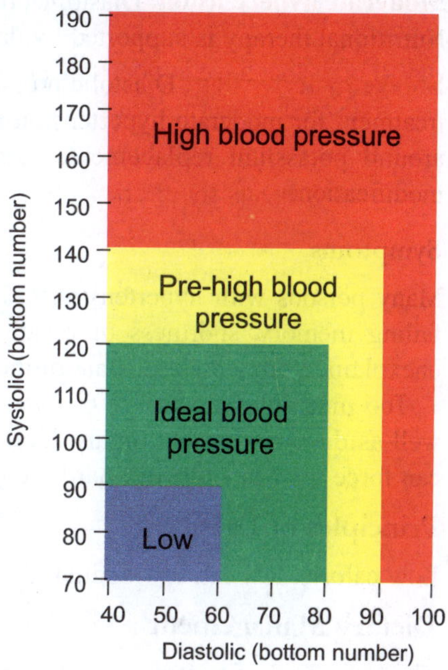

Fig. 16.9 The WHO standards of blood pressure.

Pathogenesis

Hypertension impairs the pumping function of the heart and if untreated damages the heart, brain and kidneys. Stroke occurs more often in patients with high blood pressure.

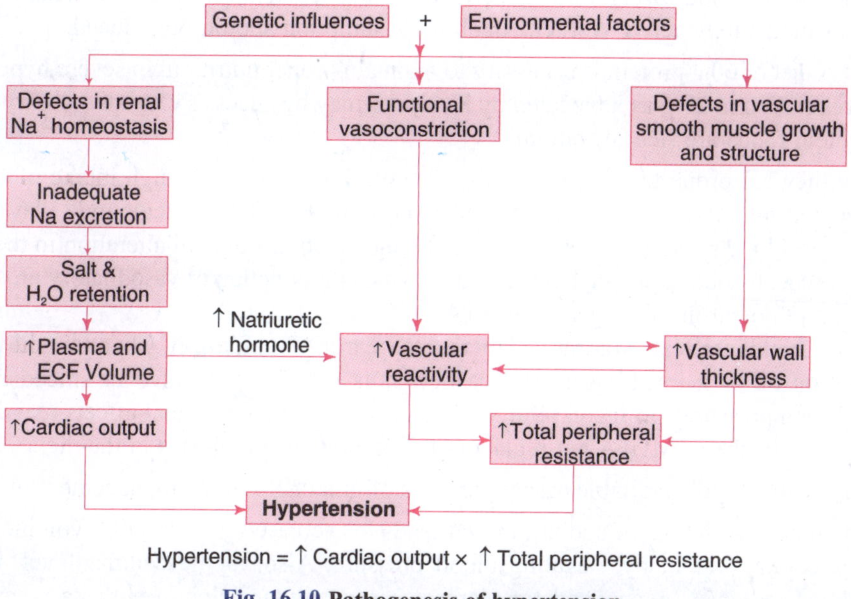

Fig. 16.10 Pathogenesis of hypertension

Types

When the cause of hypertension is unknown, it is called as essential hypertension.

Mild hypertension: Diastolic pressure is 90 to 104 mm Hg in this form. Treatment is based on weight loss, sodium restriction and behavioural techniques.

Moderate hypertension: Diastolic pressure is 105 to 119 mm Hg with moderate hypertension. Nutritional therapy is supported by drugs such as β blockers.

Severe hypertension: Diastolic pressure is 120 to 130 mm Hg and above. Apart from giving treatment for moderate hypertension peripheral vasodilators are given. Diet therapy revolves around potassium replacement, nutritional support for weight management and sodium modification.

Symptoms

Many persons with hypertension have no symptoms. Headache, dizziness, impaired vision, failing memory, shortness of breath, pain over the heart, gastrointestinal disturbance and unexplained tiredness are some of the symptoms.

Too much blood pressure can weaken blood vessel wall. It causes bulges and ruptures as well as damage delicate organs like heart, eyes or the kidney that receive the blood flow. It can force the heart to work harder contributing to eventual heart failure.

Principles of Diet

Low calorie, low fat, low sodium diet with normal protein intake is prescribed.

Dietary Management

The main goal of treatment for hypertension is lower blood pressure to less than 140/90.

Energy: An obese patient must be reduced to normal body weight with low calorie diet. About 20 kcal/kg of ideal body weight are prescribed for a sedentary worker and 25 kcal/kg of body weight for moderately active worker. Alcohol consumption should be reduced.

Protein: A diet of 60 g protein is necessary to maintain proper nutrition. In severe hypertension, protein restriction to 20 g as advocated by Kempner may be necessary as a temporary measure since protein foods are rich in sodium.

Fats: As they are prone to atherosclerosis it is advisable to avoid a high intake of animal or hydrogenated fat. About 20 g vegetable oil is permitted. ω-3 fatty acids may play a role in regulation of blood pressure. This effect may be mediated through an alteration in the balance between vacoconstrictive prostaglandins and increasing production of vasodilatory prostacyclin. DHA is more potent in this regard than EPA.

Studies conducted at Madras Diabetes Research Foundation Chennai showed that consumption of 30 g for 12 weeks of cashew nuts not fried or salted or spiced decreased systolic blood pressure and increase in HDL cholesterol. The beneficial effects may be due to the increased intake of MUFA but replacing the carbohydrate calories in the diet.

Carbohydrate: Easily available carbohydrate is of great help in the management of high B.P.

Sodium: Increased intake of sodium in diet leads to increased intravascular volume and thus increases cardiac output by elevating blood pressure. Also, at the cellular level, increased intracellular sodium is exchanged for increased intracellular calcium with its potent effects of augmented vascular tone and vascular hypertrophy with resulting persistent hypertension. Restricted sodium and a decrease in the sodium/potassium ratio in the diet is preferred. Moderate sodium restriction 2-3 g/day reduces diastolic pressure 6-10 mm of Hg and enhances the blood pressure lowering effect of diuretic therapy. American Heart Association prescribed 2 g for mild hypertension and 1 g sodium for moderate levels. Recent studies have shown that sodium restriction accompanied by weight reduction can effectively control mild or moderate arterial blood pressure. Pregnant women with toxemia need a moderate rather than low salt intake.

Salt should be reduced in the diet slowly and after sometimes one would find the normal diet tastes salty. Salt need not be added in idli batter and chapatti dough. People can avoid adding salt to plain or curd rice. Better milk can be flavoured with herbs and salt content can be reduced. Low sodium salt can be used.

Avoid these Foods High in Sodium

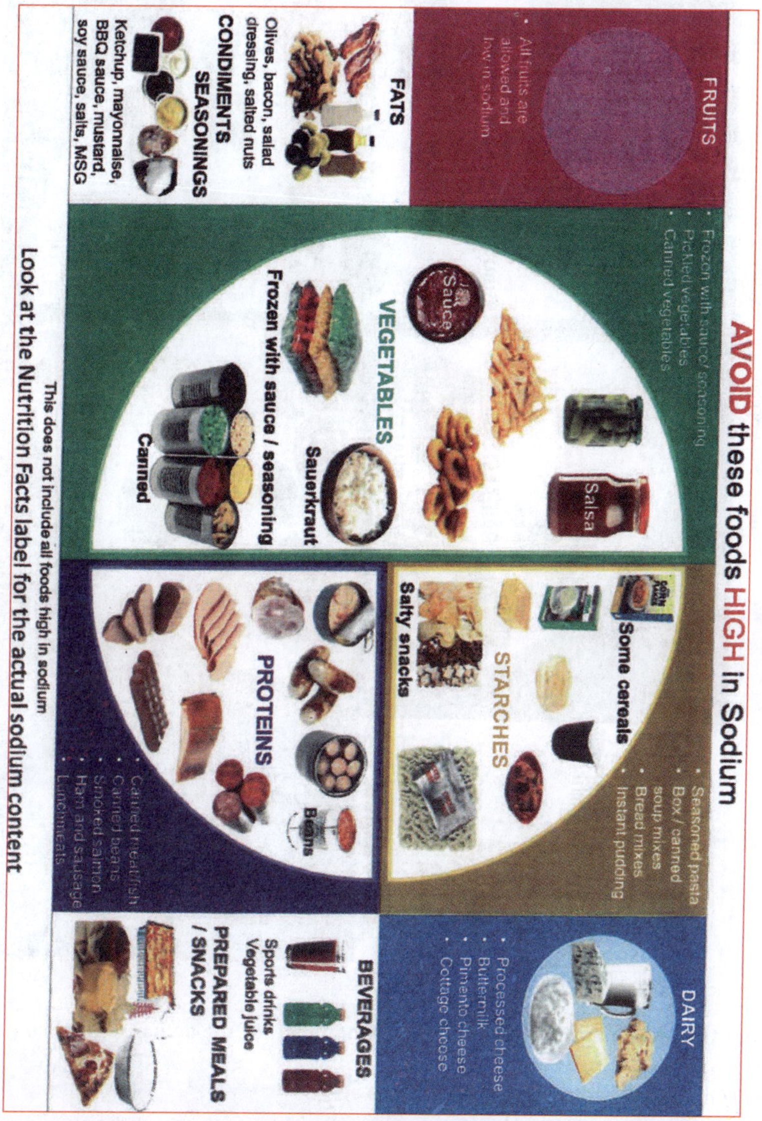
AVOID these foods HIGH in Sodium
FRUITS
All fruits are allowed and low in sodium
Frozen with sauce/ seasoning
Pickled vegetables
Canned vegetables
VEGETABLES
Sauce
Salsa
Frozen with sauce / seasoning
Sauerkraut
Canned
STARCHES
Some cereals
Salty snacks
Seasoned pasta
Box / canned soup mixes
Bread mixes
Instant pudding
DAIRY
Processed cheese
Buttermilk
Pimento cheese
Cottage cheese
BEVERAGES
Sports drinks
Vegetable juice
PREPARED MEALS / SNACKS
PROTEINS
Beans
Canned meat/fish
Canned beans
Smoked salmon
Ham and sausage
Lunchmeats
FATS
Olives, bacon, salad dressing, salted nuts
CONDIMENTS SEASONINGS
Ketchup, mayonnaise, BBQ sauce, mustard, soy sauce, salts, MSG
This does not include all foods high in sodium
Look at the Nutrition Facts label for the actual sodium content

Source: Baylor Scott and White Health 2018.

Fig. 16.11 Look at the Nutrition Facts label for the actual sodium content

CHAPTER 16

Choose these Foods Low in Sodium

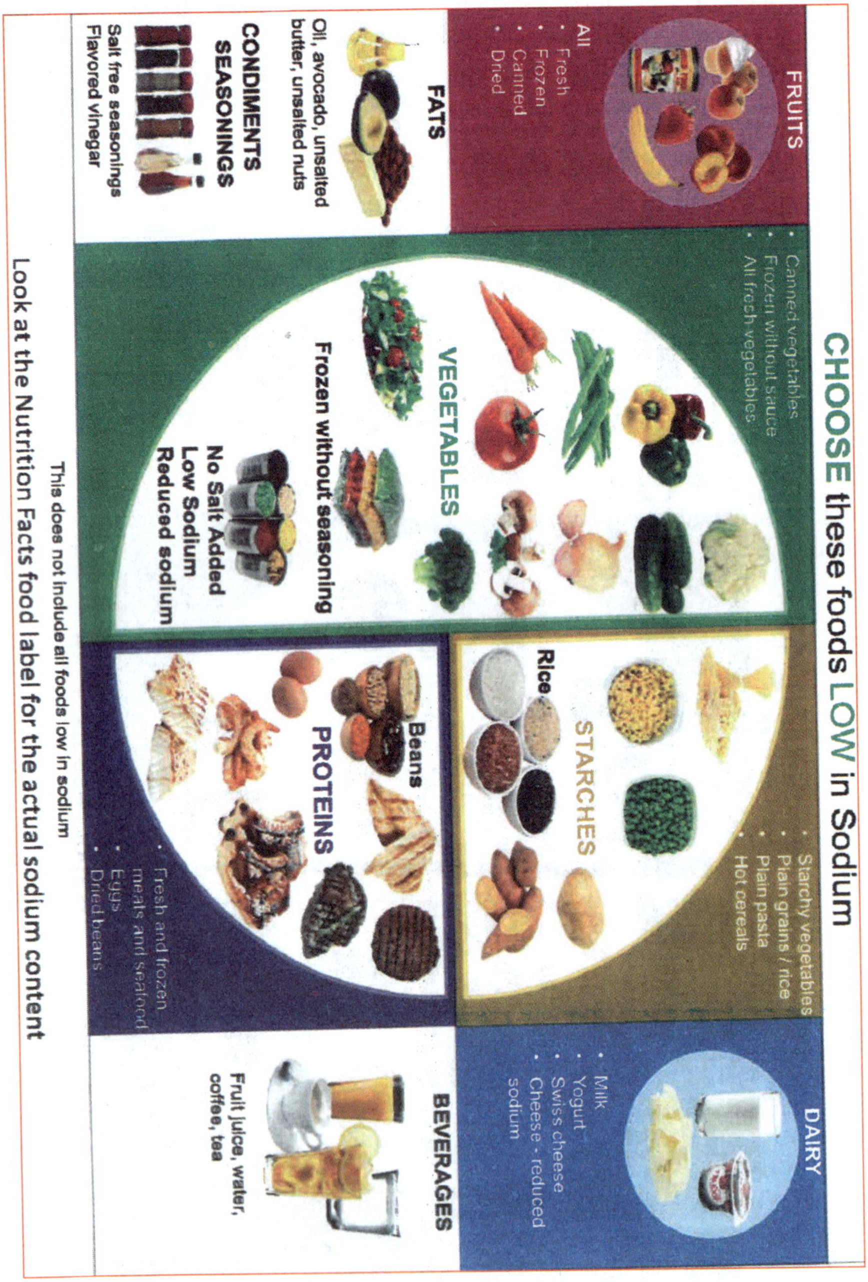
CHOOSE these foods LOW in Sodium
FRUITS
All
• Fresh
• Frozen
• Canned
• Dried
• Canned vegetables
• Frozen without sauce
• All fresh vegetables
VEGETABLES
Frozen without seasoning
No Salt Added
Low Sodium
Reduced sodium
• Starchy vegetables
• Plain grains / rice
• Plain pasta
• Hot cereals
STARCHES
Rice
DAIRY
• Milk
• Yogurt
• Swiss cheese
• Cheese - reduced sodium
FATS
Oil, avocado, unsalted butter, unsalted nuts
CONDIMENTS
SEASONINGS
Salt free seasonings
Flavored vinegar
PROTEINS
Beans
• Fresh and frozen meats and seafood
• Eggs
• Dried beans
BEVERAGES
Fruit juice, water, coffee, tea
This does not include all foods low in sodium
Look at the Nutrition Facts food label for the actual sodium content

Source: Baylor and White Health, 2018.

Fig. 16.12 Look at the Nutrition Facts food label for the actual sodium content

For salt restriction do not use the following

- Processed foods. Natural foods should be chosen instead of processed foods. Recipes should be prepared from scratch.

- Salt in cooking or at the table.
- Monosodium glutamate (Ajinomoto).
- Baking powder, sodium bicarbonate and sodium benzoate.
- Salt preserved foods—pickles, canned foods. Fresh chutneys have less salt compared to pickles.
- Hard water.
- Highly salted foods such as potato chips and papads.
- Ketchup and sauce – Soya sauce.
- Cheese, peanut butter, salted butter.
- Frozen peas.
- Shell fish and dry fish.
- Prepared mixes like ready made soups.
- Biscuits, cakes, breads, pastries.

Taste can be improved by adding herbs, garlic, mint, coriander leaves and spices and using basmati rice. Masalas should be made at home with restricted salt. Commercial masalas contain high amount of salt.

In India the nutrition label on the packet contains details about calories and transfat but not salt. Sometimes multigrain breads contain more salt to increase shelf life.

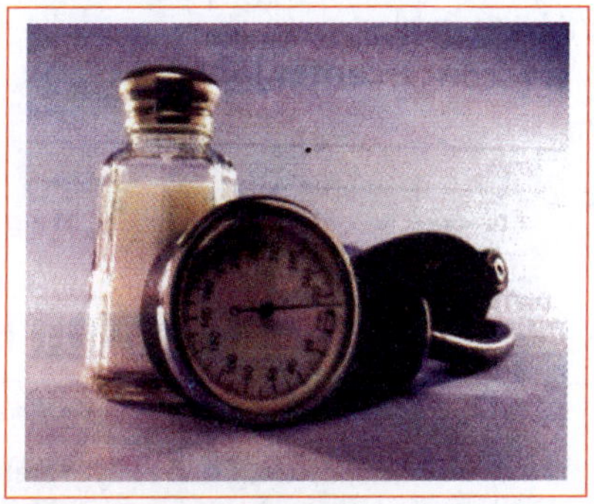

Fig. 16.13 Since taste of salt is an acquired habit, it should be possible to cut down the intake gradually without much difficulty and maintain it thereafter.

Potassium: Potassium's role in hypertension is actually the result of a complex interplay with sodium, calcium and magnesium found in all living cells and in blood. For example, low levels of potassium cause the body to retain sodium and water and this can elevate blood pressure. Research suggests that the risk of stroke, a common consequence of high blood pressure, relates inversely with the amount of potassium in the diet and the lowest risk is among the high potassium low sodium group. The requirement of potassium per day is 3500 mg. Fruits and vegetables should be taken liberally to meet potassium requirement.

Calcium: Some preliminary studies have shown that as the intake of calcium increased the incidence of hypertension declined. Calcium is involved in the control of strength with which blood is pumped by the heart and with the amount of resistances in the flow of blood in the veins and capillaries both of which contribute to blood pressure.

Magnesium: Most literature suggests that a major role for magnesium is in the regulation of blood pressure. Although data are not entirely consistent, it does appear than an inverse relationship between magnesium intake and blood pressure is strongest for magnesium from food rather than obtained via supplements.

CoQ10: This vitamin like substance is found throughout the human body. Although body synthesises natural stores may drop as one ages. CoQ10 may lower blood pressure. It can increase the effect of medications used to treat high blood pressure.

DASH, Dietary Approaches to Stop Hypertension, suggested diet is given in Table 16.13.

Table 16.13 Diet suggested by DASH

Food Group	*DASH (servings)*
Grains	7–8
Vegetables	4–5
Fruits	4–5
Milk (low fat)	2–3
Meat (lean)	2 or less

According to DASH the following diet may bring about a healthy reduction in blood pressure

- High amount of fruits and vegetables
- Inclusion of fish
- Inclusion of low fat milk
- Reducing the fat intake
- Reducing sodium.

Table 16.14 Life style modifications to manage hypertension

Modification	*Recommendation*
• Weight reduction	Maintain normal body weight (BMI - 18.5-24.9)
• Adopt Dietary Approach to stop hypertension, DASH, eating plan	Consume a diet rich in fruits, vegetables and low-fat dairy products with a reduced content of saturated and total fat
• Dietary sodium reduction	Reduce dietary sodium intake to no more than 6 g sodium chloride
• Physical activity	Engage in regular aerobic physical activity such as brisk walking (at least 30 minutes per day, most days)
• Moderate alcohol consumption	Limit to not more than 2 drinks per day, as it has a positive effect on platelet function and on the lipid profile.

Studies have shown that high intake of fruits and vegetables results in low mortality among those with stroke. Low levels of dietary flavonoids are associated with a higher risk of stroke. Fibre and folic acid have also been associated with protection against stroke. Green leafy and cruciferous vegetables and citrus fruits in particular are found to be protective.

Complications

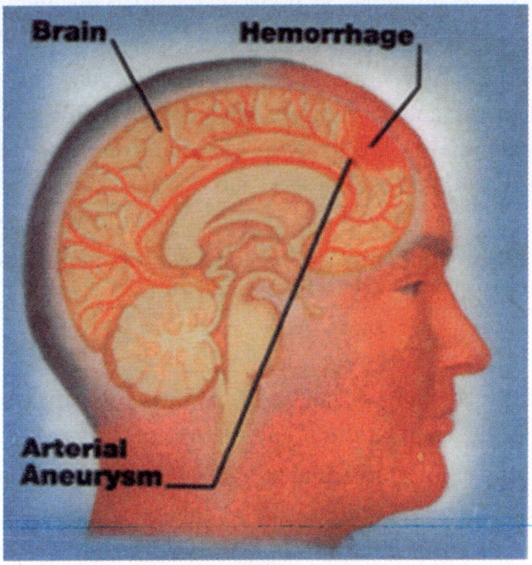

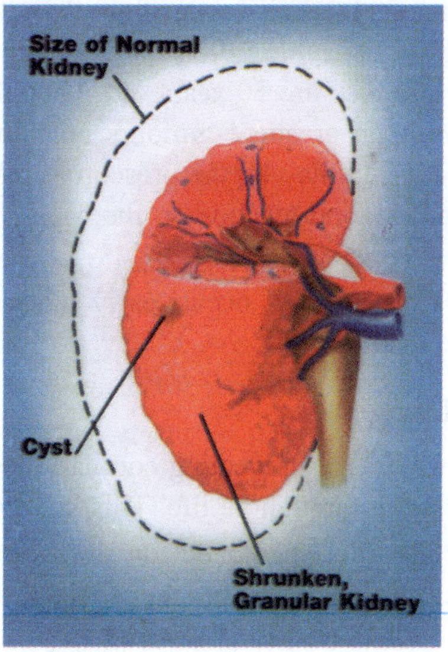

Haemorrhagic stroke **Nephrosclerosis**

Fig. 16.14 Haemorrhagic stroke and nephrosclerosis are complications of hypertension

Source: Applegate, W. (ed.), 1995, Patient Education Center, Target Media, Inc, Cincinnati, Ohio.

HYPERCHOLESTEROLEMIA

Plasma cholesterol values vary in an apparently healthy population. There is a slow rise with age starting at 20 years but ceasing at about 60 years, when it may be followed by a slight fall. The rise is less steep in women until the menopause when it may increase abruptly. After 60 years there is little or no difference between the sexes.

Mortality from CHD rises with increasing levels of plasma cholesterol. Above 210 mg/dl, the risk of death from CHD rises sharply. Below the threshold (210 mg/dl) deaths may occur but the risk is relatively low and not closely related to plasma cholesterol.

Usually only total plasma cholesterol is measured, but it is often useful to determine its distribution in the different lipoprotein fractions.

Cholesterol Intake

Dietary cholesterol has little effect on plasma cholesterol over the range of intake usual in prosperous societies (300-500 mg daily) since increasing intake inhibits endogenous production. Dietary cholesterol is much less important than dietary fat in determining plasma cholesterol.

Familial Hypercholesterolemia

This is a disorder transmitted as an autosomal polymorphic dominant gene. It consist of an increase in low density lipoproteins (LDL), the main carrier of cholesterol in the blood, and is due to genetic failure of LDL receptors. Plasma cholesterol may be over 30 mMol/litre in homozygous adult (Normal 10-20 mMol/litre.). The biochemical abnormality can be detected at birth.

CHAPTER 16

Clinical Features

There is increased risk of coronary heart disease. A heart attack due to myocardial infarction before the age of 30 is not uncommon and 50 per cent of patients present evidence of CHD before they are 50 years old. Thus the disorder greatly reduces life expectancy. Xanthomata, swellings or small tumours containing cholesterol and sometimes triglyceride, commonly occur and may be the presenting feature. Common sites are tendons, especially the Achilles tendons, and tendons on the back of the hands and skin and around the eye where they are known as xanthelasma.

Corneal arcus occurs early and when seen in someone under 40 years it is probably due to the disorder.

Management

This aims at preventing coronary heart disease by keeping plasma LDL cholesterol as low as possible throughout life. This involves lifelong dietary restriction and the use of drugs.

The diet should be low in saturated fats and cholesterol but polyunsaturated fats from vegetable oils and in other foods are permitted.

Diet is clearly a cause of hyperlipidaemia but is not the only one. It is sufficient if they follow dietary guidelines recommended for coronary artery disease.

HEART FAILURE

Heart failure is the cumulative result of all the conditions that may cause insult to the heart muscle during one's lifetime.

Heart failure represents the end result of any insult to the ventricle either acute as in myocardial infarction or chronic as in hypertension.

Diet in Heart Failure

In heart failure, the body is not able to excrete extra sodium causing swelling, fluid retention and problems related to breathing. Extra fluid increases the work of the heart and the kidneys. Thus, greatly affecting those with heart failure. Eating less sodium helps to control these problems. The daily sodium limit should be 1500-2000 mg, equivalent to two thirds to one teaspoon of salt per day. To control sodium consumption, the patients can be given the equivalent amounts of sodium in packets that can be incorporated in their diet throughout the day.

Restricting fluid intake can help to limit the build up of fluid in the body. Fluid diet is considered to be any food or beverage that is liquid at room temperature. This includes water, ice chips, beverages, ice cream and sherbets. Daily fluid limit should be 6 to 8 cups.

1 cup = 8 oz = 240 ml

To maintain sodium and water intake the patient should be weighed every morning. Sudden weight gain is a sign that fluid is building up in the body. If the gain in weight is more than 5 pounds in a week or 3 pounds in 1-2 days doctor's advice should be taken.

If the mouth is dry, hard candies, mints and gums can be used. If the patient is diabetic sugar free candies should be used. Ice chips flavoured with lemon juice can be given.

1 cup ice = ½ cup fluid.

PHYSICAL ACTIVITY AND HEART DISEASE

Physical activity is beneficial to CHD patients as it protects against the progression of CVD. Aerobic exercise increases heart size and strength. The heart's stroke volume is also increased. The heart then needs to pump fewer times per minutes to circulate the same amount of blood. This represents a long-term reduction in the heart's workload. Exercise raises blood levels of high-density lipoproteins (HDL) creating a more favourable ratio of HDL to low-density lipoproteins. This effect is more marked in men, although exercise will have the same effect in women if it is of high intensity. Exercise enhances the circulatory system by increasing the oxygen carrying capacity of the blood and increases the blood volume. Regular physical exercise increases lipoprotein lipase concentration which in turn reduces CHD risk.

Physical activity maintains desirable body composition. It improves survival rate. Specific physiological benefits derived from exercise include

- ↓ blood pressure
- ↑ HDL cholesterol levels
- ↓ triglyceride levels
- ↑ weight reduction
- ↑ glucose tolerance
- ↓ platelet aggregation
- ↑ endothelial function
- ↓ depression and anxiety

An optimal exercise programme has four phases:

Warm-up	–	5 to 10 mn	
Aerobic	–	20–60 mn	Brisk walking, cycling, swimming and slow jogging
Resistive	–	10–15 mn	
Cool down	–	5–10 mn	

The coexistence of type II diabetes and hypertension is especially damaging to cardiovascular health. Apart from controlling blood sugar and blood pressure, exercise improves endothelial vasodilator function and left ventricular diastolic function. Exercise also reduces total and abdominal fat. Regular exercise fights heart disease regardless of body weight.

ALCOHOL

Numerous epidemiological studies indicate that drinking small to moderate amounts of alcohol can reduce the risk of CVD. It decreases LDL cholesterol oxidation and reduces blood fibrinogen and other antithrombotic actions. Red wine consumption has been associated with a lower risk of CVD compared with other types alcohol. Wine contains phytochemicals, resveratrol, procyamidius and quercetin which are cardio protective. Wine is antiinflammatory, positive effect on endothelial layer and decrease LDL oxidation.

Alcohol increases blood pressure and heavy drinking weakens the heart muscle-cardiomyopathy. Alcohol is a source of empty calories. It increases the level of blood triglycerides. It does not increase the protective fraction HDL. The non-alcoholic components in wine prevent LDL oxidation.

STRESS MANAGEMENT

Stress may be acute, chronic or intermittent. Stress can be physical, social or emotional. Stress causes the heart to be faster, the blood pressure to go up, the muscles to become tense and the arteries to go into spasms.

Occupational and family stress increase blood pressure. Stress often forces one to adopt unhealthy habits like drinking, smoking and over eating.

One should master to come out of stress and try to accept the reality. Stress management varies from individual to individual. Yoga in which mind and body is controlled plays a prominent part in maintaining health. The function and state of the mind has it repercussions upon physical well being. Several chronic diseases including heart and blood vessel diseases where many factors are known to interact can be modified by yogic practice.

Stress can also be managed by stretching, relaxation, breathing exercises and meditation. One should have positive mental attitude.

Social support is built by spending more time with friends and family and bring part of group having similar interests and problems.

FAT SUBSTITUTES

Fat substitutes have been developed to impart the functional and sensory qualities of fat and decrease the quantity of fat in foods to assist in decreasing fat intake. Usually fat substitute is not fat. They are carbohydrate, proteins or combinations of guar, carrageena and xanthin which are used to substitute cream toppings and certain candies. Proteins such as gelatin or whey have often been used to provide stability and improve mouthfeel. Modified starches are used in low fat spread as thickener and temperature stability. A butter substitute, developed by National Dairy Research Institute, Karnal has butter flavour made from low fat soya. The AHA (American Heart Association) discourages the use of fat substitutes for children as they do not encourage healthful eating patterns. Within the context of a healthy diet that meets contemporary dietary recommendations, fat substitutes, used appropriately may provide some flexibility with diet planning.

PREVENTION

The Mediterranean diet is now recommended to reduce the incidence of coronary artery disease. It is appetising, and is not restrictive. The mediterranean dietary pattern is low in saturated fats and trans fats. It is high in monounsaturated and polyunsaturated fats. It has a large proportion of complex carbohydrates.

There is rising trend in the consumption of processed food. Urgent steps are to be taken to limit salt levels in processed food. Public need to be aware on the need to take less salt.

Increasing evidence supports the benefits of maintaining normal plasma lipoprotein levels, body weight and blood pressure for reducing the risk of cardiovascular disease. Adoption of these recommendations, together with other healthy practices such as regular physical exercise and abstinence from smoking can reduce the risk of CVD in the general population.

HDL-cholesterol can be increased by lifestyle modification like smoking cessation, exercise, mild to moderate alcohol consumption, weight loss and by increasing consumption of fish oils.

Drinking at least three cups of green or black tea per day can significantly reduce the risk of stroke.Consumption of olive oil reduces chances of getting stroke.

Nutraceuticals like α glucan, γ-tocopherol, tocotrienol, MUFA, quercetin, ω-3 PUFAs, resveratrol, tannins, β-sitosterol, saponins, guar and pectin have positive influence on blood lipid profile. Indigenously prepared curd with combination of *lactobacillus bulgaricus* and *streptococcus thermophilus* showed significant changes in the lipid profile parameters up on supplementation of probiotics in obese subjects.

Trans fats - 2018

WHO released REPLACE a step-by-step guide for the elimination of industrially produced trans fatty acids from the global food supply.

Review, Promote, Legislate, Assess, Create and Enforce – 'Replace' the first global initiate to eliminate a risk factor for cardiovascular disease.

WHO recommends to consume less than 1 per cent of the energy from transfat that is 2.2 g for 2000 kcal diet.

Government should ensure that transfat is out of food supply. Through FSSAI, government should make sure that transfat content should be reduced to 5 per cent in all oils. The global best practice is a maximum of 2 per cent in all oils, fats and in all foods.

Heart attacks are more common among smokers. The risk increases with the number of cigarettes a patient smokes and how long he has been smoking. The risk decreases if one stops smoking. After an attack if the patient stops smoking, the chances of second attack are reduced.

The vast body of scientific evidence shows that diet plays a primary role in the prevention of CVD. Various protocols for nutrition intervention support increased itnake of fruits and vegetables (9-11 servings per day) and dietary fiber (25 g/d) as well as regular consumption of ω-3 fatty acids from cold-water fish at least 2 times per week, plant sterol/stanols (2 g/d) and nuts (30g/day). Substituting soy protein for animal protein to reduce saturated fat in the diet may be cardioprotective. In addition, moderate alcohol intake of 1-2 drinks per day with meals is recommended (for individuals who choose to consume alcoholic beverages). Overall lifestyle behaviours, such as energy balance, weight status, BMI and waist circumference are important risk factors that deserve consideration in the scope of cardiovascular health and wellness.

May 17th is World Hypertension Day

September 30th is World Heart Day

October 29th is World Stroke Day

SUGGESTED READINGS

- Berdanier D. Carolyn, Trans-fatty acids: Good or Bad? Nutrition Today 2011; **46**.
- Evaluation of herbal and nutraceutical product for antioxidant and antiinflammatory activity, Annual report 2010–2011, NIN, Hyderabad.
- Retelny Victoria Shanta et al., Nutrition protocols for the prevention of cardiovascular disease Nutrition in Clinical Practice, 2008; **23**.
- American Heart Association. www.americanheart.org.
- DASH Research Home Page. www.dash.iwh.harvard.edu.

QUESTIONS

1. Describe the risk factors of heart attack.
2. Describe the role of fat in the cause of atherosclerosis.
3. Explain the objectives and principles of planning a diet for atherosclerotic patient.
4. Write a note on role of unsaturated fatty acids in the diet.
5. Explain why sodium is restricted in hypertension.
6. What is hypercholesterolemia? Discuss the causes and treatment.
7. Plan a day's diet for a 52-year-old-executive who had a heart attack three months ago.
8. Give three foods to be included and three foods to be avoided for an atherosclerotic patient stating the reasons.
9. List five foods low in cholesterol and five foods high in cholesterol.
10. Briefly outline the dietary advice for a patient suffering from Ischaemic heart disease.
11. What dietary advice should be followed or given in modifying the diet of a patient with hypertension?
12. Explain the role of fruits and vegetables in the prevention of heart diseases.
13. Describe the role of fat in the treatment of atherosclerosis.
14. What is DASH?
15. What are the clinical effects of CVD?
16. Explain the role of functional foods in the prevention of atherosclerosis.

TOPICS FOR ACTIVITY

- Discuss the factors involved in the development of coronary heart disease as shown in Fig. 16.1.
- Plan and prepare a diet for an atherosclerosis patient who is retired from services. List the foods to be included and avoided.
- Plan and prepare a diet for an obese hypertensive patient whose salt intake should not be more than three grams.

17

Diet in Gastrointestinal Diseases

Digestive disorders are among the most common problems in health care. Approximately 30 to 40 per cent of adults claim to have frequent indigestion. Dietary habits and specific food types can play a significant role in the onset, treatment and prevention of many GI disorders. In many cases, diet can also play a role in improving patient's sense of well-being.

UPPER GASTROINTESTINAL DISEASES

Figure 17.1 shows the location of upper gastrointestinal diseases.

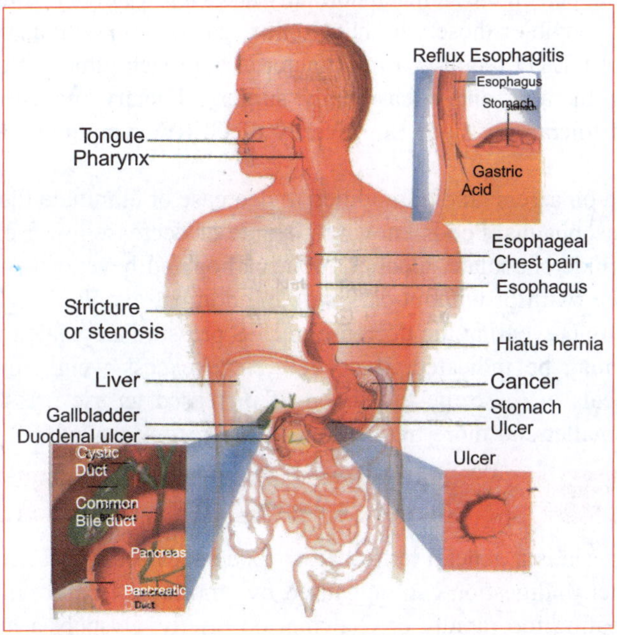

Fig. 17.1 Location of upper gastrointestinal diseases

Source: Patient Education Center, 1995, On Target media Inc. Cincinnati, Ohio, USA.

GASTRO ESOPHAGEAL REFLUX DISEASE (GERD)

Reflux is a condition where the consumed food regurgitates. It is more common among people in the age group 20–40.

Causes: Poor diet with its huge increase in the consumption of sugar, fat, soft drinks and processed foods may cause GERD. Late eating accompanied by over indulging meal is the cause of acid reflux in many. Chaotic eating patterns, stress and long hours of starvation interspersed with consumption of oily foods leads to GERD. Smoking and excess alcohol intake exaggerate the problem.

Chronic reflux permits prolonged contact of gastric contents with the lower esophagus leading to the symptoms of GERD. In general the following underlying conditions are associated with GERD.

- Irritation of the esophageal mucosa by gasteric acid, pepsin, bile and pancreatic secretions.
- Delayed gastric emptying
- Abnormal esophageal acid clearance rate
- Decreased lower esophageal sphincter pressure in severe GERD.

Symptoms: The symptoms include heartburn or cramping pain in the chest and regurgitation of food consumed. Acid reflux affects the throat, sinuses and lungs without digestive symptoms like heart burn. Reflux can lead to esophageal cancer.

Treatment: After eating in the evening it is important to stay upright because gravity helps keep food in the stomach. Reflux is the result of acid spilling out of the stomach; lying down with a full stomach makes reflux much more likely.

In a healthy young person the stomach normally takes a few hours to empty after a moderate size meal. In older people or those who have reflux, gastric emptying is often delayed.

The treatment of GERD requires a multifactorial approach aimed at dietary and lifestyle modification, drug therapy, and occasionally surgery. Dietary management is influenced by individual food tolerances, since the severity of GERD symptoms varies greatly among individuals.

The diet is based on a general diet modified to decrease or eliminate foods that cause reflux and/or irritate the esophagus. Foods known to irritate or decrease lower esophageal sphincter (LES) pressure include chocolate, alcohol, mint, carbonated beverages, citrus juices, tomato products, and coffee (with or without caffeine). In addition, avoiding high-fat foods may aid in reducing reflux by preventing the decrease in LES pressure associated with high-fat foods. Weight reduction may be indicated, if needed, since excess weight increases intragastric pressure. Large meals increase the likelihood of increased gastric pressure and subsequent reflux; therefore, smaller and more frequent meals are recommended.

INDIGESTION

Indigestion or dyspesia is a general term that is frequently used to describe discomfort in the upper digestive tract. Indigestion can be caused by emotional tension, malnutrition, disease, eating too much, eating too rapidly or chewing too briefly. Dyspepsia may be secondary to other systemic disorders such as atherosclerosis, hypertension, liver disease or renal disease.

Symptoms of dyspepsia may include vague abdominal pain, bloating, nausea, regurgitation and belching. Prolonged dyspepsia may be related to gastro-eosophageal reflux, gastritis, peptic ulcer disease, lactose intolerance delayed gastric emptying, gall bladder disease or cancer. For persistent indigestion underlying disease has to be treated.

Dietary indulgences like excessive volumes of food or high intake of fat, sugar, caffeine, spices or alcohol are commonly implicated in dyspepsia. The patients are treated by avoiding or restricting these foods.

Management of uncomplicated dyspepsia is by eating slowly, chewing thoroughly, eating at regular times and in a relaxed atmosphere. Patient should eat small and frequent meals and avoiding gas forming foods or foods known to cause indigestion.

PEPTIC ULCER

The term peptic ulcer is used to describe any localised erosion of the mucosal lining of those portions of the alimentary tract that come in contact with gastric juice. This disintegration of tissues can also result in necrosis. The majority of ulcers are found in the duodenum, although they also occur in the oesophagus, stomach or jejunum.

The defence mechanism of gastric and duodenal mucosa is incredibly efficient. The normal mechanical, thermal or chemical insults from food are well within its power to deal with.

Mechanism of Ulcer Formation

The three vital mechanisms are the mucous layer, prostaglandins and probably the urogastrone /epidermal healing factor (URO/ EHF). These mechanisms can protect the stomach against hydrochloric acid up to twice the maximum concentration which the stomach is capable of secreting.

The mucous layer, viscous gel ideally suited for its function of protection from chemical and physical hazards of water proofing and lubrication.

The second line of defence are prostaglandins. They are released locally in the mucosa and submucosa in response to any irritant stimulus. They instantly accelerate cell replacement, opening up the microcirculation to bring cell nutrients and to remove toxic metabolites. It is a mechanism which enables the gastric mucosa to withstand even absolute alcohol and boiling water and to counter a wide variety of chemical hazards even without any help from simultaneous reduction of gastric acid secretion. Their efficiency probably also depends on an adequate dietary supply of essential fatty acids for their formation.

Urogastrone (third line of defence) plays an important role by inhibiting gastric acid secretion on the one hand and by stimulation of cell proliferation and regeneration on the other hand for healing ulcer.

Usually there is a balance between acid pepsin secretion and mucosal resistance. For reasons that we still do not understand well, sometimes this balance is disturbed. As a result of excess acid production or weakening in the integrity of the stomach membrane or both, the mucosal lining is broken and the underlying layers of the stomach are exposed to the effect of the concentrated acid resulting in peptic ulcer.

The factors that influence mucosal ability to withstand destructive action are: (1) the integrity of mucosal cells; (2) the ability of epithelial cells to regenerate themselves; (3) the mucosal barrier and (4) the blood supply. Various topical irritants impair this tissue, including aspirin, alcohol, certain drugs, caffeine or bile acids that may come in contact with the mucosa.

Duodenal Ulcer

In this condition hyper secretion of acid is found although tissue resistance is normal. Acid hypersecretion is attributed to an increased number of parietal cells and impaired rapid gastric emptying with loss of buffering effect.

Gastric Ulcer

Factors that contribute to weakened mucosal resistance in patients with gastric ulcer revolve around poor nutrition, diminished mucosal blood flow and a defect in the inhibition of gastric acid and pepsin secretion.

In gastric ulcer, both the back diffusion of hydrogen ions into the mucosa and reflux of bile are believed to be involved. An abnormality in the mucosa permits penetration of hydrogen ions. Drugs such as aspirin and indomethacin (used in rheumatoid arthritis) can alter the gastric mucosal barrier. Reflux of bile acids from the duodenum due to an incompetent pyloric sphincter leads to chronic gastritis and subsequent ulceration. Gastric ulcers are more prone to develop into malignant disease.

In the development of gastric ulcers although the presence of acid is essential, the degree of tissue sensitivity seems to be the paramount factor. In a patient with duodenal ulcer, excess production of acid and pepsin is the primary factor.

Aetiology

Bacterial infection: *Helicobacter Pylori* is the chief cause of ulcer. It is spiral shaped, with gram negative unipolar flagellum. It colonises the stomach in about 50 per cent of all humans.

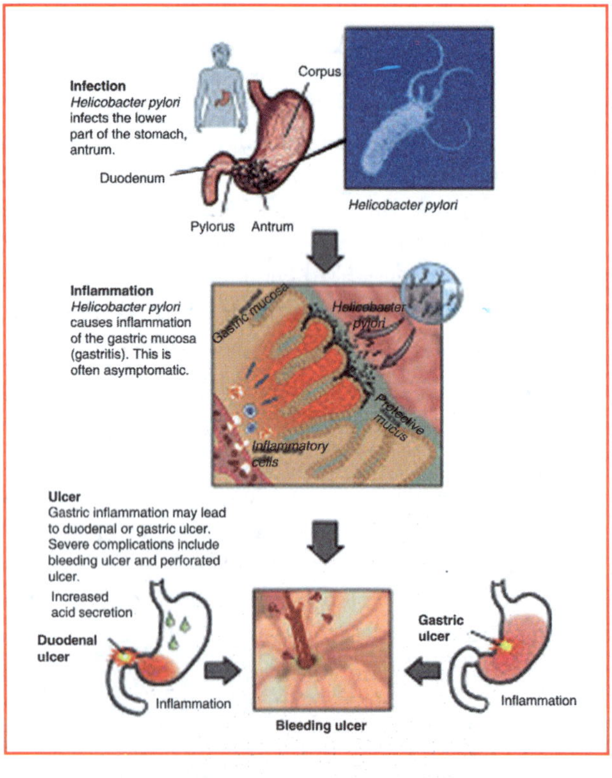

Fig. 17.2 **The infection potentiates the macrophage oxidative burst leading to tissue destruction.**

In developing countries virtually everyone may be infected. Infection is typically contracted in early childhood and remain for the rest of life. Only in one per cent of people does the infection leads to stomach cancer. In Africa infection with the bacterium is wide spread but stomach cancer levels are low. The genes that protect the African is not known. It is associated with antral gastritis and duodenitis in the presence of gastric metaplasia. If *helicobacter pylori* is cleared by antibiotic treatment especially with colloidal bismuth and ammoxycillin, the associated gastritis improves ulcer healing and recurrent rates may be lower.

Symptoms and Clinical Findings

- Epigastric pain and heart burn, due to reflux of acid into oesophagus occurring as deep hunger contraction 1 to 3 hours after meals is often the chief complaint. The pain may be described as dull, piercing, burning or gnawing and is usually relieved by taking food or alkalies.
- Discomfort and flatulence in upper part of abdomen. The basis for pain may be the action of unneutralised hydrochloric acid on exposed nerve fibres at the site of ulcer.
- Pain is also associated with hypermotility of the stomach or gastric distension following ingestion of large amounts of food or liquids.
- Low plasma protein levels are often present and delay rapid and complete healing of the ulcer.
- Weight loss and iron deficiency anaemia are common.
- The intake of iron, ascorbic acid, and B complex vitamins, particularly thiamine may be less than RDA because of self imposed limitation of leafy green vegetables and other good source of these nutrients.
- In some instances, haemorrhage is the first indication of an ulcer and requires surgical intervention. Other complications such as obstruction, perforation and carcinoma of the gastric ulcer are treated surgically.
- Bleeding ulcers can result in vomiting known as haematemesis (dark brown in colour).
- There are spasms of pyloric canal and this may give rise to a feeling of sickness, distension, and prevent taking food.

Diagnosis

Radiographic examination with Barium Meal: The technique, though simple, carries a fairly substantial risk of missing the problem.

Endoscopy: A flexible tube made of fibre optic bundles is introduced into the stomach and the endoscopist inspects the food pipe and stomach and detect any breaks in the lining membrane. It takes 15–20 minutes. If there is cancer, it can also be detected by endoscope.

Biopsy: Biopsy of lining tissue is done.

Acid secretion of the stomach: In this the acid output after stimulation by pentagastrin is measured. It is useful for further investigation if surgery is contemplated. Acid output is higher than normal in duodenal ulcer and low or absent in patients with carcinoma of the stomach.

Treatment

Therapeutic goal:

- To relieve the symptoms

- To allow healing of ulcer
- To prevent complications like surgery.

Drugs

Antibiotics against *helicobacter pylori* should be given.

It is important to neutralise the excess acid produced.

- Antacids were the earliest and most logical method of providing relief. They continue to be effective but have fallen out of routine use because they are cumbersome to prescribe; large quantities have to be taken several times a day.
- A group of chemicals are available that block certain vital steps in acid production by the stomach-H2 blockers. They are effective, devoid of major side effects and are given once or at the most twice daily.
- A third group of drugs, instead of attempting to lower or neutralise acid, they bolster the resistance of the lining of the stomach and prevent breakdown.

Dietary Management

It was customary to suggest bland diet for ulcer patients. Bland diet is a diet which is mechanically, chemically and thermally non-irritating.

Mechanically irritating foods include those with indigestible carbohydrate, such as whole grains and most raw fruits and vegetables. Foods believed to be chemically irritating because of their stimulatory effect on gastric secretion include meat extractives, caffeine, alcohol, and some spicy foods. The capsaicin present in chillies causes shedding of surface stomach cells and may cause peptic distress. Foods believed to be thermally irritating are those ordinarily served at extremes of temperatures, such as very hot or iced liquids may cause pain. Bland diet prevents irritation to the mucosa, avoids increase in acidity and aids in control of pain.

The so-called bland diets used in the past for treatment of peptic ulcer have proved to be unwarranted and ineffective. A more liberal individual approach prevails today in modern clinical practice.

Sound total nutrition: There must be optimal overall nutritional intake to support recovery and maintain healthy tissue, based on individual needs and food tolerances.

Protein foods: Milk and protein foods do have some buffering effect but they also evoke gastric secretions more than carbohydrates and fats. Milk should be included as a source of nutrient factors for healing purposes. Protein provides the necessary amino acids for synthesis of tissue protein which helps in healing ulcer.

Fat: Moderate amounts of fat help to suppress gastric secretion and motility through the enterogastrone mechanism. Fats such as cream, butter and olive oil can be particularly helpful in a thin patient. Fried foods are not advised as they are difficult to digest and often aggravate the symptoms.

Carotenoids: Reactive Oxygen Species has been considered as one of the potential toxic factors involving *helicobacter pylori* induced gastric injury. Glutathione and glutathione-S-transferase are decreased in gastric mucosa by *h. pylori* which leads to loss of gastric defence mechanism against *h. pylori* infection. These have inhibitory effect on *h. pylori* induced chemokine expression by inhibiting the activation of transcription factor NF–kB. Canoteunids help in overcoming this.

Ascorbic acid: It is assumed that low antioxidant levels predispose *h. pylori* infection. It would be prudent for people with *h. pylori* infection to increase their intake of vitamin C. It helps in wound healing. Hence citrus fruit juice and tomato juice can be given. The pH of food before ingestion has little significance. No food is sufficiently acid by itself to effect a significant pH change or cause direct irritation on an ulcer.

Vitamin B_{12} deficiency: Vitamin B_{12} deficiency is often corrected after effective *h. pylori* treatment.

Gas formers: In addition, certain foods traditionally forbidden include strongly flavoured vegetables such as cabbage, cauliflower, onions and turnips and fried foods. Restriction of these foods is based on subjective evidence from patients who experience distress following ingestion of these items. Large meals are avoided.

Fibre: A regular diet, including good food sources of dietary fibre, has proved to be beneficial.

Potentially irritant substances: Caffeine, ethanol, aspirin and nicotine may delay healing but there is little evidence to show that these substances induce ulcer. Chillies, pepper, ginger, garam masala, meat soups and strong tea or coffee and protein rich foods increase the secretion of hydrochloric acid and aggravate the condition.

Current Approach

Individualised liberal diet

1. An individual must be treated as per his tolerance. Foods that are not tolerated by an individual should be avoided. A careful initial history will have information about daily living situations, attitudes, food reactions and tolerances. On the basis of such a history a reasonable and adequate nutritional programme that can be followed may be worked out. Intolerance for a food can be for a particular form. For example, a patient who cannot tolerate green chillies, may not get any untoward reaction for chilly powder.
2. The activity of patient's ulcer will influence dietary management. During acute periods of active ulceration more modified treatment may be needed to control acidity and initiate healing. When pain disappears, feedings are liberalised according to individual tolerance and desire, using a variety of foods. Sound nutrition and improved emotional outlook would support the programme.

Dietary Guidelines

- Whether a patient is on bland diet or regular diet, he needs to know which foods are needed for a nutritionally adequate diet and the importance of including these daily.
- He should select from a wide variety of foods, omitting those foods known to be distressing to the patient.
- Moderate use of seasonings are permitted.
- Regularity of mealtimes is essential. The patient gets benefited by small and frequent meals.
- In between meals, protein rich snacks should be taken.
- Moderate amounts of food should be eaten. Heavy meals are avoided. Volume of any foods sufficient to exert antral pressure against the stomach wall stimulates gastric secretion through the gastrin mechanism.
- The diet should be planned in consultation with patient, taking into consideration his preferences, cultural pattern and economic status.
- Meals eaten outside the house will not cause any problem if good judgment is used in food selection.

- Meals should be eaten in a relaxed atmosphere and should forget personal or family problems while eating.
- A short rest before and after meals may be conducive to greater enjoyment of meals.
- Food should be eaten slowly and chewed well. How one eats is more important than what one eats because fast eating provokes gastric feeding reflux.

Smoking and Alcohol

Smoking and drinking alcohol should be avoided particularly on an empty stomach. Smoking causes pyloric incompetence and reflux of duodenal juice into stomach. Smoking also interferes with attempts to decrease gastric acid and pepsin secretion with drugs.

Rest

Good physical and mental health are essential. He should learn to cope with his or her problems constructively. Mental and physical rest are important. Modification of living and work habits is needed because overwork and physical stress cause exacerbations of the disease. The patient should remember that anxiety and worry can upset digestion.

By trial and error, patient should decide which foods to be included or avoided. Possible foods that are to be avoided and included are given below:

Foods to be Included	*Foods to be Avoided*
Dairy products like milk, cream, butter, mild cheese and eggs (not fried), steamed fish, rice, riceflakes, puffed rice, well cooked cereal, semolina, cooked green leafy vegetables, custards, malted drinks, cooked pulses (if they are not causing gas formation)	Alcohol, strong tea, coffee, cola beverages, gravies, pickles, spices, chillies, curries, condiments, all fried foods, pastries, cakes, heavy sweets like halwa, barfi, raw unripe fruits, raw vegetables like cucumber, onions, radish and tomatoes. Highly processed food should be avoided.

Modification of Diet in Bleeding Ulcer

In patients with bleeding peptic ulcer, *h. pylori* eradication and ulcer healing is done by giving proton pump inhibitor based triple therapy (reducing gastric secretion) which have efficacy to ensure long term eradication of *h. pylori* in a region of high prevalence.

The degree of dietary modification in bleeding ulcer depends on the peculiarities of the individual case. In severe haemorrhage, it is customary to give no food until the bleeding has been controlled and the patient's condition is stabilized. If haemorrhage is not severe, and if nausea and vomiting are not a problem, the patient may desire food and tolerate it well. In many hospitals initial dietary treatment consists of milk alternated at 2 hours interval with small feedings, of easily digested foods, such as egg, custards, or simple puddings, toast, and tender cooked fruits and vegetables. Gradual progression in amounts and types of foods is made as the patient improves.

Primary treatment of peptic ulcer is by giving antibiotics against *helicobacter pylori.* Liberal diet suitable to the patient is suggested. Now-a-days very rarely surgery is done for peptic ulcer.

GASTRIC SURGERY

Peptic ulcer is primarily a medical disease but surgery is advised when the ulcer is complicated by haemorrhage, perforation or obstruction.

After most types of gastric surgery, all oral intake of foods and fluids are suspended until GI tract function returns. Once function is regained, liquids are initiated, after which the patient can progress to solids, as tolerated for volume and consistency.

If the surgery requires an extended period for healing, the patient may be fed enterally through a tube, often placed as a jejunostomy. The use of total parenteral nutrition is reserved for patients with post-operative complications.

The first type of fluid allowed by mouth is usually water, typically administered in the form of ice, given in small amounts and allowed to melt in the mouth or as frequent sips of water. Later larger amounts and varieties of fluids can be offered, followed by small amounts of soft, starchy and low-fat protein foods. Highly spiced, fatty or hypertonic foods may not be well tolerated by the patient. Small, frequent meals or snacks are usually better tolerated than large meals.

INTESTINAL DISEASES

Location of intestinal diseases are given in Figure 17.3.

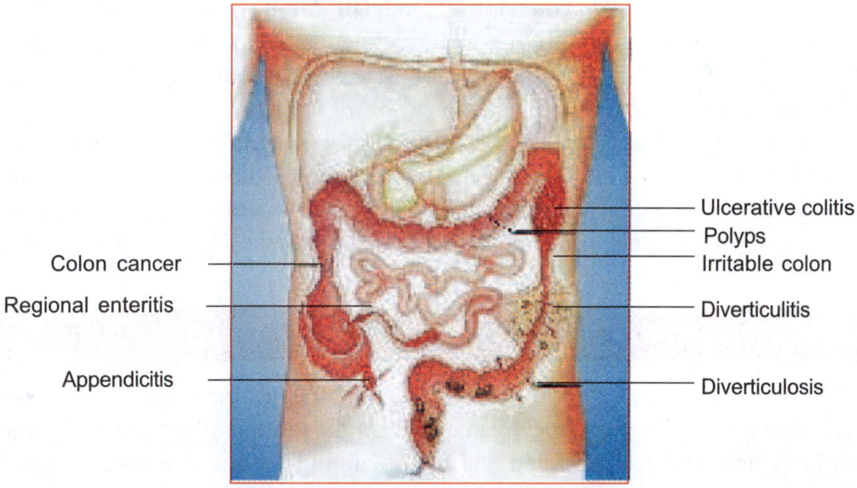

Fig. 17.3 Location of intestinal diseases

DUMPING SYNDROME

Dumping syndrome is a complex physiologic response to the presence of larger-than-normal amounts of food and liquid in the proximal small intestine. Dumping syndrome usually occurs as a result of loss of normal regulation of gastric emptying and gastrointestinal and systemic responses to a meal. The syndrome may occur as a result of total or subtotal gastrectomy.

Symptoms may occur in several stages; each is related to the 'dumping' of foods and beverages into the small intestine but the mechanisms vary.

In the first stage, patients may experience abdominal fullness and nausea within 10 to 20 minutes of eating a meal. This stage may be attributed to distention of the small bowel from foods and liquids. Also this is due to shift of fluid from systemic circulation into the small intestine as a result of ingestion of hypertonic foods or foods that are rendered hypertonic from the action of digestive enzymes. Patients may, at the same time, experience flushing, rapid heart beat, faintness, sweating and the need to sit or lie down.

In the intermediate stage, which can occur from 20 minutes to more than one hour after eating, patients may experience abdominal bloating, increased flatulence, crampy abdominal pain and diarrhoea. The 'colonic' symptoms are likely related to the increased malabsorption of carbohydrates and other food stuffs and the subsequent fermentation of the substrates entering the colon.

The late stage, occurring from 1 to 3 hours after a meal, is related to reactive hypoglycaemia. Patients may perspire; feel anxious, weak, shaky or hungry. Rapid delivery, hydrolysis and absorption of carbohydrate produces an exaggerated rise in insulin level with a subsequent decline in blood glucose level.

The resolution of dumping symptoms is achieved in most cases by dietary modifications in particular by the reduction of carbohydrate intake and the adjustment of lifestyle.

Daily food intake should be divided into at least 6 meals. Fluid intake during meals should be restricted. Drinking liquids should be avoided for at least a half-hour after a meal. Complex carbohydrates, cereals, fresh fruits and vegetables are preferred. Simple sugars like candies, cookies, sodas, sweets should be avoided. Milk and dairy products like milkshakes, sweetened yoghurt, chocolate milk are generally not well tolerated and should be also avoided. Protein, meat, fish, chicken, eggs and fat intake should be increased to meet daily caloric needs because of restricted intake of carbohydrates.

To prevent postprandial hypertension lying supine for 30 minutes after meals delay gastric emptying and improving venous return. Supplementation of dietary fibres like bran, methyl cellulose with meals has been proven effective in the treatment of hypoglycemic episodes. Five grams pectin with a meal, glucomanan and guargum have been tested with good results particularly in pediatric population.

CONSTIPATION

Constipation is a symptom and not a disease. It is passage of firm or hard pellet like stools at infrequent and long intervals with difficulty to expel. On the last leg of digestion trip food travels through colon where water is absorbed and the remaining food is transformed into waste or stools. If too much water is absorbed by the colon the result is hard dry-stool-constipation. If the colon muscles are sluggish the result is hard dry stool. In constipation there may be less than 3 motions per week or painful defaecation.

In this condition, there is resistance to movement of intestinal contents; consequently, there is distension and infrequent or difficult evacuation of feces from the intestine. The frequency of bowel movements varies greatly among individuals. For some, daily elimination is normal; in other equally healthy persons, regular evacuation occurs every second or third day.

Infrequent or insufficient emptying of the bowel may lead to malaise, headache, coated tongue, foul breath, and lack of appetite. These symptoms usually disappear after satisfactory evacuation has taken place.

Causes of Constipation

Atonic Constipation

It is the most common type of constipation. The intestinal walls lack muscular tone so that peristaltic action is impaired. The food mass thus cannot move at a normal rate down the tract.

Bacterial action may be greatly increased owing to the stagnation of material in the colon and possibly the products of this action may be responsible for at least some of the symptoms usually occurring as a result of constipation.

The chief causes of atonic constipation are selection of foods low in bulk, insufficient fluids, poor personal hygiene, lack of exercise, chronic illness, pregnancy or excessive use of enemas.

This type of constipation may be due to overuse of laxatives or poor bowel habits.

Spastic Constipation

This is characterised by increased narrowing of the colon. The contractions throughout the tract act in a spasmodic manner, causing the movement of food mass to be very irregular. Spasmodic movements cause acute pain.

Spastic constipation is caused by inactivity, immobility or obstruction. Highly, nervous people are more frequently affected by this type of constipation than by the atonic type.

Temporary or chronic constipation can be due to any one of the number of factors such as

- inadequate diet and improper lifestyle.
- failure to establish regular times for eating, adequate rest and elimination.
- faulty dietary habits, such as inadequate fluid and fibre intake or use of highly refined and concentrated foods that leave little residue in the colon.
- interference with the urge to defecate brought on by poor personal hygiene or injury to the nervous mechanism.
- changes in one's usual routine brought on by illness, nervous tension, or a trip away from home.
- chronic use of laxatives.
- difficult or painful defecation due to hemorrhoids or fissures.
- poor muscle tone of the intestine and stasis due to lack of exercise occurring especially in bed ridden patients, invalids such as arthritics, the aged and others.
- organic disorders such as diverticulosis or obstruction from adhesions or neoplasms.
- ingestion of drugs such as analgesics, anti-inflammatory agents, aluminium containing antacids, antidepressants, diuretics, iron. large amounts of sedatives or opiates; and
- spasm of intestine due to presence of irritating material or psychogenic influences.

Formula-fed infants have more chances of getting constipation than breast-fed infants.

In young child, constipation is sometimes due to emotional upset arising out of conflict with the mother over toilet training.

The cause of constipation in older children are similar to those in adults.

Pregnant women are often constipated due to pressure of gravid uterus on the colon which delays the movements of contents.

In old people sensitivity of the neuromuscular reflexes in the colon may be impaired or they may become less aware of the presence of faeces in rectum, which inturn causes constipation.

When constipation is due to low intake of dietary fibre, there is often pain in the left side of the abdomen along the side of the descending colon, and faeces may be passed as hard pellets. Passage of faeces relieves the pain. When the call to defaecate has been repeatedly ignored, a mass of inspissated (thickened), faecal matter may accumulate in the decending colon. Then fluid contents of the colon may run down the side of the mass and cause a watery diarrhoea.

The daily faecal output ranges normally from 75 to 200 g of which 50 to 75 g is water. The amount of water depends on the amount of fibre present in the diet due, to its capacity to bind water.

Determination of the cause is important so that proper treatment can be given.

Dietary Considerations

The intake of dietary fibre should be increased by eating whole grains and increasing consumption of fruits and vegetables. The most important factor is the water-holding capacity of fibre. Coarse bran has a capacity of 6 g water/g of fibre, but fine bran holds only 2–3 g water/g. Patients should be encouraged to take coarse bran as a breakfast cereal. One tablespoon of bran may be taken in the first week and two thereafter. The bran may be made more palatable by adding cooked fruits.

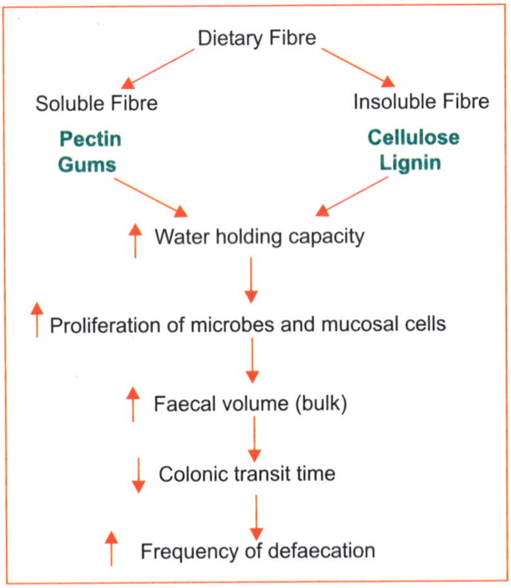

Fig. 17.4 Role of fibre in preventing and treating constipation.

Fruits and vegetables whose fibre holds water effectively are oranges, papaya, apples, carrots and the cabbage family. The diet should contain a serving of vegetables particularly in raw form and two such fruits each day preferably with skin and seed. Whole grain breads and cereals should be substituted for refined ones. Fat-containing foods such as bacon, butter, cream and oils are useful for some because of the stimulating effect of the fatty acids on the mucous membranes. Maize dry, bengal gram, onion, quinoa, curry leaves, field beans, soya beans, guava and sapota are good sources of fibre which prevent constipation. Drumstick leaves and tamarind leaves are also good sources of fibre.

Fluid intake of 8 to 10 glasses a day is useful in keeping the intestinal contents in a semisolid state for easier passage along the tract. Some individuals find that 1 or 2 glasses of hot or cold water, plain or with lemon, are helpful in initiating peristalsis when taken before breakfast.

The high sorbitol content in dried fruits such as prunes, figs and dates act as a natural laxative so does flax seed, fresh pears and apples.

Many laxatives are available. Psyllium is a popular supplement. Their continued use may lead to excessive sodium, potassium and water in the faeces hence not recommended. Laxatives become a habit and natural peristaltic movement is affected.

Correction of Faulty Habits

Regular toilet training among young children, and persistent and unhurried attempts to move the bowels at the same time each day by adults is important to overcome and prevent constipation. Worry, anxiety, fatigue and change of life style may cause stress which inturn leads to constipation. Hence stress should be avoided. Those who suffer from constipation should take more water and fibre and do more outdoor exercises. Physical activity prevents constipation.

DIVERTICULAR DISEASE

Diverticulosis refers to sac-like herniations of the colonic wall. It is a condition of having diverticula. Fecal material gets trapped in diverticula causing inflammation and infection a condition called diverticulitis (see figure 17.5). Intra colonic pressures and muscular thickening result from complete closure of colonic segments during contractions associated with attempts to propel small, dry or hard fecal material through the lumen of the bowel. In general diverticular disease is relatively rare in people who consume high fibre diet.

Overweight and obesity increase the odds of developing diverticulitis and diverticular bleeding. Total dietary fibre intake is inversely associated with the risk of diverticular disease. The combination of high total fat intake or red meat with a diet low in total dietary fibre increase the risk of disease.

Consumption of vegetarian diet and a high intake of dietary fibre are both associated with a lower risk of diverticular disease.

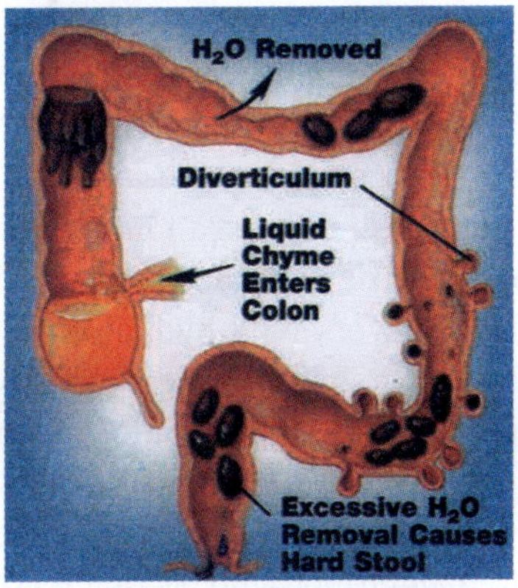

Fig. 17.5 Constipation and diverticular disease

Source: Patient Education Center, 1995, On Target media Inc. Cincinnati, Ohio, USA.

The incidence of diverticulosis increases with age.

Complications of diverticular disease range from painless, mild bleeding and altered bowel habits to diverticulitis, which may include its own clinical spectrum of inflammation.

High fibre diet promotes soft bulky stools that pass more swiftly, requiring less strain with defaecation and result in lower intracolonic pressures. High amount of coarse fibre intakes have been found to relieve symptoms for most patients.

Fibre intake should be increased gradually, as it may cause bloating or gas. However, these side effects usually disappear within 2 to 3 weeks. If needed methylcellulose and psyllium can be used. Alongwith high fibre intake, plenty of water should be consumed.

Colonic smooth muscle contraction which intensify after a high fat meal, may contribute to the discomfort felt by individuals with diverticular disease. Therefore a low fat diet is suggested. Large pieces of coarse plant matter might be restricted. Probiotics have been found to have some benefit in the treatment of diverticulosis.

DIARRHOEA

Diarrhoea in Children

Over 1,00,000 children below the age of 11 months die of diarrhea annually in India which is the second leading killer of young children globally after pneumonia.

Diarrhoea is the passage of stools with increased frequency, fluidity or volume compared to the usual for a given individual. It is a response of the bowel to infection, drugs, foods or disease. These factors can lead to the passage of unformed stools.

Three factors can lead to the passage of unformed stools

Three clinical syndromes of diarrhoea have been defined each reflecting a different pathogenesis and requiring different approaches to treatment.

Acute watery diarrhoea: It refers to diarrhoea that-begins acutely with passage of loose or watery stools without visible blood. Vomiting may occur and fever may be present. It subsides within 3–7 days. If diarrhoea occurs more than 14 days, it is called persistent diarrhoea. Most of them are of viral etiology. Persistent diarrhea may be due to giardiasis.

Dysentery: It is the term used for diarrhoea with visible blood. Dysentery may also be associated with fever and tenesmus. Causative organism is *shigella*.

Chronic diarrhoea: It is recurrent or long lasting diarrhoea due to non infectious causes such as sensitivity to gluten or inherited metabolic disorders.

Acute diarrhoea during weaning can be due to indigestion. When weaning food is introduced too early, that is, the infant's digestive system is not ready, or if there is not enough digestive enzyme secretion, diarrhoea can occur. Poor food hygiene and improperly handled food can cause infectious diarrhoea. Food intolerance or allergy can also lead to diarrhoea. Most episodes are self limiting but the condition can be fatal to children.

Thirty to forty per cent of diarrhoeal episodes are caused by viruses of which rota virus is the most common one. About 50 per cent are due to bacterial infections of the gut. Bacteria may cause diarrhoea through the action of toxin and direct invasion of the intestinal mucosa.

Osmotic diarrhoea is characterised by passage of large, frothy, explosive and acidic stools. Due to worsening hydration status of the child, there is also a serious danger of developing hypernatraemia in these cases. High osmolar solutions like carbonated soft drinks or oral rehydration solution (ORS) with high sugar content can also result in osmotic diarrhoea.

Diarrhoea has been shown to have significant impact on nutrition though most nutrients are well absorbed. Most field studies identify diarrhoea as the major determining factor leading to malnutrition in developing countries. It is the child with multiple episodes of diarrhoea and particularly chronic diarrhoea, who suffers most severely from protein energy malnutrition. If diarrhoea becomes unusually prolonged or is recurrent, the child becomes severely malnourished since he/she also loses nutrients through stools. The appetite is impaired and food is often withheld from the child by the mother due to an erroneous belief that starvation rests the bowel and promotes early recovery from diarrhoea. Atrophy of the intestinal epithelium in case of malnutrition causes malabsorption and accentuates malnutrition. A vicious cycle of diarrhoea-malnutrition-diarrhoea sets in.

Problems due to acute diarrhoea are dehydration and electrolyte imbalance due to vomiting and diarrhoea. The child may feel anorectinc. Poor cultural practice like over dilution of milk with contaminated water and withholding of breast milk are added problems.

Treatment

Fluid Management: The key to effective fluid management in childhood diarrhoea is early replacement of fluid losses, starting with the first sign of liquid stool. Plenty of fluid should be given to the child early in the illness to prevent dehydration. As long as renal function is maintained, profound electrolyte and pH disturbances do not occur.

Initial Management with any Fluid Available: The child is offered fluids as much quantity as the child can take orally without vomiting. Coconut water, butter milk, rice kanji with salt, lemon-sugar-salt beverage, light tea, etc. may be given in unlimited quantity either with a teaspoon or in small drips from a tumbler. In mild cases, diarrhoea and vomiting are generally controlled within a short period and dehydration does not develop.

Oral Rehydration Therapy with Home Made Solution: For one glass of boiled cooled water one pinch of salt and one tsp sugar can be added, to prepare ORS at home.

Oral Rehydration Salts solution: If the diarrhoea is prolonged and dehydration becomes evident, it is desirable to rehydrate the child orally by administering a solution with the composition approved by the World Health Organisation.

Table 17.1 Composition of WHO oral rehydration salt solution

Components	*Amount g/litre*
Glucose	20
Sodium chloride	3.5
Sodium bicarbonate	2.5
Trisodium citrate*	2.9
Potassium chloride	1.5

This solution provides 90 mEq of sodium, 20 mEq/L of potassium, 80 mEq/L of chloride and 30 mEq/L of bicarbonate.

Using zinc alone with oral rehydration salts to treat diarrhea not only helps children get better and faster and save lives.

It is administered in small sips or with a teaspoon, to prevent rapid passage of stools due to hyperactive gastro-colic reflex. Usually one year old infant needs about 1000 ml of ORS in 24 hours.

Since children with diarrhoea develop protein energy malnutrition, the diet should be easily digestible and nutritionally balanced. Presence of nutrients in the gut promotes absorption of sodium and water and hastens recovery of the intestinal epithelium because food in the intestine stimulates rapid cell turnover and renewal of intestinal lining.

Table 17.2 Amount of ORS to be given in the first 4 hours

Age	*<4 months*	*4–11*	*12–23*	*2–4 years*	*5–14 years*
Wt. kg	*<5*	*5–8*	*8–11*	*11–16*	*16–30*
ORS ml	200–400	400–600	600–800	800–1200	1200–2000
Measure, glass	1–2	2–3	3–4	4–6	6–11

Note: More ORS can be given in case the child requires. For infants under 6 months who are not breastfed additional 100–200 ml boiled water can be given during this period.

Source: Gnanavasundaram, A manual of pediatric nutrition. Institute of child health and hospital for children Chennai.

Dietary Guidelines

The infant should continue to be breast fed during diarrhoea. Breast milk contains viable phagocytes and other protective substances such as secretory IgA and specific IgM which protect against most enteropathogens except rotavirus infection. Thus breast milk helps the infant to recover from an attack of diarrhoea both in terms of the nutrients it supplies and its rehydrating effect and it also helps to prevent further infection because it has protective properties.

The bowel should not be 'rested' during episodes of diarrhoea but intake of milk and other lactose containing products should be avoided for a day or two because lactose malabsorption is often a result of transient lactase deficiency due to enteropathogens that have damaged the intestinal lining.

Milk should be diluted with equal volume of water and fed along with ORS till the diarrhoea stops. Mothers should be reassured that although a temporary increase in the frequency of motions might occur initially, eventual recovery will be faster if the patient continues to be fed.

They consistently show a statistically significant benefit and moderate clinical benefit of a few, well-identified probiotic strains—mostly *lactobacillus* GG and *s. boulardii*, but also *l. reuteri*—in the treatment of acute watery diarrhoea, primarily rotaviral, in infants and young children of developed countries. Such a beneficial effect seems to result in a reduction of diarrhoea duration of little more than 1 day, and to be exerted mostly on diarrhoea due to rotavirus. The effect is not only strain-dependent but also dose-dependent, with doses of at least 10 billion/d being necessary.

Fermented milk (buttermilk) with a culture of *streptococcus haemophilus* and *lactobacillus bulgaricus* has a beneficial effect. It discourages the growth of pathogenic bacteria.

Rice based solutions, potato, millet, maize and other cereal flours reduce the number and volume of stools. There is no danger of producing osmotic diarrhoea as when given sugar. Dextrins are larger molecules than sucrose or glucose and have less osmotic effect weight for weight and less likely to cause osmolar diarrhoea. The cereal provides some potassium and a little protein; amino acids have a synergetic effect with carbohydrate in promoting the absorption of water and salt.

For older infants, milled cereals are preferred to whole cereals. A well cooked gruel of rice and lentil is usually well tolerated. Mashed bananas are also good. The diet should be iso-osmolar. These foods should be started within 4 to 6 hours of starting the treatment. Sugary soft drinks, fruit juices and tea are not suitable for use because they contain high osmolites due to carbohydrate concentration which may exacerbate diarrhoea. Most children tolerate small quantities of fats and oils which are rich source of energy and the diarrhoea does not get worse. Solid foods should be offered as soon as the child is able to eat. Caffeine should be avoided. Fibre, fruits and vegetables are avoided.

Precooked ready to mix cereal pulse mixture prepared from roasted and powdered rice, wheat, black gram and powdered sugar in the ratio 1 : 1 : 1 : 2 can be given. Amylase rich food is found to be beneficial in children with diarrhoea and malnutrition.

Various step-wise diets are given in Table 17.3. Low milk, followed by milk free and starch free diet can be tried in succession to chronic diarrhoea.

Table 17.3 **Dietary management of chronic diarrhoea**

Type of diet	*Composition*
• Diet A/Level I Diet	Low milk diet (50 ml/kg/day) Curd rice/Sooji gruel with milk
• Diet B/Level II Diet	Milk free diet-Cereal-pulse mix/gruel, amylase rich food
• Diet C/Level III Diet	Lactose-Sucrose/starch Free Diet Soya based or chicken based, and Egg

Source: Elizabeth, K.E, 2005, *Nutrition and Child development* , Paras Publishing, Hyderabad/Bangalore.

Any programme for diarrhoeal disease control must include provision of potable water. Parents must also be educated regarding storage of water and foods in clean utensils, continuance of breast feeding, using only freshly prepared weaning foods and thorough washing of hands with soap before handling foods.

Usage of ORT, continued feeding and avoiding inappropriate antibiotics are all that are needed to prevent chronic diarrhoea. Vitamin A, folic acid and zinc supplementation are also found beneficial. Zinc treatment for diarrhea could reduce the risk of death.

During recovery atleast 125 percent normal caloric intake should be attempted until the child reaches pre illness weight.

Better food hygiene, improvement of nutritional status of children and food environmental sanitation are important strategies for lowering the incidence of diarrhoea.

Diarrhoea in Adults-Nutritional Care

Nutritional care for adults with diarrhoea includes the replacement of lost fluids and electrolytes by increasing the oral intake of fluids, particularly those high in sodium and potassium such as broths and electrolyte solutions. Pectin from cooked apples or other soluble fibre may also help in controlling diarrhoea.

Patients should be encouraged to avoid caffeine because it increases cyclic adinosine monophospate levels, promoting secretion of fluid.

When diarrhoea stops starchy foods like rice, potato and plain cereals can be given followed by protein foods. Fat need not be limited if the individual is otherwise healthy. Sugar, alcohols, lactose, fructose and large amounts of sucrose may worsen osmotic diarrhoea and may need to be limited.

In chronic diarrhoea, nutrients should be replaced parenterally and enterally. The loss of potassium alters bowel motility, encourages anorexia and can introduce a cycle of bowel distress. Loss of iron from gastro-intestinal bleeding may be severe enough to cause anaemia. The nutritional deficiencies themselves cause mucosal changes, such as decreased villi height and reduced enzyme secretion, further contributing to malabsorption. As the diarrhoea begins to resolve, the addition of more normal amounts of fibre to the diet may help to restore normal mucosal function, increase electrolyte and water absorption and increase viscosity of the stool.

Probiotics strengthen epithelial junctions to protect against intercellular invasion by pathogens. In addition, probiotics can enhance the mucosal immune response to specific pathogens, thus strengthening the protective effect at the mucosal surface. Probiotics help prevent and can be used to treat conditions that are related to the disruption of the ecologic balance of colonising gut flora *e.g.*, antibiotic induced infection.

Proper balance in colonising bacteria with an abundance of probiotics can modify such diverse conditions as lactose intolerance and *clostridium difficle* diarrhoea. Probiotics use can enhance the immunoglobulin A response against diverse pathogens such as viruses and bacteria.

Barley, bananas, curd, rice and potatoes may lessen diarrhoea whereas caffeine containing beverages, fried foods and food rich in fibre may worsen diarrhoea.

MALABSORPTION

Malabsorption can result in poor nutrition due to reduced intake (abdominal pain, anorexia, indigestion, nausea) or excessive nutrient losses (bacterial overgrowth of the small intestine, diarrhea) or due to raised nutrient needs (drug therapy, infection).

Malabsorption of any nutrient is possible but most commonly, it is fat that is malabsorbed. The excretion of unabsorbed fat in the stools causes the type of diarrhea known as streatorrhea.

STEATORRHOEA

It is a consequence of malabsorption in which unabsorbed fat remains in the stool. In contrast to the 2 to 6 g of ingested fat that is normally excreted each day, as much as 60 g may be lost in this condition.

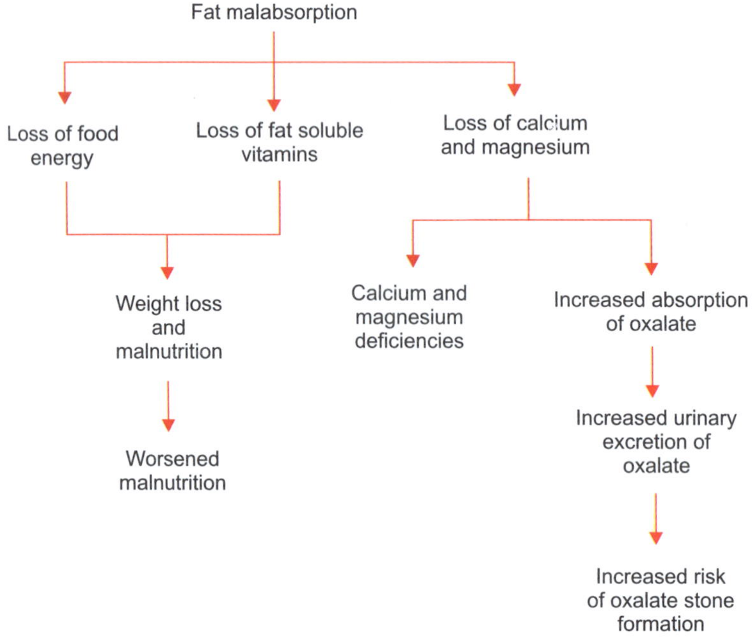

Fig. 17.6 The effects of fat malabsorption

Source: Whitney Eleanor *et al.*, 1995. Nutrition for health and health care West Publishing Company, Minneapolis US.

Excessive fat excretion may result from biliary insufficiency or biliary obstruction or pancreatic insufficiency or failure of normal absorption owing to mucosal damage (sprue).

Since steatorrhoea is a symptom and not a disease, the underlying cause of malabsorption must be treated. The presence of weight loss requires an increased energy intake. Dietary protein and carbohydrate should be high and fats may need to be added as tolerated. Fat soluble vitamins in water miscible form, and minerals such as calcium, zinc, magnesium and iron should be supplemented.

Medium-chain triglycerides are hydrolysed more rapidly and can rely on the small amount of intestinal lipase available, rather than on pancreatic lipase for digestion. The products of hydrolysis are easily dispersed and absorbed in the absence of bile acids, which is often the cause of fat malabsorption. Short-chain fatty acids and medium-chain fatty acids are able to enter the portal venous blood for direct transport to the liver without being resynthesised into triglycerides.

Initially fat restricted diet is suggested. Fat is tolerated best when given in frequent small doses.

LACTOSE INTOLERANCE

Three main types of lactase deficiency have been described: congenital, secondary and primary. Congenital lactase deficiency is extremely rare and requires a lifelong lactose-free or very low-lactose diet. Secondary lactose intolerance or lactase deficiency is transient in nature and develops secondary to illness or disease involving mucosal injury. Regional enteritis, ulcerative

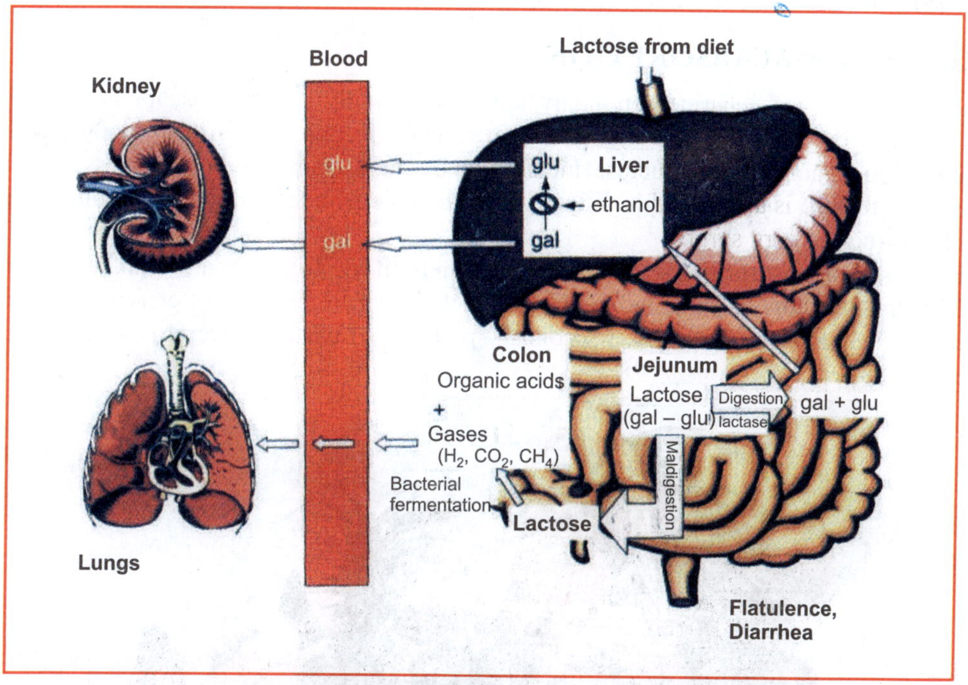

Fig. 17.7 Metabolic background for understanding the diagnosis of lactose maldigestion and intolerance. Abbreviations: glu, glucose; gal, galactose.

Source: **(Edi)** Coulston Ann M and Carol J Boushey, 2008, Nutrition in the prevention and treatment of disease Elesevier, US.

colitis, Crohn's disease, gluten-induced enteropathy, parasitic infections, antibiotic therapy, and surgical procedures including gastrectomy, extensive bowel resection, and gastric bypass are conditions associated with secondary lactase deficiency. Individuals with secondary lactose intolerance often require temporary limitation or avoidance of lactose from a few days to several months.

Primary lactase deficiency, also known as late onset or lactase nonpersistence, is the most prevalent type of lactase deficiency, which usually occurs with increasing age. Individuals exhibit tolerance to various levels of lactose. Primary lactase deficiency is most commonly seen in African Americans, Hispanics, Native Americans, Asians, and people of Jewish decent. Adult lactase deficiency is the most common of all enzyme deficiencies.

The milk sugar lactose is digested by infants and children by the enzyme β-glucosidase lactase. Lactose is supposed to enhance calcium absorption in children. However, the activity of this enzyme decreases in adults which results in a poor tolerance of milk.

Lactose intolerance can lead to bloating, cramps, flatulence and diarrhoea after taking milk and milk products.

Small quantities of dairy foods with 10–15 g of lactose can be taken rather than large amounts at one time. Dairy foods can be had with meals rather than between meals. Curd and butter milk may not produce any discomfort to the patient. Lactose free and lactose reduced milk, cheese and ice cream can be consumed if available. Lactase tablets can be taken along with high lactose food.

FRUCTOSE MALABSORPTION

Fructose is a monosaccharide commonly found in naturally sweet foods, foods with added sugar and as part of an oligosaccharide chain called a fructan. Foods that naturally contain relatively high amounts of fructose include honey, fruit, fruit juices, molasses and sweet potatoes. Fructose is also found in refined sugars commonly added to food, including sucrose and high fructose corn syrup.

Fructose malabsorption is different from hereditary fructose intolerance. Fructose malabsorption occurs when an individual does not absorb all the fructose present in the small intestine. This is exacerbated by a secondary problem of bacterial overgrowth in the small intestine.

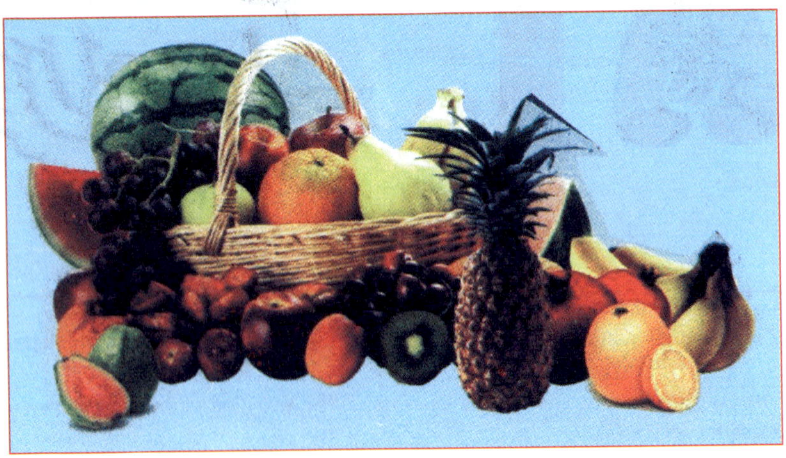

Fig. 17.8 Fruits are good sources of fructose.

People with Fructose malabsorption can tolerate some amount of fructose each time they eat but if the amount they consume is greater than the number of transporters available, a portion of the fructose continues on to the large intestine. This unabsorbed fructose creates an osmotic load and is fermented by bacteria in the large intestine, causing wide range of primarily gastrointestinal symptoms.

Diet therapy begins with removing any foods high in added sugar and restricting fruits and vegetables. Once symptoms subside slowly foods can be reintroduced beginning with the fruits and vegetables.

If an individual has significant bacterial overgrowth in the small intestine, fermentation may occur regardless of whether there are enough transporters for the fructose load. In this case all fermentable carbohydrates are a potential problem for the individual not just fructose. Limiting of broader group of carbohydrates known as Fermentable. Oligo-Di and Monosaccharides and Polyols - FODMPPs should be done.

CELIAC DISEASE

It is a debilitating autoimmune disorder that affects an estimated 1 per cent of the world's population. Celiac disease is an inherited, immune mediated intolerance to dietary gluten. Gluten is the collective term for the amino acid sequences found in wheat, barley, rye and to a lesser extent oats which trigger an immune reaction.

When gluten is ingested susceptible individuals mount a specific, intense inflammatory response within the small intestinal mucosa that damages the lining and interferes with digestion and absorption.

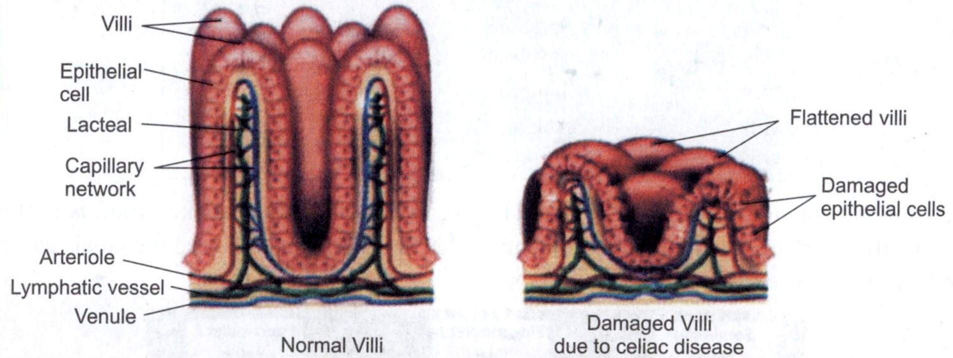

Fig. 17.9 In celiac disease villi get atrophied and there is increased chronic inflammatory cells on the surface epithelium resulting in malabsorption.

Gluten sensitivity is lifelong and cannot be outgrown. While gluten itself is the environmental cause for development of antibodies, certain stresses can trigger active disease including gluten overload, pregnancy, viral or bacterial infection, surgery, overexercise and severe stress.

It is characterized by atrophy of the villi and damage to the microvilli in the deudenum and jejunum in response to the ingestion of gluten.

The disease is accompanied by a marked reduction in absorptive surface area of the small intestine and a decreased uptake and transport of nutrients.

In celiac disease all foods containing prolamins like wheat, rye, barley and oats are avoided. The specific names of cereal prolamins that are toxic in celiac disease are gliadin in wheat, secalin in rye, hordein in barley and avenin in oats.

According to FAO/WHO guidelines a gluten free food may contain no more than 200 ppm prolamin on a dry weight basis.

In severe untreated cases of celiac disease, malabsorption of fat, calcium, magnesium, fat soluble vitamins A, D, E and K, folate, iron and vitamin B_{12} can occur. Some times the initial symptoms are severe such as nausea, weight loss, weakness, flatus, abdominal pain, bloating and diarrhea. Extra intestinal symptoms such as iron deficiency anaemia, reduced bone mineral density, chronic fatigue, irritable bowel and dyspepsia can occur. Avoidance of lactose containing foods in addition to gluten free diet, may be beneficial until the intestinal mucosa has recovered.Villi recovery can take several months to years in an adult with celiac disease. Patients who suffer from celiac disease can try millets like little millet (samai), fox tail millet (thinai), barnyard millet (kuthiraivali), kodomillet (varagu), prosomillet (pani varagu), finger millet (ragi), sorghum (cholam) and pearl millet (kambu).

Foods allowed and foods not allowed in celiac disease

Allowed		Not allowed
Amaranth seeds	Nuts	Barley
Beans	Potato	Bran
Cheese	Pea	Wheat of all kinds
Corn	Quinoa	Semolina
Egg	Rice	Malt
Fish	Sorghum	Triticale
Flax seed	Soyabean	Oats
Meat	Tapioca	Semolina
Milk	Aninoa	Rye
Millets		

Quinoa is a popular gluten free grain. It is rich in protein. Home cooked food is preferred in celiac disease as one knows the ingredients added to it. One need to read the labels carefully to prevent the sensitivity.

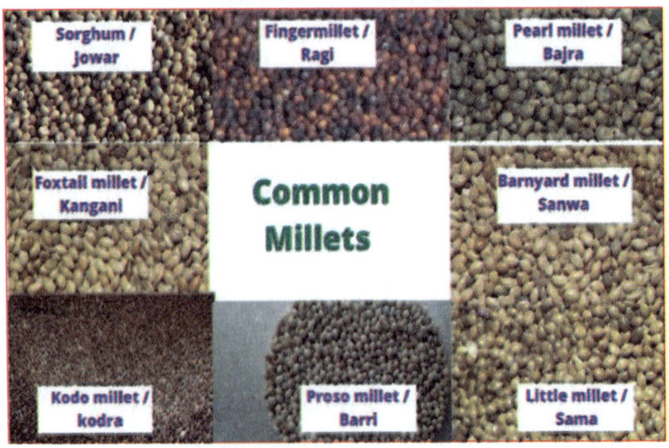

Fig. 17.10 **Millets are free from gluten and can be given in celiac disease**

Untreated celiac disease is associated with a number of complications, including nutritional deficiencies, bone disease, and lymphoma. Since a strict gluten free diet can fully restore health and improve quality of life, early detection and proper education about the disease and diet are essential.

TROPICAL SPRUE

Tropical sprue is a syndrome of unknown etiology that occurs in most tropical areas. It may be the sequala of an acute infections diarrhoea, with subsequent contamination of the bowel by bacteria. The intestinal villi are shortened. The gastric mucosa may be atrophied and inflamed with diminished secretion of hydrochloric acid and intrinsic factor.

Symptoms include diarrhoea, anorexia and abdominal distention as well as symptoms of nutritional deficiency.

Treatment involves restoration of fluids, electrolytes and nutrients. Tropical sprue often responds promptly to antibiotics and folate therapy. Along with other nutrients as needed, folate is given orally, 5 mg/day, along with intramuscular vitamin B_{12} (1000 μg/month).

INFLAMMATORY BOWEL DISEASES

Inflammatory bowel disease refers to any type of inflammatory disorder involving the small and/or large intestine including those caused by infections and immunologic or toxic agents. Crohn's disease and ulcerative colites are the two most common forms of idiopathic inflammatory bowel disease.

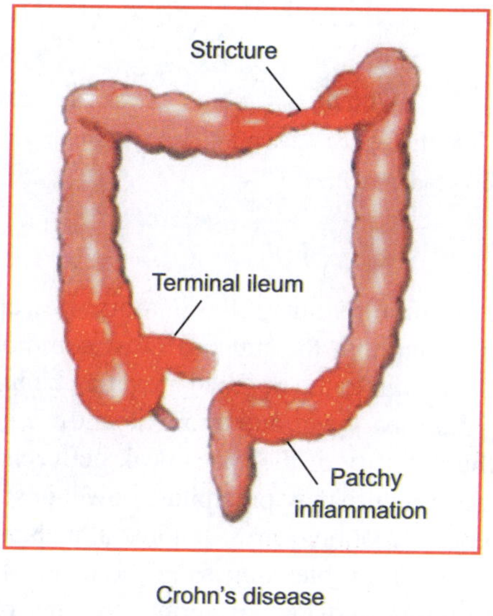

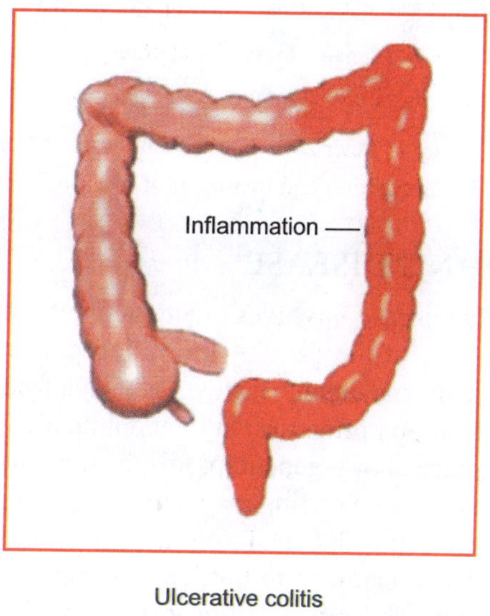

Fig. 17.11 In Crohn's disease inflammation skips certain areas. In ulcerative colitis inflammation starts in the rectum and progresses in a retrograde fashion.

Table 17.4 Characteristics of Crohn's Disease and Ulcerative Colitis

A. Features common to both Crohn's disease and ulcerative colitis
• Chronic episodes of relapse and remission
• Diarrhea
• Extra intestinal manifestations to varying degrees
• Fever
• Increased risk of colorectal cancer
• Weight loss, growth failure
B. Characteristics more common with Crohn's disease
• Any area of the GI tract but more commonly involves the distal small bowel and colon
• Segments of normal mucosa interrupted by diseased bowel
• Transmural involvement, thickening of the intestinal wall
• 70% have surgery in their lifetime; surgery does not guarantee a cure
• Abscesses, sinus tract, fistulas
• Strictures
• Hyperoxaluria, oxalate stones
C. Characteristics more common in ulcerative colitis
• More superficial mucosal disease involvement
• Confined to the colon
• Surgical resection of the colon eliminates the disease
• Normally originates in the distal colon and migrates proximally
• GI bleeding more common

Source: Beyer L. Peter 2008 Nutrition in inflammatory bowel disease and short bowel syndrome Nutrition in the prevention and treatment of disease Elsevier Academic Press US.

CROHN'S DISEASE

Crohn's disease involves acute and chronic granulomatous inflammatory bowel. With progression of the disease, ulceration develops throughout the mucosa most commonly the distal ileum and colon. However any area from the mouth to the perianal area may be involved. This ulceration often results in abdominal pain, diarrhea, fever and anorexia and weight loss. The disease shows genetic predisposition and the majority of the cases peak between 15 and 30 years of age. Scarring may narrow the intestine, stricture may precipitate bowel obstruction.

The person with Crohn's disease often experiences emotional stress, anorexia, malabsorption all of which can lead to nutrient deficiencies. In addition, bleeding from the ulcers can lead to anaemia and inflammation can cause the secretion and loss of serum proteins resulting hypoalbuminemia

If the person requires surgery or develops an infection, nutrient needs become even greater. Surgery removes a portion of the bowel, the procedure itself contributes to malabsorption. Therapy for Crohn's disease may include broad-spectrum antibiotics to reduce symptoms. Corticosteroids and immunosuppressive therapy are often used during the acute phase.

Some patients may require complete bowel rest and nutrition support. Oral or enteral elemental diets or parenteral nutrition can be given in such cases. Use of elemental diets has led to improvement in patients' body weight and serum albumin decrease in inflammatory parameters and remission rates as high as 90 per cent. When enteral nutrition aggravates pain and diarrhea, when the bowel is obstructed or the risk of obstruction is present complete bowel rest might help a fistula to close

Dietary Guidelines

- Nutritional requirements are estimated according to current BMI. BMI of 20–29 may require 25–30 kcal/kg
- With strictures or fistulas low fibre diet that is high in energy and high protein diet 1–1.5 g/kg is given
- Tube feeding with added glutamine is suggested. Enteral nutrition is effective in more than 50 per cent cases.
- Fat intake is limited if steatorrhoea is present in which case MCT, Medium Chain Triglycerides may be better tolerated.
- Use of ω-3 fatty acids and oleic acid and increased intake of diet rich in antioxidants could decrease inflammation.
- Diet need to be supplemented with multivitamin and minerals.
- Lactose and wheat intolerance need to be checked.
- Small frequent meals may be better tolerated.
- Probiotics may be beneficial.

A recent study showed that a semi vegetarian diet put Crohn's disease in 100 per cent remission for first years.

ULCERATIVE COLITIS

In Ulcerative Colitis ulceration of mucosa occurs and causes crampy abdominal pain, explosive or bloody diarrhea, pus or mucus discharged between stools, anaemia, fatigue and anorexia. Onset of ulcerative colitis is usually between 15 and 35 years of age. Children who present with ulcerative colitis may have growth failure. Blood in the stool is the most common symptom. Treatment is given to reduce inflammation.

Objectives

- In acute stages, short chain fatty acids and glutamine are used to prevent decline in nutritional status
- Fluid and electrolyte balance is corrected.
- Nutritional Status need to be improved
- Fibre is restricted to prevent obstruction
- Diarrhea is to be corrected
- Probiotic bacterial mixtures provide relief in mild and moderate ulcerative colitis.

Dietary Guidelines

- Energy requirements are based on current BMI— 30–35 kcal/kg
- Low fibre diet is needed to minimize faecal volume.

- By taking balanced diet and including fish oil, soluble fibre and antioxidants, the requirement of steroid doses can be reduced.
- TPN is useful when needed
- As the patient progresses, a high protein diet, 1–1.5g/kg should be given with high energy intake.
- Persons with the condition often have lactose, wheat or gluten intolerance. Diet should be altered accordingly.
- Vitamin and mineral supplementation may be needed.
- Medium chain triglycerides may be helpful.

Diet and nutrition play an important part in the management. Energy needs of patients with Inflammatory Bowel Diseases are not greatly increased but protein requirements may be increased by 50 per cent. Supplemental vitamins and minerals may be needed because of avoidance of foods or malabsorption or to correct drug-nutrient interactions.

A minimal-residue diet may be effective for reducing diarrhoea. Small frequent feedings may be tolerated better than large meals. In fat malabsorption, MCTs may be valuable.

For Inflammatory Bowel Diseases, the treatment should be life long and can be prevented with healthy diet, exercise and giving up on smoking.

IRRITABLE BOWEL SYNDROME

The most common symptoms are alternating diarrhoea and constipation, abdominal pain and bloating, but perception of excessive flatulence, sensation of incomplete evacuation, rectal pain and mucus in the stool may also occur.

In addition to stress and dietary patterns, factors which worsen symptoms are excess use of laxatives, antibiotics, caffeine, previous gastro-intestinal illness and lack of regularity in sleep, rest, and fluid intake. In patients with a strong family history of allergy, hypersensitivity to certain foods may be the cause of irritable bowel syndrome.

The aim of nutritional care is to ensure adequate nutrient intake, to guide the patient towards a diet that is not likely to contribute to symptoms, and to explain the role of ordinary dietary practices in producing or avoiding gastrointestinal symptoms. A normal diet is recommended, with emphasis on high-fibre foods that will add bulk to the stool, thus relieving the constricting pressure and promoting normal bowel motility. A daily fibre intake of 20–30 g is recommended. Additional fibre in the form of bulk laxatives (e.g. psyllium) may also be necessary. An excess of wheat bran may exacerbate mild cases, commercial fibre supplements are generally beneficial.

Studies have shown probiotics help the symptoms of IBS regulating motility, constipation and diarrhea but not overall the syndrome. Excesses in dietary fat, caffeine, sugars and alcoholic beverages should be avoided. Along with these measures, use of anticholinergic or antidiarrhoeal agents may be necessary. Relaxation and stress reduction techniques may also be useful.

Low FODMAPS, fermentable oligo-di and mono saccharides and polyols diet should be the first dietary approach in patients with IBS.

Melatonin may be helpful in irritable bowel syndrome, anxiety, depression, sleeping disorders. Melatomin can modulate bowel motility.

Individualization is key in the nutrition therapy of IBS.

INTESTINAL GAS OR FLATULENCE

Intestinal gases include N_2, O_2, CO_2, H_2 and in some individuals CH_4 (methane). The gases may be taken in or produced in the gastrointestinal tract. They may be absorbed into the circulation and lost in respiration, expelled through eructation (belching) or passed rectally. Patient may complain abdominal distention or cramping pain associated with the accumulation of gases in the upper or lower GI tract. Inactivity, decreased GI motility, aerophagia, diet and GI disorders can all contribute to the amount of intestinal gas and the individual's gas-related symptoms.

Gas in the upper intestinal tract results primarily from swallowing air (aerophagia). Aerophagia can be avoided by eating slowly, chewing with the mouth closed and refraining from drinking through straws.

Increased amounts of H_2 and CO_2 and sometimes CH_4-in rectal gas indicate excessive bacterial fermentation and suggest malabsorption of a fermentable substrate. Consumption of large amounts of dietary fibre (especially soluble fibre), resistant starch, lactose in persons who are lactase deficient or modest amounts of alcohol sugars such as sorbitol may result in increased gas production in the colon and increased flatulence. Consumption of unusual amounts of fructose or even sucrose may also result in increased amounts of faecal substrate. Legumes produce flatus or gas due to the presence of stachyose and raffinose.

High fibre foods should be introduced gradually. Sufficient fluids should be taken atleast 8-12 glasses a day-because high fibre intake increase fluid needs. Foods cooked or caused are better toluated than raw ones.

Health benefits of probiotics is limited to particular strains. Table gives specific probiotic products that are useful in different condition.

Table 17.5 Probiotics Products Supported by Published Human Studies

Indication	*Genus, species, strain*
Infant diarrhea	*L rhamnosus GG* *L casei*
Inflammatory bowel conditions (primary evidence in pouchitis)	8-strain combination of 3 *Bifidobacterium* strains, 4 *Lactobacillus* strains and *S. thermophilus*
Antibiotic associated diarrhea; *C difficile*	*S cerevisiae [S. boulardii]* *L rhamnosus GG* *L casei* *L acidophilus plus L casei*
Gut transit time	*B animalis* (Bifidus regularis)
Lactose intolerance	Most strains L-*bulgaricus* and/or *S thermophilus*
Colic in infants	*L reuteri*
Immune support	*B lactis* *B lactis* *L casei*
Irritable bowel syndrome symptoms	*B infantis*

Source: Palmer Sharon, Happy entrails; A close look at digestive health chains today's dietitian, 2008.

Myths and facts of gastrointestinal diseases

Myths	*Facts*
• Excessive restrictions are necessary and forever in GI diseases	• Initially dietary restrictions may be necessary and once the patient comes back to 'normal' slowly more foods can be added depending on the tolerance of food.
• Spicy foods are the cause of peptic ulcer	• *H Pylori* is the cause and spicy foods are restricted to reduce the irritation of stomach/duodenum.
• In diverticular disease, nuts and seeds are avoided	• No need to eliminate nuts and seeds from the diet, only patient should chew food well.
• Dietary restrictions are common for all IBS patients.	• Food sensitivities are individualistic hence same dietary advise cannot be suggested for all IBS patients
• Consuming more fibre is always better	• All cannot tolerate fibre-insoluble or soluble fibre. One should consume 40g/d or whatever is the tolerable limit.
• Avoiding FODMAPs (Fermentable, Oligo-Di- and Monosaccharides and Polyol) is a cure for IBS.	• Certain carbohydrates can aggregate the condition of uncontrolled IBS. Sometimes restriction of these carbohydrates prove unnecessary.
• One must detox or clean gut.	• Popular detox programmes involve diets, fasts, supplements and enemas claim that the body needs help in detoxifying of toxins. But the human body is well equipped with its own detoxification system: the lungs, kidneys, colon, lymphatic system and liver.
• Weight loss and digestive problems always accompany celiac disease	• Prolamin containing foods are avoided and the patient may lead a normal life
• Digestive health supplements are superior to whole foods	• Whole foods have not only fibre but also vitamins, minerals and phytonutrients which may also provide health benefits. Fibre supplements are helpful for many people with intestinal problems.
• Gluten containing diet is not good for health and should be avoided.	• Gluten causes problems in people who are sensitive to gliadin and not for all.
• Fibre is not essential to the body	• Fibre is as essential as any other nutrient and has many functions to perform in addition to preventing constipation

Source: Palmer Sharon Cracking myths, today's dietitian, April 2016.

A day in October first week is ulcer awareness day.

July 29th is Oral Rehydration Salt Day.

SUGGESTED READINGS

- Maura Keller, The gluten-free journey, today's dietitian, 2013.
- Health implications of dietary Fiber Position of the Academy of Nutrition and Dietetics J. Acad. Nutr. Diet. 2015: **115**.
- Schwartz Emily, Perioperative parenteral nutrition in adults with inflammatory bowel disease. A review of the literature, Nutrition in Clinical practice, 2016; **31**.
- Patient Care www.patientcareonline.com.
- International foundation for functional gastrointestinal disorders: www.iffgd.org.

QUESTIONS

1. What is dyspepsia? How do you treat it?
2. Explain the causative factors of peptic ulcer.
3. Define bland diet and flatulence.
4. Write a note on bleeding ulcer.
5. Give causes and treatment of irritable bowel syndrome.
6. Give dietary treatment of steatorrhoea.
7. Explain diet in diverticular disease.
8. Describe the recent concepts in dietary treatment of peptic ulcer.
9. What is dumping syndrome?
10. How do you prevent constipation?
11. Explain causes and treatment of diarrhoea in children.
12. Explain lactose intolerance.
13. Explain the role of 'fibre' in the prevention of intestinal diseases.
14. Describe cause and treatment of ulcerative colitis. How is it different from Crohn's disease?
15. What is celiac disease? What are the foods avoided in this condition?
16. What is GERD? Give dietary advise to such patient.

TOPICS FOR ACTIVITY

- Plan and prepare a bland diet.
- Plan and prepare a diet low in FODMAP diet.
- Plan and prepare gluten free diet.
- Plan and prepare a diet for an adult who is lactose intolerant.
- Plan and prepare a high fibre diet.

18

Diet in Diseases of Liver and Pancreas

Liver is body's chemical workshop. It is mainly responsible for the metabolism of the nutrients essential for life.

FUNCTIONS OF LIVER

Liver is the most metabolically active and at any given moment, 36,000 functions are being carried out in liver. The ducts of gallbladder, liver and pancreas are shown in Figure 18.1.

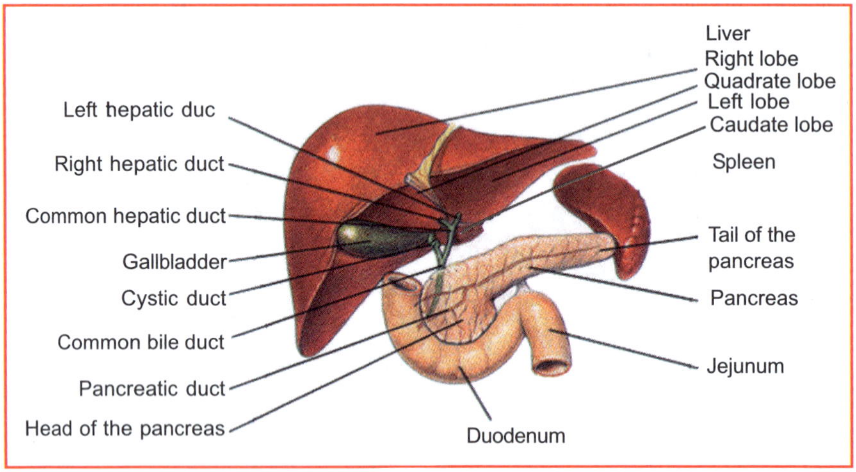

Fig. 18.1 The ducts of the gallbladder, liver, and pancreas.

Table 18.1 gives functions of liver.

Table 18.1 Major Nutrition-Related Functions of the Liver

Carbohydrate metabolism
Converts galactose and fructose into glucose
Performs glycogenesis, glycogenolysis, and gluconeogenesis
Protein metabolism
Performs transamination and deamination
Converts ammonia to urea
Forms blood-clotting factors, serum proteins, and lipoproteins
Fat metabolism
Converts fatty acids to acetyl-coenzyme A via β-oxidation
Produces ketone bodies
Synthesizes and hydrolyzes triglycerides, phospholipids, cholesterol, and lipoproteins
Forms and excretes bile to aid in fat digestion
Vitamins and minerals functions
Stores
Vitamins A, D, E, K, and B_{12}
Iron, copper, zinc and manganese
Activates
Thiamine (vitamin B_1) to thiamine pyrophosphate
Pyridoxine (vitamin B_6) to pyridoxal phosphate
Folic acid to tetrahydrofolic acid
Vitamin D to 25-hydroxycholecalciferol
Synthesises
Carrier proteins for vitamins A and B_{12}
Lipoproteins and transport vitamin E

Source: Hasse M. Jeanette, Nutrition in liver disease, Nutrition in clinical practice, 2013; **28**.

AGENTS RESPONSIBLE FOR LIVER DAMAGE

Dietary imbalances

Fatty changes in the liver in kwashiorkor may be attributed to a low protein intake and reduced capacity to produce lipoproteins.

The liver is often grossly enlarged in children with kwashiorkor, containing 30–50 per cent fat by weight, in the form of triglyceride. The intrahepatic accumulation of fat results due to excess delivery of fatty acids to the liver and/or enhanced lipogenesis. This is combined with impaired lipid transport from the liver secondary to apoprotein deficiency. When protein is supplied fat clears from the liver within a short time.

When the diet is rich in calories liver works overtime to process all that extra fat. When liver contains more than 5–10 per cent of the weight of the liver, it can lead to complications. An overload of iron can cause fatty liver. Fatty liver can lead to stones to form in the gall bladder. Surgical intervention is required to remove the stones.

Fatty changes in the liver are common whenever there is a high proportion of fat in the metabolic mixture, for example, in uncontrolled diabetes, in starvation, in some cases of obesity and when too much carbohydrate has been infused during intravenous feeding. In these cases, as in kwashiorkor, the changes are easily reversible and not followed by fibrosis.

A healthy liver can readily handle a lifetimes worth of dietary fat, but a failing liver cannot. The liver can be overtaxed by excess dietary fat. Triglycerides can build up in hepatocytes in the liver mitochondrial β-oxidation and very low density lipoprotein production are insufficient to handle the fatty acid load. Over a time, this fat accumulation can lead to scarring, inflammation, fibrosis and cirrhosis – the progressive stages of NAFLD Nonalcoholic Fatty Liver Disease. NAFLD is directly proportional to the degree of obesity particularly truncal obesity. On a molecular level, metabolic syndrome has strong clinical association with NAFLD.

The current body of research suggests that the best way to prevent and treat NAFLD is to combine a healthful diet rich in antioxidants with regular exercise to achieve a healthy weight.

Infective Agents

Virus can cause infection and damage the liver. Types A, B, C, D, E and G can cause hepatitis. Type E can be deadly during pregnancy. Hepatitis A and E virus are excreted in the stools and spread by the faecal-oral route. The patient suffers from jaundice and the liver is enlarged and tender. Recovery from a typical infection is complete and not followed by fibrosis and cirrhosis.

Hepatitis B, C, D and G virus produce a disease known as homologous serum jaundice which arises after transfusion of blood or blood products obtained from a donor who is a carrier. Improperly sterilised needles can also cause this hepatitis infection. Most patients recover. In 10 per cent of people the disease may reach a chronic stage. Types B and D can cause extreme jaundice.

Hepatitis B vaccination is now part of the routine immunisation programme. Vaccinations are available for Type A and B.

Yellow fever, like the hepatitis viruses, has a specific affinity for hepatocytes. Many other infections may impair liver function like typhoid abscesses (localised infection), Weil's disease (a type of jaundice with fever caused by a small spirochaete voided in the urine of rats and it is a disease of miners, sewer workers and who work in dirty water) and amoebiasis.

Toxic Agents

Alcohol: In malnourished patients consumption of alcohol produces acute liver damage and jaundice that resembles viral hepatitis. Alcohol is also known to have direct action on the lipid metabolism in the liver by enhancing fatty acid synthesis, decreasing fatty acid oxidation and producing specific stimulation to triglyceride formation.

Lipids accumulate, because of the increased direct channelling of ethanol as a substrate to acetate via acetaldehyde with the subsequent conversion of acetyl CoA to fatty acids. The increased NADH/NAD ratio overwhelms the cell's ability to maintain redox homeostasis and contributes to this conversion. About half the increase in liver size in heavy drinkers is explained by the excess fat.

The changes depends on amount of alcohol drunk, genetic predisposition, nutritional state, the diet eaten along with alcohol drinking and pre-existing organ damage will also alter the spectrum of changes and disease.

The increase in ethanol metabolism in the cytoplasm accelerates free radical generation and a fall in the protective concentrations of glutathione. If the dietary provision of the precursors for glutathione, that is, cysteine, a glycine and glutamate are not provided and a poor quality diet lacking in vitamin A, β-carotene and vitamin E and C by heavy drinkers and liver disease is exacerbated.

A recent study by NIN has found alcoholism to be the predominant cause of death among adults of primitive tribal group chenchus in Andhra Pradesh and Telangana, cirrhosis of liver was the major killer.

Drugs and Chemicals: Every drug that is consumed reaches the liver and its chemical nature is altered before being eliminated from the body. Drugs like paracetamol (fever) INH (TB) and oestrogen (contraceptive) may damage the liver. Workers in chemical industry like organic hydrocarbons may develop liver damage. Toxicity due to liver damage has also been observed with several commercially available herbal preparations.

Excess stores of iron, copper, galactose and glycogen may accumulate in the liver and in time lead to cirrhosis.

Cheap plastic has several layers and when this melts and is consumed, it can pose a serious hazard to the health of liver.

There is a species of wild mushrooms that can cause liver failure.

In Born Errors of Metabolism

Children with hereditary tyrosinaemia, galactosaemia and hereditary fructose intolerance may develop liver damage. Successful management depends on early diagnosis and exclusion of the offending substances from the diet.

DAMAGE CAUSED TO LIVER

Liver has a self-renewing ability and falters only when more than 80 per cent is damaged. It takes only 15–20 days to regrow in a normal individual.

Fatty globulation: The fat gets deposited in the liver. The fat present in healthy cells is not visible because the water insoluble triglycerides are present linked to phospholipids and other substances to form amphipathic molecules that are dispersed as micelles in the cell water. The complex physicochemical environment that permits micelle formation is readily disturbed by any factor affecting the nutrition of the cell. Droplets of triglycerides are formed and the function of liver is impaired. This process is readily reversed if the damaging factor is removed by changing lifestyle in diet and exercise.

Fatty liver is third leading cause of chronic liver disease and liver cancer. Obesity, diabetes, hypertension are the main causes of fatty liver.

Fatty liver can lead to unnatural levels in the enzymes, presenting with the same condition that alcoholics report with.

Necrosis: Due to excessive alcohol intake, the liver may become tender and enlarged. This is due to an inflammatory reaction provoked by necrosis or death of hepatocytes due to excessive fatty globulation or to a direct toxic effect.

Cirrhosis of liver: Cirrhosis refers to the colour of nodules of hepatocytes regenerating between strands of fibrous tissue. It is used now to refer to any diffuse chronic disease of the reticulin framework that supports each acinus (minute saccules combine to form lobules), and its replacement with fibrous tissue. Fibrous tissue contracts with time and then may obstruct the branches of the portal vein and bile duct within the liver.

Intrahepatic obstruction causes a rise in pressure in all branches of the portal vein (portal hypertension). Venous congestion leads to enlargement of the spleen which can usually be detected by palpation. It leads to varicosities which may bleed. Oesophageal bleeding is a common and a serious consequence of cirrhosis of liver. Increased venous pressure impedes the return of interstitial tissue fluid into the capillary circulation; it leaks into the peritoneal cavity where it accumulates in large amounts, up to 10 litres or more, and this is known as ascites. Ascitic fluid contains large amount of sodium.

Jaundice: Damage to liver cells leads to increase in bilirubin resulting in jaundice.

It is a symptom common to many diseases of the liver and biliary tract and consists of a yellow pigmentation of conjunctiva, skin and body tissues because of the accumulation of bile pigments in the blood.

After 120 days of life, RBC are broken and through a complex chemical reaction, bilirubin is produced. This is excreted in stools and urine along with bile. Problems like increased destruction of red blood cells, decreased functioning of the liver or obstruction to the flow of bile from the liver can result in jaundice. Figure 18.2 shows the production of jaundice due to haemolysis, hepatitis and due to obstruction to bile passage.

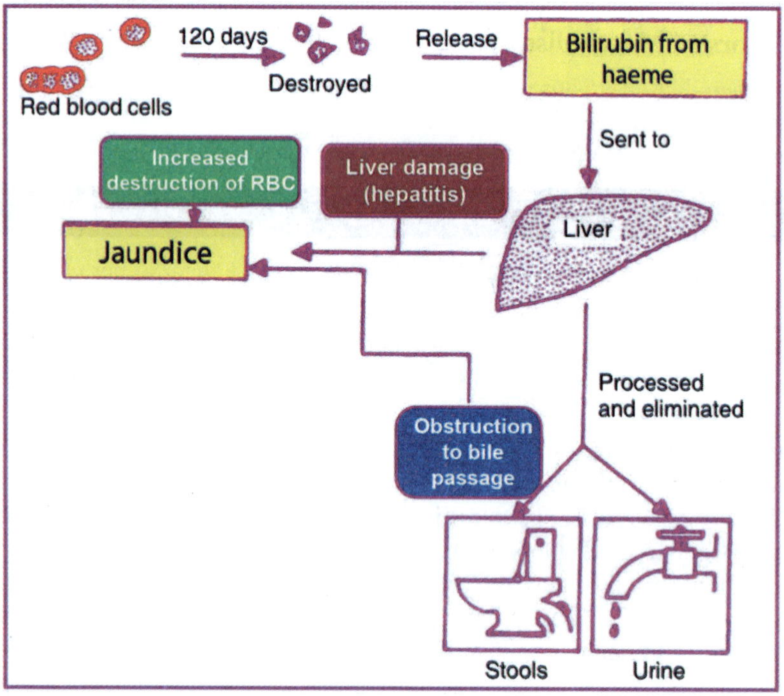

Fig. 18.2 **Causes of jaundice**

INFECTIVE HEPATITIS

Infective hepatitis is otherwise known as viral hepatitis. This is the common cause of jaundice. Hepatitis can be due to type A and E or due to B, C, D and G virus.

Symptoms

The symptoms of infective hepatitis are anorexia, fever, headache, rapid weight loss, loss of muscle tone, nausea and vomiting and abdominal discomfort. The colour of urine changes from dark yellow to red and the faeces become whitish. These develop into jaundice. The symptoms may continue for 4–8 weeks. Neglected viral hepatitis leads to cirrhosis of liver.

Acute hepatitis B, C, D and G may lead to chronic hepatitis. Hepatitis A and E are self-limiting.

Dietetic Management

A high protein, high carbohydrate and moderate fat is recommended. Small attractive meals at regular intervals are better tolerated. Overfeeding should be avoided.

Energy: In nasogastric feeding stage about 1000 kcals are supplied. In severe cases 1,600 to 2,000 kcals are suggested.

Proteins: For the liver cells to regenerate, an adequate supply of proteins is needed. Protein requirements vary according to the severity of the disease. With severe jaundice, 40 g while in mild jaundice 60–80 g of protein is permitted. With hepatic precoma and coma, protein containing foods are withheld as liver cannot metabolise protein and only high carbohydrate containing foods are recommended.

Fats: Fats make the food more palatable and increase calorie intake. During hepatic precoma and coma, due to severe liver failure, fats are not metabolised by the liver and so fat is restricted. In severe jaundice 20 g and in moderate jaundice 20-30 g of fat are recommended. In other cases of jaundice, fat needs to be restricted only if there is obstruction to bile flow that does not permit fat digestion and produces fatty diarrhoea.

Carbohydrates: High carbohydrate content in the diet is essential to supply enough calories so that tissue proteins are not broken down for energy purpose. When fever, nausea and vomiting are present, intravenous glucose is suggested. As soon as the patient can take oral feeds, intravenous feeding should be stopped and fruit juices, sugar, jaggery and honey are given not only to provide carbohydrate but also to supply adequate electrolytes.

Vitamins: They are essential to regenerate liver cells. About 500 mg of vitamin C, 10 mg of vitamin K and supplements of B complex are essential to meet the daily needs. If anorexia, nausea or vomiting is present, vitamins may be given intramuscularly.

Minerals: If food is not taken orally then a careful watch should be kept on the serum sodium and potassium levels. Oral feeds of fruit juice, vegetable and meat soups with added salt are given orally or through a nasogastric tube, maintaining the electrolyte balance. Normal serum level of sodium and potassium must be maintained through supplements.

Intravenous feeding: It may not be possible to take oral feeds with severe nausea and vomiting, intravenous administration of 10 per cent glucose solution is recommended.

Foods Included

Cereal porridge, soft chapathis, bread, rice, skimmed milk, tapioca, potato, yam, fruit, fruit juices, sugar, jaggery, honey, soft custards without butter cream and non-stimulant beverages.

Foods Avoided

Pulses, beans, meat, fish, chicken, egg, meat soups, sweet preparations where ghee, butter or oil are used, bakery products, dried fruits, nuts, spices, papads, chutney, alcoholic beverages, fried preparations, whole milk and cream.

Patients should be given enough fluid to prevent dehydration. As patients with severe hepatitis may not be able to excrete a water load, very careful monitoring of fluid balance is necessary. Patients tend to prefer small meals and these should be given frequently throughout the day.

CIRRHOSIS OF LIVER

Cirrhosis is a condition in which there is destruction of the liver cell due to necrosis, fatty infiltration, fibrosis and nodular regeneration. It is a serious and irreversible disease. Vitamin A deficiency favour the formation of cirrhosis.

The cirrhotic process may commence many years before it becomes clinically obvious and usually the patient when first seen is at a very late stage with complications, such as ascites, ruptured oesophageal varices or hepatic coma. Almost 85-90 per cent of liver damage also do not produce symptoms. The initial change in cirrhosis is widespread liver cell necrosis due to viral hepatitis, alcohol, etc. This necrosis results in collapse of the liver cells and intrahepatic shunts, due to the proximity of the hepatic artery and portal vein to the central vein. The necrosis and collapse also stimulate nodular regeneration and fibrosis. Cirrhosis of liver is the structural and functional end result of nutritional, infective or toxic changes in the liver.

Aetiology

Viral infection: The hepatitis viruses B, C, D and G are more likely to produce cirrhosis.

Alcohol: It has a direct toxic effect on the liver. It occurs after years of excessive alcohol intake in individuals whose diets are less than optimal in a number of nutrients. It is estimated that 60 g alcohol for men and 20 g for women taken daily over a prolonged period of time increases the risk of cirrhosis. A chronic alcoholic is often deficient in proteins, carbohydrates and vitamins. These make the liver highly vulnerable to any infection or toxin. Alcohol is also known to have direct action on the lipid metabolism in liver by (1) enhancing fatty acid synthesis; (2) decreasing fatty acid oxidation; (3) producing specific stimulation to triglyceride formation leading to fatty liver; (4) decreased release of lipoproteins and (5) enhanced uptake of circulating lipids.

Alcohol can cause 'deadly' damage to the liver. It enhances B and C hepatitic infections and exacerbates drug toxicity.

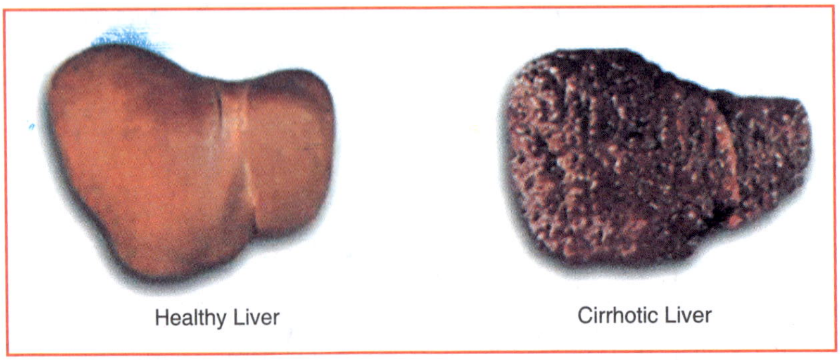

Fig. 18.3 Normal liver in comparison to liver in alcoholic cirrhosis, showing the characteristic diffuse nodularity induced by the underlying fibrous scarring

Nutrition: Malnutrition aggravates any injury to the liver particularly vitamin A, β-carotene and vitamins E and C.

Toxins of food: Aflatoxin may be one of the causes of cirrhosis. Chillies and spices are irritant foods which when absorbed are likely to damage the liver cells. However, the effect of such substances on the liver is as yet unknown. Metabolic disturbances such as haemochromatosis (no control on iron absorption) or Wilson's disease (disturbance in copper metabolism) can lead to cirrhosis of liver.

Indian childhood cirrhosis is a common disease in India. The clinical and histological features are similar to those of adult cirrhosis. Usually they are seen between the age of 1 to 3 years but even babies less than a year old may show an advanced stage of the disease.

Symptoms and Clinical Findings

The onset of cirrhosis may be gradual with gastrointestinal disturbances such as anorexia, nausea, vomiting, pain and distension. The patient may also suffer from weakness, muscle cramps, weight loss and fever. As the disease progresses jaundice and other serious changes occur.

Ascites is the accumulation of abnormal amounts of fluid in the abdomen. It may develop as a consequence of portal vein hypertension, obstruction of the hepatic vein, a fall in plasma colloid osmotic pressure due to impaired albumin synthesis, increased sodium retention or impaired water excretion.

Oesophageal varices or varicose veins in the oesophagus and upper part of the stomach may develop as a complication of portal hypertension. Haemorrhage is then an ever present danger and may be provoked by roughage of any kind.

The haemorrhage itself may be fatal or the blood may provide for the accumulation of ammonia and subsequent hepatic coma. Greater prevalence of PEM is found in alcoholic patients.

Principles of Diet

A high calorie, high protein, high carbohydrate, moderate or restricted fat, high vitamin diet helps in regeneration of liver and helps to prevent the formation of ascites. Low fat with supplementation of fat soluble vitamins and minerals should be given. Sodium should be restricted only when there is ascites.

Fibre should be restricted when there is danger of oesophageal varices and portal hypertension. The diet should be attractive and palatable.

Dietary Treatment

Energy: Consumption of food is difficult because of anorexia and ascites. The patients are usually emaciated by the time cirrhosis of the liver is diagnosed. The patient requires highly nutritious food i.e., high calorie diet is necessary because of prolonged undernourishment. The calorie requirement should be between 2000–2500 kcals.

Proteins: The serum albumin which is exclusively synthesised by the liver cells, is low in cirrhosis and aggravated by the loss of a considerable amount of albumin into ascitic fluid. A high protein diet is helpful for regeneration of the liver. In the absence of hepatic coma a high intake of proteins about 1.2 g/kg of body weight can be given. If the patient is in precoma or coma, proteins should be withheld till the patient tides over the crisis. In cirrhosis there is rapid breakdown of liver cells. The protein content of the diet varies according to the symptoms. The increased amounts of proteins can be met by the addition of casein (milk protein concentrate) which can be added in milk, soups and ice creams. Vegetable proteins containing more valine is beneficial in preventing encephalopathy.

Fats: About 20 g of fat is given. Even if fatty changes are present in the liver, fats should be given provided adequate amounts of protein is supplied. Medium chain triglycerides containing C_8 to C_{10} fatty acids can be given as these are digested and absorbed in the absence of bile salts. Coconut oil contains medium chain fatty acids.

Carbohydrates: Should be supplied liberally so that the liver may store glycogen. Liver function improves when an adequate store of glycogen is present in liver cells. Sixty per cent of the calories should come from carbohydrate so that liver damage is minimised.

Vitamins and Minerals: The liver is the major site of storage and conversion of vitamins into their metabolically active form. In cirrhosis, the liver concentration of folate, riboflavin, nicotinamide, vitamin B_{12} and vitamin A are decreased which may be due to decreased synthesis of retinol binding protein. Since vitamin D is converted to calcidiol in the liver, oral administration or injection of vitamin D in biliary cirrhosis is not successful in raising the serum level of calcidiol. Vitamin supplementation especially of B vitamins is required to prevent anaemia. Choline and methionine are useful if fatty infiltration is present. Sodium is restricted in oedema and ascites.

In all patients with cirrhotic ascites dietary sodium intake may initially be restricted to 400–800 mg/day. Restriction of fluid intake (800–1000 ml/day) is required for patients with hyponatremia (serum sodium < 125 mEq/l). If there is no ascites very little salt is permitted to make the food more appetising. Potassium salt is administered for ascites and oedema to prevent hypokalaemia. Anaemia is common among cirrhosis patients hence iron supplementation is essential. Ferrous sulphate 0.3 g tablet 3 times daily after meals should be given. Folic acid 1 mg/d orally is indicated in the treatment of macrocytic anaemia.

If patient cannot maintain a sufficient intake by eating, supplementation with sip feeding should be considered. If this is inadequate, enteral supplementation should be considered. Parenteral nutrition should be reserved for patients in whom enteral nutrition is unsuccessful and to be given only for short time. Due to risk of catheter sepsis and poor resolution of ascites parenteral nutrition is not the best choice of feeding.

Hepatic herbal supportives, antioxidants and maintenance of adequate calorie, fluid and electrolytes, fat soluble vitamins are routinely recommended.

NON ALCOHOLIC FATTY LIVER DISEASE

With increasing global prevalence of pedeatric obesity, non-alcoholic fatty liver disease has been increasing. NAFLD is a chronic liver disease that ranges from simple fatty liver to fatty liver with inflammation and fibrosis to cirrhosis. The prevalence of NAFLD has been estimated to approximate 25-30% in overweight and obese children. Most children with NAFLD who are obese with central obesity are male with cutaneous signs of insulin resistance (acanthosis nigricans) and hyperinsulinemia.

The body habitus– visceral fat/centrally located subcutaneous fat– appears to be correlated with an increased risk of liver disease and altered insulin, fat, lipoprotein and cytokine expression that may contribute to chronic liver disease in obese children and adolescents.

It is the fatty infiltration and oxidative injury to hepatocytes that results in progression of fibrosis and chronic hepatitis. Although diet and exercise are the hallmark of preventing further complications, limiting carbohydrate intake and increasing coffee consumption can also be beneficial in the long run. Fat soluble antioxidants should be given. Avoidance of products containing high fructose corn syrup in NAFLD is advisable.

HEPATIC ENCEPHALOPATHY

Complex syndrome characterised by neurologic disturbances which may develop as a complication of severe liver disease. It results from entrance of certain nitrogen containing substances such as ammonia into the cerebral circulation without being metabolised by the liver. It may be a consequence of shunting of the portal blood into the systemic circulation in cirrhosis or of severe damage to liver cells in hepatitis.

Precipitatory factors

Gastrointestinal bleeding, severe infections, surgical procedures and excessive dietary protein and sedatives may precipitate hepatic coma. Plasma aromatic amino acid levels, (phenylalanine and tyrosine) and methionine are elevated while branched-chain amino acids (isoleucine, leucine and valine) are lowered. It has been postulated that alterations in the plasma amino acid pattern may be usually related to encephalopathy.

Symptoms

Confusion, restlessness, irritability, inappropriate behaviour, delirium and drowsiness are present. There may be incoordination and a flapping tremor of the arms and legs when extended. Electrolyte imbalance occurs. The patient may go into coma and have convulsions. The breath has a faecal odour. Prompt treatment is imperative or death occurs.

Treatment

The treatment of hepatic encephalopathy is empirical and based on preventing the formation and absorption of gut-derived toxins/principally ammonia.

The prevalence of protein energy malnutrition in patients with liver disease varies according to severity of hepatic damage.

Factors that contribute to malnutrition are poor dietary intake, nutrient malabsorption excessive protein losses, impaired protein synthesis and difficulty in utilization of fuel source.

Efforts should be made to maintain normal dietary intake in patients with stable chronic liver disease. Patients with more severe liver dysfunction will require dietary modifications and nutritional supplementation.

Caloric intake: During the first 24 to 48 hours of admission with encephalopathy intra gastric or IV infusion of 100 per cent dixtrose in water can be given. The goal is to provide a source of energy that can prevent protein catabolism. Most patients improve with lactulose and with elimination of precipitating cause. They can resume oral diet which contains 30–40 kcal/kg/d.

Protein intake: A low sodium isomolar formula containing glucose, polymers, casein or soya protein hydrolysates and medium chain triglycerides is well tolerated by critically ill patients. Standard amino acids can be used. Normalization of the ratio of branched chain amino acids to aromatic amino acids improves encephalopathy, nutritional status and short term survival.

Daily protein intakes in patients with cirrhosis should be 1.0 to 1.5 g/kg. Protein restriction should be avoided in patients with hepatic encephalopathy. Some patients may require a transient restriction of daily protein intake to 0.5 g/kg. In protein intolerant patient, nitrogen should be provided in the form of an amino acid supplement.

Fuel utilisation and nitrogen economy are optimised in these patients by provision of four to seven small meals. A late-night snack of complex carbohydrate should be given. The feeding pattern should ensure even distribution of protein throughout the day thereby avoiding protein loading.

Dairy protein and vegetable proteins are better tolerated. The increased tolerance to vegetable protein diets reflects their high dietary fibre content. Fibre effects on colonic function, namely decreased transit time, increased intraluminal pH, stimulation of microbial growth and increased faecal ammonia excretion. Plama arginine and citrulline concentrations tend to be higher in patients on vegetable protein diets. This may facilitate ammonia removal via the Krebs-Henseleit cycle.

In general, patients should be encouraged to take 30–40 g of vegetable protein. Branched chain amino acids can be given to malnourished decompensated cirrhotic patients with hepatic encephalopathy who are intolerant of dietary protein.

One of the causes of hepatic encephalopathy is hyperammonemia along with other pathological conditions. Besides the urea cycle of liver, BCAA supplementation is proven to enhance detoxification of ammonia in skeletal muscles. Thus, BCAA may have therapeutic effects in hepatic encephalopathy patients and help to improve the efficacy in treatment.

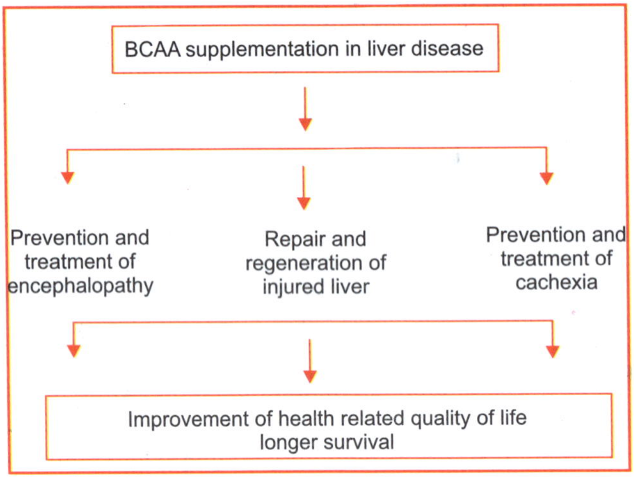

Fig. 18.4 Three possible targets of BCAA supplementation in treatment of liver disease.

Dietary Guidelines

A wholesome well-balanced diet maintains the health of liver and minimise further damage. It can also help immune system and fight off illness.

- A healthy calorie intake should be maintained.
- Vegetable and dairy proteins are preferred.
- If needed dietary supplements containing certain types of amino acids can be included.

- Diet should include whole grains at least five servings of fruits and vegetables of varying colours.
- Salt, sugar and fatty foods should be restricted.
- A minimum of 6–8 glasses of fluids per day should be taken. In addition to water, juices, tea, milk and soups can be taken.
- Small and frequent meals should be taken and long periods of fasting is avoided.

LIVER TRANSPLANTATION

Liver transplantation is now a viable alternative for patients with end-stage hepatic failure. Obesity is a major risk factor in the development of NASH, Nonalcoholic steatohepatitis, a precursor to cirrhosis. Diabetes and hyperinsulinism may also play a role in the development of NASH. Alcohol is a major contributor to cirrhosis and the need for transplantation.

Pretransplantation and Nutrition Recommendations

The following factors to be considered.

- Malnutrition, oedema and ascites to be corrected.
- Electrolyte imbalance to be corrected.
- Nutritional support need to be provided to normalize nitrogen balance and other nutrients.
- Blood glucose to be normalised
- Abnormal amino acid metabolism to be corrected. Serum ammonia to be corrected.
- Protein – 1-1.5 g/kg; Energy 35-45 kcal/kg. vitamins and minerals RDA levels should be given

Pretransplant diet

Foods to be included	*Food to be restricted/avoided*
High protein foods – lean cuts of meat, poultry and egg white. Low fat milk and milk products.	Saturated and transfat – ghee, butter, vanaspathi.
Soya protein – flour milk, tofu chunks, Brown rice, Nuts and seeds, Avocado and rolled oats, Lentils, chickpeas.	Foods rich in sodium – Table salt (3g/day). Salted snacks
High intake of complex and simple carbohydrate vegetable oils.	Pickles, papads
	Ajinomoto
	Bakery items.

Post transplantation Nutrition and Diet Recommendations

Early postoperative nutrition is clearly beneficial following liver transplantation in terms of morbidity. Nutrition should be given preferably by the enteral route as early as possible.

With the exception of potentially elevated nitrogen requirements transplanted patients do not differ from surgical patients in general with regard to macronutrient requirements. Micronutrient and electrolyte status should be monitored in order to identify and correct deficiency.

High calorie, high protein diet is given after transplant. Nutritional deficiencies are to be corrected immediately after transplant phase. Excessive weight gain is avoided. Hyperlipidemia can be controlled by statins and fibrates taking into consideration comorbidities and drug interaction. Close monitoring may be required.

Nutrition aspects are important both for patients awaiting liver transplantation and for those who live or with a liver graft. While pre-transplant patients are those in the immediate post-transplant period usually require correction of numerous nutritional deficiencies to improve their overall condition, post transplant liver patients have to be followed up to ensure they do not develop over nutrition.

- Diet should be low in cholesterol and saturated fat.
- Adequate calcium and vitamin D intake to be given as transplant medications interfere with absorption of calcium.
- Blood sugar levels need to be controlled.
- High drug levels are to be avoided and water is the best liquid to use after medications.
- Magnesium blood levels need to be maintained as absorption of it affected by transplant medication.
- High blood potassium need to be prevented.
- Safe food handling practices need to be emphasised to reduce risk of infection.

Good nutrition is an important part for complete recovery following transplant.

CHOLECYSTITIS AND CHOLELITHIASIS

Cholelithiasis or gallstones are rare in rural areas of developing countries. Although genetic factors are involved, environmental factors seem to be important. Hypertriglyceridaemia is strongly associated with cholelithiasis, independently of obesity.

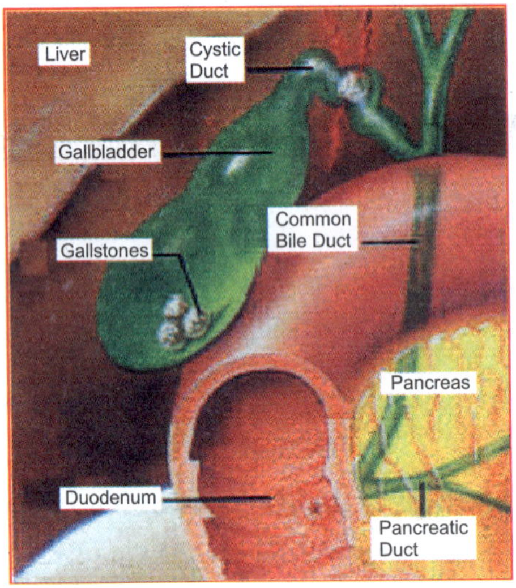

Fig. 18.5 Gallbladder with Gallstones

Inflammation of gall bladder, cholecystitis, occurs usually from a low grade chronic infection. When mucosal changes occur in cholecystitis, the absorptive powers of the gall bladder may be altered, affecting the solubility ratios of the bile ingredients. Excess water or excess bile acid may be absorbed under abnormal absorptive conditions. Cholesterol may precipitate causing gallstones called cholelithiasis. High dietary fat intake over a long period predisposes to gallstones. Dietary deficiency of fibre may cause gallstones. Sugars and rapidly digestible starch operating via hyperinsulinemia may cause gallstones. There is no evidence that a high intake of cholesterol promotes gallstones.

Table 18.2 Conditions and probable causes of Cholelithiasis

Conditions	*Probable cause*
Obesity	Hypersecretion of cholesterol into bile
Hypertriglyceridaemia	Hypersecretion of cholesterol into bile
Constipation (slow colonic transit)	Altered composition of bile salts pool
Multiparity	Gallbladder stasis
Cirrhosis of liver	Hyposecretion of bile salts
Resection of disease of terminal ileum	Hyposecretion of bile salts (which escape reabsorption) and/or gallbladder stasis
Abdominal surgery	Gallbladder stasis
Total parenteral nutrition	Gallbladder stasis
Oestrogen, progesteron and fibrates	Hypersecretion of cholesterol

Source: Garrow J.S. *et al.*; 2000, Human Nutrition and Dietetics, Churchill Livingstone, Edinburgh.

Diabetes, obesity, cholesterol lowering drugs, rapid weight loss, fasting, being female and over 60 are some risk factors of cholelithiasis. An expansion in a woman's waistline of 36″ or more are at risk of suffering from gallstones and would require surgery. Waist to hip ratio > 0.86 has more chances of developing gallstones than those with a ratio of 0.70 or less. Fat which is abdominally distributed is the risk factor for gallstones. Crash slimming diets are a potent cause of gallstones.

When inflammation, and/or stones are present in the gallbladder, contraction from the cholecystokinin mechanism causes pain, sometimes the pain is severe. There is fullness and distension after eating and particular difficulty with fatty foods.

Hepatic herbal supportives, antioxidants, liver cell membrane protectives and maintenance of adequate calorie, fluid and electrolytes, vitamins, especially fat soluble vitamins are routinely recommended. A moderate intake of alcohol protects against cholelithiasis.

Removal of gall bladder by surgery, cholesystectomy, is usually indicated. If patient is obese, some weight loss before surgery is advisable. Thus the supportive therapy is largely nutritional. Fat is the principal cause of contraction of the diseased organ and consequent pain. It must be greatly reduced to 20 g/day and energy should be derived chiefly from carbohydrate.

Foods included are cereals in a soft form, cooked rice, chapathi, bread and idli, milk pudding, milk shakes, curds, cooked or pureed vegetables, kichidi and porridge. Pulses, beans, meat, fruit, fruit juices, fish and chicken, soft cooked eggs can also be given. These foods are high in energy and protein and help in regeneration of liver cells.

PANCREATITIS

Pancreatitis is inflammation in the pancreas. The pancreas produces enzymes that help digestion and hormones that regulate body processes. Pancreatitis can occur as acute – lasting for days or can occur as chronic which may last over many years.

Pancreatitis occurs when digestive enzymes become activated while still in the pancreas irritating the cells of pancreas and causing inflammation.

Conditions that lead to pancreatitis are alcoholism, gallstones, abdominal surgery, certain medications, cigarette smoking, hypercalcaemia due to overactive parathyroid gland, hypertriglyceridemia, infection and pancreatitis can also occur due to family history.

Both acute and chronic pancreatitis can cause pancreas to produce fewer of the enzymes that are needed to breakdown and process nutrients. This can lead to malnutrition, diarrhoea and weight loss inspite of eating normally.

Acute Pancreatitis

In acute pancreatitis there is upper abdominal pain, fever, nausea and vomiting. In the mild form, care includes withholding food and drink and administering IV fluids and parenteral analgesia. Bowel rest reduces pain. When there is pain and abdominal tenderness, small meals composed primarily of carbohydrate may be attempted. Carbohydrate causes less pancreatic stimulation than protein or fat. Advancement of oral diet prolongs length of stay in the hospital due to relapse of symptoms.

When initiating specialized nutrition therapy, enteral nutrition is the preferred route over parenteral nutrition for patients admitted with acute severe pancreatitis. In comparison to PN, use of EN may hasten the resolution of the disease process and favourably affect the patient outcome.

Impaired microcirculation may be a major factor contributing to pancreatic necrosis; thus aggressive fluid resuscitation is needed.

Eighty per cent of patients with acute pancreatitis who are admitted to a hospital recover with a few days of IV fluids and bowel rest. These patients are often not malnourished and resume an oral diet within 5 to 7 days. IV lipid emulsions are safe in acute pancreatitis provided triglyceride levels are monitored and remain below 400 mg/dl.

Chronic Pancreatitis

Chronic pancreatitis is defined as a continuing inflammatory disease of the pancreas characterized by the irreversible morphological changes that typically cause abdominal pain and/or permanent impairment of pancreatic function.

Chronic pancreatitis present as repeated attacks of mild to moderately severe abdominal pain or persistent and intractable abdominal and back pain. Both diabetes and steatorrhoea occur commonly with calcified pancreatitis. Weight loss may also be caused by avoidance of food, as pain is frequently exacerbated after eating.

Chronic pancreatitis causes hypermetabolism. The nutrition therapy of such patients should be of high calorie (35 kcal/kg) high protein (1.0 to 1.5 g/kg) and rich in carbohydrates with moderate amounts of fats in order to minimise symptoms of underlying disease. The intake of carbohydrates should be monitored when it is evident that diabetes is present. Normally vegetable fats are better tolerated than animal fats. Medium chain triglycerides may be used to increase fat absorption because they need minimal digestion and do not require lipase, colipase and bile salts.

Medium chain triglycerides have a lower energy density than long chain triglycerides and quite foul-tasting. Associated adverse effects can include cramps, nausea and diarrhoea. MCTs should be increased slowly according to the tolerance of the patient.

Oral nutrition therapy should be low in fibre because fibre may absorb pancreatic enzymes and delay the absorption of nutrients. Fat-soluble vitamins (A, D, E and K), vitamin B_{12} and micronutrients including antioxidants should be replaced as clinically indicated. Calcium and vitamin D supplements within the physiologic dosage range are recommended for vitamin D deficiency to prevent bone disease even in the face of pancreatic calcifications.

Elemental formulas or enteral formulas consisting of predigested products and low-fat content are beneficial for patients with chronic pancreatitis. These products generally cannot be consumed because of their taste.

Lipase supplements reduce steatorrhoea in chronic pancreatitis patients. Nutrition therapy has always been considered part of the treatment of chronic pancreatitis because of the frequent malnutrition associated with the disease. Jejunal feeding improves weight, reduces narcotic use and improves patient's quality of life.

To keep pancreas healthy, high cholesterol, high calcium diets and excess consumption of alcohol should be avoided.

World Liver day is on 19th April.

World Hepatitis Day is on 28th July.

SUGGESTED READINGS

- Eibl Guido *et al.*, Diabetes Mellitus and obesity as risk factors for pancreatic cancer, J. Acad. Nutr. Diet. 2018; **118**.
- Mager R Diana *et al.*, Anthropometric Measures of Visceral and Subcataneous Fat are important in the Determination of Metabolic Dysregulation in Boys and Girls at Risk for Nonalcoholic Fatty Liver Disease, Nutrition in Clinical Practice aspen, 2013; **28**.
- Kawaguchi Tutenmi *et al.*, Effect of oral BCAAs on hepatic encephalopathey. Nutrition in Clinical Practice, 2013; **28**.
- Rahini S. Robert and Carmeu Landavede, Non-alcoholic fatty liver disease and the metabolic syndrome: Clinical implications and treatment. Nutrition in Clinical Practice 2013; **28**.

QUESTIONS

1. Mention three basic functions of liver that are affected in cirrhosis.
2. State the factors that cause obstructive and infective jaundice.
3. List three basic symptoms in a jaundice patient.
4. State the principles involved in planning diets for patients suffering from (*a*) infective hepatitis (*b*) cirrhosis of liver.
5. Write a note on hepatic encephalopathy.
6. Give a day's diet for a patient with infective hepatitis.
7. Explain the agents responsible for liver damage and discuss the damage caused to the liver.
8. Bring out the relationship between alcohol and cirrhosis of liver.
9. Write a short note on cholecystitis.
10. Give in detail nutritional support required in acute and chronic pancreatitis.
11. Explain dietary treatment in nonalcoholic fatty liver disease.

19

Diet in Diabetes Mellitus

Diabetes mellitus is a chronic metabolic disorder that prevents the body to utilise glucose completely or partially. It is characterised by raised glucose concentration in the blood and alterations in carbohydrate, protein and fat metabolism. This condition can be due to failure in the formation of insulin or liberation or action. Insulin is produced by the β cells of the islets of Langerhan of pancreas, any decrease in the number of functioning cells will decrease the amount of insulin that can be synthesised. Many diabetics can produce sufficient insulin but some stimulus to the islets tissue is needed. It is an autoimmune disease.

The hormones of the anterior pituitary, adrenal cortex, thyroid and α cells of the islets of Langerhans are glycogenic, that is, they increase the supply of glucose. Possibly they could increase the demand, decrease the secretion or antagonise and inhibit the action of insulin. The body releases hormones that raise blood glucose levels to provide a quick source of energy for coping with stress. During stress conditions diabetes mellitus may precipitate if genetically predisposed.

PREVALENCE

Indians get diabetes mellitus at a lower body weight and the onset of the disease is much earlier than other countries. Around 20–25 per cent of Indian diabetes are not over weight. More than 90 per cent of all diabetics belong to type 2 diabetes.

TYPES

Type 1

Type 1 diabetes mellitus, also known as juvenile onset diabetes or insulin dependent diabetes. There is usually sudden onset and occur in the younger age group. It is an autoimmune disease, as a result of an overactive immune response of the body against substances and tissues normally present in the body. In type I diabetes body's immune system, which normally helps in fighting infection, attacks and destroys the insulin producing β-cells of pancreas. As a result there is little or no production of insulin and hence such individuals require daily insulin injections. This may be caused by virus or due to autoimmunity. The child is usually underweight. Acidosis is fairly common. In older group there is slower onset of the disease which is referred to as latent auto immune diabetes of adults-LADA.

Type 2

Type 2 diabetes mellitus, adult onset diabetes, is called non-insulin dependent diabetes. It is the most common form of diabetes and develops slowly and is usually milder and more stable. Insulin may be produced by pancreas but action is impaired. This form occurs mainly in adults and the person is usually overweight. Acidosis is infrequent. The majority of patients improve with weight loss and are maintained on diet therapy. Women who have had large babies or large families are also prone to develop this type of diabetes later in life.

By far the majority of people world wide have type 2 diabetes mellitus. This is characterised by insulin resistance with relative insulin deficiency. Centrally distributed abdominal body is known to increase insulin resistance.

Prediabetes

Prediabetes is defined as a state of abnormal glucose homeostasis in which glucose levels are elevated above those considered normal but not high enough to meet the criteria required for the diagnosis of diabetes.

It is charecterized by impaired fasting glucose (IFG) and/or impaired glucose tolerance. In obsesity prediabetes occurs.

The pathophysiologic defects underlying prediabetes include insulin resistance, β-cell dysfunction, increased lipolysis, inflammation, suboptimal incretin effect and hepatic glucose overproduction.

These metabolic dearrangements associated with concomitant obesity cause endothelial vasodilator and fibrinolytic dysfunction, leading to increased risk of macrovascular and microvascular complications. Prediabetes has also been associated with increased risk of cancer and dementia.

Lifestyle interventions including diet and exercise are first-line treatments. Medications have shown benefits.

According to WHO guidelines for prediabetes $HbA1_C$ is 5.7 to 6.4 for diabetes it is ≥ 6.5 percent.

AETIOLOGY

Pattern of inheritance and the environmental factors differ in type 1 and type 2 diabetes mellitus. Type 1 and type 2 can coexist in the same family and in the same individual.

Type 1 diabetes mellitus

Genetics

The inheritance of human type 1 diabetes mellitus is polygenic. It has been estimated that over 50 per cent of the heritability is contributed by the HLA class II genes (chromosome 6).

Environmental Factors

Infections: Infections cause a non-specific outpouring of catabolic hormones which antagonise insulin action and then may trigger the onset of the disorder.

There is increasing evidence that type 1 diabetes, especially in the younger patients, follows a coxsackie or other virus infection. There is sometimes a long interval between infection and the onset of symptoms. The virus may trigger an autoimmune reaction in the pancreatic islets and this impairs insulin secretion and ultimately destroys the β cells.

Acute stress: The normal glucose homeostasis in the body is achieved by a delicate interplay of various hormones. The body releases adrenaline, noradrenaline and cortisol hormones that raise blood glucose levels to provide a quick source of energy for coping with stress. In acute cases of stress, blood glucose levels may rise quite profoundly and in extreme cases diabetic ketosis and coma also may result particularly among those with a genetic predisposition.

Physical injury, surgery and emotional distress sometimes precede the first symptoms of diabetes. Like infection, these cause a sudden increase in secretion of catabolic hormones which may precipitate the disorder.

Immunological Factor: Type 1 diabetes mellitus is a slow autoimmune disease and is associated with other autoimmune disorders. Hyperglycaemia accompanied by classical symptoms of diabetes occurs only when 90 per cent of insulin secreting cells are already destroyed.

Type 2 diabetes mellitus

Genetics

Indians have a high genetic risk for diabetes. Genetic factors are more important in the development of this type of diabetes than in type 1 diabetes.

Type 2 diabetes mellitus is commonly associated with obesity, hypertension and hyperlipidemia. In all this, insulin resistance being the primary defect known as syndrome X or metabolic syndrome. Type 2 diabetes occurs in subjects who are obese insulin-resistant accompanied by impaired β cell function. Therefore, it seems likely that type 2 diabetes represents a combination of major and minor genes affecting insulin secretion, insulin action and obesity.

Environmental Factors

Life style: Type 2 diabetes is associated with people who are obese, underactive who overeat. The majority of middle aged diabetic patients are obese but only a few obese people develop diabetes. Obesity probably acts as a diabetogenic factor through increasing resistance to the action of insulin among those genetically predisposed to develop type 2 diabetes. Recently, resistin, a cysteine rich secretory protein has been implicated at the molecular link between obesity and type 2 diabetes.

Higher intake of refined grains which have high GI such as white rice, combined with sedentary activity could be major reason for the incidence of obesity, diabetes and cardiovascular disease epidemic in India. The diet of South Indian adult is high in refined cereals low in fibre, fruits and vegetables compared to the standards set by FAO/WHO.

The thrifty phenotype, 'small and thin' Indian babies possess relatively more body fat. A combination of poor intrauterine nutrition and subsequent obesity is strongly associated with Insulin Resistant Syndrome (IRS).

Life style factors modulators of inflammation:

- High carbohydrate intake and high glycaemic load
- High saturated and transfatty acids
- High intake of caffeine
- Alcoholic stress
- Insufficient intake of micronutrients and antioxidants
- Low fibre diet
- Sedentary life style
- Overweight

Age: Type 2 diabetes is principally a disease of the middle age and elderly. Half of all new cases of type 2 diabetes occur among people over age 45.

Abdominal fat: People with a high waist/hip ratio—indicating that fat is largely in the abdomnial cavity—have a greater risk of diabetes than people with a similar amount of fat distributed peripherally. This probably relates to the insulin insensitivity which is caused by a high flux of free fatty acids in the portal circulation, since intra-abdominal fat cells can release fatty acids very rapidly. Diabetes can be predicted in people who have waist circumference ≥ 90 cms.

Insulin Resistance

Insulin resistance is a characteristic feature of Indians. Insulin resistance, the inability of the body to control blood glucose with normal levels of insulin is associated with obesity and non-insulin dependant diabetes mellitus. Insulin resistance may be due to an abnormal insulin molecule, an excessive amount of circulating antagonists and target tissue defects. The last is the common cause of insulin resistance in NIDDM and seems to be the predominant abnormality among those with more severe hyperglycaemia. Insulin resistance is associated with a high amount of refined grain consumption leading to higher dietary glycaemic load.

Subclinical zinc deficiency could be prevalent in India which might be contributing to insulin resistance. There seems to be a role of subclinical micronutrient deficiency in this phenotype of central obesity and increased insulin resistance among Indians. Of the micronutrients, zinc has been shown to promote insulin sensitivity, protein synthesis and also reduce fat deposition apart from modulating chemokine response.

Pollution, pesticide residues, radiation, textile dyes jeopardize human health and endocrine disruption.

Table 19.1 gives comparative clinical features of type 1 diabetes and type 2 diabetes.

Table 19.1 Comparative features of type 1 and type 2 diabetes mellitus

Factor	*Type I diabetes mellitus*	*Type II diabetes mellitus*
Age of onset	Juvenile onset (< 20 years)	Maturity onset (> 30 years)
Sex	M:F = 1:1	India M > F
Incidence	10% of Diabetics	90% of Diabetics
Genetic Locus	chromosome 6	chromosome 11
Genetic predisposition	Mild or moderate	Very strong
Mode of onset	Abrupt	Usually gradual
Body weight	Normal or underweight	Obese (80%) or non-obese
Defect	Insulin deficiency due to destruction of β-cells	Impairment in the production of insulin by β-cells and/or resistance of target cells to insulin
Ketoacidosis	Prone	Resistant or rare
Plasma insulin	Low or absent	Usually depressed but may be raised
Islet auto-immune disease	Present at onset (50–85%)	Absent or very low (10%)
Insulin need	Dependent (ketosis without insulin)	May be required by 20 to 30 per cent to control hyperglycaemia
Oral hypoglycaemic agents Treatment	Rarely efficacious treatment Insulin is mandatory	Efficacious Can be controlled by diet, exercise and hypoglycaemia agents

To maintain normal blood glucose if the requirement of insulin decreases it is an indication of reduction in insulin resistance or greater insulin sensitivity.

SYMPTOMS

A deficient supply of functioning insulin affects the metabolism of carbohydrates, fats, proteins, electrolytes and water and the consequences of impairments are complex.

Hyperglycaemia: When insulin is not being produced or is ineffective, the formation of glycogen is decreased and the utilisation of glucose in the peripheral tissues is reduced. As a consequence, the glucose that enters the circulation from various sources is removed more slowly and hyperglycaemia follows. This is further accentuated by gluconeogenesis.

Glycosuria: When blood glucose level exceeds the renal threshold i.e., 160 to 180 mg per 100 ml glycosuria occurs.

Fluid and electrolyte imbalance: The loss of glucose in the urine represents a wastage of energy and entails an increased elimination of water and sodium.

Table 19.2 Consequences and clinical features of change in metabolism

Metabolism	*Consequences*	*Clinical features*
Carbohydrate metabolism Diminished uptake of glucose by tissues such as muscle, adipose tissue and liver	Hyperglycaemia	Polyuria, polydipsia polyphagia, fatigue, muscle weakness
Over production of glucose glycogenolysis and glyconeogenesis	Hyperglycaemia	Pruritis, blurred vision, diminished mental alertness
Protein metabolism		
Diminished uptake of aminoacids and diminished synthesis of protein	Negative nitrogen balance, Elevated levels of branched chain amino acids, elevated blood urea nitrogen level	Loss of muscle mass, weakness
Increased proteolysis level	Elevated potassium	
Fat metabolism		
Increased lipolysis	Elevated plasma fatty acid level, Elevated plasma glycerol level	Loss of adipose tissue, nausea and vomiting
Decreased lipogenesis	Elevated plasma ketones	Abdominal pain Acetone in breath xanthoma
Increased production of triglycerides	Hypertriglyceridaemia	Exudative (skin lesions) lipaemia, retinitis, pancreatitis (abdominal pain)
Decreased removal of triglycerides	Metabolic acidosis	Hyperventilation Rapid breathing

Acidosis: With a deficiency of insulin, lipogenesis decreases and lipolysis is greatly increased, these effects being of both immediate and long-range consequences. The fatty acids released from adipose tissue or available by absorption from the intestinal tract are oxidized by the liver to form 'ketone bodies' including acetoacetic acid, β-hydroxybutyric acid and acetone. The liver utilises only limited quantities of ketones and releases them to circulation.

In diabetes mellitus the ketones are produced at a rate that far exceeds the ability of tissues to utilise them and the concentration in blood is greatly increased. Acetone is excreted by the lungs and gives the characteristic fruity odour to breath. Acetoacetic acid and β-hydroxy butyric acid are excreted in the urine (ketonuria). Being fairly strong organic acids these ketones combine with base so that the alkaline reserve is depleted and acidosis results.

Polyuria and Nocturia: Glycosuria occurs when the blood glucose level is 180 mg/dl. Glucose increases the osmolality of the glomerular filtrate and thus prevents the reabsorption of water as the filtrate passes down the renal tubules. In this way the volume of urine is markedly increased in diabetes and polyuria and nocturia occur.

Polydipsia and Polyphagia: Polyuria leads to loss of water and electrolytes which results in thirst and polydipsia. Patient feels excess hunger as glucose is lost in urine and tissues are starved of glucose.

Dehydration: As the blood glucose rises, the extracellular fluid becomes hypertonic and water leaves the cells. If the loss of water and electrolytes continue, depletion of extracellular fluid leads to the clinical features of severe dehydration.

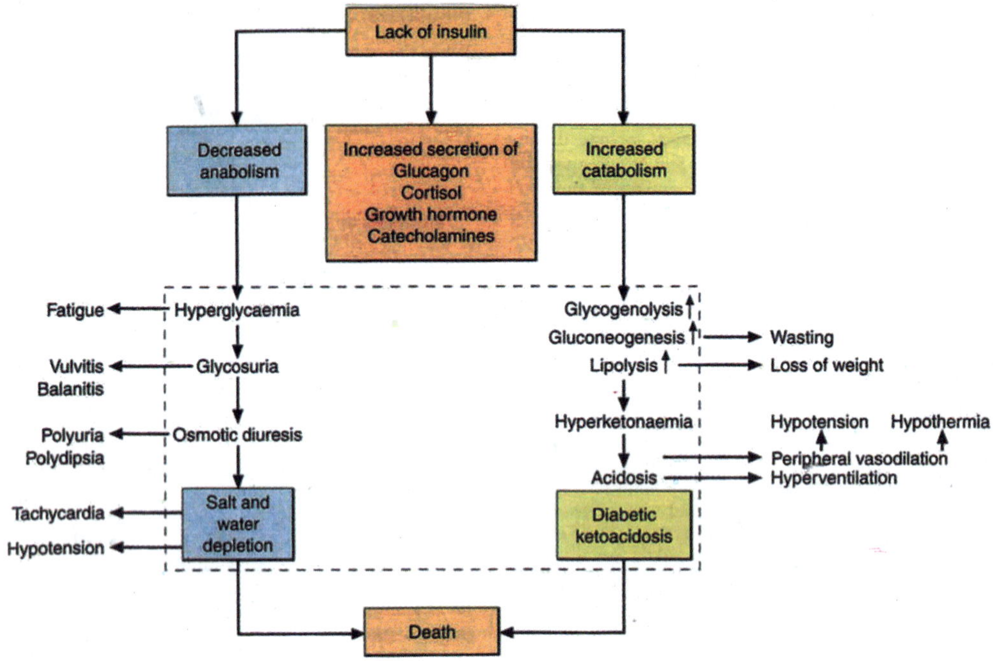

Fig. 19.1 **Pathophysiological basis of the symptoms and signs of untreated or uncontrolled diabetes mellitus**

Source: Edwards, C.R. W. lan A.D. Bouchier *et al.*, 1995, Davidson's principles and practice of medicine, Churchill Livingstone, Edinburgh.

Fatigue and loss of weight: Impaired utilization of carbohydrate results in a sense of fatigue and two compensatory mechanisms operate to provide alternative metabolic substrate. This leads to loss of body tissue and wasting which may occur inspite of a normal or even increased intake of food. This is added to any loss of weight resulting from loss of fluid.

Increased excretion of potassium, magnesium and phosphorus: Glycogen and protein present are associated with water and intracellular electrolytes. As glycogen and protein are catabolised, glucose, water and electrolytes, particularly potassium are released into the extracellular space. An increased urinary excretion of potassium, magnesium and phosphorus therefore occurs in uncontrolled diabetes.

DIAGNOSIS

Several tests are used for diagnosis of diabetes.

Glycosuria

The presence of an abnormal amount of sugar in the urine, should be regarded as evidence of diabetes until proved otherwise. It is necessary to observe the following procedure to detect early diabetes:

- Urine is voided just before the meal.
- Breakfast or lunch is taken with usual helpings of carbohydrate rich foods such as bread, chapathis, rice, fruits and sweets.
- Urine is voided two or three hours after the meal and examined for sugar.

Glucose specific dip-stick methods are the best. Diastix (Ames and Co) consists of a paper stick impregnated with an enzyme preparation which give a semi-quantitative estimate of glycosuria (0.25 to 2.0%) when dipped in urine containing glucose.

Some undoubtedly diabetic people have a negative test owing to a raised renal threshold and non-diabetics with a low renal threshold may give rise to a false positive test.

Interpretation of Benedict's test is given in Table 19.3.

Table 19.3 Interpretation of Benedict's test

Colour	Report	Approximate sugar in Urine g %	Approximate sugar in Blood mg %
Green discolouration	0 to trace	—	< 200
Green precipitate	+	0.25	200–250
Greenish-yellow precipitate	++	0.5	250–300
Yellowish-orange precipitate	+++	1.0	300–350
Brick red precipitate	++++	> 2.0	> 350

Ketonuria

The amount of ketone bodies normally excreted by healthy persons are not detected by routine methods. High amounts excreted can be detected in the urine by nitroprusside reaction which is conveniently carried out using Acetest tablets or Ketostix paper sticks (Ames and Co).

If both ketonuria and glycosuria are found, the diagnosis of diabetes is practically certain.

Random Blood Sugar

In many cases, diabetes can be diagnosed by a single blood estimation, which may be used as a confirmatory test when a classical symptom suggest the diagnosis. A random blood glucose exceeding 200 mg/dl is almost certain to indicate diabetes.

According to WHO recommendations, in a patient with overt symptoms of diabetes, a fasting or random plasma glucose measurement is often sufficient for the diagnosis of diabetes. If the fasting plasma glucose is greater than 126 mg/dl or the random plasma glucose is greater than 200 mg/dl on more than two occasions, diagnosis of diabetes may be made.

Glucose Tolerance Test

Oral glucose tolerance test is a confirmatory test. Expert committee on diabetes of the WHO recommends for the test that 75 g to be used as the glucose load for adults and 1.75 g/kg body weight for children with maximum of 75 g.

All medications should be stopped for at least three days before the test.

- The fasting blood sample is drawn.
- 75 g of glucose dissolved in 250–300 ml of water is given. Lemon juice may be added for flavour and to prevent nausea.

- Blood and urine specimens are collected every 30 minutes for 2 hours after the administration of glucose.

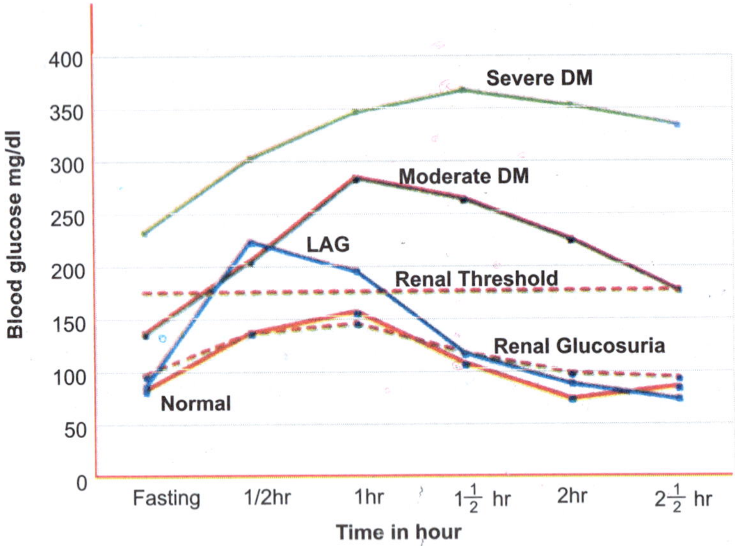

Fig. 19.2 Oral Glucose Tolerance Test (OGTT)

Note initial blood sugar levels, peak values and values after two hours in normal and diabetic patient. Also note the diabetic curve goes beyond renal threshold.

Impaired Glucose Tolerance

When the glycaemic response, after the administration of 75 g of oral glucose load, is intermediate between normal and diabetic, that condition is described as impaired glucose tolerance. Individuals with impaired glucose tolerance are generally free from symptoms of diabetes. However, they have the potential to develop diabetes at a later stage; they should be more careful in their diet and avoid obesity. In addition, they should undertake regular exercise.

Criteria set down by the WHO expert committee on diabetes mellitus for blood glucose levels is given in Table 19.4.

Table 19.4 Criteria for the diagnosis of diabetes and intermediate hyperglycaemia, WHO

	Fasting plasma mg/dl	*2 hrs after glucose load mg/dl*
Diabetes	≥ 126	> 200
Impaired glucose tolerance, IGT	126	140–200
Impaired fasting glucose, IFG	110–125	< 140
Normal	< 110	< 140

TREATMENT

Diabetes can be treated by diet alone or diet and hypoglycemic drugs or diet plus insulin depending on the type and severity of the condition. Regular exercise is essential for all diabetics.

Clinical Criteria

- Relief from symptoms.
- Reduction in obesity (overweight) and maintenance of normal body weight depending upon height and built.
- Prevention or reduction of both acute and chronic complications of diabetes.
- Adequate energy and endurance for work performance.
- In childhood diabetes, normal or near normal growth and development including physical, mental, emotional and sexual development.
- In gestational diabetes, delivery of a normal baby without any medical complications for the mother.

Bio-chemical Criteria

- Urine sugar testing.
- Repeated blood glucose estimation is the most effective and reliable method to assess the degree of control of diabetes.
- Urine should be tested for ketones in insulin dependent diabetics.

Table 19.5 Degree of control of diabetes

Status	*Degree of control*		
	Good	*Fair*	*Poor*
	Blood glucose in mg/dl		
Fasting	< 110	110–130	> 130
2 hours after meal	< 130	130–150	> 150

- 24 hours urinary glucose excretion is a useful test for assessing control of diabetes in children.
- $HbA1_C$ (Glycosylated Haemoglobin) estimation, gives an excellent indication of overall control over preceding 3 months period. As the concentration of glucose in blood rises, more of it gets attached to haemoglobin and the combined molecule is chemically estimated as glycosylated haemoglobin. In a normal population, the glycosylated haemoglobin concentrations vary from 4–7 per cent, while in diabetes it is in the range of 8–18% of the total haemoglobin depending on the blood sugar level.
- Serum lipid profile should be maintained within normal range.

$HbA1_C$ reflects average blood glucose concentrations over ~2–3 months, it does not address glycemic variability or hyperglycemic and hypoglycemic events.

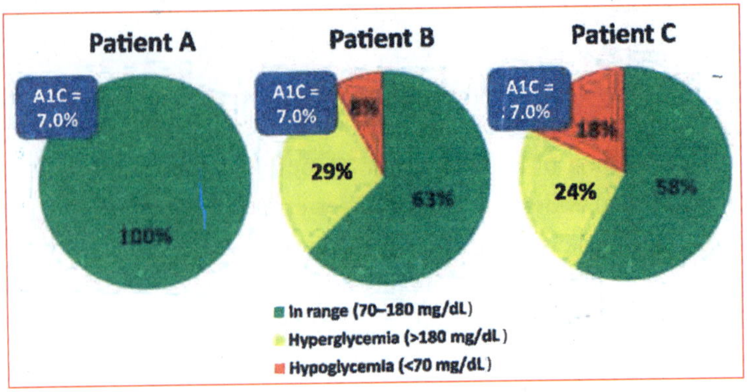

Fig. 19.3 **A depiction showing how patients with the same $A1_C$ value may experience different levels of blood sugar.**

Source: clinicaldiabetesminerals.org

Blood Glucose Monitoring

The overall goal of diabetes management is to achieve as near normal physiological or ideal plasma glucose values as possible without having detrimental effect on quality of life. Glucose control should be achieved without causing significant hypoglycaemia.

This helps in checking the effects of food, activity and insulin on blood sugar. Blood glucose monitoring technology measures the glucose content of a blood sample by means of an electrical current produced in the test strip and sent to the meter for measurement.

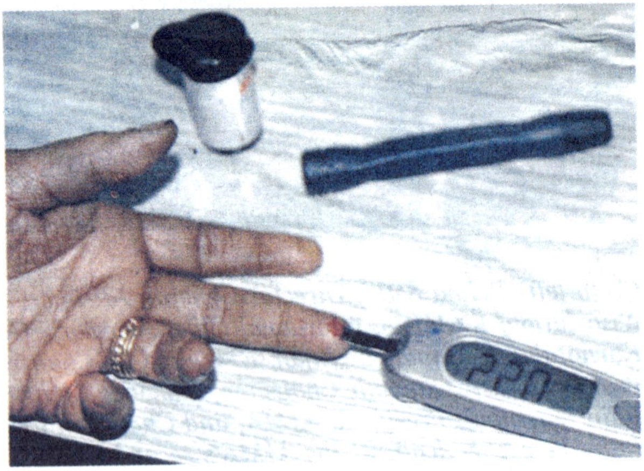

Fig. 19.4 **Blood glucose meter**

Continuous glucose monitoring (CGM) provides comprehensive assessment of daily glucose measurements for patients with diabetes and can reveal high and low blood glucose values that may occur even when a patient's $A1_C$ is adequately controlled.

Monitoring of metabolic parameters, including glucose, A1C, lipids, blood pressure, body weight, and renal function is essential to assess the need for changes in therapy and to ensure successful outcomes.

Management of Diabetes

Objectives

- To improve blood glucose and lipid levels. Blood glucose levels should not go too low or too high.
- To promote consistent day-to-day intake for people with insulin dependent diabetes and weight management for people with noninsulin dependent type.
- To encourage healthy eating habits.

The main modes of treatment of diabetes are

- Diet
- Oral hypoglycaemic drugs
- Physical activity
- Education.

DIET

Dietary measures are an essential part of the treatment of diabetic patients, whether they are on diet alone or on sulphonylurea drug or insulin. If a fixed daily intake is to be achieved an exchange system is necessary.

There should be of weight and waist circumference. Significant weight loss > 15 percent is accompanied by diabetes remission. Life style intervension at early stage reverses type 2 diabetes and has long term health benefit.

Food Exchange Lists

The diet for diabetic patient is prescribed in terms of exchange lists. Food exchange lists are groups of measured foods of the same calorific value and similar protein, fat and carbohydrate and can be substituted one for another in a meal plan. All foods of exchange make a specific contribution to a good diet. None of the exchange groups can itself supply all the nutrients needed for a well balanced diet.

The food exchange lists help the patient (*a*) to restrict the food intake according to the insulin prescription so that both hyperglycaemia and hypoglycaemia can be prevented (*b*) to have variety in the diet so that he can adhere to it always and (*c*) easy learning of the principles of diet. Since diabetes is a chronic disease patient need to be educated regarding diet prescription and food exchange list helps in this. By following the food exchange list, the patient can also maintain body weight.

Diet and Insulin

The philosophy of diet therapy for the juvenile diabetic is that while in a healthy child, the insulin secretion matches the food intake, in a diabetic the food intake has to match the injected insulin. A child unlike an adult, is still in the process of growth and development and is bound to have more activity and exercise. Hence, the requirement of insulin has to be adjusted for the element of growth and activity. Dietary measures should be used to control blood glucose and to minimise the risk of hypoglycaemia and to reduce the long-term complications.

Table 19.6 gives types of insulin and their action.

Table 19.6 Types of insulin and their action

Insulin	*Onset of action (Hr)*	*Peak of action (Hr)*	*Total duration of action (Hr)*
Short acting			
Regular	0.5 – 1	2 – 4	4 – 6
Semilente	1 – 2	3 – 6	
Lispro (Humalog)	within min.	1	4
Intermediate acting			
NPH	3 – 4	10 – 16	20 – 24
Lente	3 – 4	10 – 16	
Long acting			
Glargine (Lantus)	–	peak less action	24
Premixed			
Novamix	–	peak less action	24
Humalogmix			
30/70 (Regular/NPH)			

Insulin Dose is Adjusted For Normal Eating (DAFNE)

The doctor will decide the type of insulin that the diabetic requires. A person who is on short acting insulin has to be more careful with the timing of his meals. The quantity of calories/ carbohydrates also should match the dose of insulin given. Measured diets using household measures or weighing scales are used by type 1 diabetes patients. In addition to a regular schedule of breakfast, two meals and evening tea, patients with type 1 diabetes may require bedtime snacks to prevent hypoglycaemia during the night. Patients with type 2 diabetes also require insulin under certain circumstances, such as inadequate response to oral hypoglycaemic drugs and during ketoacidosis, acute infections, surgery and pregnancy.

The use of acarbose in combination with insulin reduces post prandial blood glucose level in patients with type 1 diabetes who are not satisfactorily controlled by the use of insulin alone. It prevents long term diabetic complications. It is safe and effective agent.

Insulin dose need to be adjusted according to the individual's physical activity. The patient has to maintain a set pattern for the quality and quantity of meals, timing of the meal and type of physical activity he does to control blood glucose level.

Nutritional Requirements

Energy: Hospitalised patients are given 25 kcal/kg body weight.

Table 19.7 The recommended calorie intake (kcal/kg body wt/d) for diabetics based on body weight and activity level.

Category	*Sedentary activity*	*Moderate activity*
Overweight / obese	20	25
Ideal weight	30	35
Underweight	40	40

Source: Raghuram TC *et al.*, 2012 Diet and diabetes National Institute of Nutrition, Hyderabad.

Carbohydrate: Carbohydrate restriction impairs insulin sensitivity and reversed by high carbohydrate diet. High carbohydrate and high fibre diet improve insulin binding and increase in monocyte insulin receptor binding. Carbohydrate is maintained about 45-60 per cent of total calories. Most carbohydrate should be in the form of polysaccharides such as whole grains. Rapidly absorbed mono and disaccharides such as sweets, chocholates and sweetened drinks should be avoided. High fibre and low glycaemic index foods are preferred. Consuming whole apple is better than apple juice because of its high fibre and low ghycremic index.

Several studies have shown that raising the carbohydrate intake does not adversely affect the fasting blood glucose levels, glucose tolerance or insulin requirements provided that total calories are not increased. Insulin needs are more closely correlated with the carbohydrate intake than with the total calorie intake.

Indian diet is cereal based. Hence when calorie intake is increased in the traditional diet carbohydrate intake also increases correspondingly. If one follows the principles of balanced diet and takes good carbohydrate and avoids simple sugars, diabetic diet is not different from the diet of normal individual. Only complex carbohydrates should be included in the diet.

Carbohydrates should be distributed in accordance with the one's daily needs, particularly type 1 diabetics, who are on short acting insulin. One carbohydrate exchange is equal to 15 g of carbohydrate.

Proteins: A diet high in protein (15–20% of total intake) is good for the health of diabetics because it supplies the essential amino acids needed for tissue repair. Protein does not raise blood sugar during absorption as do carbohydrates and it does not supply as many calories as fats.

In patients with type 2 diabetes, consumption of protein along with carbohydrate will lower the blood glucose concentration due to amino acid stimulation of insulin secretion; this helps to compensate for the defect in glucose mediated insulin secretion seen in patients. Protein also promotes satiety and helps both types of diabetic patients to adhere to the carbohydrate allowance.

When hyperglycaemia is present, protein intake may be > 0.8 g/kg body weight. One gram of protein per kilogram body weight is adequate but more may be given and the amount of fats and carbohydrates proportionately reduced. In type 1 diabetic children, 1-1.5 g/kg body weight is recommended. In diabetes with renal problems, protein is restricted to 0.6g/kg body weight. However the biological value should be high.

Pulses like beans, peas and lentils are high in protein and fibre, low in fat foods and have low GI and GL. Proteins from vegetarian sources are better than from flesh foods. Vegetarian sources do not contribute to cholesterol and are rich in fibre.

Fat: Low fat diet increases insulin binding and also reduces LDL and VLDL levels and reduce the incidence of atherosclerosis which is more common in diabetics. Fat content in the diet should be 15–25 per cent of total calories and higher in polyunsaturated fatty acids. Saturated fat should be < 7 per cent of total calories. Diabetics can take 20–25 g/d visible fat.

Total quantity as well as the type of fat influence the serum lipids and could increase the risk for heart disease. Since serum lipids are generally raised in diabetes, daily dietary cholesterol should be less than 300 mg/d. Diabetics can consume fish or chicken without skin, instead of mutton, liver and brain.

Diabetics should also focus on taking protective fats from nuts, seeds, cold pressed oils and fatty fish.

ω-3 fatty acids are anti-inflammatory, antithrombotic, hypolipidemic and vasodilatory. Fish, mustard, soyabean, walnuts, flaxseed, green leafy vegetables, fenugreek seeds and spirulina are rich in ω-3 fatty acids and should be included in the diet of diabetics. *Trans* fat should be avoided. Blended vegetable oils should be consumed.

Vitamins and minerals: When patient takes balanced diet vitamin and mineral supplementation is not required. Routine supplementation with antioxidants such as vitamins E and C and carotene is not advised because of lack of evidence of efficacy and concern related to long term safety. Metformin is a frequent cause of low serum vitamin B_{12} levels.

Diabetics should consume a diet rich in foods which naturally contain significant quantities of dietary antioxidants, especially fresh fruits and vegetables.

Diabetics who consume < 1200 kcal/day require supplementation of micronutrients.

Supplementation of vitamin B_{12}, calcium and iron can be given to vegans, pregnant and lactating patients. Patients who take medications that affect micronutrient status should be given supplementation.

Consumption of diet rich in vitamin C and E and antioxidants should be encouraged. Foods rich in minerals especially magnesium and zinc need to be taken.

Diabetic patients should have the same recommendations for calcium intake as for the general population and guard against low intakes. Vitamin D deficiency may contribute to impaired glucose tolerance hence special care should be taken in the elderly or institutionalised.

Chromium: Most diabetics are not chromium deficient but severe chromium deficiency can lead to glucose intolerance and insulin resistance. Chromium prevents loss of lean muscle, promotes weight loss and lower cholesterol and triglycerides. Chromium supplementation decreases the requirement for insulin or oral hypoglycaemic agents in patients with type 2 diabetes.

Zinc: Studies have shown zinc deficiency is associated with reduced insulin secretion and increased insulin resistance. Very high or very low plasma levels impair the secretion of insulin.

Pregnancy related diabetic complications are seen more often in women with zinc deficiency compared to women with normal zinc levels. Zinc supplementation may have a beneficial effect on healing of venous ulcers in elderly patients, especially diabetics. Diabetics with poor control are at a high risk of zinc deficiency.

Sodium and potassium: Dietary sodium may have a role in the development of insulin resistance apart from its role in maintaining blood pressure. Moderate dietary sodium restriction is beneficial. A new study claimed that consuming diet rich in potassium may help protect the heart and kidney health of patients with type 2 diabetes.

Although the emphasis in diabetes mellitus is on intake of macronutrients there is an abnormal metabolism of several micronutrients in diabetic individuals.

Dietary fibre: Dietary fibre and complex carbohydrates benefit type 1 and type 2 diabetics. Such diets lower

- insulin requirements,
- increase peripheral tissue insulin sensitivity,
- decrease serum cholesterol and triglyceride values,
- aid in weight control, and
- lower B.P.

Soluble fibres such as pectin, gums, hemicellulose (in fruits) increase intestinal transit time, delay gastric emptying, slow glucose absorption and lower serum cholesterol. About 20–30 g of soluble fibre should be taken.

Insoluble fibre such as cellulose and lignin (vegetables, grains) decrease intestinal transit time, increase faecal bulk, delay glucose absorption and slow starch hydrolysis.

Diets high in carbohydrate and fibre improve glucose metabolism without increasing insulin secretion. They lower fasting serum and peripheral insulin concentrations in response to oral glucose administration in both diabetic and non-diabetic individuals.

High fibre diets promote weight loss. They increase satiety, delay gastric emptying by releasing certain gut hormones. From high fibre foods starch, fatty acids and nitrogen may be less well absorbed. Also high fibre foods usually take longer time to eat.

Fenugreek seeds which contain high fibre are useful to diabetics. It contains mucilaginous fibre and total fibre to the extent of 20 per cent and 50 per cent respectively. In addition, it also contains trigonelline—an alkaloid known to reduce blood sugar level. Fenugreek also lowers the levels of serum lipids such as cholesterol and triglyceride.

The quantity of fenugreek seeds to be taken daily depends upon the severity of diabetes. The doses vary from 25 g to 50 g. To begin with 25 g of fenugreek seeds may be taken in two equal doses of 12.5 g each (approximately two teaspoons) along with lunch and dinner. The seeds can the taken as such after over night soaking in water or in powder form as a drink in water or butter milk, 15 min before the meal. The fenugreek seed powder can be incorporated in preparations such as chapati, sambar, dhal and vegetables. It has been observed that the requirement of antidiabetic drugs decreases with the use of fenugreek.

Consumption of brown rice in place of white rice can help reduce 24h glucose and fasting insulin responses among overweight Indians. Processed foods should be avoided.

Fluids: Fluids are essential for diabetics who are at a higher risk of dehydration. Soft drinks, sweetened fruit juices and energy and sports drinks are to be avoided.

Artificial Sweeteners

High content of sugar consumption is undesirable for diabetics and for obese individuals. Non-caloric and high intense sweeteners are available in the market as sugar substitutes. Many soft drinks contain artificial sweeteners.

Acceptable daily intake for sweeteners as per JECFA (Joint FAO/WHO Expert committee on food additives is given in Table 19.8).

Table 19.8 Acceptable daily intake for sweeteners as per JECFA regulations for normal individuals

Sweetener	*ADI mg/kg body weight*
Acesulfame k	15
Aspartame	40
Neotame	2
Saccharin	5
Sucralose	15
Stevia (as Stevia glycosides)	4

Source: Editors Sudha V. *et al.*, 2017. Perspectives on low calorie sweeteners Dr. Mohan's health care products Chennai.

Use of sweeteners by a diabetic patient is not encouraged as it does not help the patient to wean away from sweet foods.

Glycaemic Index

Glycaemic index is a ranking of foods based on the postprandial blood glucose response compared with a reference food (Jenkins, 1981). The index integrates multiple influences on glucose availability and is proposed as a means for prescribing diabetic and energy controlled diets. Consumption of a diet low on the glycaemic index influences multiple parameters of glucose and lipid metabolism.

Reduced rate of glucose absorption after the consumption of low-glycaemic index carbohydrate foods will reduce the postprandial rise in gut hormones (e.g., incretins) and insulin. Prolonged absorption of carbohydrate seen over a time will maintain suppression of free fatty acids and counter regulatory response while at the same time achieving lower blood glucose concentration. Over a time with the reduction in free fatty acid concentrations and the rise in respiratory quotient with tissue insulinisation, glucose is withdrawn from the circulation at a faster rate (Figure 19.5).

High glycaemic index forms of carbohydrate are foods that produce high concentrations of blood glucose and increased insulin demand and that therefore, could plausibly contribute to higher risk of type 2 diabetes. The individual response to a given carbohydrate load is influenced by the degree of underlying insulin resistance, which is in turn determined primarily by degree of adiposity, physical activity, genetics and other aspects of diet. Thus it might be expected that the adverse metabolic effects of high glycaemic index foods would be exacerbated in sedentary overweight or genetically susceptible persons.

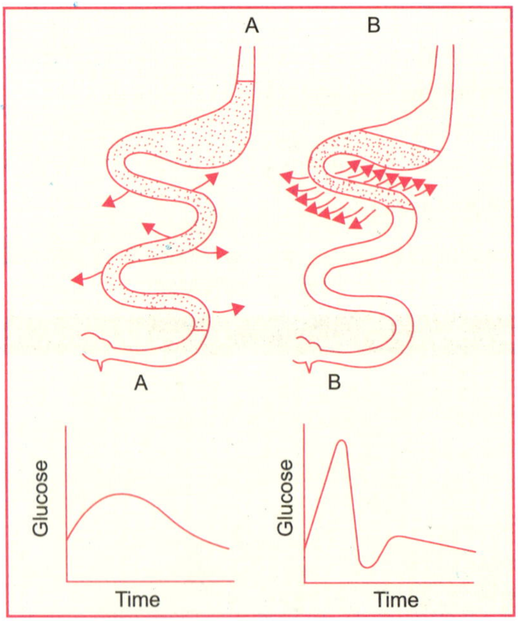

Fig. 19.5 Hypothetical effect of feeding diets with a low (A) or high (B) glycemic index on gastro-intestinal glucose absorption and postprandial blood glucose

Source: Jenkins David *et al.*, 2002, Glycaemic Index: Overview of Implications in Health and Disease, Am J Clin Nutr., 76.

The adverse effects of high glycaemic index diet appeared to be due to an increased production of free fatty acids in the late postprandial state, presumably as a result of a depression in blood glucose below base line (reactive hypoglycaemia) and possibly mediated by increase in counter regulatory hormones (cortisol, glucagon and growth hormone). (Figure 19.5) Studies have shown that the postprandial rise in glucose is consistent with depression of serum antioxidants including lycopene and vitamin E. The higher the glycaemic index the greater the postprandial depression of serum antioxidants.

Glycaemic Index and glycaemic load are positively associated with prevalence of metabolic syndrome, elevated triglycerides and low HDL-C and inversely associated with elevated glucose in men.

Glycaemic load was also inversely associated with large waist girth and elevated glucose in men.

Increased carbohydrate meal results in increased post prandial peak, longer time to return to pre prandial glucose, larger 4 hour area under the curve, higher 4 hour mean glucose.

High blood concentrations of insulin and glucose can damage the endothelium that lines coronary arteries and set the stage for the formation of plaques.

Protein rich foods are known to increase insulin secretion without augmenting glucose concentrations. Therefore as more protein is taken in conjunction with carbohydrate, the insulin response will increase, whereas postprandial glucose will not change much. Similarly, adding fat to a carbohydrate meal also enhances insulin secretion even though the plasma glucose response actually decreases. All 3 macronutrients stimulate the release of several gut peptides but to different degrees. Protein and fat are particularly efficacious in stimulating gut peptide release despite a small glucose effect. Thus, the insulin response to a carbohydrate food varies with the amount of fat, protein or both with which it is ingested.

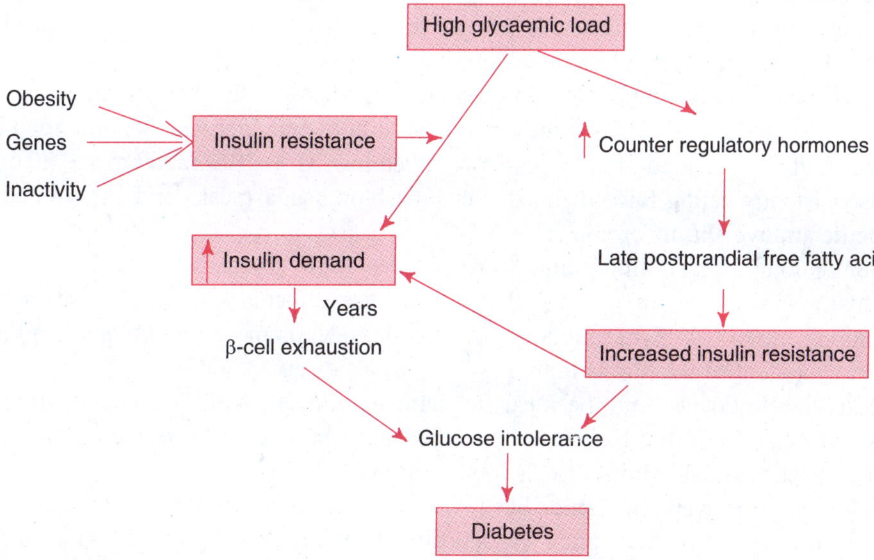

Fig. 19.6 Glycaemic index in relation to diabetes mellitus

Low glycaemic foods like whole grains, plant oils and vegetables keeps blood glucose levels relatively constant sparing the pancreas overwork. According to Willet, steady blood glucose also helps keep the appetite in check which makes maintaining a healthy weight easier. Willet plan's directives are good carbs and good fat.

Source: Willet Walter *et al.*, 2002, Glycaemic Index, Glycaemic Load and Risk of Type 2 Diabetes, Am J Clin Nutr., 76.

Factors which Influence the Glycaemic Index

- The presence of non-absorbable oligosaccharides and viscous dietary fibres such as pectins, β-glucons and gums fruits, vegetables and cereals reduce the efficiency of enzyme hydrolysis and slows the rate at which glucose enters the blood stream.
- Starch encased in its seed coat or coarsely ground is not efficiently hydrolysed to glucose because digestive enzymes are prevented from reaching the starch.
- Starch granules subjected to moist heat and subsequent cooling become dense and less available to enzyme action. Retrograded starch has low glycaemic index.
- Rice bran, which is rich in fibre and oil has low glycaemic index.
- High amylose rice varieties which are slowly digested are potentially useful in low glycaemic diets.
- Chapathis, which need chewing have lower glycaemic index compared to wheat 'kanjee'.
- Raw food has lower glycaemic index than cooked food.
- Foods rich in fat and protein have low glycaemic index.
- Phytic acid present in whole grains decrease GI.
- Natural food has low glycaemic index compared to processed foods.
- The GI for fructose is low (23) compared to lactose (46), sucrose (65) or glucose (97). Fructose produces lower risk of blood sugar than glucose. In view of its effect on serum lipid, it can be taken only in moderation.

In general, high-fibre foods with low glycaemic indices (e.g., beans, vegetables, whole fruit and whole grains) are the preferred forms of carbohydrate in a defensive nutrition plan. Meal combination is also an important factor in managing blood glucose levels. Combining protein, fat and carbohydrate at meals and snacks i.e., small serving of nuts and a piece of fruit, can lead to better control of blood glucose levels and less insulin release than meals or snacks that consist mainly of carbohydrate like bread and jam.

Soluble dietary fibre combined with low glycaemic index food is good for diabetics. While planning diets glycaemic load that is the amount of carbohydrate derived from the food is also considered. A glycaemic load of 10 or less considered low, 11 to 19 is medium and 20 or more is high. Consistently eating low GI foods evens out blood sugar peaks and valleys and helps keep appetite and weight under control.

Glycaemic load is also important. Carrots have high glycaemic index. The amount of carbohydrate is so low in a carrot that it has little effect on blood glucose or insulin concentrations due to low glycaemic load. Glycaemic index is more important when the total carbohydrate content of the diet is high.

All foods low in GI need not be ideal for diabetics. For example, ice cream, fried foods and pongal are low in GI but high in GL or other macronutrients. These are not suitable for diabetics. Diabetics should choose foods low in GI and GL.

Several dietary intervention studies have shown that increasing dietary intake of legumes including beans as well as whole grain foods positively affects blood glucose management and insulin sensitivity.

In general, low GI foods have been shown to have beneficial effects on glucose control, hyper-insulinaemia, insulin resistance, blood lipids and satiety.

Carbohydrate counting

Counting carbohydrates is one way to plan meals and keep blood glucose on target. Carbohydrates are one of the three main energy sources in food, along with protein and fat. There should be a balance between the carbohydrate intake and insulin to stay in target range. Counting carbohydrate sevings can help reach blood glucose goals and prevent diabetes complications. Carbohydrate counting helps to choose what and how much to eat. Carbohydrate counting can be easier to use than other meal planning methods.

Foods have Carbohydrate

These foods that are listed in table affect blood glucose much more than other foods such as meat and meat substitutes, vegetables, or fats.

Table 19.9 **Carbohydrate foods**

Carbohydrate foods	
• biscuits, bread, crackers	• dried beans (such as kidney or pinto beans) and peas (such as black-eyed or split peas)
• ready-to-eat or cooked cereal	• fruit (canned, dried and fresh) and fruit juice
• pasta and rice	• milk, soy milk and yogurt
• starchy vegetables such as corn, potatoes and sweet potatoes	• sweets such as cake, cookies, ice cream, jam, jelly and all Indian sweets
• pancakes and chapathis	• popcorn and potato chips

Large servings of salads or cooked vegetables (such as 1½ cups of cooked carrots) are counted as carbohydrate servings too. Some foods, such as pizza, casseroles and soups, are a combination of carbohydrate, protein and fat.

Table 19.10 **Serving sizes for some carbohydrate foods (approximately 15 grams of carbohydrate)**

apple: 1 small (4 ounces)	**milk:** 1 cup
	orange juice: 1/2 cup
banana: 1 small (4 ounces)	**pasta (cooked):** 1/3 cup
bread: 1 slice	**peas:** 1/2 cup
cake (unfrosted): 2 inch square	**pinto beans or kidney beans:** 1/2 cup
cereal (ready-to-eat): 3/4 cup	
cereal (cooked): 1/2 cup	**potato, mashed:** 1/2 cup
cookies: 2 small (about 2/3 ounce)	**potato chips:** 3/4 ounce (about 15-20)
corn: 1/2 cup	
crackers (saltiones): 6	**rice:** 1/3 cup
fruit, canned: 1/2 cup	**sugar:** 1 tablespoon
ice cream (light): 1/2 cup	**sweet potato:** 1/2 cup
jam or jelly: 1 tablespoon	

Carbohydrate exchange = 15g of carbohydrate

Distribution of carbohydrates exchange

Calories	Breakfast	Lunch	Dinner	Night time snacks
1200	3	3	2	2
1400	4	3	2	2
1500	4	3	3	2
1800	5	4	4	2
2000	5	5	5	2
2200	6	5	5	2

Dietary Guidelines

- Daily energy intake must be estimated after considering such factors as age, sex, actual weight in relation to desirable weight, activity and occupation. Adequate calories for the existing weight, gradually raised for the expected weight, due allowance for activity.
- Nutrient requirements of children relative to their body weight are generally higher than those of adults to take care of their growth and developmental needs. Children suffering from type 1 diabetes require the normal diet recommended for their age group. It can also be calculated based on their age. Calorie requirements for children are 1000 basal calories plus 125 calories for boys and 100 calories for girls for every year of age up to 12 years. For example a 10 year old boy requires 2250 kcal (1000 + 1250 for 10 years).
- The patient should maintain body weight 10 per cent lower than the ideal/desirable body weight.

  Ideal weight is calculated using Broka's index

  Broka's index = Height in cm – 100 = Ideal body weight in kg

  The BMI should be maintained at < 23.
- If he is overweight 20 kcal/kg, if he is of ideal weight 30 kcal/kg and if he is underweight 40 kcal/kg are prescribed.
- For persons engaged in greater physical activity, the recommended calorie intake may be increased as per the needs. A person above the age 50 years of age requires 10 per cent less calorie for each decade.
- The total intake of calories is more important for a diabetic than the exact proportions of protein, fat and carbohydrate in the diet.

Table 19.11 Total Free sugar content of fruits/100 g

Fruits containing ≤ 8 g	Fruits containing 8 – 10 g	Fruits containing > 10 g
Avocado – 1.6	Mango (banganapalli) – 7.7	Grapes (black seeded) – 10.0
Muskmelon – 2.3	Pineapple – 8.5	Pomegranate – 10.8
Goose berry – 3.3	Figs – 8.6	Jackfruit – 12.2
Watermelon – 3.6	Apple – 9.5	Sapota – 12.3
Guava – 4.1		Custard apple – 13.3

All dried fruits like raisins and dates are very high in total free sugar content. Diabetics should not include these in their diet. Fruits containing < 8 g/100 g total free sugar content should be preferred by diabetics. Other fruits should be consumed in restricted amounts.

Source: Longvah. T. *et al.*, 2017. Indian food composition. Tables NIN, Hyderabad.

- Dietary calories should be 55–60 per cent from carbohydrates, 15–20 per cent from protein and 15–20 per cent from fat. To prevent ketosis a minimum amount of 130 g of carbohydrate should be given.

- Percentage distribution of calories in each meal if no insulin is taken:

Breakfast Mid morning	33
Lunch Tea	33
Dinner Before going to bed	33

- Insulin is adjusted depending upon the need. Calorie distribution is adjusted according to type of insulin taken by the patient.
- Simple sugars should be restricted since they are easily absorbed and have a high glycaemic index. Glycaemic peaks should be avoided.
- Intake of polished rice and incidence of diabetes are related. When consumption of rice increases other food items are consumed less. There is a link between the type of carbohydrate and diabetes.
- Complex carbohydrates and fibre should be included in the diet. 25–40 g of dietary fibre can be included per 1000 kcal consumed. Millets should be consumed Refined cereals should be avoided.
- Soluble fibre has greatest hypoglycaemic and hypocholesterolemic effect. The diet should include legumes, whole grain and fenugreek seeds.
- A mixture of oils is preferred than single oil. Poly unsaturated fatty acids and mono-unsaturated fatty acids containing vegetable oils are preferred (sunflower oil, corn oil, ground nut, gingelly oil) to animal fat and hydrogenated fat. They contain more saturated and *trans* fatty acids. Atherogenic fat is avoided.
- Lean protein such as fish and chicken are preferred to meat.

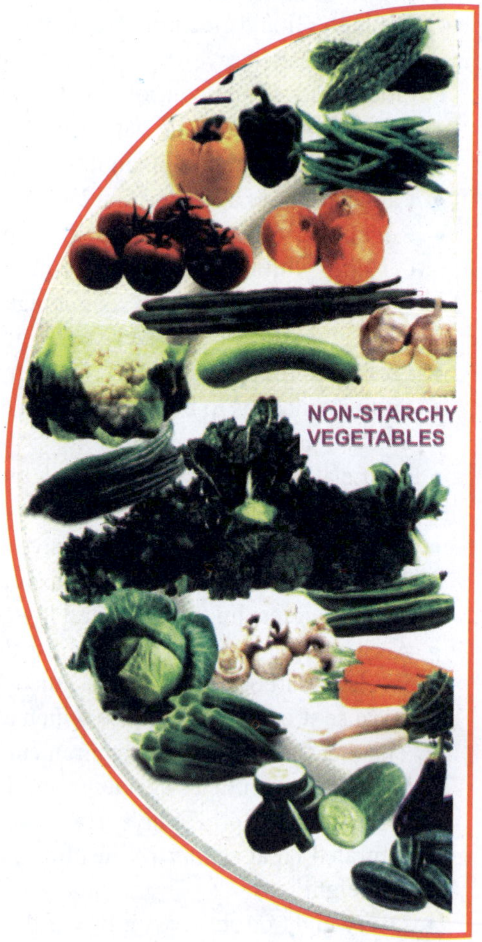

Fig. 19.7 Vegetables permitted in diabtetes.

Nonstarchy vegetables are low in carbohydrate and are high in fibre.

- Fried food should be restricted.
- High protein intake helps to increase insulin production and promotes satiety. Pulses are rich in protein and fibre. Whole grams and beans improve health and reduce cholesterol Proteins from vegetable sources are preferred to animal proteins as they are cholesterol free and fibre rich.

- Vitamins and minerals are supplemented if needed. (especially fat soluble vitamins).
- Timely intake of in between meal snacks should be stressed to avoid hypoglycaemia. Three main meals and three in between meal snacks can be taken.
- Food exchange lists should be followed to prevent hypo and hyperglycaemia. The exchange systems should be followed to avoid monotony and to get dietary constancy and flexibility.
- Influence of chew count, glycaemic indices, type and form of food in altering the blood sugar level should be recognised. Both the source (GI) and the quantity (Glycaemic load) of carbohydrate influence the metabolic response to the ingestion of carbohydrate. Rice has high GI and rice bran has low GI due to high content of fibre and fat.
- Mixed unsalted raw or dry roasted nuts have benefits for both blood glucose control and blood lipids. They control diabetes without weight gain.
- Patient should eat wide variety of foods.
- Patients should avoid alcohol.
- Patients should avoid fasting and feasting.
- Regulating of meals is needed for persons taking insulin. Meals should be spaced to consider with the availability of insulin.
- If insulin or oral hypoglycaemic agents are not used, marked obesity is not present or hyperglycaemia is relatively mild, general balanced diet principles must be followed.
- Probiotics may help improve insulin sensitivity and reduce inflammation.
- Sodium intake is to be no more than 6 g daily. Sodium is restricted to 3 g in hypertensive diabetic patients.
- Artificial sweeteners can be taken by patients, occasionally.
- Junk foods should be avoided by patients. Diabetics should use less added fat, sugar and salt.
- Special diabetic foods are expensive and may not have health benefits over normal foods.
- The slowing of small intestinal absorption by increased meal frequency (nibbling) results in reduced insulin secretion and lower low density lipoprotein cholesterol concentration.
- Antihyperglycaemic agent acarbose delays and reduces rise in postprandial blood glucose levels. Acarbose is an alpha-glucosidase inhibitor. Whole wheat is preferred to rice because it contains acarbose which allows carbohydrate to be absorbed slowly.
- The diet should meet the requirement of antioxidants, micronutrients and phytochemicals, by taking permitted vegetables and fruits in the prescribed quantity.
- Increased intake of whole grains and legumes and reduced intake of fat specially the saturated fat also improve insulin sensitivity and reduce the risk of diabetes independent of weight loss.
- Overweight or obese with type 2 diabetes, a weight loss of 5 per cent improves glucose and lipid levels and blood pressure.

Foods to be avoided	*Eaten in moderation*	*Foods permitted*
Simple sugars (glucose, honey, syrup) sweets, dried fruits, cake, candy, fried foods, jaggery, brown sugar, sweetened juices, roots and tubers, bananas, pineapple, mango ripe, grapes, sapota, tamarind pulp	Fats, cereals, pulses, meat, egg, musk melon, jack fruit, orange, papaya, artificial sweeteners	Green leafy vegetables, lemon, clear soups mint, curry leaves, spices vegetable salads with carrots cucumbers, tomatoes, and onions, plain butter milk , gooseberry, mango. Plain coffee and tea without sugar, skimmed milk, butter milk goose berry avocado, guava (whitl flesh) Mango green, water melon, wood apple

Myths and Facts

Myths	*Facts*
Diabetics can eat wheat but not rice.	Calorie value of wheat and rice are similar. Many diabetics feel it is convenient to count and limit the number of chapathis and chew count is more and satiety is better. Wheat flour rotis have a GI of 45 and those made from multigrain flour have a GI of 27.3 while the GI of white rice is about 64. Wheat is more nutritious as it is richer in protein, fibre, B-vitamins and acarbose. Brown rice can be consumed in restricted amounts.
Any amount of wheat can be consumed.	Large quantities of wheat increases GL and blood sugar.
Fasting can be compensated by the next meal.	Fasting can lead to hypoglycaemia. It is dangerous particularly who are on oral medicines or insulin. Complications of hypoglycaemia are more common than hyperglycaemia.
Feasting can be done by fasting the next meal.	This results in hyperglycaemia and on long term complications can occur.
Diabetic diet is a special diet.	This is balanced diet eaten regularly and in moderation avoiding certain foods.
Fruits can be eaten in unlimited quantities.	Certain fruits like musk melon, sweet lime, guava, water melon, papaya and strawberry are low in total free sugars and can be consumed. Banana, grapes, custard apple, pineapple, chikoo and mango are high in fructose. When eaten in unlimited quantities cholesterol levels may increase. Dried fruits should be consumed in very small quantities.
Vegetables can be eaten in unlimited quantities.	If eaten raw or with little fat or coconut. Non starchy vegetables are preferred.
Liquids are easily digestible.	Preparations like kanjee are not preferred as they have high GI. Chapathis/rotis are preferred.
Fruit juices/cola drinks can be taken.	It is better to avoid empty calories like cola drinks. It is better to eat the fruit as such as glycaemic index and nutritive value are better than fruit juice.
Bitter foods like fenugreek and bitter gourd are good.	Fenugreek seed (not leaves) to be taken 25 g/day to have an impact. This may not apply to all other bitter foods.
Sugar is to be totally be avoided.	Sweets where concentrated sugar and fat are used like mysorpak are avoided totally. Artificial sweeteners can be added to coffee and tea. Best is to appreciate bitterness in tea or coffee.
Avoid carbohydrate and fats.	Good carbohydrate like complex carbohydrates and good fats like mono and polyunsaturated fatty acids can be consumed from the allowance.

A significantly risk of diabetes was most pronounced in those who consume processed meats such as bacon and hot dogs frequently.

Higher intake of vegetables, whole grain foods, legumes and nuts are associated with lower risk of insulin resistance and type 2 diabetes and improved glycaemic control in either normal or insulin resistant individuals. Diets rich in whole grain foods are associated with improved insulin sensitivity partially due to magnesium and cereal fibre present. Nut consumption is inversely associated with risk of type 2 diabetes. Legumes contain slowly digested carbohydrate and have a high fibre content, improve glycaemic control and reduce the incidence of diabetes. Consumption of greens and fruits lower the risk of diabetes mellitus.

Meal replacement products in diabetes

Calorie controlled meal replacement products can be used by most people with diabetes not only for safe and effective weight loss but also for a grab-and-go balanced meal or to add extra nutrients during times of special need.

According to the American Diabetic Association, "use of meal replacement once or twice daily to replace a usual meal can result in significant weight loss, but meal replacement therapy must be continued if weight loss is to be maintained."

Meal replacement products come in many different forms: multiflavoured shakes, bars, puddings and powders which can be mixed in cold water. Most are lactose and gluten free and have different types of artificial sweeteners.

Special meal replacements are available for diabetics to control the post meal rise in blood sugar and lose weight. Many also have a lower glycemic index.

Meal replacement products are good for diabetes who are leading a hectic life. Eating a healthy diet can become a challenge on days there is no time to prepare a meal or even eat it. Meal replacement products can be particularly beneficial when additional carbohydrates, protein, fat and fibre and additional nutrients need to be added.

Meal replacement products can be used safely and effectively under the advice of a physician and a nutritionist.

ORAL HYPOGLYCAEMIC DRUGS

Patients of normal weight may start oral hypoglycaemic drugs as soon as it is clear that dietary measures alone are inadequate. A number of compounds reduce hyperglycaemia in patients who would otherwise require insulin. Their action depends on supply of endogenous insulin and hence they are not substitutes for insulin.

Socioeconomic factors also impose limitations on patient and provides motivation. Middle and poorer income groups which account for the majority of diabetic patients, oral hypoglycaemic agents are most often prescribed followed by diet and exercise and lastly by insulin.

Combination of drugs is necessary for good control after a few years of having the disease. Acarbose and metformin combination therapy is more effective in reducing intraday and interday glycaemic variability without increasing duration of hyperglycaemia. There are innumerable new drugs available like GLP-1 analogs, DPP-4 inhibitor, SGLT-2 inhibitors for diabetes. They are used in combinations like insulin combinations.

Table 19.12 Glucose-lowering interventions

Nutrient	*Expected decrease in A1C with monotherapy (%)*	*Advantages*	*Disadvantages*
Initial therapy			
Lifestyle change to decrease weight and increase activity	1.0 to 2.0	Broad benefits	Insufficient for most within first year owing to inadequate weight loss and weight regain
Metformin	1.0 to 2.0	Weight neutral	GI side effects, contraindicated with renal insufficiency (eGFR < 30 mL/min/1.73 m²)*
Glinide	0.5 to 1.5$^{\Delta}$	Rapidly effective	Weight gain, 3 times/day dosing, hypoglycemia
SGLT2 inhibitor	0.5 to 0.7	Weight loss, reduction in systolic blood pressure, reduced cardiovascular mortality in patients with established CVD, improved renal outcomes in patients with nephropathy	Vulvovaginal candidiasis, urinary tract infections, bone fractures, lower limb amputations, DKA*
DPP-4 inhibitor	0.5 to 0.8	Weight neutral	Possible increased risk of HF with saxagliptin, expensive
Alpha-glucosidase inhibitor	0.5 to 0.8	Weight neutral	Frequent GI Side effects, 3 times/day dosing
Pramlintide	0.5 to 1.0	Weight loss	3 injections daily, frequent GI side effects, long-term safety not established, expensive

A1C: glycated hemoglobin; GI: gastrointestinal; eGFR: estimated glomerular filtration rate, GLP-1: glucagon-like peptide-1; CVD: cardiovascular disease; MI: myocardial infarction; HF: heart failure; SGLT: sodium-glucose co-transporter 2; DKA: diabetic ketoacidosis; DPP-4: dipeptidyl peptidase 4.

PHYSICAL ACTIVITY

In the absence of coexisting conditions which may require limitation of physical activity, exercise plays an important role in facilitating a good control of diabetes. In addition, to strengthening and toning up the muscles, it consumes more energy derived from blood glucose and sensitises the tissues to the action of insulin, which helps in keeping the blood glucose in a lower range.

Type and timing of exercise should depend on the preexercise blood sugar values, type of diabetes and associated complications.

In obese overweight diabetics, a negative calorie balance produces mobilisation of stored fat for meeting the energy demands leading to weight reduction.

Aerobic exercise means physical activity that encourages utilisation of oxygen to provide energy for exercising muscles. Efficiency of pumping action of heart improves and blood vessels open up to accommodate increased amount of blood being pumped by the heart. Walking, bicycling, stationary cycling, swimming and jumping rope are good examples of such an exercise. Walking is the most natural form of exercise.

It is recommended that diabetics should do exercise of moderate intensity for a minimum period of 150 minutes a week, that is, at least 30 minutes a day for five days a week.

Exercise should be avoided if the blood glucose is very high (> 250 mg/dl) or low (hypoglycaemia or during infections).

If the patient is obese, carbohydrate and calorie supplementation is not recommended either before or after exercising. About 15 g of carbohydrate is 'borrowed' from the next meal to prevent hypoglycaemia. Exercising either right before or shortly following a meal will often prevent hypoglycaemia.

Sudden initiation of a vigorous exercise programme in a person of sedentary habits is not desirable. This is an essential warning of those over the age of 35 years.

The short-term effects of exercise include lowering of blood glucose. This is due to increased uptake and utilisation of glucose by exercising muscle. Glucose is moved from its main storage site, liver, and is utilised by the muscle. Several hormones play an important role and facilitate this process. A small amount of insulin in circulation is considered essential for this beneficial effect. In the total absence of circulating insulin the release of glucose from liver under the influence of exercise, is not accompanied by its enhanced uptake and utilisation in the muscles. Thus exercise always results in lowering of blood glucose in those diabetics who have some circulating insulin like in type 2 diabetes. Exercise benefits diabetics by enhancing the action of insulin through an increased number of insulin receptor sites particularly in type 2 diabetes.

In the management of type 1 diabetes, the nature and scheduling of physical activity must be balanced with food and insulin to prevent hypoglycaemic reactions. It may be harmful in those with absolute lack of insulin type 1 diabetes. Exercise should not be prescribed in patients with type 1 diabetes until and unless such patients are well controlled with insulin near normalisation of blood glucose.

Physical activity influences insulin requirements and adjustments in the diet may be needed. Carbohydrate rich snacks should be taken before participating in exercise.

Physical activity also improves lipid profile and reducing blood pressure which are known risk factors for heart disease. Preliminary study conducted at M.V. Hospital for Diabetes in Chennai has shown that yogasanas may be beneficial in reducing the intake of hypoglycaemic drugs. Exercise is better than metformin. Exercise is medicine.

In addition exercise is known to reduce stress and strain and enhance quality of life.

Exercise Recommendations

The American Diabetes Association and American Heart Association provide the following exercise recommendations for individuals with type 2 diabetes:

- At least 150 minutes per week should be devoted to moderate-intensity aerobic physical activity (40% to 60% of maximal oxygen consumption [VO_2max] or 50% to 70% of maximum heart rate) and/or at least 90 minutes per week of vigorous aerobic exercise (above 60% of VO_2 max or above 70% of maximum heart rate). The physical activity should be distributed over at least three days per week and with no more than two consecutive days per week and with no more than two consecutive days without physical activity.
- In the absence of contraindications, people with type 2 diabetes should perform resistance exercises three times per week, targeting all major muscle groups and progressing to three sets of eight to 10 repetitions at a weight that cannot be lifted more than eight to 10 times. Initial supervision and periodic reassessments by a qualified exercise specialist are recommended.
- Four or more hours per week of moderate-to-vigorous aerobic and/or resistance exercise should be performed as it is associated with greater CVD risk reduction compared with lower volumes of activity.
- For long-term maintenance of major weight loss [30 pounds 13.6 kilograms or more], more exercise [seven hours per week of moderate or vigorous aerobic physical activity] may be helpful.

A thorough medical evaluation and clearance from a physician are necessary before beginning a program more vigorous than brisk walking. Previously sedentary patients should embark on any activity program cautiously.

A physically active lifestyle plays a vital role in both management of type 1 diabetes and prevention and management of type 2 diabetes. Benefits of physical activity are numerous and include aiding weight loss and weight maintenance and improving the insulin/glucose profile for people with prediabetes, glycaemic control in individuals with type 2 diabetes and quality of life for all individuals of particular importance for people with diabetes or at risk is a reduction of cardiovascular risk factors and all cause mortality.

According to a university of Florida study, a regular tai chi exercise programme may help lower blood glucose level and control the disease. Tai chi is an ancient Chinese form of meditation that combines breathing and relaxation techniques with slow deliberate movements.

Exercise Checklist for People with Diabetes

- Talk to the doctor about the right exercise.
- Check blood sugar level before and after exercising.
- Check feet for blisters or sores before and after exercising.
- Wear proper shoes and socks.
- Drink plenty of fluid before, during and after exercising.
- Warm up before exercising and cool down afterward.
- Have a snack handy in case your blood sugar level drops.

Physical activity helps in

- effective weight management
- lower blood sugar, blood pressure and blood fats
- increases oxygen level in the body
- reduces stress
- strengthening the heart, muscles and bone
- improves blood circulation
- tones the muscles
- sensitizes muscle and hepatic cells to facilitate glucose uptake and increase insulin sensitivity.

Hayes Charlotte and Kriska (2008) have given the following steps of management of diabetes.

Prediabetes

- ↓ calorie ↓ fat diet
- Regular physical activity
- Modest weight loss 5-7 per cent starting weight
- Prevent weight gain

Type 2 diabetes

- Meal planning, physical activity, plus glucose lowering medications
- Modest weight loss 5–7 per cent starting weight
- Prevent weight gain
- Extra food for increased activity should be used judiciously
- For individuals on insulin or insulin secretagogues : additional carbohydrate should be consumed if blood glucose is <100 mg |dl; 15 g rapidly absorbable carbohydrate should be available for treatment and prevention of hypoglycaemia.

Type 1 diabetes

- Carbohydrate supplementation is often necessary for maintaining target range glucose levels with exercise, if activity is spontaneous or unplanned, long duration or high intensity.
- Insulin sensitivity is altered by exercise, therefore, skill in adjusting insulin dosages can increase exercise safely and performance.
- 15–30 g carbohydrate consumed every 30–60 min of exercise.
- 1.5 g carbohydrate / kg body weight consumed 30 minutes after intense exercise and again 1-2 h later may prevent post exercise hypoglycaemia and replenish glycogen stores.

EDUCATION

Giving information is different from education, for education it should bring about a change in behaviour. The diabetics should be educated on the nature of the disease they have and the possibility of development of acute and long-term complications of the disease, if blood sugar is not kept under control. Diabetes education includes the need and importance of renal, eye, cardiac and foot care. It must help the patients understand about vital parameters, blood pressure, blood sugar, its complications, prevention and control. Patients must be educated and comply on healthy lifestyle choices, principles of dietary modifications, mental and physical health. Adequate basic information on diabetes enables the diabetic to comprehend and improve their psychological acceptance of the disease. In addition, the importance of following the doctor's instructions regarding diet, exercise and drugs should be explained.

For patients with type 2 diabetes, body weight management should be considered as a therapeutic target in addition to glycaemia. Patients should receive counselling regarding changes in diet and physical activity to achieve weight loss or to prevent weight gain.

Diabetics should be aware of the importance of monitoring urine and blood sugar and serum lipids at regular intervals to ensure overall well-being.

Diabetics should be informed about the symptoms of hypoglycaemia and the immediate need for taking sugar in such conditions. They should be aware of the acute complications such as ketoacidosis and the danger of infections which require immediate medical attention. Diabetics should maintain a diary to keep a record of their urinary and blood glucose results, body weight and alterations in their diet and drugs. They should have regular check up of their feet, eyes and kidneys.

Counselling is the key for treatment of diabetes.

COMPLICATIONS

Glycaemic variability over each 24-hour cycle is an independent risk factor for vascular complications. Glycaemic variability and sustained hyperglycaemia in diabetes eventually lead to the macro and microvascular complications.

Acute glucose fluctuations during the post prandial period trigger oxidative stress and are more predictive of atherosclerosis development than are fasting plasma glucose or HbA1c. This suggests that treatment should not only target HbA1c as a long term goal, but also aim to avoid acute glucose fluctuations as an immediate goal.

There should be an emphasis an efforts to control all aspects of blood glucose disorders including HbA1c, fasting blood glucose, post prandial glucose as well as glucose fluctuations.

It is suggested that patients with diabetes check their glycaemia at least four times a day (before meals and at bed time) with a blood glucose meter with additional measurements if they experience symptoms of hypo or hyperglycaemia.

Acute Complications

Hypoglycaemia: It is defined as a condition in which there is blood glucose concentration of less than 70 mg/dl. Sweating, trembling, hunger, confusion, drowsiness, incoordination and nausea are some of the symptoms of hypoglycaemia.

The most common causes are unpunctual or inadequate meals, unexpected or unusual exercise and ingestion of alcohol. Patients should be taught that if unusual exercise is anticipated the preceding dose of insulin should be reduced and extra carbohydrate should be ingested. All patients taking insulin should carry glucose tablets with them.

Having hypoglycaemic episodes that are severe enough to require hospitalization are associated with greater risk of dementia for older adults with type 2 diabetes.

Ketoacidosis: Any form of stress, particularly an acute infection or neglect of treatment due to carelessness can lead to ketoacidosis. There is intense thirst and polyuria. Constipation, muscle cramps and altered vision are common. Hyperventilation with low blood pressure and acetone may be smelt in the breath and finally it may lead to coma. Glycosuria and ketonuria would be present. Blood glucose levels may be as high as 360–720 mg/dl and low plasma bicarbonate and low blood pH.

Table 19.13 Distinguishing characteristics of hyperglycaemia and hypoglycaemia

Characteristics	*Hyperglycaemia*	*Hypoglycaemia*
Causes	Too much food	Too little food
	Too little insulin	Too much insulin or diabetes medicine
	Illness or stress	Extra exercise.
On set	Gradual, may progress to diabetic coma	Sudden, may progress to insulin shock
Blood sugar	Above 250 mg/dl	Below 70 mg/dl
Symptoms	Extreme thirst	Shaking
	Frequent urination	Fast heart beat
	Dry skin	Sweating
	Hunger	Anxious
	Blurred vision	Dizziness
	Drowsiness	Hunger
	Nausea	Impaired vision
		Irritable
		Weakness
		Fatigue
		Headache
Treatment	If over 250 mg/dl, call the doctor	Drink a cup of orange juice or milk or eat candy and call the doctor

The condition should be treated with utmost urgency in hospital. Intravenous fluid replacement is required since, even when the patient is able to swallow, fluids given by mouth may be poorly absorbed. If 6 to 8 units of insulin per hour is given, blood glucose level comes down. 13-20 mMol of potassium per 0.51 infusion fluid, should be started from the outset. Intracellular fluid is replaced once the blood glucose has fallen below 250 mg/dl by infusing glucose solution. Intensive medical care is needed and the blood glucose, pH, electrolytes and ketones have to be monitored, hourly at first.

Long-Term Complications

Uncontrolled diabetes may lead to complications. The elevated levels of glucose in tissues such as the nerve, kidney, retina and lenses are converted to sorbitol by aldose reductase. Accumulation of sorbitol leads to complications of diabetes mellitus.

The long term complications of diabetes includes angina, cardiac failure, intermittent claudication and gangrene due to atherosclerosis; blindness due to diabetic retinopathy; difficulty in walking with chronic ulceration of feet due to diabetic neuropathy and also diabetic microangiopathy and diabetic nephropathy due to small blood vessel disease.

Infections: In diabetics, cuts and wounds heal slowly. Wound healing is delayed in diabetics because of neuropathy, hyperglycaemia and ischaemia. They are prone to tuberculosis and infections of the skin, urinary tract and foot. Diabetics should take special precautions and keep skin and food clean to prevent infections.

Recent studies conducted in India revealed that diabetes is likely to be responsible for 15 per cent of all new tuberculosis cases and 3 per cent of AIDS.

Cataract and retinopathy: Studies indicate that diabetes increase the risk of development of cataract. Oxidative damage to the constituents of the eye lens is considered to be a major mechanism in the initiation and progression of diabetic cataract. Diabetes causes increased oxidative stress in various tissues including lens. A number of studies suggest that intake of antioxidant rich foods may slow the progression of cataract.

Yellow brown pigments accumulate in the lens with age and do so at an accelerated rate in diabetics. These pigments are capable of cross-linking proteins, a hallmark of cataract formation.Low ascorbic acid intake and low plasma vitamin C levels are associated with the increased risk of cataracts which may be seen in diabetic subjects. Vitamin C may have antioxidant role or it may participate in the oxidative modification of lens protein that is seen in ageing.

Uncontrolled diabetes can lead to ocular complications. Recent research shows that diabetic retinopathy patients have decreased plasma levels of vitamin B_6, B_{12}, cobalt and manganese. Diabetic complications can be alleviated not only controlling diabetes but also by meeting the micronutrient requirement.

Neuropathy

Diabetic neuropathy is a type of nerve damage. High blood sugar can injure nerves throughout the body. There are four main types of neuropathy:

Peripheral neuropathy affects the feet, legs, hands and arms. Symptoms are pain, burning sensation, increased sensitivity to touch, cramps and numbness. Serious foot problems such as ulcers, infections, bone and joint pain can occur.

Autonomic neuropathy affects the nerves in the areas such as heart, bladder, stomach, intestine, sex organs and eyes. Symptoms are bowel problems, slow stomach emptying (gastroparesis) that causes nausea, vomiting and loss of appetite and decreased sexual response.

Proximal neuropathy affects the nerves in the thighs, hips, buttocks or legs, abdomen and chest. Symptoms are severe pain the hips and thighs, shrinking of thigh muscles and severe stomach pain.

In mononeuropathy symptoms are difficulty in focussing, aching behind one eye, paralysis on one side of the face and weakness in the hands. Diabetic neuropathic can be prevented by consistent blood sugar management and a healthy lifestyle.

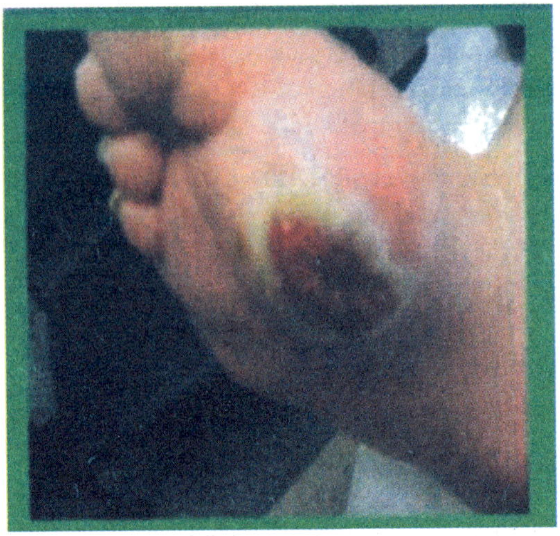

Fig. 19.8 **Sensation may be lost due to neuropathy. There is decreased blood flow to the feet which may lead to slow or non-healing of wounds**

Heart disease: High blood concentration of insulin and glucose can damage the endothelium that lines coronary arteries and set the stage for the formation of plaques. The overall mortality in diabetic people is increased around 2.6 times that of the normal population and there is a threefold rise in mortality in diabetes with cardiovascular disease. The increased mortality seen in diabetic population is mainly caused by large vessel disease which accounts for about 80 per cent of all deaths mostly from heart attack and stroke. CAD is strongly associated with type 2 diabetes.

Diabetes affects the blood vessels, the blood and the heart. Next to smoking diabetes is the major cause of heart disease. Diabetes increases the risk of heart disease by 3 to 4 fold. Diabetic patients are at great risk of developing atherosclerosis. The susceptibility of the diabetic to atherosclerosis is due to several factors. Hyperlipidemia occurs in one-third to one half of patients. HDL levels are reduced in type 2 diabetes, possibly enhancing susceptibility to atherogenesis. Non-enzymatic glycosylation of LDL renders it more recognisable by the LDL receptor while glycosylated HDL is more readily degradable than normal HDL—both these effects enhance atherogenesis. Diabetics have increased platelet adhesiveness and response to aggregating agents. These changes are also likely to favour atherogenesis. Most patients with type 2 diabetes also tend to be obese and hypertensive. All diabetics who have had the disease for at least 10 years, irrespective of the age of onset are likely to have clinically significant atherosclerosis.

Complications can be prevented by maintaining strict glycaemic control and at the same time keeping the hypoglycaemic episodes to the minimum. Post prandial glucose level should also be kept under control as elevated 2 hour post prandial glucose level is associated with increased cardiovascular mortality.

Nephropathy: Diabetic nephropathy is one of the chronic vascular complications of diabetes, which tends to develop after several years of diabetes and results in progressive loss of kidney function and face an increased risk of death.

Control of blood sugar is the most important factor in the prevention of nephropathy in both type 1 and type 2 diabetic individuals. Intensive management of blood sugar to achieve near normal levels significantly reduces the progression of diabetic nephropathy.

In general, people with diabetes should aim for blood pressure 130/80 mm Hg.

With the onset of overt nephropathy, dietary protein is to be restricted to 0.8 g of protein/kg body weight (less than 10 per cent of daily calories).

During the early stages of diabetic nephropathy, there are usually no symptoms. As the condition progresses, individuals with diabetic nephropathy may show oedema of the feet and legs. Later oedema may occur throughout the body, increase in blood pressure, larger amounts of protein leaking into the urine and elevated levels of cholesterol and triglyceride occur in the blood. Once the kidneys are severely damaged, blood sugar levels may drop because the kidneys retain insulin in the body. In late stages, patients become severely anaemic, breathless and serum potassium levels may rise, necessitating urgent dialysis.

The diet of every patient needs to be individualised based on the tendency to retain or lose salt, serum potassium, serum protein and cholesterol levels, overall nutrition status and urine volume. The dietary guidelines for management of diabetic nephropathy is given in Table 19.14.

Table 19.14 Dietary guidelines for diabetic nephropathic patients

Nutrient	*GFR > 60 ml/mn*	*GFR-30–60 ml/mn*	*GFR-15–30 ml/mn*
Calories kcal/kg	35	35	35
Protein g/kg	0.8	0.8	0.6–0.8
Salt g	5–6	5–6	5–6
Phosphorus mg/kg	no restrictions	8–12	8–12
Potassium mMol/kg	no restrictions	Individualised	1.0

Source: Sahay, R.K. *et al.*, 2009, Diabetic management of diabetic nephropathy, 41st National Conference Nutrition Society of India, National Institute of Nutrition, Hyderabad.

Strict control of hypertension in diabetic patients help in reducing the macro and microvascular complications especially nephropathy.

Diabetes being a multisystem metabolic disease needs a multi-faceted approach for its management. Diabetic patient should be made aware of the complications of diabetes and ways to prevent them and the physician / dietician should individualise the treatment options available.

"You should control diabetes otherwise it will control you".

PREGNANCY

Pregestational diabetes exists before pregnancy can be either type 1 or type 2 and is associated with significantly greater risks.

Most cases of diabetes diagnosed during the first trimester reflect pregestational diabetes as gestational diabetes occurs when insulin resistance increases in the later trimesters.

Diabetes in pregnancy increases the risk of adverse maternal, obstetric, fetal and neonatal outcomes. These risks can be reduced by optimising glycaemic control before conception and providing effective counselling on strategies to reduce the risks associated with pregnancy and diabetes.

Routine screening of reproductive-age women and diabetes should include a comprehensive physical examination and laboratory tests to identify at risk patients and begin strategic management.

The aim should be haemoglobin A1c of 6.5 per cent or lower without increasing the risk of hypoglycaemia.

Registered dietitian need to give individualised counselling about proper nutrition during pregnancy for a diabetic. Emphasis should be on regular exercise and the patient should maintain or achieve a medically optimal weight before conception.

Diabetic women who are planning pregnancy should avoid medications that have potential teratogenicity. Diabetic treatment should continue in pregnancy.

Glycaemic control should be assessed during every visit to the doctor and adjustments made to maintain or achieve optimal glycaemic control.

Reproductive age women with diabetes and high blood pressure benefit from lifestyle and behavioural modifications.

Maternal diabetes, insulin therapy and oral hypoglycaemic agents are not contraindications to breastfeeding. Breastfeeding is encouraged based on various short and long term health benefits for both breastfed infants and breastfeeding mothers. Breastfeeding decreases a woman's insulin requirements and increases the risk for hypoglycaemia especially in type 1 diabetics.

Insulin sensitivity increases immediately following delivery of the placenta. Therefore it is prudent to adjust insulin doses. Postpartum especially while a patient is breast feeding.

During pregnancy, the diabetic should be given 30–35 kcal/kg of the desirable body weight. The diet should provide 1.5–2.5 g of protein/kg body weight. The total gain in body weight during pregnancy should ideally not exceed 12 kg.

ALCOHOL

Alcohol contributes to calories and upset the dietary regulation. Alcohol damages the liver. Hypoglycaemia occurs due to impairment of glucose generating capacity of liver. Alcohol is absorbed from the stomach and reaches the liver through blood stream. It is metabolised and the capacity to release glucose from its reserve stores is blocked. Thus the danger of lowering of blood sugar, especially among those who are on insulin and oral drugs. Alcohol induced intoxication may mask the usual symptoms of low blood glucose level. Combination of alcohol and sulfonylurea may cause intense flushing of face and palpitation. Abstinence should be encouraged if obesity, hypertension or hypertriglyceridaemia is present.

The calorie value of some drinks is given in Table 19.15.

Table 19.15 Energy value of hard and soft drinks

Drink	*Amount*	*kcals*
Beer	240 ml	127
Brandy	30 ml	77
Gin	43 ml	105
Rum	43 ml	105
Whisky	43 ml	105
Wine	100 ml	105
Campa Cola	1 bottle	84
Campa Orange	1 bottle	84
Limca	1 bottle	52
Thumps Up	1 bottle	84
Colalite	1 bottle	52

Alcohol should be consumed in moderation i.e., not more than 2 equivalents one equivalent = 1 $^{1}/_{2}$ oz distilled beverage, 12 oz beer or 4 oz wine.

PREVENTION

Increased energy intake and decreased physical activity appear to have together promoted overweight and obesity, which are strong risk factors for diabetes. Several studies have demonstrated the potential for moderate, sustained weight loss to substantially reduce the risk for type 2 diabetes.

Both moderate-intensity and vigorous exercise can improve insulin sensitivity independent of weight loss and reduce risk for type 2 diabetes.

Clinical trial data from both the Finnish Diabetes Prevention study and the Diabetes Prevention program in the US strongly support the potential for moderate weight loss to reduce the risk for type 2 diabetes. The lifestyle intervention in both trials emphasised lifestyle changes that included moderate weight loss (7% of body weight) and regular physical activity (150 min/week) with dietary strategies to reduce intake of fat and calories.

In adiditon to preventing diabetes, the diabetes prevention program lifestyle intervention improves several CVD risk factors including dyslipidaemia, hypertension and inflammatory markers. Lifestyle intervention is cost-effective.

Reduced intake of fat, particularly saturated fat may reduce risk for diabetes by producing an energy-independent improvement in insulin resistance as well as by promoting weight loss.

Several studies have provided evidence for reduced risk of diabetes with increased intake of whole grains and dietary fibre. Whole grain containing foods have been associated with improved insulin sensitivity independent of body weight.

Dietary fibre has been associated with improved insulin sensitivity and improved insulin adequately to overcome insulin resistance.

Low glycaemic index foods that are rich in fibre and other important nutrients are to be encouraged.

Moderate consumption of alcohol (one drink for woman and two for men (15–30 g alcohol per day) has decreased risk of type 2 diabetes, coronary heart disease and stroke.

Carbohydrate Recommendations

- A dietary pattern that includes carbohydrate from fruits, vegetables, whole grains, legumes and low-fat milk is encouraged for good health.
- Monitoring carbohydrate whether by carbohydrate counting, exchanges or experience based estimation remains a key strategy in achieving the glycaemic control.
- The use of GI and GL may provide a modest additional benefit over that observed when total carbohydrate is considered alone.
- Sucrose containing foods should be avoided as they increase glycalmic index and energy value.
- People with diabetes are encouraged to consume a variety of fibre containing foods.
- Sugar alcohols and non-nutritive sweeteners are safe when consumed in permitted levels.
- Minimum requirement of carbohydrate is 130 g/d.

The amount of carbohydrate ingested is usually the primary determinant of postprandial response but the type of carbohydrate also affects the response. Intrinsic variables are specific type of food ingested type of starch (amylose vs amylopectin), style of preparation (cooling method and time, amount of heat or moisture used) ripeness and degree of processing. Extrinsic variables that may influence glucose response including fasting and pre-prandial blood glucose level, macronutrient distribution of the meal in which the food is consumed, available insulin and degree of insulin resistance.

Diabetics should be encouraged to consume fibre rich cereals like whole grains (greater than or equal to 5g fibre/serving), legumes, fruits, vegetables and whole grain products. Fibre intake goals for the general population is 14g/1000 kcal.

Fructose produces a lower postprandial glucose response when it replaces sucrose or starch in the diet. Fructose may adversely affect plasma lipids.

No reason to recommend that people with diabetes avoid normally occurring fructose in fruits, vegetables and other foods. Fructose from these sources usually accounts for only 3–4 per cent of energy intake.

Primary Prevention

This aims to prevent the onset of diabetes. It consists of 3 steps.

- Creating awareness about diabetes by mass media campaigns and education programmes.
- Screening programmes for diabetes and identification of high risk groups.
- Prevention of diabetes in high risk groups by diet, exercise, weight reduction and by avoiding diabetogenic drugs.

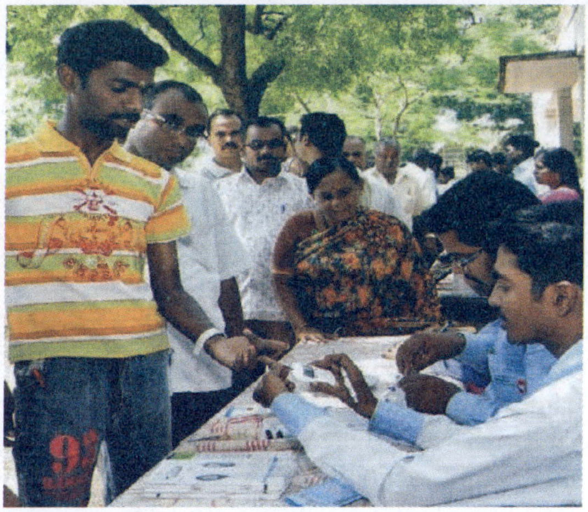

Fig. 19.9 Diabetes screening is the first step in preventing diabetes.

Primary prevention efforts will likely focus on weight management in childhood. Control of maternal diabetes and breastfeeding is potentially important in the etiology of type 2 diabetes.

Secondary Prevention

This aims to prevent the oneset of complications of diabetes in those who are already diagnosed to have diabetes. This can be achieved by

- Lifestyle modification
- Good glycaemic control
- Blood pressure control
- Lowering lipid levels

Lifestyle intervention is cost effective.

Moderate intensity and vigorous exercise can improve insulin sensitivity independent of weight loss and reduce risk of type 2 diabetes.

Reduced intake of fat particularly saturated fat may reduce the risk for diabetes by producing an energy independent improvement in insulin resistance as well as by promoting weight loss.

Whole grains and dietary fibre have been associated with improved insulin sensitivity independent of body weight. Consumption of low glycaemic index foods are to be encouraged.

Moderate consumption (15-30 g alcohol) per day decreases the risk of type 2 diabetes, coronary heart disease and stroke.

Fructose produces a low postprandial glucose response when it replaces sucrose or starch. Diabetics need not avoid naturally occurring fructose in fruits, vegetables and other foods. These foods can be taken in small quantities at a time.

Monitoring carbohydrate intake is the key strategy in achieving glycaemic control. Minimum requirement of carbohydrate is 130 g/d.

Sugar alcohols and nonnutritive sweetners can be used in permitted levels.

Tertiary Prevention

This aims to prevent, limit or reverse the complications of diabetes by regular screening and taking the necessary precautions and treatment.

DIETARY SUPPLEMENTS

A wide range of products claiming to lower blood glucose levels or prevent and treat diabetes complications and co morbidities are marketed to the public. Diabetics use supplements due to the difficulties they face with side effects from conventional treatments, a need to have control over one's healthcare, having belief in alternative therapies, due to high cost of prescription medications and dissatisfaction with traditional healthcare. Products classified now as dietary supplements are not approved by FSSAI for safety and efficacy.

Dietary supplements are pharmacologically active, it is important for healthcare providers to understand their chemical constituents, theorized mechanism of action, side effects and potential drug interactions.

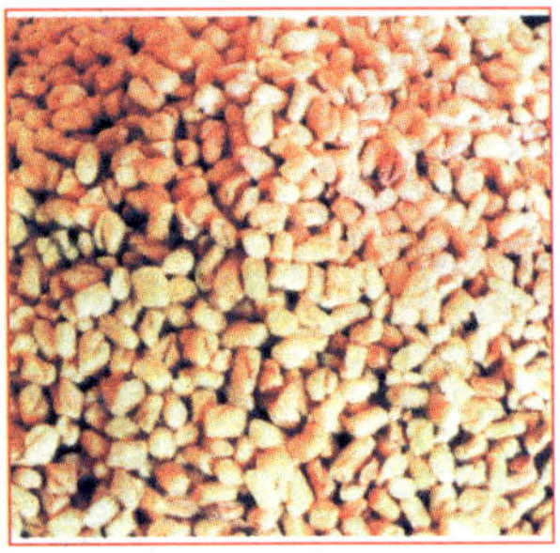

Fig. 19.10a It is scientifically proven that consumption of fenugreek 25 g/d reduces blood sugar levels.

Fenugreek: It belongs to the family leguminosae or *fabaceae*. Fenugreek contains saponins, glycosides and chemical constituents. It may have beneficial effects in pancreatic and other tissues and improve glucose and carbohydrate absorption as well as decrease insulin resistance, it delays gastric emptying, inhibits glucose transport, increases insulin receptors, improves peripheral glucose use and possible insulin secretion stimulation. It may increase anti coagulant effects of warfarin or herbs with anti coagulant activity.

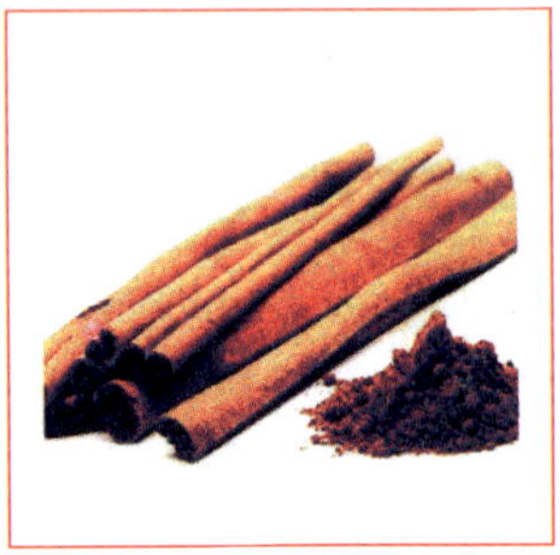

Fig. 19.10b Cinnamon may decrease blood glucose if combined with secretogogues.

Cinnamon: It belongs to the family *Cinnamomum zeylancium*. This is used for diabetes treatment. The active ingredient is related to procyanidin type A polymers which may increase insulin sensitivity. It has the potential benefit of decreasing fasting glucose and lipid levels. Dose used in studies include 1, 3 or 6 grams per day in divided doses. It promotes glycogen synthesis. Coumarin component warrants caution with anti coagulants.

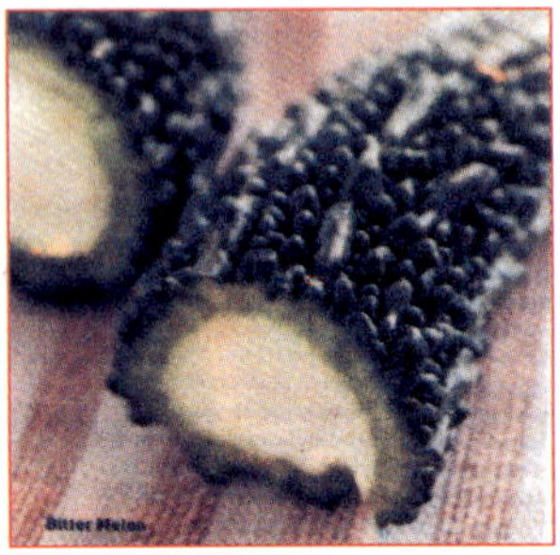

Fig. 19.10c As a food bitter melon consumption is acceptable

Bitter melon: It belongs to the family *Momordica charantia*. Bitter melon is a plant also called bitter gourd, karela or balsam pear. It may promote glucose uptake and inhibition of enzymes involved in glucose production and enhanced glucose oxidation. Different forms of bitter melon is available like powder and juice. Hypoglycemia can occur when used with sulphonylureas. As a tablet or a capsule caution should be exercised because this dosage form has not been tested in clinical studies.

Aloe Vera: Aloe is a member of the *Liliaceae* family. Aloe gel is been used to treat diabetes and hyperlipidemia. Two forms of aloe are dried leaf juice and aloe gel. Short term use may decrease fasting glucose and triglyceride levels and glycosulated hemoglobin concentration. It may cause additive hypoglycemia if combined with secretogogues.

Gymnema sylvestre: It increases enzymes that promote glucose uptake. It may stimulate β cells and increase β cell number, it may increase insulin release. Hypoglycemia is theoretically possible if combined with secretogogues.

Supplements may be considered as adjunctive agents to prescription treatments for hyperglycaemia, not something to be used instead of medications.

5th September is International Diabetes Educators' day.

14th November is World Diabetes day.

SUGGESTED READINGS

- Abbasi Jennifer, Interest in the ketogenic diet grows for weight loss and type 2 diabetes, JAMA, 2018: **319**.
- Lewis Hannah *et al.*, Diabetes and pregnancy: risks and opportunities. Cleveland clinic journal of medicine, 2018: **85**.
- Costello B. Rebecca, Do cinnamon supplements have a role in glycaemic control in Type 2 diabetes? A narrative review: J Acad Nutr Diet, 2016: **116.**
- Mohan V. *et al.*, (2014), Handbook of Diabetes Mellitus, Dr. Mohan's Diabetes Specialities Centre, Madras Diabetes, Research Foundation, Chennai.
- American Diabetes Association, www.diabetes.org.

QUESTIONS

1. Give three foods to be avoided and three foods to be included for a diabetic patient giving reasons. Explain the dietary guidelines.
2. Write a note on glucose tolerance test.
3. Differentiate between Type I and Type II diabetes.
4. What are food exchange lists? Write the importance of it in planning diabetic diet.
5. Explain how types of insulin affect modification of diet.
6. What is glycaemic index? What is the importance of it in diabetic diets? Give five foods which have low glycaemic index.
7. Discuss the principles of planning a diet for a diabetic patient.
8. Explain the metabolic changes in diabetes.
9. Describe the clinical symptoms and diagnosis of diabetes.
10. Write a note on (*a*) complications in diabetes and (*b*) artificial sweeteners.
11. Differentiate between hyperglycaemia and hypoglycaemia.
12. Write short note on pregnancy in diabetes mellitus.
13. Explain the following terms:
    (*a*) Insulin resistance (*b*) Glycaemic load
    (*c*) Ketoacidosis (*d*) Aspartame.
14. Explain the dietary supplements used in diabetes mellitus.
15. Discuss the preventive aspects of diabetes mellitus.

TOPICS FOR ACTIVITY

- Make a list of commonly consumed Indian recipes giving 15g carbohydrate.
- Plan and prepare a diet for a diabetic patient who takes long acting insulin at 9 pm.
- Plan and prepare a diet for a diabetic patient who takes oral glycaemic drugs in the morning and evening.

20

Diet in Diseases of Kidneys

The two bean-shaped kidneys sit just above the waist on each side of the spinal column.

Each kidney is only about the size of a fist yet they carry much of the responsibility of maintaining chemical homeostasis for the entire body.

Each kidney is composed of one million functional units called nephrons. Each nephron consists of a glomerulus which is a tuft of capillaries, invaginated into an epithelial sac called Bowman's capsule from which arises a tubule. Blood flow through the kidney is large, amounting 130 ml/mn which is about 1/4th of the cardiac output at rest. Figure 20.1 shows the diagram of glomerulus and glomerular capsule.

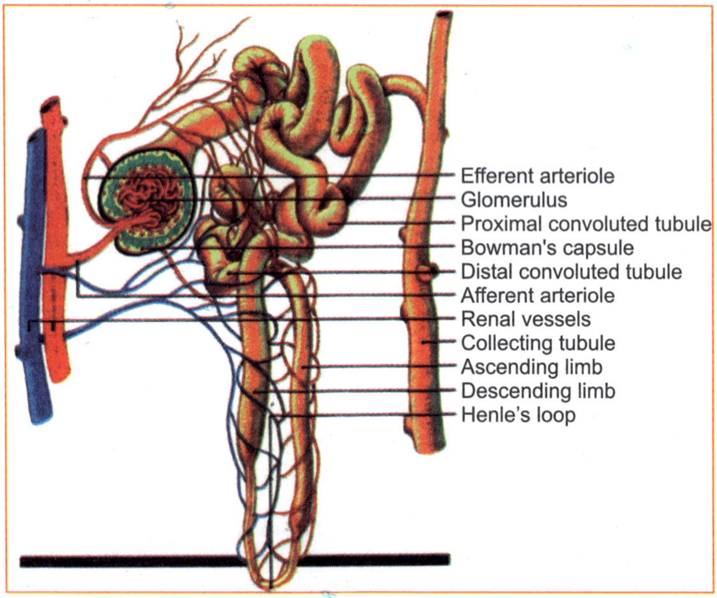

Fig. 20.1 **Nephron-Basic functional unit of kidney**

The hydrostatic pressure within the glomerular capillaries results in the filtration of fluid into Bowman's capsule. This fluid is similar in composition with plasma, except that it normally contains no fat and very little protein.

The filtrate, formed in the glomerulus is at a rate of 100 ml/min, passes first into the proximal convoluted tubule and from there, through the loop of Henle and distal convoluted tubule to the collecting ducts. The filtrate is modified according to the needs of the body by the selective reabsorption of its constituents and of water and by tubular secretion. Of the 50,000 ml of water and 22,500 mMol of sodium filtered through the glomerular capillaries during the course of a day, only about 1500 ml of water and 100–120 mMol of sodium remain to be excreted as urine.

Blood constituents which pass into the glomerular capsule: water, mineral salts, amino acids, keto acids, glucose, hormones, urea, uric acid, toxins and drugs.

Blood constituents which remain in the glomerulus: leucocytes, erythrocytes, platelets, blood proteins, globulins, albumin, prothrombin, and fibrinogen.

FUNCTIONS OF KIDNEYS

1. As excretory organs kidneys remove waste products of nitrogen metabolism. Urea, (dietary protein × 1/3 g) uric acid and creatinine as well as hydrogen ions and sulphates which arise from degradation of sulphur containing amino acids are excreted. They also excrete surplus quantities of water, sodium, potassium, calcium, phosphate and magnesium. In kidney failure, there is increased concentrations of nitrogenous waste products like urea (uraemia).
2. Kidneys regulate the amount of water, sodium and hydrogen ions in the body. By modifying the composition of urine, they maintain not only the volume of body fluids but also their electrolytic composition within narrow limits. Change in 2 per cent of water can result in the usual 1500 ml to 20 litres when kidneys fail to function. Acidosis, hypertension or hyperkalaemia can occur.
3. (*a*) Kidneys are an exclusive site for the production of 1,25 dihydroxy cholecalciferol, the active form of vitamin D. Improper function of kidneys can lead to bone diseases.
   (*b*) Kidneys also produce erythropoietin, which is essential for the synthesis of RBC
   (*c*) Renin is an enzyme released from the kidneys in response to low B.P. directly and also stimulates production of aldosterone.
4. Parathyroid hormone, calcitonin, insulin and gastrin are degraded by the kidneys.

Biochemical Assessment of Renal Function

(*a*) Measurement of plasma concentrations of urea, creatinine, sodium, potassium bicarbonate, calcium, inorganic phosphate and alkaline phosphate provide inexpensive and convenient biochemical indices of renal function. The upper limit of serum creatinine is 1.4 mg/100 ml for males and 1.3 mg/100 ml for females. Creatinine is execreted completely by glomeruli. As there is no tubular absorption, estimation of serum creatinine gives a good indicator of Glomerular Filtration Rate, GFR.

(*b*) GFR can be measured by creatinine clearance. The normal clearance level is 125 ml/min. When kidneys fail GFR would be less than 30 ml/min.

Formula for GFR = $\frac{UV}{P}$

U = Creatinine concentration in urine.

V = Volume of urine excreted in one minute.

P = Creatinine concentration in plasma.

The normal GFR is about 100–125 ml/mn/1.73 m^2.

(*c*) Potassium and phosphate increase in plasma and bicarbonate concentration also increases when there is kidney failure.

(*d*) Renal dysfunction increases alkaline phosphatase as vitamin D synthesis is affected.

(*e*) Volume of urine may be increased, decreased or normal at different stages of acute and chronic renal failure.

(*f*) Abnormal urinary constituents like blood and protein may be present in the urine when kidneys fail to function.

(*g*) In the disorder of renal tubules, excess loss of sodium, potassium or magnesium can occur.

GLOMERULONEPHRITIS

Glomerulonephritis is an inflammatory process affecting the glomeruli, the small blood vessels in the head of the nephron. It is most common in its acute form in children 3 to 10 years of age although it can also occur in adults past age 50. The onset is sudden and lasts a short time and proceed to either complete recovery or development of chronic nephrotic syndrome. The most common presentation follows a streptococcal infection and is usually although not always self-limiting. Renal infarction, acute pyelonephritis and metallic poisoning also cause glomerulonephritis. Other causes include primary kidney diseases such as IgA nephropathy and hereditary nephritis.

Mothers who are undernourished during pregnancy could have premature or low birth weight babies. Research has shown that these babies could have fewer glomeruli which later in life could lead to kidney problems. Individuals who consume a diet high in sodium or artificially sweetened drinks are more likely to experience a decline in kidney function. Secondary nephritis can occur due to systemic lupus erthematosus.

Clinical Symptoms

Haematuria and proteinuria are the classical symptoms. Oedema and shortness of breath can occur as a result of sodium and water retention and circulatory congestion. Tachycardia and elevated blood pressure may be present. The patient is generally anorexic which may contribute to feeding problems. There may be oliguria or anuria and uraemia which signals development of acute renal failure.

Figure 20.2 is a schematic diagram showing the sequence of reactions leading to kidney failure.

Principles of Dietary Management

The dietary management provides optimal nutritional support. Adequate proteins should be given unless there is oliguria or anuria. Salt is restricted if there is oedema, hypertension or oliguria. In most patients with acute uncomplicated disease, children with post-streptococcal glomerulo nephritis, diet modifications, are not crucial. Bed rest and antibiotic drug therapy are the main treatment. The fluid intake will be adjusted to output including losses in vomiting or diarrhoea.

Antibody response to bacteria, viruses, chemicals, and antibiotics—antigen (*streptococcal* infection)

↓

Excess Antigen-Antibody Complex (AAC) in circulation

↓

Antigen-Antibody Complex trapped in glomeruli

↓

Antigen-Antibody Complex binds components of complement

↓

Activated complement provide chemical factors that attract leukocytes

↓

The lysosomal enzymes of leukocytes cause injury to the glomerulus

↓

Lumps of AAC deposit between the epithelial cell of nephron capsule and the basement membrane of glomerui

↓

Lesions develop, fibrinogen leaks into Bowman's capsule

↓

Scar tissue is formed and obstruct the circulation through glomeruls

↓

Fatty degeneration, necrosis and destruction of nephrons

↓

Reduction in the number of functioning nephrons

↓

Nephrits

↓

Kidney failure

Fig. 20.2 Sequence of reactions leading to kidney failure

Dietary Treatment

Fluid: During the first stage of treatment the fluid should be decreased to allow for dispersal of oedema fluid. Daily weighing is needed to monitor overall fluid balance. In later stages the fluid intake is based on the volume of fluid excreted and an allowance (500 ml/day) is given for insensible water loss. The fluid is calculated taking into account the water consumed with drugs, water present in milk, curds, butter milk, tea, coffee, fruit juice and water used in sambar, rasam and curries. Small cups can be used for beverages. Daily fluid replacement should be 500 ml plus daily amount excreted in urine.

Insensible water loss is

– 30 ml/kg body weight for infants

– 20 ml/kg body weight for older children

– 10 ml/kg body weight for adults.

If liquids are limited, controlling thirst may be a problem. This can be overcome by sucking on a lemon wedge or eating sour candy or chew gum to moisten the mouth. Diabetics should choose sugar-free types. Blood sugar should be controlled in diabetics. Salt should be restricted to feel less thirsty. Mouth can be rinsed with water without swallowing it. To quench the thirst a few chips of ice can be sucked.

Water allowance should be put in a container and the patient should take from the allowance only. Water should be taken from a small 100 ml cup.

Energy: For children 80 kcal/kg body weight and 10 per cent for infection is suggested. Sufficient calories is given without increasing the protein intake by means of sugar, honey, glucose, sago, fats and oil and starchy foods. By giving carbohydrates liberally, protein catabolism and starvation ketosis are reduced. Above mentioned foods are not only rich in calories but also poor in sodium and potassium. Requirements are calculated based on age and weight and additional allowance of 10 per cent is given for infections. Cereals in all forms and sago are allowed.

Protein: If blood urea nitrogen is elevated and oliguria is present, dietary protein must be restricted. Usually the diet contains 0.5 g of protein/kg of ideal body weight for older children and 1 to 1.5 g/kg per day for younger children. The intake of proteins is reduced to a minimum by excluding protein rich foods. A low protein diet is recommended so as to give rest to the kidneys. Complete proteins are better, to ensure maximum utilisation. If anuria develops proteins should be stopped.

An intake of 20–40 g/day is considered sufficient. Out of the recommended protein, 50 per cent should be from animal protein. While prescribing high quality protein foods, it should be remembered that they are also good source of sodium. Foodstuffs containing high amount of poor quality protein should be restricted, for example, pulses and groundnuts increase urea levels in blood. Rice is preferable as it has low amount of protein but better quality of protein than wheat. Sago can be included as it does not contribute to protein. Fruits and vegetables which are usually low in protein can be prescribed provided they are also poor source of sodium and potassium.

Calcium: The intake should be roughly 1 g/day. When kidney function is impaired the body is unable to use calcium efficiently. When there is too little calcium and too much phosphorous in the blood the body tries to correct this by taking calcium from bones. Then bones become weak.

Sodium: The restriction of sodium varies with the degree of oliguria and hypertension. If renal function is impaired, the sodium will be restricted to 500 to 1000 mg/day. As recovery occurs, sodium can be increased. If oedema is present, sodium is restricted.

In sodium restricted diets, the following foods are avoided.

- Salt during cooking or on the table.
- Baking powder and soda bicarbonate which are added to cakes and pastries.

- Sodium benzoate, potassium metabisulphite which are added as preservatives in pickles, squashes and canned foods.
- Papads, cheese, salted chips and nuts, popcorn and biscuits. Processed foods are rich in sodium.
- Commercial soft drinks and proprietary drinks where sodium or potassium is present.
- Dried foods like fish, fruits and soup cubes.

Foods containing moderate amounts of sodium like milk, curds, pulses, vegetables (broad-beans, cauliflower, green mango, fenugreek leaves, spinach), coriander seeds, cumin seeds and jaggery should be taken in restricted amounts. Cereals, all gourds, brinjal, capsicum, peas fresh and fruits do not contain much sodium.

Use of herbs and spices like dash of lime, garlic, vinegar, nutmeg, bayleaf, coriander and cinnamon enhance flavour of foods.

Potassium: When the kidneys do not work properly, potassium builds up in the body and causes the heart to beat unevenly and stop suddenly. All renal patients should remember that too little potassium can also be dangerous. Potassium is restricted to 1 mmol/kg/day.

Table 20.1 gives potassium content of vegetables.

Table 20.1 Potassium content of vegetables mg/100 g

Vegetable low in potassium < 200 mg		*Vegetables high in potassium > 200 mg*	
Tinda	56	Spinach	625
Snake gourd	104	Amarnth	572
Parwar	117	Coriander leaves	546
Ridge gourd	118	Potato	541
Chocho marrow	120	Colocassia	514
Bottle gourd	124	Drumstick	419
Mango green raw	147	Ash gourd	372
Capsicum green	154	Broad beans	362
Tomato ripe	167	French beans	324
Cucumber	183	Brinjal	302

Source: Longvah, T. *et al.*, 2017, Indian food composition tables, National Institute of Nutrition, Hyderabad.

Potassium is found naturally in almost all foods particularly in fruits, vegetables and meats. Potassium content can be reduced in vegetables by cooking in excess water and discarding the water. Spices and condiments can be used in small quantities as they are rich in potassium. When urine formation is reduced potassium is also restricted.

Foods high in potassium are nuts, jaggery, instant coffee, chocolate and cocoa powder.

Foods low in protein and potassium and high in calories are sugar, honey, arrow-root, sago, unsalted butter, vegetable shortenings, vegetable oils and ghee can be consumed in unrestricted amounts.

Table 20.2 gives potassium content of fruits.

Table 20.2 Potassium content of fruits mg/100 g

Fruits low in Potassium < 200		*Fruits high in Potassium > 200*	
Lemon	113	Musk melon orange flesh	206
Apple	116	Pomogranate	206
Watermelon	126	Goose berry	223
Mango	143	Custard apple	278
Pineapple	143	Jack fruit	279
Litchi	161	Sapota	280
Plums	162	Guava	283
Orange	164	Dates processed	289
Grapes	171	Banana	335
Papaya	173	Tamarind pulp	836

Source: Longvah, T. *et. al.*, 2017, Indian food composition tables, National Institute of Nutrition, Hyderabad.

Salt substitutes may contain potassium salts which are contra-indicated for patients with kidney problems.

Phosphorus: Phosphorus is a mineral found in almost all foods. Large amounts are found in cheese, nuts, dried beans and peas. The balance between dietary intake and excretion of phosphorus can be impaired in patients with decreased renal function, leading to hyperphosphatemia. Eating foods high in phosphorus will raise the phosphorus in blood and this can cause calcium to be pulled from bones. This will make bones weak and cause them to break easily. Hence these foods should be restricted in the diet. Phosphorus intake should be restricted to 8-12 mg/kg/d.

Foods to be included: rice, sugar, leached vegetables, sago, honey.

Foods to be restricted: milk, curd, jaggery, pulses, fruits.

Foods to be avoided: salts, greens rich in sodium like amaranth, bakery products, pulses, meat, chicken and egg.

Table 20.3 gives a model diet for acute nephritic patient.

Table 20.3 Model diet for an acute nephritic patient

Patient's age: 5 years, wt.—15 kg., B.P. 130/90, urine output—300 ml.

Requirement: Calories 15 × 80 = 1200 + 120 (10%) = 1320.

Renal failure: Absent.

Protein: 1.5—1.75 × 15 = 25 g/day.

Sodium: Moderate hypertension 10 mMol = 500 mg NaCl.

Fluid: 300 ml. + 25 ml/kg body weight = 300 + 25 × 15 = 675 ml.

Food	*Fluid*	*Energy kcal*	*Protein g*	*Sodium mg*
Idlis 2		100	4	90
Sugar 20 g		80	—	—
Ghee 5 g		45	—	—

(*Contd...*)

Table 20.3 (Contd...)

Food	Fluid	Energy kcal	Protein g	Sodium mg
Milk 100 g	100	65	3.5	15
Sugar 10 g		40	—	—
Rice 2 cups		200	4	5
Dal 4 tsp		60	2	3
Ghee/oil 10 g		90	—	—
Vegetable 50 g		25	1	20
Buttermilk 300 ml	300	60	3	15
Sugar 15 g		60	—	—
Rice 2 cup		200	4	5
Dal 4 tsp		60	2	3
Ghee/oil 2 tsp		90	—	—
Vegetable 50 g		25	1	20
Buttermilk 300 ml	300	60	3	15
Sugar 15 g		60	—	—
Total	700	1320	27	191

Source: Gnanasundaram, S., 1988, II Annual Conference of Nutrition India (Tamil Nadu chapter).

NEPHROTIC SYNDROME (NEPHROSIS)

Nephrotic syndrome can be caused due to progressive glomerulonephritis, diabetes mellitus, systemic lupus erythematosus, amyloidosis, quartan malaria, resulting due to drugs, heavy metals and toxic venom. Medical treatment of the nephrotic syndrome requires diagnosis and management of the underlying disorder responsible for proteinuria.

Clinical Symptoms

Nephrosis is distinguished clinically from glomerulonephritis by the consistent absence of hypertension and haematuria and the usual absence of anaemia and nitrogen retention. Like in glomerulonephritis, proteinuria is present but to an even more marked degree, along with oedema.

Nephrotic syndrome usually starts between the age of 2–6 years; 60–70 per cent are boys. The onset is insidious with swelling around the eyes and facial puffiness. The swelling gradually increases to involve the extremities and abdomen and if untreated may become massive.

There is heavy proteinuria, hypoalbuminaemia and peripheral oedema. Proteinuria develops when the leakage of protein from the glomeruli exceeds the reabsorptive capacity of the renal tubules. Daily losses up to 5 g in adults and up to 0.1 g/kg in children can usually be tolerated. Plasma albumin is in small molecules and escapes most readily through a leak in the glomerular membrane. Plasma globulins which have higher molecular weight appear in urine in much smaller amounts. Proteinuria leads to oedema. Figure 20.3 shows the role of protein in maintaining fluid balance between capillaries and intercellular spaces and Fig. 20.4 shows the sequence of glomerular inflammation leading to oedema.

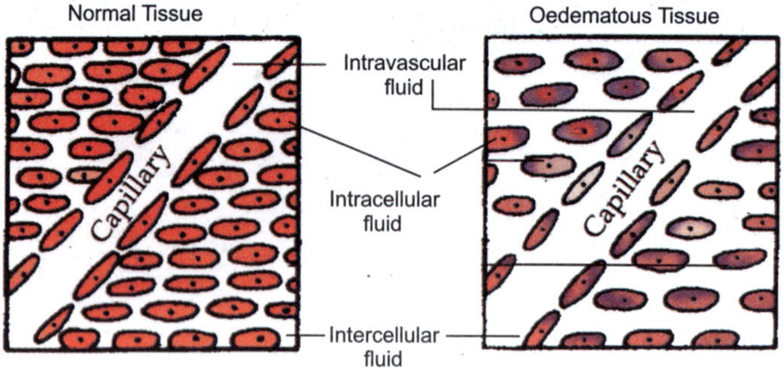

Fig. 20.3 **Distribution of fluids in normal and oedematous tissue**

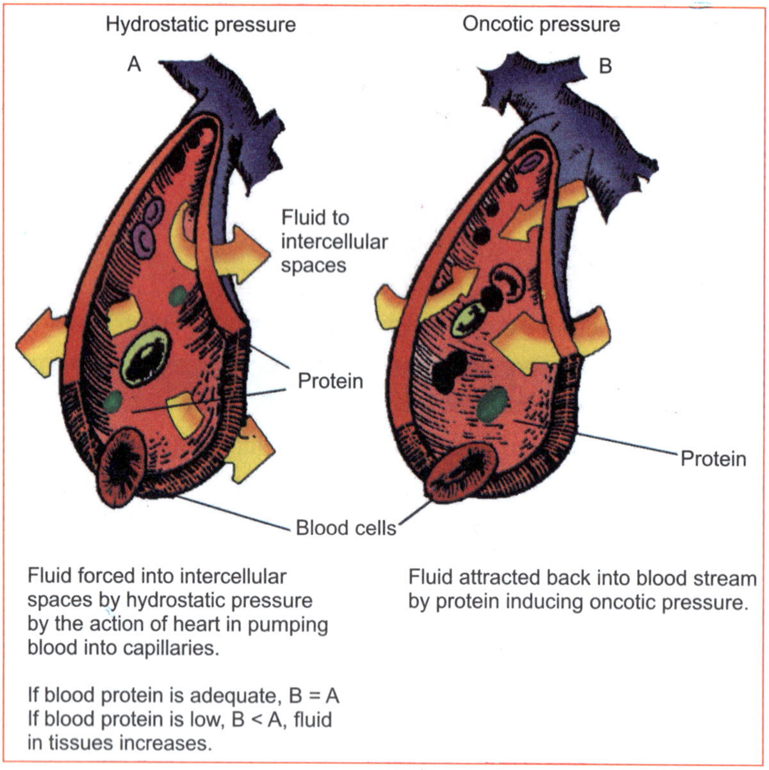

Fig. 20.4 **Role of protein in maintaining fluid balance between capillaries and intercellular spaces**

Large urinary losses of albumin and other plasma proteins lead to tissue wastage, fatty liver, malnutrition and increased susceptibility to infection. Lipoproteins and other proteins such as fibrinogen and other coagulation factors are increased while antithrombin 3 is lost in urine. This may help to account for the increased incidence of atherosclerosis and thrombosis in patients with nephrotic syndrome. Plasma cholesterol is increased in them.

Principles of Diet

Restricted protein, high carbohydrate, restricted salt, moderate fat with restricted fluid are recommended for a nephrotic patient. Vitamin supplements especially vitamin C should be given.

Patients with severe and persistent hyperlipidemia should maintain a normal weight for height. The diet should be low in fat and cholesterol.

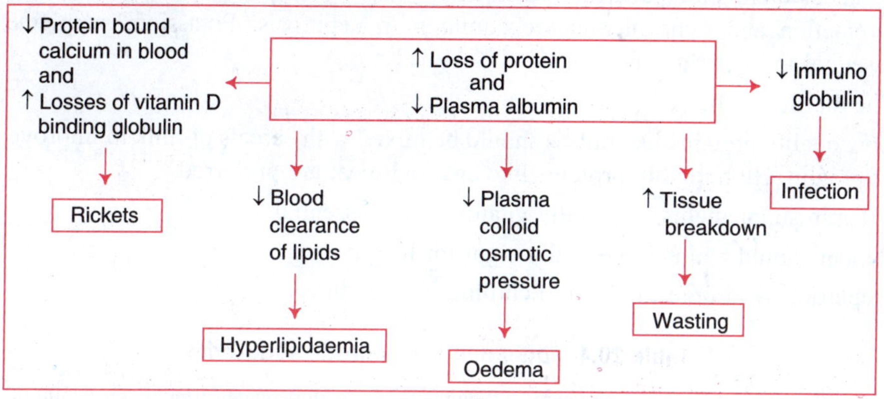

Fig. 20.5 Effects of protenuria in nephrotic syndrome

Dietary Treatment

To ensure protein use for tissue synthesis, sufficient kilocalories must always be provided; 2000 kcals is suggested. Since appetite is usually poor, much encouragement is needed and food must be appetising. Weight loss or infection indicates the need for additional calories.

Moderate protein restriction 0.8–1.0 g/kg is often employed. Restriction is often advocated since increased protein intake may have an adverse effect on renal function in some diseases. In patients whose renal function is already impaired, there is evidence that an increased intake of protein is associated with hyperfiltration in the remaining nephrons which may result in glomerulosclerosis and renal failure. The daily total dietary protein intake should replace the daily urinary protein losses so as to avoid negative nitrogen balance. Protein malnutrition often occurs with urinary protein losses greater than 10 g/day.

To allow for optimal protein use, three fourth's of the protein should be from sources of high biologic value.

Diet should be low in saturated fat, cholesterol and refined sugars to control elevated blood lipids.

Hypocalcaemia in nephrotic syndrome is due to a reduction in protein bound calcium secondary to hypoalbuminaemia. Occasionally, low ionised calcium levels are seen, which result from urinary loss of vitamin D binding globulin and 25-hydroxy vitamin D_3 and may cause tetany. An adequate calcium intake is necessary and if symptoms of hypocalcaemia occur, supplement of vitamin D should be given.

Diuretics are of great value when controlling oedema. Diuretic induced losses of potassium may be replaced by potassium supplement.

Sodium is restricted to prevent further accumulation of oedema fluid and prevent hypertension. Modest restriction may be used to prevent recurrence of oedema. But severe sodium restriction may be carefully selected as it may affect the potassium elimination. Salt is restricted to around 2–3 g per day. No salt is to be added while cooking or on table. Low sodium foods can be consumed liberally. Restriction of fluid is necessary if oliguria is present, that is, urine output is less than 25 ml/kg/24 hours and when the kidney is affected in its functions accompanied by oedema.

Special Instructions

- Since calcium and potassium deficiency may accompany severe proteinuria, bone rarefaction and hypokalemia are common in nephrosis. Potassium supplements are essential in the treatment.
- The diet has to be soft.
- Low quality proteins like pulses should be mixed with cereals or milk to improve quality of protein. High quality proteins like egg and meat are preferred.
- Vitamin supplements, especially vitamin C are essential.
- Patient should maintain normal weight for height.

  Nephrotic syndrome can lead to chronic renal failure.

Table 20.4 Model diet in nephrotic syndrome

Age: 5 years Weight - 15 kg with oedema (urine output – 500 ml)
Serum albumin: 1.8 g No Hypertension*
Calories: 15 × 80 = 1200 + 10% extra = 1320 – 1400 kcal
Protein*: 15 × 3* = 45 g (Since he is undernourished)
Fluid: 550 + 325 = 825
Salt: Restricted.

	Allowance	*Fluid ml*	*Protein g*	*Energy kcal*	*Sodium mg*
Idlis	4	–	8	200	180
or					
Bread slices	4	–	8	200	600
Butter g	12.5	–	–	112	100
Milk ml	750	750	25	510	105
Rice (cooked 3 cups) g	100	–	6	300	7.5
Dhal g	25	–	6	90	9
Vegetable g	100	–	1	30	40
Egg	1	–	6	70	70
Plantain	1	–	0.5	30	36
Orange	1	–	0.5	40	5
	Total	750	53	1382	732

*If the child is normal 1.5–2 / kg body weight is sufficient

Source: Gnanasundaram S. 1988, 11th Annual Conference of Nutrition Society of India (Tamil Nadu Chapter).

ACUTE RENAL FAILURE

There is a sudden shutdown of renal function following metabolic insult or traumatic injury to normal kidneys. There is high mortality and the condition needs a medical emergency in which the nutritionist plays a supporting role.

Causes

- Loss of blood can cause acute renal failure, as the blood flow to kidney decreases during accidents, ulcers, internal haemorrhage or at the time of delivery.
- Loss of plasma as in burns and crush injuries.
- Loss of fluid in diarrhoea, vomiting, diabetic coma (excessive urination and excessive sweating).
- General anasthesia and surgical operation reduce renal blood flow and may precipitate renal failure.
- Serious infections produce shock and reduce renal blood.
- Acute haemolytic disorders (RBC are destroyed due to some disease).
- Nephrotoxins like paracetamol and some variety of mushrooms.
- Nephritis or nephrosis can also result in acute renal failure.

Symptoms

- Low urine volume (anuria or oliguria). The urinary output may be as little as 20 to 200 ml/day.
- Accumulation of waste products of protein metabolism in blood. Serum urea nitrogen and creatinine levels are increased.
- Excretion of potassium is diminished. The rise in serum potassium is due to its release from tissue protein during breakdown to provide calories.
- There is also increased phosphate and sulphate with decreased sodium, calcium and base bicarbonate.
- The patient may be lethargic, anorexic and may suffer from nausea and vomiting. There may be elevation of blood pressure and signs of ureamia. Oral intake is difficult during this period.
- Death is caused not because of rise in blood urea but potassium intoxication or water intoxication due to over treatment with fluids to stimulate urine excretion.

Dietary Management

Energy: A minimum of 600–1000 kcal is necessary. A high calorie intake is desired mainly from carbohydrates and fats.

Proteins: All foods containing protein are stopped if the patient is under conservative treatment and blood urea nitrogen is rising. However, 40 g is allowed during haemodialysis or peritoneal dialysis as it will reduce endogenous protein breakdown. Usually the protein content of diet varies depending upon the urea content of the blood.

Carbohydrates: A minimum of 100 g/day is essential to minimise tissue protein breakdown. Two litres of 5 per cent glucose meets this. If the patient is not fed by mouth, a nasogastric tube feeding of 700 ml of 15 per cent glucose is administered. If orally given, 700 ml of glucose with lime juice can be given.

Fluid: The total fluid permitted is 500 ml + losses through urine and gastrointestinal tract. With visible perspiration, an additional 500 ml may be necessary.

Sodium: Sodium loss through urine is measured and replaced. Dilutional hyponatremia occurs due to water retention. Restriction of water than salt administration is indicated. Therefore, sodium restriction is also judged based on sodium loss in the urine.

Potassium: Potassium intoxication (hyperkalemia) occurs with a daily rise of 0.7 mEq serum potassium. It has deleterious effects on heart. A bowel wash may remove 100 mEq of potassium. Potassium sources like tomato juice, coffee, tea, cocoa and potassium rich vegetables are avoided.

Haemodialysis or peritoneal dialysis may be considered when blood urea level is over 200 mg/100 ml. The diet may then be raised to 2000–3000 kcal and 40 g protein. If patient cannot take oral feeds, intravenous fat and amino acid solutions are given.

Foods allowed/restricted	*Foods avoided*
Bread, salt free butter, low protein pudding	Protein concentrates, pulses, excess consumption of milk, egg and meat.

Table 20.5 gives model diet for a patient suffering from acute renal failure.

Table 20.5 Model diet for a patient suffering from acute renal failure

Age: 5 years, weight—15 kg B.P. normal.

Fluid: output 125 + 25 × 15 = 500 ml.

Energy: 15 × 80 = 1200 + 20% more = 1450-1500 kcal.

Protein: 1–1.25 g/kg body weight = 15 – 18.75 g.

Sodium: Salt free.

Food	*Amount g*	*Fluid g*	*Energy kcal*	*Protein g*	*Sodium mg*
Milk	500	500	340	17	75
Custard powder	25	—	90	1	—
Sugar	100	—	400	—	—
Butter (unsalted)	75	—	675	—	—
		500	1505	18	75

Source: Gnanasundaram, S., 1988, II Annual Conference of Nutrition Society of India (Tamil Nadu chapter).

CHRONIC KIDNEY DISEASE

Chronic kidney disease is a permanent progressive loss of kidney function characterised by a decline in glomerular filtration rate. Chronic kidney disease is defined as abnormalities of kidney function or structure that persist for > 3 months and have health implications.

The primary causes of chronic kidney disease are diabetes and hypertension. The major outcomes of chronic kidney disease regardless of cause include progression to kidney failure, metabolic complications of decreased kidney function, and cardio vascular disease.

Decreased Kidney Function

Glomerular Filtration Rate Categories in CKD			
Stage		***Description***	***Glomerular Filtration Rate (GFR) ml/min***
At increased risk		With risk factors for CKD (diabetes, high blood pressure, family history, older age, etc)	More than 90
1		Kidney damage (protein in the urine) and normal GFR	More than 90
2		Kidney damage and mildly decreased GFR	60–89
3	3a	Mildly to moderately decreased GFR	45–59
	3b	Moderately to severely decreased GFR	30–44
4		Severely decreased GFR	15–29
5		Kidney failure	Less than 15

As kidney disease worsens, the glomerular filtration rate (GFR) goes down. At Stage 5, renal replacement therapy (dialysis or transplant) is commonly initiated. Urine albumin to creatinine ratio (ACR) is an additional marker for CKD. When the ACR is > 30 mg/gm, albuminuria is present. Higher levels of albuminuria indicate more severe kidney damage and are associated with increased risk of progression to End-Stage Kidney Disease (ESKD) and mortality.

The prevalence of protein energy wasting (PEW) in patients with CKD remains high. In experience spite of complexity and multi-factorial etiology of PEW, many of these factors are related to decreased dietary intake of energy and protein. Nutrition support therapy can improve many signs of PEW.

The immediate strategy should be the use of oral nutrition supplements to replenish and avoid further depletion of protein and energy stores.

Only when these fundamental steps fails to improve nutrition status should be more invasive approaches should be considered for patients with CKD who have been diagnosed with PEW such as enteral tube feeding, partial parenteral nutrition and total parenteral nutrition therapies.

Nutrition management remains among the most important interventions for slowing CKD progression and delaying or preventing ESKD end stage kidney disease. Healthy lifestyle habits and the maintenance of a healthy weight play a key role in preventing type 2 diabetes and hypertension, the two major causes of CKD. Once kidney disease is established, dietary modifications such as decreasing intake of animal protein, phosphorous additives and salt and increasing intake of fresh fruits and vegetables may slow kidney disease progression. However dietary modifications for slowing kidney disease progression require patient education and close monitoring due to risks of malnutrition and hyperkalemia. Medical nutrition therapy (MNT), is individualized.

The urine volume depends upon GFR. Once chronic renal disease occurs, the normal functions of kidney like regulation of body fluids, electrolytes, pH and excretion of metabolites are disrupted and the following symptoms occur.

Symptoms

- Clinical symptoms result from the progressive loss of nephrons and the consequent decrease in renal blood flow and glomerular filtration.
- Dehydration or water intoxication, sodium depletion, high serum potassium, acidosis and increased susceptibility to infection are the most general manifestations.
- When GFR falls below 5 ml/min., oedema, high blood pressure, irregular heart beats and pericarditis occur.
- The symptoms of gastrointestinal system may be loss of appetite, vomiting and hiccups.
- Neurological symptoms like peripheral neuropathy, twitching, convulsions and coma can also occur.
- Haemopoietic system may be affected leading to anaemia resulting in tiredness and breathlessness and tendency to bleed due to abnormal platelet function.
- Skin changes like pigmentation, itching and purpura.
- Renal osteodystrophy metastatic calcification and dwarfism and ricket growth failure can also occur.

Acidosis: Non-volatile acids are excreted by kidneys. Chronic kidney disease therefore produces acidosis that increases calcium resorption from bones leading to osteomalacia and renal osteodystrophies. In chronic kidney disease, the activation of vitamin D and the action of parathyroid hormone in controlling serum calcium and phosphorus levels cannot proceed at normal levels. The impaired vitamin D metabolism results in a bone disease called osteodystrophy in which there is bone pain, various bone deformities, and awkward gait and in children it impairs growth. There may be calcification of soft tissues further hindering renal function.

These metabolic impairments may cause hyperphosphataemia and hypocalcaemia. Failure of renal tubular reabsorption results in hyperphosphataemia which in turn produces rickets. Phosphate intake has to be restricted. Aluminium hydroxide 1 ml/kg/day should be given. Serum phosphate levels should be maintained at 4–6 mg/100 ml in children. Calcium and active form of vitamin D supplementation should be given.

Anaemia: Kidneys release an enzyme called renal erythropoietic factor. The enzyme acts on one of the plasma proteins, a globulin to split the glycoprotein molecule. When kidneys are damaged there is depressed red blood cell production, red cells survive a shorter time but have their usual size and haemoglobin content.

Anaemia can also occur due to blood loss through nose bleeding, haematuria, ecchymosis or gastrointestinal bleeding due to deficient coagulatory factors and increased vascular fragility. Hemolysis may also contribute to anaemia. Those on haemodialysis lose blood due to blood sampling and in dialysis machine.

Deficiency of iron, vitamin C and folic acid may result in anaemia.

Objectives of Treatment

- To prevent protein catabolism and minimise uraemic toxicity.
- To avoid dehydration or overhydration.
- To carefully correct acidosis.
- To correct electrolyte depletion and avoid excesses.
- To control fluid and electrolyte losses from vomiting and diarrhoea.
- To maintain optimal nutritional status.
- To maintain appetite and stimulate morale and a sense of well being.
- To control complications such as hypertension, bone pain and control nervous system abnormalities.
- To retard progression of renal failure, thus postponing the ultimate necessity of dialysis.

Management varies according to the stage of illness. In mild cases, active steps should be taken to control hypertension, salt and water imbalance. During the course of illness in which oral feeding cannot be maintained, fluids and electrolytes should be given intravenously. Protein restriction may not be necessary in the absence of symptoms.

As renal failure progresses, the patient develops symptoms of uraemia and the patient may be treated by dietetic measures alone or by regular haemodialysis or peritoneal dialysis or by renal transplantation.

Nutrient recommendations

Table 20.6 gives nutrient recommendations for CKD patients who are in stages 1–4.

Table 20.6 Nutrient recommendations for CKD (stages 1-4) for adults

Nutrient	*Recommendations*
Energy (kcal/kg/day)	> 60 Years of age: 25–35 < 60 Years of age: 35
Protein (g/kg/day)	0.55 to 0.75 High biological value
Fat (% total kcal) ω-3 fatty acid	25%-35%; Cholesterol < 200 mg/day; saturated fat < 7% 1.3–4 g/d
Sodium (mg/day)	2400
Potassium (mg/day)	Generally unrestricted unless serum potassium level is > 5 mg/dL or potassium-sparing medications are used
Calcium (mg/day)	< 2000 Including binders and dietary intake
Phosphorus (mg/day)	800–1000 If serum phosphorus level is > 4.6 mg/dL
Fluid (ml/day)	Generally unrestricted and dependent on medical status
Vitamins/minerals	Individualised. Deficiency of folic acid, B_{12} and vitamin D to be corrected
Vitamin C	90 mg/for men and 75 mg for women

Source:
- Kent S. Pamela, Integrating clinical nutrition Practice guidelines in chronic kidney disease, J. Amer, Diet, Asso. 2005; **20**.
- Handu Deepa et al Executive Summary of the 2020 Academy of Nutrition and Dietetics and National Kidney Foundation. Clinical Practice guidelines for Nutrition in CKD J Acad Nutr Diet 2021:121.

Energy: Adequate kilocalories are mandatory. Carbohydrate and fat must supply sufficient non-protein kilocalories to spare protein for tissue protein synthesis and to supply energy. Patients are encouraged to consume all the carbohydrate and fats they can, since the end products of their metabolism, carbon dioxide and water, do not impose a burden on the progressive renal failure. If energy intake is inadequate endogenous protein tissue catabolism takes place to supply energy and will further aggravate the existing uraemia. Requirements of calories is similar to the normal requirements

Infancy	–	100–120 kcal/kg body weight
Childhood	–	80–110 kcal/kg body weight
Adults	–	25–35 kcal/kg body weight

Protein: Failing kidneys need to be given rest. Protein intake can be reduced to 0.5 g/kg of body weight per day. There is then a parallel fall in urea production and fall in blood urea and anorexia and vomiting are relieved. This may result from a reduction in the diffusion of urea from the plasma into the intestinal lumen, where it is hydrolysed by bacteria to ammonium carbonate. The ammonium ion is a well-known gastrointestinal irritant and could thus mediate the potentially toxic effects of increased blood urea. The ammonia released in the gut is reabsorbed and taken to the liver by the portal circulation where it is either recycled to urea or used for synthesis of non-essential amino acids. This provides an important metabolic pathway which is exploited in patients on very low protein diets in the treatment of severe chronic kidney disease. To prevent endogenous losses protein intake should be 0.25 g/kg body weight or 15–20 g daily in older children and adolescents. Very low protein diets are advised during severe degree of chronic kidney disease.

With these dietetic measures, a patient in whom the GFR has fallen to 2 to 4 ml/min can sustain. Otherwise dialysis would be necessary.

In chronic kidney disease, the protein intake can be adjusted according to creatinine clearance. If the patient has a creatinine clearance of 40 ml/min or higher, no protein restriction should be required.

$$\text{Creatinine clearance (for male)} = \frac{140 - \text{Age} \times \text{wt in kg (present body weight)}}{\text{Serum creatinine mg/dl} \times 72} = - \text{ ml}$$

$$\text{Creatinine clearance (for female)} = \frac{140 - \text{Age} \times \text{wt in kg (present body weight)}}{\text{Serum creatinine mg/dl} \times 72} \times 0.85 = - \text{ ml}$$

Table 20.7 gives relationship between creatinine clearance and protein intake.

Table 20.7 Relationship between creatinine clearance and protein intake

Creatinine clearance ml/mn	*Nitrogen intake g/day*	*Protein intake g/day*
10–40	9.6	60
5–20	6.4	40
2–10	2.5–3	20

In general, a patient with creatinine clearance below 8 ml/min requires dialysis and will probably require transplantation.

Fluid and electrolytes: In patients with less than 5 per cent of the original functioning kidney tissue, other steps have to be taken in addition to protein restriction to preserve fluid and ionic balance. Oedematic diuresis is secondary to plasma hyper osmolarity. Thirst controls fluid intake. Increase in fluid intake often increases the excretion of urea. If fluid retention occurs, patient should be given diuretics and sodium should be restricted especially if weight increases in the presence of hyponatraemia. If all the above measures fail, dialysis is considered. The usual fluid permitted is, volume of daily urine plus 500 ml.

Sodium: Excretion of sodium is more or less constant in chronic kidney disease. Ideal intake: 1 to 2 mMol/kg of body weight for infants 40–60 mMol/day for older children.

Strict restriction is necessary only if hypertension and oedema are present. 0.2 mMol/kg of body weight/day + diuretics are given until crisis is over.

In chronic kidney patients, salt intake is restricted to 2.4 g/day.

Potassium: Potassium excretion varies appropriately with intake, a response that is mediated by a hormone aldosterone and according to plasma potassium concentration. The kidneys are able to maintain near normal levels of potassium excretion as long as the distal tubule in kidneys are responsive to aldosterone. Thus dietary restrictions are necessary only in potassium retention status. Up to 4 g/day potassium intake is recommended in these patients. This has to be restricted to 1 mMol/kg of body weight/day. If not possible, calcium, potassium exchange resin is given. Hypokalemia can occur at any time in chronic kidney disease. If it occurs, small dose of potassium should be given and serum levels are monitored.

Hyperkalaemia occurs only in severe glomerular filtration failure. Treatment is same as in acute renal failure. Double boiling and draining excess water reduces potassium content.

A combination of high potassium, low calcium and high magnesium have an adverse effect on heart.

In renal failure there is a reduction in the phosphate excretion. If intake remains constant, the net effect will be phosphate retention and an increase in the plasma phosphate concentration. This leads to abnormalities in the metabolism of calcium, vitamin D and high parathyroid hormone levels finally leading to renal bone disease. The dietary phosphate restriction early in the renal disease is able to reverse many of the abnormalities in mineral metabolism. Guidelines recommend restricting the dietary phosphorus levels to 800–1000 mg/day. Maintaining the calcium intake within the RDA is reasonable.

Dietary flavonoids contribute to beneficial antioxidant properties and should include in the diet of chronic kidney disease patients. Dietary flavonoids decrease the risk of death from coronary heart disease because of their oxidative properties. Flavonoid rich foods include fruits and vegetables as well as tea, red wine and dark chocolate.

Effective management of CKD improves survival, decreases morbidity, and improves quality of life. The clinical implications associated with CKD are numerous and challenging. Recent studies have shown that intensive nutrition intervention can control modifiable risk factors like diabetes, high blood pressure, dyslipidemias, anemia, obesity, bone disease, and prevent or delay the onset of kidney disease. In the early stages of CKD, the objective is to preserve renal function and limit accumulation of nitrogenous waste products. This is accomplished with a moderately low-protein intake. Prevention of malnutrition is paramount, and an adequate caloric intake is essential. Most patients with CKD have multiple risk factors for progression of kidney disease and for development or worsening of CVD. Optimal management of CKD requires the integration of available clinical guidelines and life-style modifications.

DIALYSIS

Dialysis is a procedure that replaces some of the kidney's normal functions. It is performed when a person experiences more than 95 per cent kidney failure. Like healthy kidneys, dialysis keeps the body in balance by removing waste products including salt and excess fluids, maintaining a safe level of blood chemicals such as potassium, sodium and chloride in the body and controlling blood pressure.

In general, dialysis becomes necessary at a creatinine clearance of 4 to 8 ml per minute or a serum creatinine of about 10 mg/dl. If anorexia due to uraemia is a predisposing factor, initiation of dialysis is mandatory.

There are two basic kinds of dialysis—haemodialysis and peritoneal dialysis.

Haemodialysis: In this, an artificial kidney, haemodialyser is used to remove the waste products from the blood and restore the body's chemical balance.

Plastic tubing attached to the needles connects the patient to the artificial kidney. Artificial kidney contains, two compartments, one for the patient's blood and one for a cleaning solution called dialysate. A thin porous membrane separates these compartments. Blood cells, proteins and other important substances in the blood remain in their compartment because they are large to pass through while smaller waste products like urea and creatinine in the blood and excess water pass through the holes of the membranes and are washed away. The clean blood now enters the patient's body. Needed substances like calcium or dextrose can be added to dialysate. Haemodialysis is done approximately for 3–4 hours and is usually three times a week.

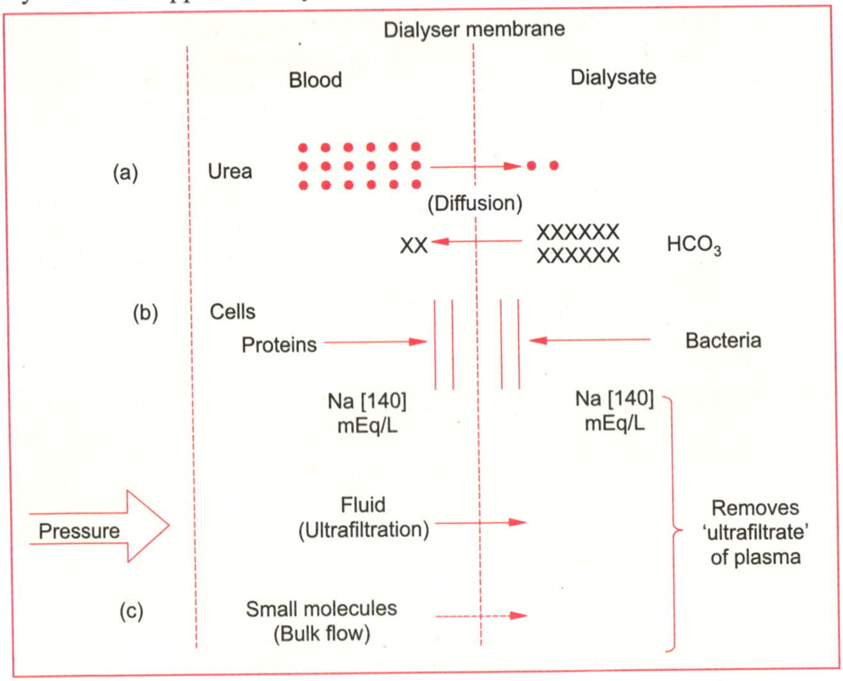

Fig. 20.6 Mechanisms of removal of solute and fluid during dialysis

(*a*) Diffusion of urea from high concentration in blood into dialysate and of bicarbonate from higher concentration dialysate into lower concentration in the blood of patient with renal failure. (*b*) The dialysis membrane is impermeable to red blood cells and plasma proteins and to bacteria in the dialysate (but not to endotoxins). (*c*) The dialysate sodium is freely diffusible and determines the plasma sodium; fluid is removed by application of a transmembrane pressure (in peritoneal dialysis by increased glucose and hence osmotic pressure in dialysate). The fluid is accompanied by small molecules such as sodium and chloride by convection (solvent drag).

A blood vessel with a rapid flow of blood that is also close to the skin is needed for haemodialysis. Since it does not exist naturally, an access has to be made. It is made during a short surgery using one of the two methods as shown in Fig. 20.7.

A fistula is made by connecting a vein to a nearby artery. Blood flows rapidly into the vein making it larger. It takes weeks to months before a fistula is ready for use.

A graft may be sewn between the artery and vein. Blood flows rapidly through the graft from the artery to the vein. A graft is usually ready to be used during treatment after a week or two.

Blood flow rates of 200 to 300 ml per minute are usual. Heparin is given intermittently or infused continuously to prevent clotting of blood in the dialyser during three to six hour procedure.

Adequate clearances can usually be achieved by a total of 12 hours of haemodialysis per week on a thrice-weekly schedule.

For haemodialysis patients unable to take oral supplements, inter-dialytic parenteral nutrition is a means of providing alternate calories and proteins.

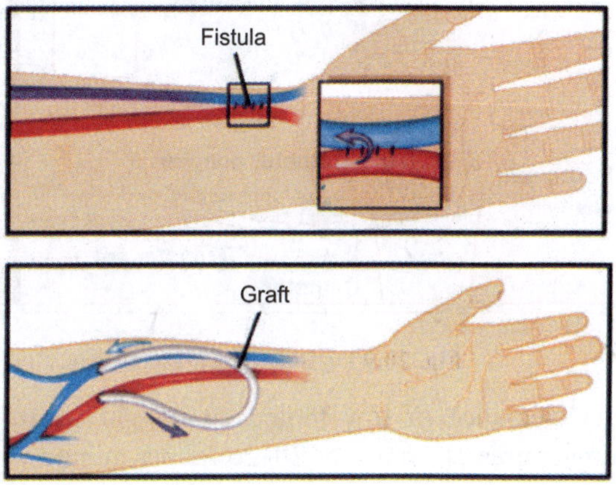

Fig. 20.7 **Fistula and graft between artery and vein**

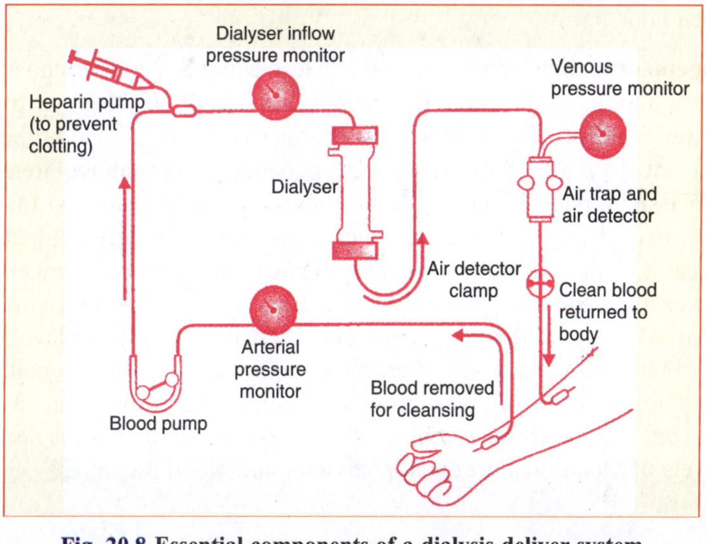

Fig. 20.8 **Essential components of a dialysis deliver system**

Peritoneal dialysis: In this type, the patient's blood is cleaned continuously within the body, the blood stays in the blood vessels which line the patients abdominal (peritoneal) space. The lining of the space acts like a membrane in the artificial kidney. Catheter is surgically placed to create an access. The dialysate is slowly filled through the catheter. The exchange of waste products and chemical balancing takes place. Once exchange is completed, the used dialysate is drained from the peritoneal cavity.

Figure 20.9 shows the connections for peritoneal dialysis.

Peritoneal dialysis is mostly performed by the patients themselves. There are three types. CAPD (Continuous Ambulatory Peritoneal Dialysis) is done for 4–5 hours and usually 4 to 5 times a day. CCPD (Continuous Cycling Peritoneal Dialysis) lasts about 1½ hours and is done several times a night. IPD (Intermittent Peritoneal Dialysis) is the oldest form and lasts about 10 to 12 hours, three times a week. Person can work and travel but should avoid physical strain.

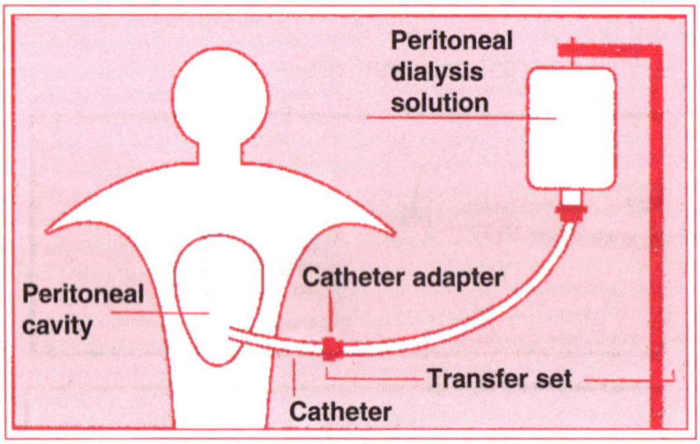

Fig. 20.9 **Peritoneal dialysis**

In peritoneal dialysis clearance of low molecular weight substances are less than for haemodialysis (for example, urea clearance of 20–25 ml per minute versus 150 ml per minute for haemodialysis). But clearance of some larger perhaps also toxic substances is greater because of the greater permeability of the peritoneal membrane to these larger molecules and the longer duration of treatment. Exchange volumes during peritoneal dialysis are commonly 1 to 3 litres each hour.

Dietary management: Patients on haemodialysis lose about 8–9 g of amino acids along with 2–3 g of peptides during each session, leading to a net loss of 10–13 g per dialysis.

The energy requirement of a haemodialysis patient is about 35 kcal/kg body weight and protein requirement is 1.1 g/kg for CAPD/CCPD patients, the protein requirement is 1.3 g/kg. Dietary salt, potassium, phosphorus and water intake should be restricted to: salt 3–4 g; K+ 50–70 mEq/day, phosphorus 1 g/day and water according to the urine output of the patient. Vitamin A increases in dialysis patients and supplementation is not recommended.

Patients approaching end-stage renal disease but not yet initiated on haemodialysis should consume protein at the rate of 0.6 g/kg. If protein is restricted to a lower level, the diet should be supplemented with keto analogues of essential amino acids to prevent malnutrition.

Patients on chronic haemodialysis usually require a slightly reduced protein intake (0.8 to 1.0 g/kg) but a more stringent control of salt and potassium intake is needed to maintain satisfactory levels of blood urea nitrogen, potassium and blood pressure.

Characteristics of Haemodialysis

- Takes only 3 to 5 hours per treatment.
- Requires only three treatments weekly.
- Requires surgical creation of vascular access between circulation and dialysis machine.
- Requires complex water treatment, expensive dialysis equipment and highly trained personnel.
- Requires large doses of heparin.
- Confines patient to special treatment unit.
- Risk of complications.

Characteristics of peritoneal dialysis

- Can be performed immediately.
- Requires less complex equipment and less specialised personnel.
- Requires small amount of heparin or none at all.
- Can be performed by patient anywhere without assistance.
- Allows patient independence without long interruption in daily activities.
- Allows for more liberal diet.
- Costs less.

Oral iron is given because there is a chronic small loss of blood that cannot be returned to the patient at the end of each dialysis. The major cause of anaemia appears to be lack of erythropoietin together with depression of erythropoiesis by azotemia or uraemia.

Vitamin supplementation is prescribed for renal failure patients including dialysis patients because restricted diets, uraemic toxins and effects, the process of dialysis increases the risk of frank and subclinical vitamin deficiency.

Correction of anaemia is done by using erythropoietin, supplemental iron, folic acid and vitamins B_{12} and C. This improves the overall well being and appetite of the patient. Vitamin B_6 may be given 80–160 mg per week.

Dialysis contributes to loss of ascorbic acid and folic acid. During dialysis the requirements for B-complex and C vitamins increase while the requirement for vitamins A and D decrease.

In malnourished patients, supplementation of carnitine helps to improve the general well being. A rise in serum creatinine to 2.4 mg/dl produces a 25 per cent fall in the normal level of serum bicarbonate. This should be corrected by giving oral alkali such as sodium bicarbonate or sodium citrate to increase the bicarbonate level to 20–23 mEq/dl.

Hyper lipidemia may manifest when the GFR falls to 15–30 ml/min. Dietary manipulation and drug therapy may help prevent atherosclerotic complications.

However there are some limitations of dialysis.

Drawbacks

- Dialysis can only control the kidney failure and does not cure the diseased kidneys.
- Patients with chronic kidney failure need to continue dialysis throughout their lives or until they receive a kidney transplant.

- Discomfort is seen when needles are inserted for haemodialysis.
- Patients may also experience a drop in blood pressure accompanied by nausea, vomiting, headaches and cramps.
- Dialysis is very expensive.

Nutritional requirement during various stages of renal failure is given in Table 20.9.

Prevention

Treating diabetes mellitus and hypertension with lifestyle modification is essential to prevent kidney damage. Patients should be encouraged for annual check up and test for the presence of protein in urine. Proteinuria can be treated. In the hyper active or diabetic patient proteinuria is the first sign of a problem. By treating immediately the number of dialysis patients could decrease. For those who have impaired renal function, the treatment protocol must follow. The value of such prevention is inestimatable because only about one per cent of patients with end stage renal disease in India can afford treatment.

Table 20.8 Nutritional requirement during various stages of renal failure

Nutrient	*Acute renal failure*	*End-state renal disease predialysis*	*Haemodialysis*	*Peritoneal dialysis*
Energy	30–50 kcal/kg of present body weight	35 kcal/kg ideal body weight	35 kcal/kg ideal body weight	35 kcal/kg ideal body weight
Protein	0.5 g/kg of present body weight (but not less than 40 g/day)	GFR ml/min 15–20 – <1.0, 10–15—0.7 4–10—0.55 0.6 (But not less 35–30 g/day)	1.0 to 1.2 g/kg ideal body weight	1.2 to 1.5 g/kg of ideal body weight
Sodium	Anuric-oliguric phase 500–1000 mg Diuretic Phase—Replace loses	2–3 g/day or no added salt	2–3 g/day or no added salt	2–3 g/day or no added salt
Potassium	Anuric-oliguric phase 1000 mg Diuretic phase– Replace losses	Not restricted unless serum potassium is elevated and urine output is less than one litre/day	2–3 g (individualise)	2–3 g (individualise)
Fluids	Anuric-oliguric phase–replace output minus 500 CC from the previous day Diuretic phase–large amount of fluid	Generally unrestricted Balance fluid intake with urine output to avoid oedema	1000 CC and urine output	1000 CC and urine output
Phosphorus	—	600–800 mg/day or 15 mg/g of protein prescribed	800–1200 mg or 15 mg/g of protein prescribed	1200–1600 mg

RENAL TRANSPLANT

Renal transplant is done in End Stage Renal Disease, when GFR drops to 10 ml/min. It is the second commonest transplant surgery after the corneal grafts.

The diet is usually less restrictive than the one followed during dialysis treatment.

Post transplant Nutrition

- Infection need to be prevented and healing is promoted.
- Diet is modified according to drug therapy.
- Abnormalities in calcium or phosphorous metabolism with hyperparathyroidism is prevented.
- Blood pressure need to be controlled and cardiac problems prevented.
- Normal electrolyte balance need to be maintained.
- Input and output fluid should be balanced.
- Weight gain should be minimum.

Dietary recommendations

- Progress should be made from clear liquids to solids as quickly as possible.
- Fluid status is monitored and adjusted accordingly.
- While on steroids 1.5 g/kg protein is given.
- Calorie intake should be 30–35 kcal/kg.
- Sodium intake should be 2–4 g. Potassium levels should be adjusted.
- Calcium should be 1–1.5 times RDA to offset poor absorption. Daily intake of phosphorous should be balanced with calcium intake.
- Diet is supplemented with vit D, magnesium and thiamine.
- Calories from fat should be 30–35 per cent of total calories.
- Hyperlipidemia should be prevented.
- Special diet is discontinued when drug therapy is reduced to maintenance levels.
- Exercise and weight control should be planned.

UROLITHIASIS OR URINARY CALCULI

Urolithiasis or calculi are found to be lodged in the urinary tract namely, kidney, ureters, bladder or urethra.

Small foci are formed and supersaturated urinary salts are precipitated around the foci of mucoid structures. Mucopolysaccharides and mucoprotein combine with chemicals bound to form the foci. The end products of protein metabolism leaves uric acid, phosphate and oxalates of sodium, calcium and magnesium. Urine concentrated with calcium phosphate and ammonium phosphate predisposes stone formation. A patient with acidic urine tends to form uric acid or calcium oxalate crystals. A patient with alkaline urine tends to form triple phosphate, calcium carbonate or calcium phosphate crystals.

Renal stones are prevalent between 30–45 years of age, with the incidence rate declining after the age of 50. Relapse of kidney stones is common.

Symptoms

Sometimes there is blood in the urine and the stones can cause intense pain. The pain comes in waves. Patient may feel nauseated and vomit. Frequent and painful urination can also be a symptom.

Causes

The occurrence of urolithiasis may be an outcome of different nutritional status, dietary habits and environmental factors such as temperature and humidity. The incidence is high in north, northwest and central India, moderate in deccan plateau and far less in South India.

- *Climate:* In warm climates, the urine volume is low and concentrated with urates, oxalates and calcium salts. In India, a higher incidence of renal stones is found in people residing in Rajasthan, Saurashtra and Punjab. This may be related to excessive heat or water scarcity prevailing in the region.
- *Occupation:* People who work directly under the sun and perspire a lot may pass concentrated urine.
- *Infection of urinary tract*: Frequent infection of urinary tract may be contributory in that pus cells and epithelial cells may form a focus around which the stone may be formed.
- *Dietary habits:* Persons consuming foods rich in oxalates, calcium, purines and phosphate may predispose to formation of renal calculi. Excessive consumption of tea may also be a contributing factor. A diet rich in sodium, fats, meat and sugar and low in fibre, vegetable protein and unrefined carbohydrate increase the risk of renal stone disease.
- *Heredity:* Family history may show that some of the blood relations of a patient with kidney stone had similar problem. Inherited metabolic disorders, inherited or congenital renal condition predispose to renal stone formation.
- *Gender*: Three times more common in males.
  Medications: Triamterene, indinavir and azetazoalmide are associated with urolithiasis.

Types of Calculi

The majority of urinary calculi are made up of calcium phosphate, calcium oxalate, uric acid or magnesium ammonium phosphate. In India, the most common type of calculi is calcium oxalate.

Figure 20.10 shows formation of different type of stones in different parts of kidney.

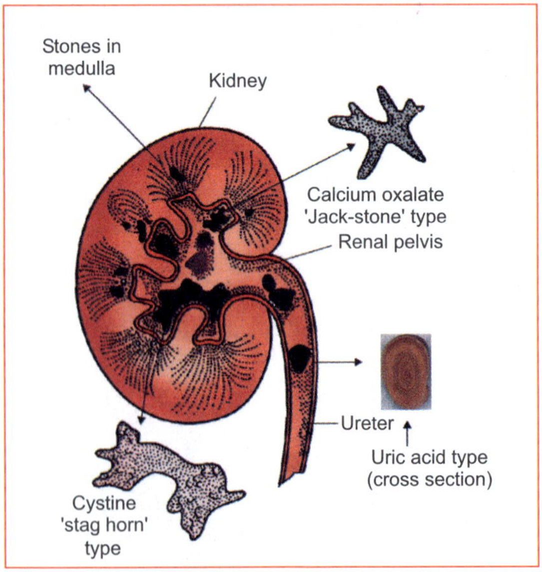

Fig. 20.10 Renal calculi: Stones in kidney, renal pelvis and ureter

Contributing Factors of Calculi

In mammals, only about 5–15 per cent of urinary oxalate is derived from exogenous sources like tea, spinach, cocoa and sesame seeds. The major portion is produced endogenously from ascorbic acid, amino acids—especially glycine, carbohydrates and proteins. To a negligible extent, stones are known to occur in certain metabolic and genetic disorders. Formation of calculi depends upon the balance between the concentration of precipitating substances like calcium phosphate, oxalic acid, uric acid, magnesium and the solubility of their salts and crystal inhibitors in urine. Volume and pH of urine are two other important determinants.

- It is also reported that high intakes of animal proteins like meat, fish, and poultry might augment the risk of stones.
- Pyridoxine deficiency is known to increase the production of oxalic acid in the body and its excretion in urine, hence may be one of the contributory factors. As a cofactor for the enzyme transaminase, vitamin B_6 helps in the metabolism of glyoxylate to glycine. Deficiency of this vitamin results in increased pools of glyoxalate and oxalate in the blood. This in turn increases the urinary excretion of oxalate.
- Excess intake of vitamin C, high intake of foods rich in oxalates like spinach, cabbage, and tomatoes are common causes of supeoxaluria.
- People living in rocky areas are more prone to urolithiasis because drinking water is likely to be either hard or may contain some elements. Studies conducted at NIN, Hyderabad reported that in Punjab the incidence of urolithiasis is higher where fluoride content of drinking water is high resulting in increase in the incidence of urinary calculi.

Treatment

When stones are composed of calcium and magnesium phosphates and carbonates, the urine is alkaline and hence acid-ash diet is used. When calcium phosphate urolithiasis is associated with hyperparathyroidism or hyperthyroidism the acid ash is of little value.

The acid ash diet should maintain the urine pH between 4.5 and 5. If an alkaline ash diet is prescribed, a urinary pH of 7.6 to 8 is maintained.

Table 20.9 gives a list of foods rich in acid producing, alkali producing and neutral foods.

Table 20.9 Acid producing, alkali producing and neutral foods

Acid producing	*Alkali producing*	*Neutral producing*
Bread, especially Whole wheat	Milk	Butter
Cereals	Fruits	Coffee
Cheese	Vegetables	Fats
Corn	Almonds	Sugar
Eggs	Apricots dried	Tapioca
Lentils	Beans	Tea
Macaroni, spaghetti,	Beet greens	
Noodles	Dates	
Meat, fish, poultry	Figs,	
Walnuts	Peas dried,	
Chocolate	Raisins,	
	Spinach	
	Foods prepared with baking powder or baking soda.	

Source: Robinson, H.C. Marilyn. R. Laeler, 1990, *Normal and Therapeutic Nutrition*, Oxford and IBH Publishing Company, New Delhi.

Planning acid ash diet

A liberal fluid intake is important. Salt may be used in moderation. The fruits and vegetables so selected should not contribute more than 25 cc of base daily. The reaction of the food is expressed as the number of cubic centimeters of normal hydrochloric acid to which it is equivalent.

Planning alkaline-ash diet

If stones of uric acid or cystine type occur, the diet should give alkaline ash, such a regimen stresses the use of alkaline producing foods such as fruits, vegetables and milk while acid producing foods like meat, eggs and cereals are restricted. The diet must contain all essentials of good nutrition.

Planning low oxalate diets

An acid or alkaline reaction of the diet is of little value for oxalate urolithiasis. However foods that are a significant source of oxalates should be omitted which include beans, beet greens, chocolate, cocoa, dried figs, plums, potatoes, spinach, tea and tomatoes.

Table 20.10 summarises foods to be included and excluded in renal calculi.

Table 20.10 Foods to be included and excluded in renal calculi

Diet	*Type of stone*	*Foods to be included*	*Foods to be excluded*
Acid ash diet	Ca and Mg phosphates and carbonates	Cereals, non-veg. foods, protein rich foods like nuts	Bakery products, milk, fruits and vegetables
Alkali ash diet	Uric acid and cystine stones	Bakery products, milk, fruits and vegetables	Cereals, non-veg. foods, protein rich foods like nuts.
Low oxalate diet	Calcium oxalate stones	Other than the foods excluded Skim milk and curd. Moderate intake of protein	Beets, greens, spinach, tea, nuts tomatoes, potatoes, chocolates, cocoa, coffee, cola

Dietary Management

Fluids: The fundamental principle in the treatment of kidney stone is to supply adequate fluids. Water, coconut and barely water, fruit juice and light tea should ensure the passage of over 2000 ml of urine per day. Dilute urine avoids concentration of solids and also tend to make the urine neutral, thus preventing the strong acid or alkaline which predisposes the individual to precipitation of crystals. The simplest guide to patient is to drink enough fluids to see that the urine when voided is very light in colour. Extra fluid intake is needed by those who live in hot and dry conditions and those who exercise and perspire significantly.

Foods: Moderate protein intake decreased calcium excretion mainly through a reduction in bone resorption and renal calcium loss probably due to decrease in exogeneous acid load. It is advisable to restrict foods which are rich in calcium, oxalate or uric acid according to the type of stone formed. Thus, a person who has passed calcium oxalate stone should avoid a diet rich in calcium and oxalate.

Studies conducted at National Institute of Nutrition, Hyderabad showed that L-tartaric acid, a component of tamarind is an inhibitor of urolithiasis while wheat based diets are considered conducive to uric acid and calcium oxalate crystalluria.

Prevention

An acid or alkaline ash diet is not very effective in bringing about solution of stones already formed but may serve to prevent the recurrence of stones.

The diet should be low in oxalic acid and purine contents. The intakes of calcium and phosphates should also be reduced to moderation. Correction of B_6 deficiency may be helpful.

Vitamin C is a precursor to endogeneous production of oxalates. A normal diet with sufficient vitamin C is suggested.

The subject should consume large amounts of fluid to increase urine output to 2–2.5 litres per day. Dilute urine prevents the precipitate formation around the matrix. Lemonade is good for the patient. Acidity of urine must be regulated. Table 20.11 gives foods rich in calcium,

Table 20.11 Foods rich in calcium, phosphates, oxalates and purines

Calcium	*Phosphates*	*Oxalates*	*Purines*
Leafy vegetables, milk and milk products, small fish with bones, prawns, crabs, ragi.	Whole cereals, bran, legumes, nuts, oil seeds, banana, carrot, meat, fish, egg, milk products, cheese, organ meat, soft drinks.	Leafy vegetables, grapes, tea, chocolates, cocoa, coffee, cola drinks, beef, cashewnuts, beetroot, yam.	Meat, fish, animal tissues and organs (kidney, liver, brain, heart).

phosphates, oxalates and purines. A balanced diet, high ratio of magnesium to calcium foods such as brown rice, bananas and oats should be taken. Magnesium supplementation may decrease the size of an existing stone and prevent further formations. Alcohol, antacids, excessive protein, dairy products, salt, carbonated beverages, caffeine and refined white flour are to be avoided. Coffee, iced tea and colas contain caffeine which can cause dehydration. Colas contribute to the build up of calcium oxalate. Fast foods containing salt should be avoided.

Schools have to play a role in making bottled water available, limiting soft drinks and allowing children to visit the rest room as needed.

15th March is World Kidney Day.

SUGGESTED READINGS

- Augustine Joshna, Kidney transplant, New opportunities and challenges, Cleveland Clinic Journal of Medicine, 2018: **85**.
- Sekar Arjun *et al.*, Phosphorus binders: The new and the old and how to choose, Cleveland Clinic Journal of medicine 2018: **85**.
- Chan winnie Chronic kidney disease and nutrition support, Nutrition in Clinical Practice, 2021; **36**.
- U.S. National Library of Medicine: PubMed Health.www.ncbi.nlm.nih.gov/pubmedhealth.

QUESTIONS

1. Define glomerular filtration rate.
2. Differentiate between nephritis and nephrosis.
3. Explain the dietary modifications for treatment of glomerulonephritis.
4. How are kidney stones formed?
5. What are the foods included and avoided in the diet planned for a nephrotic patient?
6. Explain the reasons for dietary restrictions in kidney disorders. Plan a day's diet for a school boy suffering from nephrosis.
7. What are the foods included and avoided in the diet planned for a nephritic patient? Give reasons.
8. What is acute renal failure? Explain the causes and treatment.
9. What is dialysis? Discuss diet control in dialysis.
10. Write a note on peritoneal dialysis.
11. What are acid ash diets? In which conditions would you suggest these? List the foods to be included and excluded.
12. Discuss the factors contributing to oxalate stones. How do you prevent it?
13. Write short note on Nutrition and Renal Transplantation.
14. What is CKD? Explain causes, symptoms and nutritional recommendations.

TOPICS FOR ACTIVITY

- Plan and prepare a diet for chronic kidney disease who is in fourth stage.
- Plan and prepare a diet for a child recovering from nephrosis.

21

Diet in Cancer

Cancer is a term used to refer malignant neoplasms or tumours. Neoplasia means cells in a tissue proliferate without the normal controls on growth. In malignant neoplasms the cells spread to adjacent tissues and interfere with the function and often has undesirable systemic effects. Benign tumours represent the accumulation of cells which have been transformed to reproduce in abnormal numbers but remain within the tissue of origin.

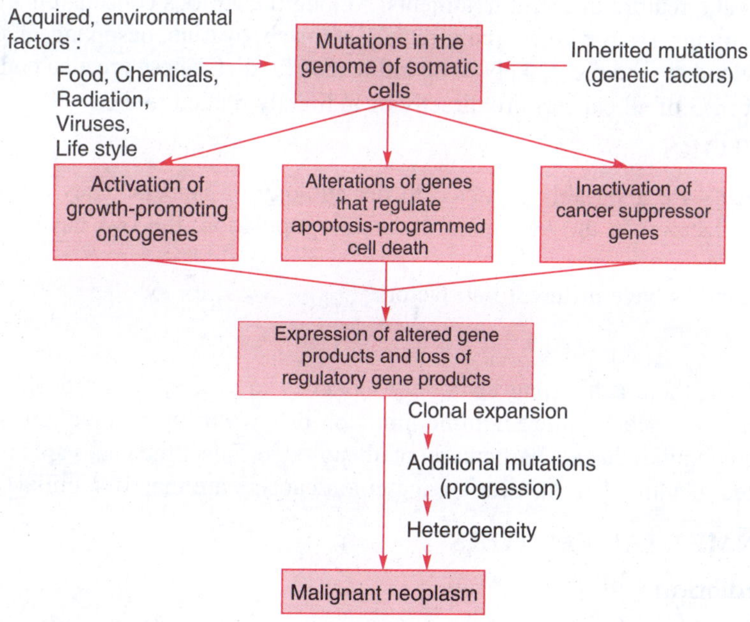

Fig. 21.1 Flow chart depicts a simplified scheme of cancer pathogenesis

Cancer is caused by mutation or abnormal activation of cellular genes that control cell growth and cell mitosis. The abnormal genes are called oncogenes. It is now recognised that there exists regulatory genes known as tumour suppressor genes whose normal function is to prevent malignant transformation. The latter might be triggered by exposure to a carcinogen (e.g., tobacco) or by a spontaneous mutation. Conversely normal cells contain growth promoting genes known as proto-oncogenes where inappropriate activation (by a carcinogen or mutation) to produce oncogenes that could result in malignant transformation. The probability of mutations can be increased manifold when a person is exposed to certain chemical, physical or biological factors. Cancer can occur at any age and in any part of the body.

Cancers are classified into four major groups.

Table 21.1 Classification of cancers

Type	*Tissue or cell of origin*	*Example*
Carcinoma	Endoderm or ectoderm	Epithelial lining of gut (*e.g.*, adenocarcinoma of colon) or bronchus (*e.g.*, squamous cell) or small cell carcinoma of bronchus
Sarcoma	Mesoderm	Osteosarcoma Fibrosarcoma
Leukaemia	White blood cell	Acute lymphoblastic leukaemia
Lymphoma	Monocyte, macrophage	Hodgkin's disease

Source: Edwards, C.R.W *et al.*, 1995, Principles and practices of medicine ELBS with Churchil/ Living stone

Cancer is not a single disorder. There are many different kinds of cancers which take different courses and require different treatments. Among the various cancers, the uterine cervix, breast, oro-pharyngeal, large bowel (colo-rectal), stomach, ovarian, oesophageal, endometrium and prostate gland are the most likely to be influenced by diet. These are also common type of cancers. About 1/3 of all cancers are directly or indirectly related to diet.

RISK FACTORS

Two components are invariably involved in the etiology of cancers. They are a genetic and environmental factors. In the vast majority of the population, the two have to synergise to induce cancer.

Different cancers have different risk factors.

HEREDITY

In many families there is a strong hereditary tendency to cancer. This probably results from the fact that most cancers require not one mutation but two or more mutations before cancer occurs. In those families that are particularly predisposed to cancer the genes are already mutated in the inherited genome. Breast, ovarian and colon cancers are mostly familial.

ENVIRONMENTAL FACTORS

Ionising radiation

X-rays, gamma rays and particle radiations from radio-active substances, even ultraviolet rays can predispose to cancer by rupturing DNA strands, thus causing mutations.

Chemical substances

Chemical substances that can cause mutation are called carcinogens. Benzene and asbestos are considered as carcinogens.

The carcinogens that cause by far the greatest number of deaths are those in cigarette smoke. Tobacco is the most clearly identified cause of cancer. In India, tobacco use causes a million deaths every year. Cancers associated with tobacco are lung, mouth, larynx, oesophagus and bladder. According to National Cancer Registry Programme of the Indian Council Medical Research, nearly a third of all cancer incidents in the country are attributable to the use of tobacco. Consuming pan with tobacco causes leukoplakia and erythroplakia which are precancerous lesions that occur among 70 per cent of tobacco users. Persistent use of such

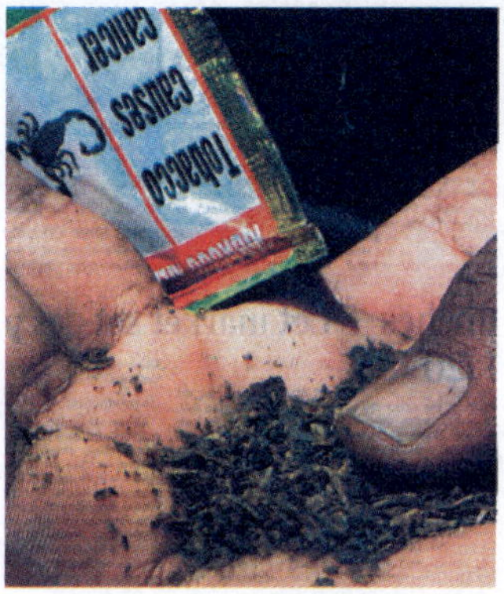

Fig. 21.2 **Smokeless tobacco is a strong cause of oral cancer**

Tobacco smoke contains carcinogens like nicotine, hydrogen cyanide, formaldehyde, lead, arsenic, ammonia, benzene, carbon monoxide, nitrosamine.

products could also cause genetic deformities. Cancers of head and neck correlate strongly with use of alcohol and tobacco. Beedi smoking from younger age related to higher risk of gastric cancer. Risk increases with the number of beedis smoked and duration.

The carcinogenic effect of red meat is mainly from the chemical residues in meat passed on through the food preservatives rather from the natural meat.

Dietary Factors

Interaction of genes with food components can affect carcinogen metabolism, regulation of hormones, DNA repair, apoptosis, cell differentiation, cell growth cycle and inflammatory response.

Foods may cause cancer by being direct carcinogen or carcinogen may be produced by cooking. Sometimes microorganisms may produce carcinogens in stored foods. Food stuff may also act as substrate for the formation of carcinogen in the body or food stuff may alter the bacterial flora of the bowel thereby producing carcinogen.

Meat: Meat intake has been positively associated with risk of digestive tract cancers and breast cancer and renal cell carcinoma. Intake of red meat (beef, lamb and pork), and processed meat (ham, salamn and bacon) increase the risk of colon cancer. Cancers of prostate are significantly more likely in nonvegetarians and frequent beef consumers also have higher risk of bladder cancer. High intake of fish sauce is a risk factor for gastric cancer. Intake of red meat cooked by broiling or barbecuing tend to be positively related to risk of non-Hodgkin's lymphoma. Cooking meat, poultry and fish at high temperatures causes carcinogens to form on food surfaces.

Energy balance: The relationship between body weight, body mass index or relative body weight and site-specific cancer has been widely investigated. In most epidemiologic studies, a positive association has been seen with cancers of the breast, endometrium, gall bladder and kidney. In breast cancer, a positive association with weight gain and increased waist/hip ratio is seen in post-menopausal women, especially those who do not use hormone replacement therapy.

Physical inactivity, high energy intake and large body mass are associated with increased risk of developing colon cancer in men and women.

Insulin Resistance: The glycaemic index may have relevance to cancer prevention. In addition, insulin resistance and insulin like growth factors have been implicated in the diet related cancers at colon, breast and prostate. Studies showed that there is a direct association between dietary

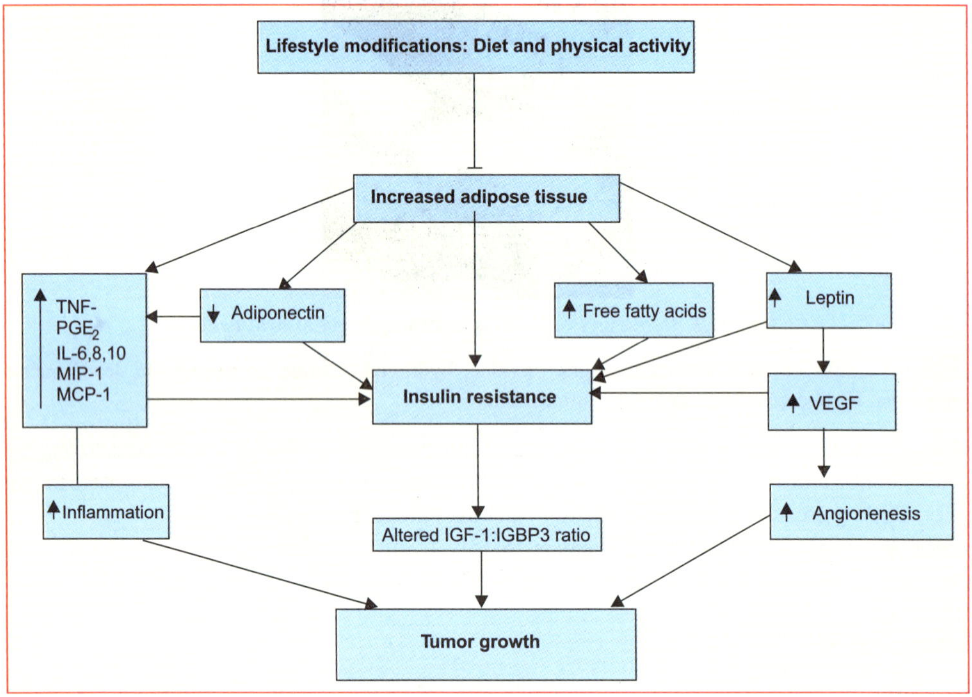

Fig. 21.3 Potential mechanisms of obesity, insulin resistance, and related biomarkers in cancer progression. This figure illustrates how adipocyte-derived cytokines (adipokines), inflammatory factors, insulin, and the insulin-like growth factor-1 (IGF-1) axis, might work in concert to promote tumor growth. Insulin resistance seems central to the pathway promoting tumor growth.

TNF-α = tumor necrosis factor 'α'; PGE2 = prostaglandin E=2; IL-6, -8, -10 = interleukin-6, -8, -10; MIP-1 = macrophage inflammatory protein 1; MCP-1 = monocyte chemoattractant protein 1; VEGF = vascular endothelial growth factor; IGF-1; IGBP3 = insulin-like growth factor 1:insulin-like growth factor binding protein 3.

Source: Parekh Niyati *et al.*, Obesity, insulin resistance and cancer prognosis J Amer Diet Assoc. **109**, 2009.

glycaemic index and colon cancer risk. A sedentary lifestyle in conjunction with a high glycaemic index diet increases the risk of colon cancer.

Sugars: Consumption of simple sugars (mono and disaccharides) may be related to colorectal cancers. Excessive starch foods may predispose to gastric cancers.

Fat: Dietary fats have been known to play a significant role in the etiology of cancer. A positive association between high intake of fat and the incidence of breast, colon, pancreatic and prostate cancers has been shown Such an association may be independent of the energy content of the fats. Diets high in animal fat and ω-6 fatty acid intake contribute to an increased risk of colorectal cancer and breast cancer.

Studies have shown that intake of saturated fat tended to be positively related to risk of non-Hodgkin's lymphoma.

Protein: Increased meat intake has been found to be associated with an increased risk of colon cancer and possibly with advanced prostate cancer.

Vitamins and Minerals: Low blood carotenoid levels and lung cancer, low dietary vitamin C and oro-pharyngeal, stomach and esophageal cancer and low dietary vitamin E and lung, cervix and colorectal cancer have been shown to be related in several studies. Deficiency of folic acid and vitamins A and C have been associated with the development of cervical dysplasia and cervical cancer. Homocysteine levels which increase due to folate deficiency, increases the risk of colon cancers. Selenium and zinc deficiency may also increase the risk of cancer.

Cohort Studies on breast cancer survivors showed that most women had low serum concentrations of 25(OH)D, the primary biomarker used to assess vitamin D status.

Studies have shown that people who consume low amounts of fruits and vegetables have more chances of getting cancer.

Table 21.2 Food related cancers

Type of cancer	*Increases risk*	
	Convincing	*Probable*
Breast cancer, premenopause	Alcoholic drinks	Height which is affected by genetic, environmental, hormonal and nutritional factors. Greater birth weight
Breast cancer, postmenopause	Alcoholic drinks, Body fatness, Adult attains height, sedentary living	Abdominal fatness, Adult weight gain
Colon, rectum cancer	Red meat, processed meat, high intake of fat, body fatness, abdominal fatmess, sedentary living, adult attained heights.	Alcoholic drinks
Endometrium	Body fatness	Abdominal fatness
Lung	Arsenic in drinking water	β-carotene supplements.
Stomach	—	Salt, salted and salty foods.
Liver	High intake of alcohol	Iron over load, toxins of mould
Mouth, pharynx, larynx, oesophagus	Alcoholic drink, Body fatness	—
Pancreas	Body fatness	Abdominal fat, Adult attained height
Prostate	Diet high in calcium	—
Skin	—	Arsenic in drinking water
Gall bladder	Foods containing fat	Alcoholic drinks
Ovary	Body fatness	High lactose intake from milk products
Cancer in any part of the body	Sedentary living	Energy dense foods, sugary drink, fast foods, Body fatness
Cervical cancer	Folate deficiency	—
Kidney cancer	—	High intake of red meat

Alcohol: Epidemiologic studies indicate that alcohol has a causal role in carcinogenesis, especially for cancers of the mouth, throat, breast, pharynx and oesophagus. Alcohol appears to have an increased effect on those tissues directly exposed to it during its consumption and tends to act synergistically with tobacco. Alcoholism often damages the liver and precedes the development of liver cancer.

Alcohol, especially beer consumption, has been associated with an increased risk for colorectal cancer.

Nitrates: Nitrates are present in a variety of foods, but the main dietary sources are vegetables and drinking water. Sodium and potassium nitrates are used in the processes of salting, pickling and curing foods; they are also added to hot dogs and meat to get pink colour. Nitrosamines are present in tobacco and tobacco smoke. Nitrosamines related to nitrates which are potent carcinogens and may cause naso-pharyngeal, stomach and colorectal cancers.

Aflatoxins: The fungi which grows on cereals and groundnuts can cause liver cancer.

β-carotene supplements: Research has shown that when lung cancer patients are supplemented with β-carotene, severity of disease increases.

Oestrogens

These have been given extensively for the relief of post-menopausal symptoms and for the prevention of osteoporosis. A major uncertainty concerns the role of estrogens in the production of cancer of the breast and endometrial cancer.

Leptin, an adipokeine found among obese individuals at higher concentration, is the key player in energy balance and appetite control. Laboratory evidence shows that leptin promotes proliferation and invasiveness of endometrial cells. It interferes with insulin signalling and is associated with higher concentrations of circulating insulin which has proliferative properties.

Viruses

Indirect evidence suggests that viruses may act as cofactors in the development of some malignant diseases. Epidemiological studies have suggested a possible role for Hepatitis-B virus in human primary liver cancer. Human papillomavirus and the Epstein Barr virus are considered oncogenic. Vaccines for cervical cancer are under trial.

Stress

Stress may cause damage to the thymus gland and the immune system and hormonal effects mediated through the hypothalamus, pituitary and adrenal cortex. This 'Cascade of Physiologic events' may provide the neurologic currency that converts anxiety to malignancy. Stress may also influence the integrity of the immune system, food behaviour and the nutrition status.

Metabolic Syndrome

It is associated with a higher risk of colorectal pancreatic in males and breast cancers in females.

Age

The risk of developing colorectal cancer (incidence) increases with age. The incidence is 6 times higher among persons aged 65 years when compared with those persons aged 40–64 years. It has been suggested that the increasing risk of cancer with age reflects the accumulation of critical genetic mutations over a time that ultimately culminate in neoplastic transformation. Factors that have been associated with an increased likelihood of cancer include exposure to exogenous mutagens, altered host immune function and certain inherited genetic syndromes and disorders.

Physical Activity

Men and women whose lifestyles include regular, vigorous physical activity have the lowest risk of colon cancer. Physical activity may also protect against breast cancer by reducing body weight and the other mechanisms unrelated to body weight.

Immune Factors

A healthy immune system recognises foreign cells and destroys them. Ineffective immune system may not recognise tumour cells as foreign, thus allowing unchecked growth. Ageing affects immune function. There is increased cancer risk when immune system suppressed. Patients who take immuno suppressants are at risk of developing cancer.

Cancer is a complex multifactorial disease state. There are more than 200 different types of cancers each with its own etiology and symptoms.

SYMPTOMS

Malignant diseases manifest themselves in a variety of ways resulting in general symptoms like fever, loss of appetite, fatigue or malaise. Specific cancers give rise to symptoms different for each one.

Oral Cancer: Ulcers, white or red patches inside the oral cavity or difficulty in swallowing or opening the mouth wide, thickening of the tongue.

Lung/Throat Cancer: Persistent cough, chest pain, blood in sputum, shortness of breath, weight loss or loss of appetite, hoarseness, repeated bouts of pneumonia or bronchitis, difficulty in swallowing.

Stomach Cancer: Early satiety, indigestion or heartburn, pain in the abdomen, bloating of stomach after meals, loss of appetite, weakness, tiredness; diarrhoea or constipation, blood in vomit.

Colon Cancer: Diarrhoea, constipation or any other change in bowel habits, frequent gas pains, blood in faeces.

Breast Cancer: A lump in the breast or under-arm area, change in shape, size or colour of the breast, discharge from the nipple, dimpled, puckered or scaly surface of the breast (like an orange peel).

Cervical/Uterine Cancer: Unusual vaginal bleeding, pain in the pelvic area, foul smelling or unusual discharge.

Kidney Cancer: Blood in urine; frequent fevers, weight loss or loss of appetite, tiredness, pain in the side, anaemia or high blood pressure.

Bladder Cancer: The need to urinate frequently, painful urination, blood in urine.

Prostate Cancer: Urination problems.

Melanoma (Skin Cancer): Change in size, shape or colour of a mole or wart.

Danger Signals of Cancer

- Sore that does not heal.
- Change in the colour of a wart or mole.
- Chronic indigestion or difficulty in swallowing or early satiety.
- A lump or thickening in the breast or any part of the body.
- Abnormal bleeding or discharge from any body opening.
- Change in normal bowel habits.
- Persistant hoarseness of voice.

GENERAL SYSTEMIC REACTIONS

Neoplastic disease is commonly associated with three basic systemic effects: anorexia, hypermetabolic state, and negative nitrogen balance, often accompanied by increasing weight loss.

Abnormalities in Metabolism

The extreme weight loss and weakness is caused by abnormalities in glucose metabolism, in which cancer patients cannot produce glucose efficiently from carbohydrates and instead 'feed off' their own tissue protein and convert it to glucose instead. Gluconeogenesis increases, further straining the supply of body proteins. Many patients develop insulin resistance. Drugs can be used to correct this metabolic error.

Glucose intolerance occurs in cancer patients due to increased insulin resistance and due to inadequate insulin release. There is increased lipolysis, free fatty acids and glycerol turnover and decreased lipogenesis and hyperlipidemia. Fat oxidation rates are higher.

Tumours derive protein at the expense of the host. The rates of whole body catabolic rate exceeds that of synthetic rate, depletion of body protein occurs. Albumin is depleted in cancer. Branched chain amino acid infusions can decrease protein catabolism in cancer patients.

These metabolic abnormalities may be the cause for the failure to gain lean body mass or maintain healthy body weight inspite of receiving adequate energy and nutrients.

Anorexia

Anorexia is frequently accompanied by depression or discomfort from normal eating. This contributes further to a limited nutrient intake at the very time the disease process causes an increased metabolic rate and nutrient demand. Often this imbalance of decreased intake and increased demand creates a negative nitrogen balance, an indication of body tissue wastings. Such a vicious cycle can lead to 'cancer cachexia'. This occurs in as many as 80 per cent of people with cancer.

Loss of appetite can occur due to systemic effect of malignant tumour per se. It may often be intensified by fatigue, pain, fear, depression, sepsis or can develop as a consequence of such treatments as surgery, radiation, chemotherapy and other drug treatments. Anorexia leads to weight loss and malnutrition.

Wasting

Many factors appear to play a role in the wasting associated with cancer. Cytokines, released by both tumour cells and immune cells involved in the inflammatory response induce a hypermetabolic, catabolic state. The combined effects of a poor appetite, accelerated and abnormal metabolism and diversion of nutrients to support tumour growth result in a lower supply of energy and nutrients at instances when demands are high.

Malabsorption

This can occur due to blind loop syndrome. The associated overgrowth of bacteria in the upper small bowel may result in steatorrhoea and vitamin B_{12} deficiency. Direct interaction of bacteria with certain nutrients result in abnormalities of the intestinal epithelium which cause malabsorption. Protein-losing enteropathy can occur not only in intestinal lymphoma and gastric carcinoma but now is known to occur with tumours arising outside the alimentary tract (malignant melonoma).

If the malignancy involves the pancreas, the pancreatic duct or the common bile duct, normal secretory function of digestive enzymes and related materials such as bile salts is subsequently limited. Biliary obstruction can also produce a deficiency of prothrombin, leading to blood clotting problems and a deficiency of bile flow. This inturn interferes with normal digestion and absorption and lead to further decreased calcium absorption and metabolism with subsequent osteomalacia. Protein and electrolyte absorption as well as that of other nutrients may also be diminished by solid tumor infiltration of the small intestine or dissemination to lymphnodes.

Abdominal tumours may also cause either gastrolic or jejunocolic fistulas. This results in a bypass of the small intestine and contributes to the subsequent malabsorption. Diarrhoea and steatorrhoea as well as protein loss follow. Extensive protein may also be lost in exudates associated with various gastrointestinal enteropathies.

Fluid-Electrolyte Imbalances

Gastrointestinal lesions leading to general malabsorption can also contribute to fluid and electrolyte losses. Continuous vomiting and diarrhoea not only bring loss of water but also cause loss of minerals and water-soluble vitamins.

Villous adenoma and adenocarcinomas of the colon can contribute to severe electrolyte imbalance.

Anaemia

The underlying problem of anaemia may be compounded by a number of factors, including anorexia with curtailment of dietary nutrients necessary for haemoglobin synthesis, iron, protein, folic acid, vitamin B_{12} and vitamin C as well as malabsorption of these materials. Additional contributory factors may be increased hemolysis, bleeding of ulcerated lesions or presence of gastrointestinal fistulas.

Taste and Appetite Changes

These may be due to psychosomatic factors, fear, pain and side-effects of medications. Diet prescribed should be according to the preferences and likes of the patient.

Chemotherapy or head and neck radiation may cause taste blindness and inability to distinguish the basic tastes of salt, sweet, sour or bitter with consequent food aversions. Since the aversion is often toward basic protein foods, a high-protein liquid supplement may be needed while preparation of foods.

Learned Food Aversions

Psychologic factors undoubtedly play a role in appetite. The fear and uncertainty engendered by the diagnosis of cancer and its uncertain outcome and the stress of diagnostic procedures are exacerbated by the physiologic and metabolic effects of various antitumor intervention. Those stresses can cause learned food aversion. This behaviour is the unconscious association of the consumption of a particular food with a concurrent or subsequent unpleasant reaction such as nausea and vomiting. The result is subsequent avoidance of that food. In cancer patients, unpleasant reactions may occur in association with antitumour therapy such as a chemotherapeutic drug or ionising radiation.

Hypercalcaemia

It is one of the most common metabolic complications of cancer. Approximately 20 to 40 per cent of patients with breast, squamous, bladder and renal carcinoma develop hypercalcemia at some point of their disease.

Osteomalacia

Certain tumours reduce plasma calcitriol concentration in conjunction with hypophosphatemia, thereby inducing an oncogenic osteomalacia. Gastrointestinal malabsorption of calcium and phosphate has been observed. Resection of the tumour corrects the bone disease.

Most neoplasms, however, obstruct slowly and progressively resulting in anorexia, dysphagia, nausea, vomiting, pain, diarrhoea or anaemia, leading to weight loss and weakness. Fluid and electrolyte and acid-base balance result from persistent vomiting or diarrhoea or as a consequence of dehydration and/or malnutrition.

All the methods of treating cancer involves killing cancerous cells. In this process, some healthy cells are also damaged. That is what causes the side effects of cancer treatment.

NUTRITIONAL PROBLEMS OF CANCER THERAPY

Problems Related to Surgical Treatment

Beyond the regular nutritional needs surrounding any surgical procedure and its healing process, gastrointestinal surgery poses special problems for normal ingestion, digestion and absorption of food nutrients. Head and neck surgery or resections in the oropharyngeal area are sometimes necessitated by cancer. Food intake is greatly affected in such cases and a creative variety of food forms and semiliquid textures as well as modes of feeding must be devised. Often the mechanical problems of food ingestion make long-term tube feeding necessary.

Gastrectomy may cause numerous post-gastrectomy ‘dumping’ problems requiring frequent, small, low-carbohydrate feedings.

Vagotomy contributes to gastric stasis. Pancreatectomy contributes to loss of digestive enzymes, induced insulin dependent diabetes mellitus and general weight loss.

Problems Related to Radiotherapy

Radiation to the oropharyngeal area often produces mucositis, dysphagia, a loss of taste sensation with increasing anorexia, nausea, diarrhoea and consequent decreased appetite.

Other means of tempting appetite through food appearance and aroma, as well as texture must be developed. Abdominal radiation may cause intestinal damage with tissue oedema and congestion, decreased peristalsis or endarteritis (inflammation of the intima or lining coat of an artery) in small blood vessels. In the intestinal wall there may be fibrosis, stenosis (narrowing), necrosis or ulceration. If this condition continues over time, it may lead to haemorrhage, obstruction, fistulas, (abnormal communication between two body surfaces) diarrhoea or malabsorption, all contributing to nutritional problems. The liver is somewhat more resistant to damage from radiation in adults, but children are more vulnerable.

High energy (1 kcal/ml) and protein (50 gms/litre) containing oral liquid nutrition supplements are given. Two glasses of supplements per day with a total amount of 480 ml should be taken for three months.

Adequate nutrition support during radiotherapy can decrease the impact of side effects, minimize weight loss, improve quality of life and help patients recover from radiotherapy quickly.

Problems Related to Chemotherapy

These problems are related to:

- The gastrointestinal symptoms caused by the effect of the toxic drugs on the rapidly developing mucosal cells.
- The anaemia associated with bone marrow effects.
- The general systemic toxicity effect on appetite.

Table 21.3 Some side effects of cancer therapy and suggested dietary management

Nausea and Vomiting	Clear, cold and carbonated beverages with added polycose; Sipping beverages slowly through a straw; small, frequent meals low in fat. Dry crackers or toast before arising, tart or salt foods liquids 30 to 60 minutes before eating.
Dry mouth	Drinking at least 2 litres of liquid daily. High calorie beverages are preferable to water.
	Sauces, gravies broth to moisten foods and to make them easier to swallow. Chewing sugar-free gum or sugar free candy to stimulate salivation. Artificial saliva is given.
Taste alterations	Experimenting with different flavours and seasonings.
	Substitution of other proteins for red meats.
Loss of appetite	Small, frequent feedings, high calorie, high protein snacks and beverages.
Sore mouth and throat	Soft, non acid foods, blended or liquefied foods.
	Foods and beverages at room temperature using straw with liquids.
Swallowing problem	Avoiding highly seasoned foods. Liquid feedings or pureed foods; frequent feedings. Tube feeding.
	Adding butter and sauces to foods.
	Finely chopped foods.
Early satiety	Small frequent meals, chewing foods well and eating slowly.
	Avoiding foods excessively high in fat.
	Liquid 30 to 60 min. before meal not at meals.

Source: Robinson, C.H., Marilyu R. Lawler, 1982. *Normal and Therapeutic Nutrition*, Oxford and IBH Publishing Company, New Delhi.

The stomatitis, nausea, diarrhoea and malabsorption contribute in many food intolerances. Prolonged vomiting seriously affects fluid and electrolyte balance especially in elderly persons and needs to be controlled. Anti-depressant drugs which are used for pretreatment to relieve mental depression cause well-known pressor effects when used with tyramine rich foods thus these foods should be avoided when using such drugs.

Malnutrition during treatment can lead to negative consequences such as increased risk of infections, treatment toxicity, increased health care costs and decreased response to treatment, quality of life and life expectancy.

NUTRITIONAL REQUIREMENTS

Weight loss is often evident at the time cancer is diagnosed and severe malnutrition often seen in the later stages of cancer may be the ultimate cause of death in many cases. Studies have shown that once lean body mass is significantly depleted, regardless of the cause, death will follow. Without adequate energy and nutrients, the body is poorly equipped to maintain immune defenses, support organ function, absorb nutrients and mend damaged tissues.

Objectives of Nutritional Therapy

- To meet the increased metabolic demands of the disease and prevent catabolism as much as possible, and
- To alleviate symptoms resulting from the disease and its treatment through adaptation of food and the feeding process.

Energy

To prevent excessive weight loss and to meet increased metabolic demands, the total energy value of the diet must be increased. Calorie density sufficient to counter catabolic or hypermetabolic states and to support necessary anabolism is necessary. Of this total dietary kilocalorie value, there must be sufficient carbohydrate to spare protein for vital tissue synthesis. For an adult patient with good nutritional status about 2000 kcal will provide for maintenance needs. A malnourished patient may require 3000 to 4000 kcal depending on the degree of malnutrition and body trauma.

Calorie requirements are

- 20–25 kcal/kg - non-ambulatory or sedentary patients.
- 30–35 kcal/kg - slightly hypermetabolic; for weight gain/anabolism.
- 40–45 kcal/kg - hypermetabolic or severely stressed patients; significant malabsorption.

Use of carbohydrate and/or fat to achieve caloric levels (type and amount consistent with patient's condition) is often helpful. Patients who are stressed, initiating cancer therapy or have history of diabetes mellitus should be monitored for hyperglycaemia.

Many breast cancer patients gain weight during treatment. Body composition often changes during treatment–muscle tissue is lost while fat is gained. Physical activity is decreased and intake may be increased. Studies show that weight gain during breast cancer treatment is associated with increased risk of recurrence and death from breast cancer. Current strategy is to work on physical activity to maintain muscle mass. Healthy eating is encouraged.

Protein

Protein energy malnutrition is common in cancer patients. Additional protein is required to provide essential amino acids and nitrogen necessary for tissue regeneration, healing and rehabilitation. Branched-chain amino acid infusions can decrease protein catabolism in cancer patients. An adult patient with good nutritional status will need about 80 to 100 g to meet maintenance needs and to ensure anabolism. A malnourished patient will need more to replenish tissues and to ensure positive nitrogen balance.

- 0.5 g/kg - minimal daily requirement
- 0.8 – 1.0 g/kg - normal maintenance level
- 1.5–2.5 g/kg - if increased protein demands exist, e.g., protein losing enteropathy, hypermetabolism or extreme wasting.

Glutamine is suggested for clinical use of oncolory patients. In patients with cancer, marked glutamine depletion develops over a time. Cancer cachexia is due to massive depletion of skeletal muscle glutamine. This can have a negative impact on the function of host tissues that are dependent on adequate stores of glutamine for optimal functioning *e.g.*, intestinal epithelial cells and lymphocytes. Furthermore, the extent of normal tissue damage from radiation or chemotherapy may be influenced by the presence of adequate tissue glutamine stores.

Micronutrients

Tumours located in the digestive tract have the potential of causing obstruction resulting in poor intake. Deficiency of B vitamins can arise from prolonged general malnutrition. Normal metabolism of micronutrients may also alter the disease process. Reaction of the lower gastrointestinal tract may result in malabsorption and micronutrient deficiencies. In all these circumstances supplementation may be required.

Radiation and chemotherapy induced side effects like nausea, vomiting, diarrhoea can lead to electrolyte imbalance.

A daily multivitamin and mineral supplement may be recommended for patients whose intake is limited for a a prolonged period.

In addition, dietary supplements are given to improve the nutritional status. There is mounting evidence that vitamin D (400–800 IU) helps to protect against several types of cancer including breast cancer.

Fluid

Fluids are increased to compensate losses from gastrointestinal problems as well as any additional loss caused by infections and fever. Also sufficient fluid intake is necessary to help the kidneys rid the body of the breakdown products from destroyed cancer cells and drugs themselves. Increased fluid also helps to protect the urinary tract from irritation and inflammation.

DIETARY MANAGEMENT

Oral and other enteral feeding modes pose fewer problems than do alternative means.

The spectrum of feeding modalities

- Oral diet amplified with nutrient supplement for increased protein, calories, vitamins and minerals.

- Enteral tube feeding with several routes of entry.
- Parenteral nutrition through central and peripheral veins.

Feeding the patient by normal ingestion of food and nutrient supplements is most desirable. Based on individual nutritional assessment, a personal food plan is developed with the patient, incorporating desired food forms and family food patterns. Often the diet of the hospitalised patient can be supplemented with familiar foods from home as the clinical nutritionist plans with the family. A number of adjustment in food texture, temperature, amount, timing, taste, appearance and form can be made to help alleviate symptoms. With support, the patient and family are better able to build a positive mental attitude toward the diet as an integral part of the treatment.

Food should be nutrient dense. Texture can be varied as tolerated, with appeal to sensory perceptions of colour, aroma and taste to enhance the desire to eat. Often a series of mini meals using a wide variety of food items is better tolerated than regular large meals. If appetite is better in the morning, a good breakfast should be emphasised. Getting some exercise before meals and maintaining surroundings that reduce stress may also help in the eating process appealing in aroma and appearance and in small amounts should be continued. Since zinc deficiency is related to diminished taste, sometimes a zinc supplement may be indicated.

Salivary secretions are also affected by cancer therapy, so foods with a high liquid content should be used.

Nausea is often enhanced by foods that are hot, sweet, fatty or spicy. So these can be avoided according to individual tolerance. Frequent small feedings of cold foods, soft to liquid in texture can be given. Eating dry foods such as crackers and dry toast on waking in the morning may be helpful.

Sore mouth often results from chemotherapy or radiation to the head and neck area. It is increased from any state of malnutrition or from infections such as candidiasis (thrush) with numerous ulcerations of the oral and throat mucosa. Frequent small meals and snacks, soft in texture, bland in nature and cool to cold in temperature are often better tolerated.

Cancer patients can be benefitted from early and continued individualised nutrition intervention. The intervention may start before therapy begins, continuing throughout therapy and after completion for atleast 3 years.

The diet should be supplemented with medium chain triglycerides if there is fat malabsorption. When an adequate intake cannot be achieved orally, enteral or parenteral support may be necessary to prevent or respond to malnutrition.

Dietary Guidelines

Whole grains are rich in many components, including dietary fibre, starch, fat, antioxidant nutrients, minerals, vitamins, lignans and phenolic compounds, all of which have been linked to reduced risk of cancer. Most of these components are found in the germ and bran which are removed in the refining process.

- Whole grains to be included and refined and processed foods should be avoided.
- Five to nine servings of coloured vegetables and fruits which have cancer fighting phytochemicals should be included in the diet.
- Legumes such as soyabean to be consumed. Red meat is avoided or reduced as they contain high amounts of inflammatory saturated fat and ω-6 fatty acids.

- Sufficient milk is to be included.
- Refined sugars to be avoided. If needed stevia can be used.
- Total intake of fat should be restricted. Foods rich in ω-3 and ω-9 fatty acids can be included. Fish, nuts, avocados, flax and olives can be taken. Trans fats should be avoided.
- Plenty of water should be consumed. At least 3 cups of tea to be included as it provides antioxidants.
- More number of meals to be included to meet increased requirement of calories and protein.
- Fish can be included in the diet.
- Diet can be supplemented with medium chain triglycerides.

NUTRIENT SUPPLEMENTS

Supplements supplement a healthy diet. Supplements cannot counter act a poor diet. Emphasis should be on diet with plenty of whole grains, vegetables, legumes with soya bean, fish and ω-3 fatty acid.

Most of the cancer patients with advanced cancer suffer from anorexia and there is need for supplements.

Commercial nutrition supplements may be useful for increasing energy and/or protein intake in individuals unable to meet their nutritional requirements through natural foods. Commercial nutritional supplements can be suggested when there is impairment in the ability to consume or prepare conventional nutrient-dense foods and fluids and when there is dysgeusia and lactose intolerance.

Patient need to be educated about the potential harmful effects of herbal preparations and megadoses of vitamins and minerals. Usually there is risk of contamination, adulteration, fake products and having ingredients which are not permitted. They may have possible interactions that interfere with radiotherapy and chemotherapy regimes.

Whey protein is given to prevent clinical malnutrition, preventing cancer patients dying due to malnutrition.

Some mushrooms boost immunity and help in preventing and/or treating cancer. Reishi mushroom, *ganoderma lucidium* is immunostimulant, anti-inflammatory and act as anti-tumour. It is known as mushroom of immortality. Maitake, *grifola frondosa's* key component is β-glucan. It is immune stimulating activate certain cells and proteins that attack cancerous cells.

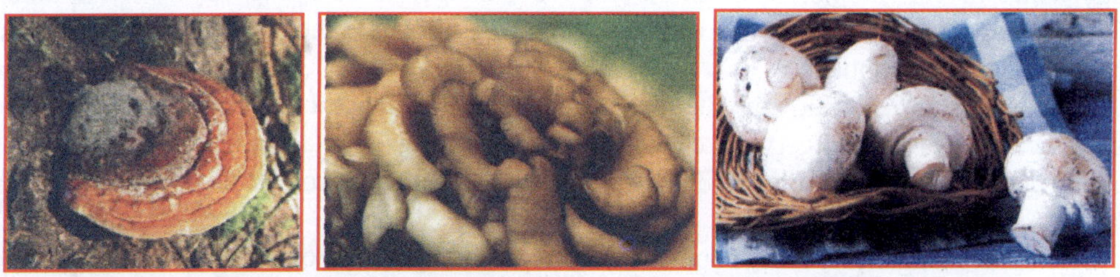

Reishi mushroom — Maitake — Button mushroom

Fig. 21.4 Mushrooms used in the prevention and treatment of cancer.

White button mushrooms, *agaricus bisporous* has phytochemicals which block the activity of the aromatase enzyme would decrease the production of estrogen, which in turn helps control and possibly prevents the growth of hormone dependent breast cancer cells.

Nutrient supplements in a variety of forms and flavours may be used in different ways to enhance nutrient density. When the patient is unable to eat but the gastrointestinal tract can still be used, tube feedings may be needed to provide the necessary nutritional support.

PREVENTION

Role of Food

Diet is an important area of intervention for primary cancer prevention. Foods containing anti-initiators and antipromoters of cancer are recommended. Consumption of vegetables and fruits (more than 400 g/day) can prevent at least 20 per cent of all cancer incidence.

Nutrients as Cancer Preventing Agents

Diets rich in monosaturated fats, ω–3 fatty acid-fish/flax seed oil - high in ω-3 fatty acid contents in erythrocyte membranes are inversely correlated with the development of colorectal cancer and breast cancer. ω-6 to ω-3 ratio seems to play a major role.

Epidemiological studies strongly suggest that high intakes of food rich in β-carotene as well as those rich in vitamin E or C decrease the risk of some cancers.

The beneficial effects of nutrient antioxidants is given in Table 21.4.

Table 21.4 Beneficial effects of nutrient antioxidants

Nutrient	*Beneficial effect*
β-Carotene	Reduced risk of various cancers especially lung cancer and also stomach, cervix, oesophageal and throat cancers.
Vitamin C	Reduced risk of upper gastrointestinal tract, cervix cancer, cardiovascular disease.
Vitamin E	Significant decrease in the risk of oral and pharyngeal cancer, cardiovascular disease
Selenium	Reduced risk of oesophageal and stomach cancers

Vitamin E or tocopherol occur widely in nature and help to stabilise most of the oils derived from plants. The antioxidant activity decreases from delta to alpha tocopherol. Vegetable foods contain considerable amounts of different tocopherols and tocotrienols in their lipid fraction. In soyabean oil the active antioxidant is tocopherol. Whole grains are concentrated sources of antioxidant nutrients, vitamin E. It is an intracellular antioxidant that protects polyunsaturated fatty acids in cell membranes from oxidative damage. It also inhibits the formation of nitrosamines, especially at low pH levels. Vitamin E prevents the formation of carcinogens from precursor compounds.

Deficiencies of folic acid and vitamins A and C have been associated with the development of cervical dysplasia and cervical cancer. Dark green leafy vegetables and some citrus fruits are also good sources of folic acid. This may have a protective role at the molecular level in cancer development.

Selenium, manganese, zinc, copper and iron are components of the antioxidant enzymes. Glutathione peroxidase (GSH-Px) is selenium dependent. Manganese superoxide dismutase, copper-zinc superoxide dismutase (SOD) and catalase are enzyme antioxidants. Selenium prevents development of bladder cancer in women.

Copper, like iron is generally considered as a prooxidant. It is an essential nutrient and a part of copper, zinc-SOD and also ceruloplasmin. Nutritional copper deficiency may impair antioxidant status by decreasing the activity of these enzymes.

Levels 25–35 per cent below these thresholds predict atleast 2-fold high risk. Suboptimal levels of any single antioxidant may increase the relative risk independently.

Dietary deficiencies of selected antioxidant micro-nutrients (β-carotene and vitamins A, C and E) are known risk factors in the pathogenesis of cancer to stop further development. Concurrent correction of suboptimal plasma antioxidant levels is an important part of optimal nutrition at the early stages of cancer.

Phytochemicals as Anticancer Agents

Biologically active substances present in plants are known as phytochemicals. A wide range of epidemiologic studies demonstrate a consistent dose-response relationship between fruit and vegetable intake and the prevention of cancers; higher intake is associated with lower risk. A consistent finding among various studies show that fruit and vegetable consumption is inversely associated with oropharyngeal cancer. The association appears to be most marked for epithelial cancers, particularly those of the alimentary and respiratory tracts, a weaker to nonexistent relationship has been noted for hormone related cancers.

Terpenes

Terpenes: Carotenoids are one subclass of terpenes that are present in tomatoes, parsley, oranges and spinach. Terpenes are plant foods that act as antioxidants, α-carotene inhibits tumour growth.

Table 21.5 Phytochemicals and their sources

Phytochemical	*Source*
Carotenoids	Dark yellow and orange and deep green vegetables and fruit
Diallyl sulfide	Onions, garlic, scallions, leeks, chives
Flavonoids and phenols	Parsley, carrots, citrus fruits, broccoli, cabbage, cucumbers, squash, yams, tomatoes, egg plant, peppers, soya products, berries, potatoes, broad beans, peapods, coloured onions, radishes, tea, onions, apples
Isoflavones	Soyabeans and soyabean products
Isothiocyanates	Cabbage, cauliflower, broccoli, brussels sprouts, mustard, radishes
Lignans	Whole grain products
Limonone	Citrus oil
Lycopenes	Tomatoes, red grape fruit, guava, dried apricots
Organosulfuric compounds	Garlic, onions, chives, citrus fruits, broccoli, cabbage, cauliflower, brussels sprouts
Terpenes and monoterpenes	Citrus fruits, parsley, carrots, celery, broccoli, cabbage, cauliflower, cucumbers, squash, yams, tomatoes, egg plant, peppers, mint, basil, caraway seeds.

Lycopene: This carotenoid found in tomatoes is most effective biological singlet-oxygen quencher. This is two times as powerful as β-carotene in the destruction of free radicals. Research has shown that lycopene rich foods like tomatoes reduce the risk of prostate cancer development; lutein and zeaxanthin other forms of carotenoids reduce the risk of lung cancer and breast cancer.

Limonoids: These are found in citrus fruits like grape fruit and orange juice. They have chemopreventive agents that induce enzymes in the liver's phases I and II enzyme detoxification system. This system detoxifies carcinogens by making them more water-soluble for excretion from the body.

Citrus fruits may reduce the risk of stomach cancer.

Phenols

Phenols: These phytochemicals include the subclass flavonoids. Grape juice and red wine are good sources. Apples, chocolates and tea are good sources of flavonoids. Flavonoids scavenge free radical compounds. By scavenging activated mutagens and carcinogens, flavonoids may also decrease the risk of cancer. Tea has been shown to contain several polyphenolic compounds and their derivatives which are reported to possess antioxidant activity. Colon cancer appears to show a negative association with tea consumption. Cherry tomatoes have more flavonols than the ordinary variety.

Flavonols are not easily destroyed by cooking. Peanuts are rich in the antioxidant flavonols.

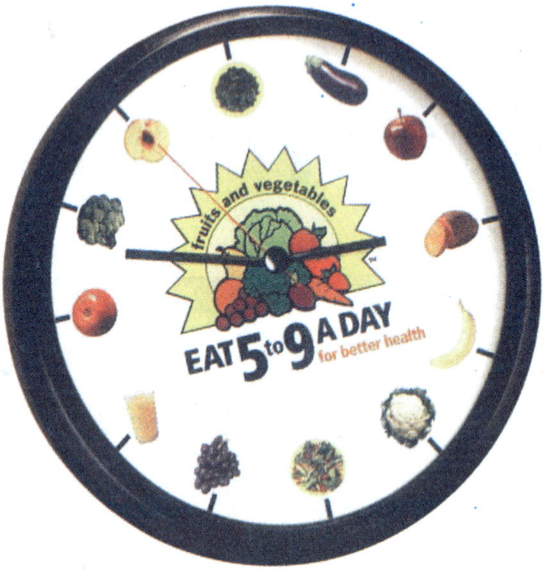

Fig. 21.5 **Eat 5 to 9 A day. Eating fruits and vegetables not smoking and drinking in moderation can have a big impact on a person's risk of getting cancer. Now it appears that these factors also impact survival after diagnosis.**

Source: Department of Health and Human Services, National Institutes of Health, National Cancer Institute, US.

Phenolic compounds: Caffeic and ferulic acids present in whole grains have been classified as cancer inhibitors. They act by preventing the formation of carcinogens from precursor compounds and by blocking the reaction of carcinogens with critical cell macromolecules. The potentially anticarcinogenic mechanism of these phenolic compounds involves the induction of detoxification systems in the cell. Phenolic acids possessing antioxidant activity have also been found in soyabean. The antioxidant activity of oats is supposedly based on its high content of dihydrocaffeic acid.

Isoflavones: These are found in beans and other legumes especially soyabeans and soya foods. Genistein, phytoesterogens found in soya foods act as antioxidants, carcinogen blockers and tumour suppressors which may exert a protective effect against hormone related cancers like breast cancer and prostate cancer. Recent studies suggest that isoflavones may mitigate the harmful effects of radiation treatment for cancer.

Thiols

Thiols: It is a sulphur containing phytonutrient found in cruciferous vegetables, such as broccoli, cauliflower, brussels sprouts and cabbage. Cruciferous vegetables contain subclasses of thiols identified as indoles, dithiolthiones and isothiocyanates. These organosulphuric compounds upregulate enzymes involved in the detoxification of carcinogens and other foreign compounds.

A study conducted at Rutgers the USA, shows that certain vegetables—broccoli and cauliflower have sulphoraphane which may reduce the risk of developing hereditary cancers. Indole-3-carbinol is a phytochemical found in cruciferous vegetables such as broccoli, kale and cauliflower. It prevents or slows breast, colon, prostrate and cervical cancer.

Organo sulphur compounds are also found in the allium or onion family which includes garlic, shallots and leeks. Allyl sulphides increase the production of glutathione S transferase, a phase II enzyme of the liver's detoxification system. They inhibit mutagenesis and increase the activity of macrophages and T lymphocytes. The allyl sulphur compounds reduce the activation of many procarcinogens to active carcinogen by lowering the activity of microsomal cytochrome P_{450} enzymes.

Lignans

Lignans: These are phytochemicals found in flax seeds, wheat bran and barley. Lignans are phytoestrogens that may have a protective effect against hormone-sensitive cancers by virtue of the interference with sex hormone metabolism.

Phytic acid: Phytic acid chelates with various metals which suppress damaging iron-catalysing redox reactions. Colonic bacteria produce oxygen radicals in appreciable amounts and dietary phytic acid may suppress oxidant damage to intestinal epithelium and neighbouring cells.

Fruits and vegetables intake has been examined in relationship to the incidence of various types of cancers. Raw and fresh vegetables, fruits, leafy green vegetables, cruciferae (cabbage), lettuce and carrots are protective against cancer. Vegetable intake is associated with a substantial reduction of risk for several epithelial cancers. Persons with low fruit and vegetable intake have been found to experience twice the risk of cancer compared to those with high intake. Fruits in particular were significantly protective in cancers of the oesophagus, oral cavity and larynx and urinary tract neoplasm. Strong evidence of a protective effect of fruit and vegetables has been seen in cancers of pancreas, stomach, cervix, ovary, endometrium, colon, bladder and breast. The biochemical and biological rationale for an effect of these foods is extremely strong. This is because fruits and vegetables are rich sources of antioxidant nutrients and other phytochemicals. They are also rich in phytochemicals such as dithiolthiones, glucosinolate and indoles, lycopene, isothiocyanates, flavonoids, phenols, phytates, protease inhibitors, plant sterols, allium compounds and lignans.

These agents have both complementary and overlapping mechanism of action, including the induction of detoxification enzymes, inhibition of nitrosamine formation, provision of substrate for formation of antineoplastic agents, dilution and binding the carcinogens in the digestive tract, alteration of hormone metabolism and antioxidant effects. It appears extremely unlikely that any one substance is responsible for all the associations seen.

Whole grains contain phytic acid. Whole grains can also alter development of disease process of its ability to bind carcinogens.

Ways to Increase Fruits and Vegetables in the Diet

- Trying a new fruit or vegetable each week
- Doubling the normal serving size for vegetables
- Eating fruit with curd
- Making recipes where vegetables are incorporated in cereals and pulses
- Consuming all vegetables based meals on a regular basis
- Eating fruit as a snack
- Adding vegetables to favourite recipes.
- Eating greens and green herbs like curry leaves and mint every day in some form.

Prebiotics and Probiotics

Two factors that influence intestinal integrity are the bacterial populations in the gut and the health of the gut mucosa, both of which are influenced by nutrition.

In an optimally functioning gut, there is a balance between beneficial and pathogenic bacteria in the large intestine. Researchers found that potentially carcinogenic agents (food dyes, aflatoxins, pesticides, nitrites) and cancer-causing agents in non-foods (smokeless tobaccos, medications) are bioactivated by enzyme systems in gut bacteria. These bioactivations which can lead to cancer are promoted at a higher rate in GI systems with imbalanced floral populations.

Healthy microflora can be supported by two interventions: prebiotics and probiotics. Prebiotics include foods that contain substrates that nourish beneficial gut microbiota. These substrates include dietary fibre and fructo oligosaccharides (FOS). Food sources of these FOSs include honey, beer, onion, banana and oats.

The probiotics support intestinal health by inhibiting the over growth of toxic bacteria. By competing for attachment sites and nutrients these beneficial bacteria inhibit the proliferation of non-beneficial organisms. Lactobacillus and bifidobacteria also produce organic acids that reduce intestinal pH and retard the growth of pathogenic bacteria. Fermented dairy products like curds contain live culture which prevent cancer, particularly colorectal cancer.

Resistant Starch

A strong correlation exists between high intake of resistant starch present in substances like beans and lower risk of colorectal cancer. Resistant starch increases the production of short chain fatty acids. Butyrate may slow the growth of colon tumour cells.

Dietary Fibre

Several mechanisms have been proposed to explain the protective action of dietary fibre against colon cancer.

- The fibre dilutes bile acids or binds to it thereby preventing its role in mutation or cell proliferation.

- Fermentation of dietary fibre results in production of short chain fatty acids lowering the intestinal pH. This inhibits conversion of primary bile acids to secondary bile acids. The secondary bile acids are believed to promote mutation in intestine.
- At low pH the solubility of free bile acids is reduced, diminishing their availability for carcinogenic activity.
- Fermentation of dietary fibre results in production of butyrate which has been shown to be antineoplastic.
- Dietary fibre exerts its beneficial effect by speeding the passage of faeces through the large intestine so that carcinogens are in contact with the intestinal wall for much shorter period of time.
- Additionally the bulk and water of faeces may dilute the carcinogen to a nontoxic level.

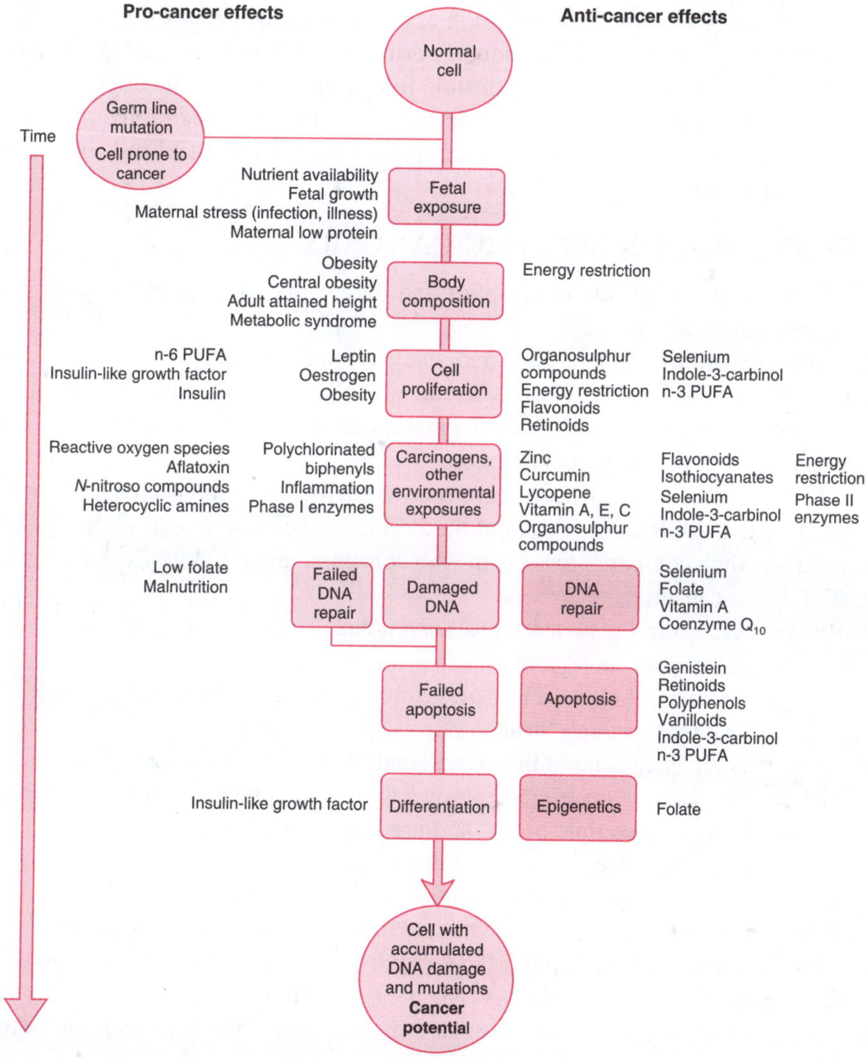

Fig. 21.6 Factors involved in pro-cancer and anti-cancer

Source: World Cancer Research Fund, American Institute for Cancer Research.

CHAPTER 21

- Dietary fibre also influences the colonic microbial metabolism, influences fermentation in the colon and the production and distribution of short chain fatty acids in the colon. It modifies pH, increases the faecal nitrogen and influences mutagens and faecal enzymes in the colon.
- Many human studies find that the consumption of fructo oligo saccharides (FOS) increases beneficial bifidobacteria in the gut, while decreasing concentrations of potentially harmful *E. coli*, clostridia and bacteroids.

A large number of potentially anticarcinogenic agents are found in fruits and vegetables including antioxidant vitamins, fibre and other agents such as dithiolthiones, glucosinolates and indoles, isothiocyanates, flavonoids, phenols, protease inhibitors, plant sterols, allium compounds, and limonene. These agents have both complementary and overlapping mechanisms of action, including the induction of dectoxification enzymes, inhibition of nitrosoamine formation, provision of substrate for formation of antineoplastic agents, dilution and binding of carcinogens in the digestive tract, alteration of hormone metabolism and antioxidant effects. It is unlikely that any one substance is responsible for the anticarcinogenic effect, it is the range of agents in fruits and vegetables that together may offer the observed protection. Thus, fruits and vegetables act through the micronutrients and phytochemicals and influence carcinogen metabolism and maintain DNA integrity.

RECENT STUDIES ON SPECIFIC CANCERS

Studies indicated that a high fat consumption like butter in adolescence was correlated with breast carcinoma in adulthood.

Studies from Japan which is a low frequency region for breast cancer has shown that reduction in risk was associated with milk and green/yellow vegetable consumption in pre and post menopausal woman. Traditional Japanese diet with fish was more beneficial in post menopausal women so did fruit consumption.

Early life (adolescence) diets also influence adult onset of breast caner. Studies from Harvard showed that adolescent consumption of eggs, vegetable fat and fiber was associated with a lower risk when compared to woman who consumed more butter. Consumption of dairy products and breast cancer.

Phytoestrogens are natural plant substances and are of 3 main classes isoflavone, coumestans and lignans. Phytoestrogens have anti cancer properties but also have significant estrogenic properties. Their benefits in breast cancer prevention would again depend on how early in age were the subjects exposed to them through regular plant food consumption.

Endometrial cancers or cancers of the uterine body are mostly seen in postmenopausal obese woman. It is attributed to the oestrogens produced post menopausally from the peripheral fat tissue. Plant estrogens oppose this action and are beneficial.

Colorectal tumors have been found to be inversely related to a high ω-3 fatty acid to arachidonic acid ratio in tissue. Fish consumption would be beneficial. Physical inactivity, high energy intake and obesity are associated with rectal cancer and there is probably a synergistic effect among the 3 risk factors. Animal fats are not only associated with large bowel cancers but also with benign tumors or adenomas. The greater the animal fat intake, greater is the size of adenomas. Food derived polycyclic aromatic hydrocarbons play an important role in colon cancers. These carcinogens are formed by endogenous drug metabolizing enzymes which are genetically determined, which account for the individual variations in susceptibility.

Stomach cancers have been largely narrowed down to an infection due to *helicobacter pylori* which is quite common in the population. Its interaction with a high salt and pickled diet is responsible for most gastric cancers. Capsaicin in chilli peppers are also considered as human carcinogens for stomach cancers in studies. No association was seen with safrole, the spice principle in black / white pepper.

When 30 per cent of cancers are diet related and diet is well within an individual's reach to modify, it is probably the best approach to minimize cancer incidence. Recent evidences indicate ω-3-PUFA to be a major favorable determinant of several cancers like oral, oesophageal, large intestine, breast and ovary. On the other hand too much on ω-6 fatty acid is not found beneficial. The presence of insulin like growth factors as an indicator of cancer risk is also being recognized. This too is modifiable to a certain extent with diet. Thus independent of what new research is bringing out, the final conclusions of avoiding being obese, avoiding alcohol, exercising regularly and eating more of fruits and vegetables does not change. Micronutrients like vitamins and minerals not only help protect against cancer but are also involved in getting better reponses to treatment and therby a better long term disease free survival.

Table 21.6 Recent findings in specific cancers

Type of cancer	*Dietary modification*	*Action involved*
Breast cancer	Mediterranean diet	Lowered risk, due to reduced endogenous, oestrogens, provide flavonoids, olive oil rich in antioxidants which prevent damage to DNA.
	Milk, green/yellow vegetables, Fish	Lowered risk
	Eggs, vegetable fat and fibre	Lowered risk
Colorectal cancer	High ω-3 to ω-6 ratio	Lowered risk
	High energy intake and obesity	High risk
	High animal fats	High risk
	High dietary folate	Lowered risk due to lowered risk of colon polyps.
	High intake of dairy products	Lowered risk
	Fermented milk products	Prevent colorectal cancer
Stomach cancer	*Helicobacter Pylori* and high salt and pickled diet	–
Prostate cancer	ω-3 fatty acids	Protective against cancer variant *rs4647310* in *cox2* is a known inflammatory gene. Reversed by ω-3 fatty acid taking half a gram/day
Renal cell carcinoma	Dark green leafy vegetables, cruciferous, vegetables, Tomatoes	Protective role
	Meat, white bread and potatoes	Increased risk
General	Turmeric	Inhibits the formation of nitrosomine which may be carcinogen Nitrates/Nitrites with secondary amines can be prevented.

PHYSICAL ACTIVITY

Life time total physical activity reduces the risk of post menopausal breast cancer. Exercise can have significant benefits for breast cancer survivors during and after treatment. The general aerobic prescription is for moderate intensity activity (50–75% heart rate reserve) 3–5 days per week, 20 to 60 minutes per session. Resistance training should also be incorporated into the programmes. Men who have been treated for colorectal cancer can reduce their risk of dying from the disease by engaging in regular exercise. They live longer.

Studies show higher levels of HDL seem to be protective for all cancers. Avoiding obesity, avoiding alcohols, exercising regularly and eating more fruits and vegetables are beneficial for preventing cancer. Limiting consumption of salt and avoiding mouldy cereals or pulses can prevent the incidence of cancer. Meeting the nutritional requirement through diet alone is the best way to prevent cancer.

Thus, as a dietary guideline, a judicious inclusion of foods in our daily diet, rather than pills containing nutrients is suggested. In addition, participation in regular physical activity may reduce a person's risk for developing cancer.

February 4th is World Cancer Day.

May 31st is World Anti-tobacco Day.

September 22nd is Rose Day or Cancer Day.

October is Breast Cancer Awareness Month.

November 7th is National Cancer Awareness Day.

SUGGESTED READINGS

- Eibl Guido *et. al.*, Diabetes Mellitus and Obesity as risk factors for pancreatic cancer, J Acad Nutr Diet. 2018: **118.**
- Getz Lindsey, Nutrition therapy during breast cancer treatment, today's dietitian, 2010.
- Bioactive phytochemicals in Indian foods. Annual report 2014-15, NIN, Hyderabad.
- Thomson Cynthia, A. *et al.*, Association between dietary energy density and obesity – Associated Cancer J Acad Nutr Diet. 2018: **118.**
- American Cancer Society. www.cancer.org>.

QUESTIONS

1. What is cancer? Give classification.
2. Explain the risk factors of cancer.
3. Discuss the systemic reactions of neoplastic disease.
4. Describe the nutritional problems of cancer therapy.
5. What are the dietary modifications required while treating cancer patient?
6. Describe the role of food in the prevention of cancer.
7. Explain the relationship between antioxidants and the incidence of cancer.
8. Give the risk factors for the following cancers:

   (*a*) Breast (*b*) Large intestine (*c*) Stomach.
9. What are the seven danger signals of cancers?
10. What are the recommendations for preventing cancer?
11. Explain the factors involved in precancer and anticancer.
12. Explain the relationship between insulin resistance and cancer.
13. Describe recent findings in specific cancers.

TOPICS FOR DISCUSSION

- Discuss procancer effects and anticancer effects as given in Fig. 21.6.
- Plan and prepare a diet for an elderly man who wants to prevent cancer as he is genetically predisposed.

22

Inborn Errors of Metabolism

Inborn errors of metabolism are genetic disorders occurring due to lack of an enzyme in the metabolic cascade in the body. This disrupts a biochemical pathway, leading to symptoms and signs due to accumulation of toxic metabolites prior to the block or deficiency of the end product beyond the block. Nearly all the inborn errors of metabolism are inherited recessively, mostly autosomal and some X-linked. They are individually rare but collectively common. They are increasingly being recognized in the neonatal period because of the advances in diagnostic facilities, like blood gas analysis and automated biochemical tests, and the reduction in mortality related to infections and perinatal asphyxia. Other factors that lead to an increased frequency of inborn errors of metabolism in our country are the large number of births and the custom of consanguineous marriages among many communities.

Classification of inborn errors of metabolism

These can be broadly categorized into three groups. The enzyme defects occurring in the metabolism of amino acids, carbohydrates, and fatty acids or in the mitochondrial energy metabolism are referred to as 'small molecule disorders'. Examples for these disorders are phenylketonuria, tyrosinemia and homocystinuria. Clinical manifestations of these disorders are severe and non-specific, and occur early in life. In contrast, in large molecule diseases (also called storage disorders) the symptoms develop gradually due to accumulation of substrates. For example, fabry disorder, alpha -galactosidase-A deficiency. This results in progressive organomegaly and coarse body features A third group consists of miscellaneous disorders of metals (Wilson and Menkes' disease), lipoproteins, congenital adrenal hyperplasia and hyperinsulinism.

Table 22.1 gives details of genetic disorders having nutritional implications.

PHENYLKETONURIA

It is a group of autosomal recessive (other than sex chromosome) inherited disorders of phenylalanine metabolism. It is caused by impaired activity of liver enzyme, phenylalanine hydroxylase which oxidises phenylalanine to tyrosine. Several other types of phenylketonuria result from defects in the synthesis of tetrahydrobiopterin. In addition to functioning as coenzyme for phenylalanine hydroxylase, tetrahydrobiopterin is also required by tyrosine hydroxylase and tryptophan hydroxylase. Because these enzymes produce essential neurotransmitters, defects in biopterin synthesis are associated with progressive neurologic disease unless tetrahydrobiopterin L-dopa and serotonin are replaced.

Table 22.1 Inborn errors of metabolism having nutritional implications

Name of the disorder	*Enzyme Affected*	*Nutrient Involved and Therapy*
Phenylketonuria	Phenylalanine hydroxylase	Low protein (phenylalanine) adequate energy
Maple syrup urine disease	Branched chain α ketoacid dehydrogenase complex	Low protein (leucine, isoleucine, valine) adequate energy, and supplemental calcium.
Homocystinuria	Cystathonine betasynthase	Low protein (methionine) and adequate energy and calcium.
Citrullinemia	Arginiosuccinic acid	Low protein, adequate energy, supplemental calcium, vitamin and minerals
Tryrosinemia	Fumarylaceto-acetate hydrolase	Low protein (tyrosine and phenylalanine) adequate energy
Galactosaemia	Variant forms, 3 different enzymes	Galactose restricted diet and supplemental calcium.
Fructosuria	Fructokinase	Sucrose and fructose are avoided
Hypoglycaemia and acidosis	Fructose-1,6 biphosphatase	Cane-sugar, honey, and fructose should be avoided.
Fatty acid oxidation	Long chain hydroxyacyl-CoA dehydrogenase deficiency	Very low fat (replacement with medium chain triglycerides).
	Medium chain hydroxyacyl-CoA dehydrogenase deficiency	Prevent fasting, avoid high fat intake routine nutrition care
	Very long chain hydroxyacyl-CoA dehydrogenase deficiency.	Very low fat (replacement with medium chain triglycerides)

Prognosis

The accumulation of phenylalanine or its catabolic products, a deficiency of tyrosine or its products or all four circumstances will produce central nervous system damage. The pathologic consequence varies with the time in brain development at which the chemical insult occurs. Deficient myelination and abnormalities in brain proteolipids and/or proteins occur in late gestation and during the first 6 to 9 months of life. During this period, oligodendroglia migration may also be impaired, resulting in irreversible brain damage later in childhood. Protein synthesis is inhibited by high phenylalanine on blood-brain barrier transport with consequent imbalance in intraneuronal amino acid concentrations. In the mature brain neurodegeneration, behavioural difficulties and prolonged performance times may result from depressed neurotransmitter synthesis. Impairment of these neuropsychologic functions in mature brain may be reversible when phenylalanine returns towards normal concentrations in cells and blood.

Symptoms

The disease is expressed at 3 to 6 months of age and is characterised by developmental delay, microcephaly, abnormal electro encephalogram, eczema, musty odour and hyperactivity. If not treated before 3 weeks of age, the metabolic imbalance produces irreversible mental retardation. The IQ of affected persons is usually below 50. The central nervous system damage causes increased motor irritability, hyperactivity, convulsive seizures and bizarre behaviour. Because tyrosine, normally produced from phenylalanine is used in the production of the pigment melanin, the untreated PKU children usually have blonde or light brown hair and blue eyes and a fair skin susceptible to eczema. Tyrosine is also involved in the production of epinephrine by the adrenal gland.

Diagnosis

Newborns with blood phenylalanine concentrations greater than 2 mg/dl on the screening test is restudied. Guthrie (microbiological) test is used worldwide.

If the initial or follow-up screening test is greater than 8 mg/dl plasma amino acids should be quantitated by ion exchange chromatography with the infant on a known phenylalanine intake from natural protein sources. A precise diagnosis is necessary to establish the mode of therapy.

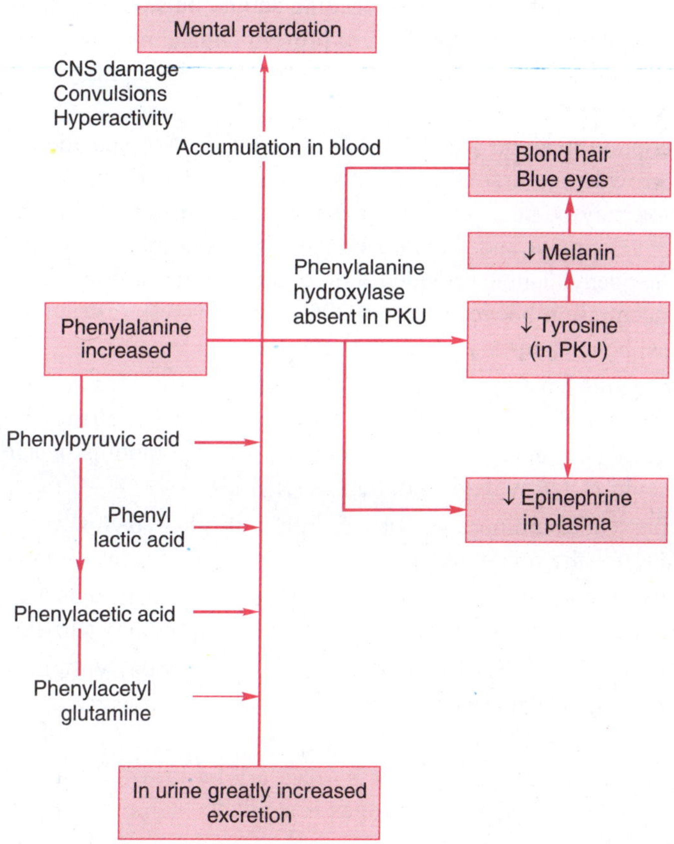

Fig. 22.1 The metabolic error in phenylketonuria

Source: William, S.R., 1985, *Nutrition and Diet Therapy*. Times Mirror/Mosey College Publishing, St. Louts.

Nutrition and Dietary Management

The objective of nutrition support in the child with classic phenylketonuria is to maintain blood phenylalanine concentrations that will allow optimum growth and brain development by supplying adequate energy, protein and other nutrients while restricting phenylalanine and supplementing tyrosine intake.

Phenylalanine restricted diet with isoleucine, leucine and valine have found improvement in behaviour and decreased plasma phenylalanine. This may be related to inhibition of phenylalanine transport by competition at either the intestinal or blood-brain barrier uptake steps.

Therapy of the child with biopterin-deficient forms of hyper phenyl-alaninemia requires administration of tetrahydrobiopterin and use of phenylalanine restricted, tyrosine-supplemented diet in combination with 'L-dopa and carbidopa'. Serotonin that is derived from tryptophan may also improve behaviour if tryptophan hydroxylase is secondarily impaired by the absence of tetrahydrobiopterin.

As soon as the diagnosis is made, breast feeding should be stopped and the infant is bottle fed with a low phenylalanine milk substitute, to prevent clinical manifestations. Within 4 days, the infant is fed 67 kcal/dl low phenylalanine formula. Then blood phenylalanine concentration drops to treatment range.

A formal prescription must be written that is individualised to specific degree of impaired enzyme activity, growth rate and consequent needs of each patient. Weekly adjustments in the diet prescription may be necessary, particularly during the first 6 months of life based on hunger, growth, development and laboratory analysis of plasma phenylalanine and tyrosine concentrations. The phenylalanine provided should maintain the 3–4 hours post-prandial blood phenylalanine concentration between 50 and 300 μ mol. Excess restriction produces growth failure, skin rashes, bone changes and mental retardation.

Phenylalanine required for growth by the infant with classic phenylketonuria is 20 to 70 mg/kg of body weight with the younger infant requiring the larger amount. Phenylalanine requirement declines rapidly between 3 and 6 months of age as growth rates plateau. Intake should match with growth rate.

Tyrosine is an essential amino acid for children with phenylketonuria. Tyrosine is given 180–200 mg/kg/day for the infant and 120 to 150 mg/kg/day for the child and adult.

Recommendations for protein for nutrition support are greater than the RDA. Recommendation for energy and fluid intake are the same as those for normal infants and children.

Adequate protein cannot be obtained from natural foods without ingesting excess phenylalanine. Low-phenylalanine and phenylalanine free chemically defined medical foods can be given.

Energy, the first requirement of the body is necessary for growth. When energy is provided as carbohydrate and fat and if adequate nitrogen is available, non-essential amino acids may be synthesised from the keto acid metabolites. Carbohydrate ingestion leads to insulin secretion and insulin promotes amino acid transport into the cell and consequent protein synthesis. The mechanisms by which insulin regulates amino acid uptake in muscle changes with increasing age. When energy intake is inadequate, tissue catabolism occurs to meet energy needs. Such catabolism releases phenylalanine leading to elevated blood phenylalanine concentrations. Provision of sufficient energy through generous use of non-protein and low protein foods is important to assure a normal growth rate. In acute infections with concomitant tissue catabolism high carbohydrate and fluids should be given.

Prescription for phenylalanine can be increased by addition of measured amounts of milk and/or solid foods. Concentrated chemically defined medical foods are frequently used without any untoward side effects.

Extra fluid must be offered between feedings to maintain appropriate water balance.

A mother has to prepare a low phenylalanine diet for her child from the five lists of foods. She needs continuing help from a dietitian. The lists are:

- Basic foods containing negligible phenylalanine which can be used freely—sugar, jams, sweets, solid vegetable oils and cooking oils.
- Fruits and vegetables which can be taken freely, since they provide negligible phenylalanine and protein in a normal helping. Excess amounts may contribute some phenylalanine.
- A basic list of 50 mg phenylalanine exchanges of foods.
- Manufacturers' foods of negligible phenylalanine content.
- Exchanges of foods containing one gram of protein equivalent to 50 mg of phenylalanine.

Certain clinicians have suggested that the diet might be discontinued at 4, 6 or 12 years of age with no adverse effects. The goal is to maintain serum phenylalanine level between 3–15 mg %.

Aspartame, artificial sweetener contains aspartic acid and phenylalanine. It should not be used in phenylketonuria because phenylalanine is released during its metabolism.

It is extremely important to maintain normal plasma phenylalanine concentrations in the reproductive female before and after conception.

Assessment of Nutrition support: The child needs to be assessed periodically as given here.

- Biweekly assessment of growth : height, weight, head circumference.
- Evaluation of development : developmental scales
- Adequacy of phenylalanine and tyrosine, twice weekly : blood phenylalanine and tyrosine concentration

The first year is the period of most rapid growth and of greatest vulnerability to nutritional insult. Therefore, twice weekly blood tests are suggested during the first 3 months and weekly thereafter until the child is 1 year of age. After 1 year of age, weekly blood tests are sufficient for monitoring diet.

GALACTOSAEMIA

Lactose is the principal carbohydrate and energy source for infants and young children. Galactose maintains a central metabolic role in human nutrition.

Galactosaemia may occur because deficient functioning of any of the three enzymes-galactokinase, galactose-1-phosphate uridyl transferase or UDP galactose-4-epimerase.

$$\text{Galactose} \xrightarrow{\text{Galactokinase}} \text{+ATP Galactose-1-phosphate + ADP.}$$

In galactokinase deficiency cataract occurs without mental retardation or aminoaciduria. Definite diagnosis is made by demonstrating deficiency of galactokinase activity in erythrocytes. Cataract can be prevented if galactose free diet is given to the infant. The prognosis is good. Other than cataract children are normal.

$$\text{Galactose-1-phosphate UDP glucose} \xrightleftharpoons[\text{uridyl transferase}]{\text{Galactose-1-phosphate}} \text{UDP galacose + glucose-1-phosphate} \xrightleftharpoons[\textit{galactose-4-epimerase}]{\textit{Uridine diphospho}} \text{UDP glucose}$$

Galactosemia can occur due to a deficiency of galactose-1-phosphate uridyl transferase which metabolises galactose to glucose. This produces an accumulation of galactose-1-phosphate in tissues and erythrocytes.

It can be an acute fulminating disorder associated with an infective agent such as *Eschrichia coli* and death can occur within 24 hours without a diagnosis being made. More usually there is failure to thrive, with vomiting, diarrhoea, jaundice and hepatomegaly. If the infant survives without treatment, the child will be mentally retarded and have cirrhosis of the liver and cataracts.

If the condition is suspected, lactose-free milk should be given. Early dietary management prevents renal and hepatic damage and cataracts but overall results are disappointing. Unfortunately, although severe mental retardation is usually prevented, these patients often only achieve intelligence in the low normal range and have speech problems, growth failure and ovarian dysfunction. It seems likely that the prenatal accumulation of galactose-1-phosphate and galactitol leads to some brain damage and eye changes in utero. The diet should exclude galactose and therefore lactose.

Dietary management: The infant should receive a nutritionally complete lactose-free milk substitute and this should be used to replace normal milk thereafter. If less than 500 ml is taken in children over the age of 1 year it may be necessary to give a calcium or even vitamin and mineral supplement. Some manufactured foods may have milk and some tablets may have lactose in it and these should be excluded from the diet.

Milk and milk products should be avoided. 'Non-dairy creams' prepared from soyaprotein may be used. Non-fat milk solids and lactose are added to baked foods to improve texture and nutritive value and for its browning properties. Hence baked items should be avoided. Galactose is present in some complex starches (stachyose, raffinose) in peas, soyabean and some vegetables. Hence formulas prepared from soyaprotein isolate can be given whereas whole soya flour preparations are avoided. Among fleshy foods, organ meat like liver is avoided. Strict dietary restriction is necessary in early years which can be somewhat relaxed during school age.

Galactose-Restricted Diet

Foods allowed	*Food excluded*
Beverages: Isomil, prosobee, carbonated drinks	All products containing milk
Fruit drinks free of apple, grape, pear and papaya	Milk products
Breads without milk	Bread with milk
Cheeses none	All excluded
Desserts: water and fruit ices, gelatin	Commercial cakes
Eggs all	Omelettes and souffles containing milk
Fats oil shorting not butter	
Fruits: canned, fresh, frozen that do not contain galactose figs grapes, kiwi fruit, papaya,	Any fruits processed with lactose apple, apple sauce banana, dates, pears, watermelon.

FRUCTOSURIA

It is a rare hereditary condition in which about 10–20 per cent of the fructose taken in food is excreted in the urine. It is postulated that in normal individuals, about 80 per cent of the ingested fructose is converted to glucose and glycogen when the rest is broken down to form lactic acid. It is suggested that in fructosuria, there is lack of fructokinase the enzyme fructose-1-phosphate aldolase B required for the conversion of fructose to fructose-1-phosphate. This leads to accumulation of fructose in blood and its excretion in urine.

In fructosuria, infants are free of symptoms unless sugar (sucrose) is given. Then there may be vomiting and hypoglycaemic fits and a series of episodes may lead to jaundice and enlargement of the liver. It is potentially fatal as liver failure may develop if the condition is not recognised and treated.

Treatment

Sucrose and fruit should be excluded from the diet. This is easy in an infant, but is a formidable problem for a mother as her child grows up. Fortunately the condition is very rare.

Vitamin C supplements should be given.

It has been noted that the teeth of patients with fructose intolerance do not show caries.

FRUCTOSE-1, 6, BIPHOSPHATASE DEFICIENCY

This condition, which affects gluconeogenesis presents in infancy with hypoglycaemia and with signs and symptoms of acidosis due to the accumulation of acetate and ketones. These patients do not like sweet foods. They should receive regular feeds or meals preferably using glucose or glucose polymers especially during infections. Although the diet does not have to be too strict and small amounts of fruit are allowed. Added canesugar, fructose and honey should be avoided.

MENKES' DISEASE

Copper deficiency is rare in humans. It occurs mainly in infants resulting in psychomotor retardation, hypotonia (low osmotic pressure of blood) hypopigmentation, pallor, anaemia, osteoporosis, low concentrations of plasma copper and ceruloplasmin.

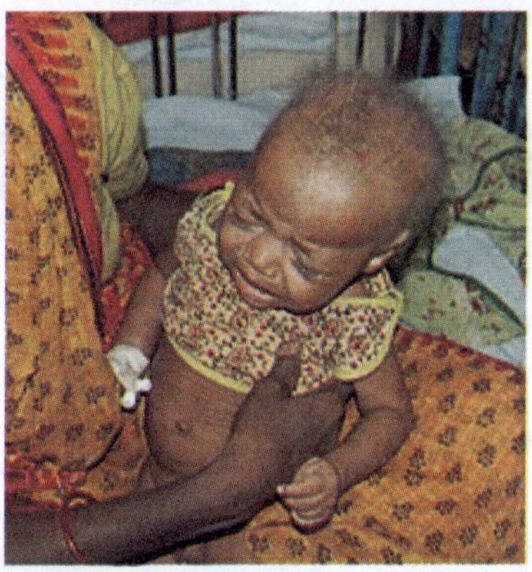

Fig. 22.2 Menkes' kinky hair syndrome is copper absorption disorder.

Low serum copper and ceruloplasmin levels are also found in an inherited condition known as Menkes' kinky hair syndrome as shown in Figure 22.2. This is characterized by slow growth, degeneration of brain tissue, hypothermia, seizures, defective arterial walls, depigmentation of skin and hair and peculiarly stubby white hair (pili torti). The syndrome results from defective absorption of copper, abnormal transport of copper and increased excretion of copper through urine.

WILSON'S DISEASE

Copper poisoning occurs from contamination of food with copper from containers or ingestion of higher quantities of copper salt. Symptoms of acute copper poisoning include excessive salivation, epigastric pain, nausea, vomiting and diarrhea. Consumption of milk based formula foods or weaning foods stored in brass containers may prove harmful. Liver failure is often associated with massive accumulation of copper.

Chronic copper toxicity is relatively rare but occurs in the hereditary condition called Wilson's disease. In this disease a failure to excrete copper in bile leads to accumulation of copper in the liver, brain, kidneys and cornea of the eyes, where it causes brown or green rings to appear. Pathway of copper metabolism leading to Wilson's disease is shown in Figure 22.3. D-penicillamine, a penicillin derivative that forms a chelate with copper in a way that promotes its excretion, has been used to help reduce the copper levels of people with Wilson's disease. Zinc is also used to treat Wilson's disease.

A genetic defect inherited from both parents causes those with the disease to produce abnormal epithelial secretions throughout the body that impair lung function, digestive enzyme production, electrolyte balance, and nutrient absorption, among other effects. The disease's pathophysiology increases the metabolic rate and caloric needs of both children and adults, often resulting in malnutrition.

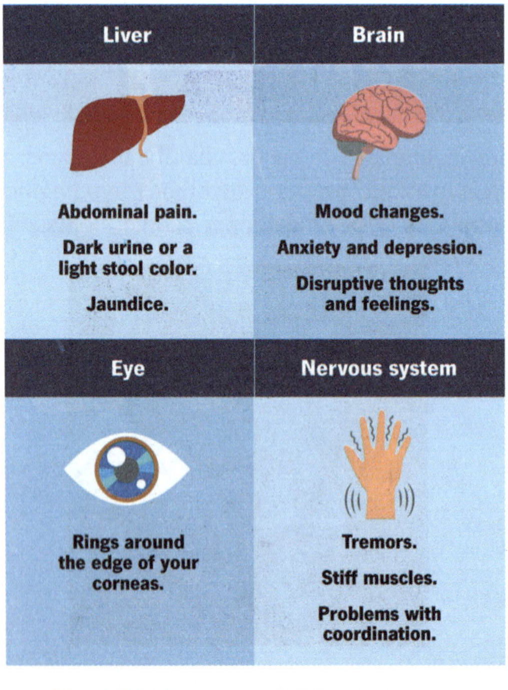

Fig. 22.3 Symptoms of Wilson's disease.

For children with CF, optimizing nutrition can be esepecially challenging. High caloric requirements for growth and development, combined with behavioral issues surrounding food common to all kids, necessitates intervention from skilled practitioners who understand both behavioral management theory and nutrition therapy for chronic disease.

SUGGESTED READINGS

- Manta – Vogli D. Penelope, Phenylketonuria dietary management and an emerging development, J. Acad. Nutr. Diet, 2018; **118**.

QUESTIONS

1. What is phenylketonuria? Explain the dietary management.
2. What kind of exchange lists are used in phenylketonuria?
3. Name five foods rich in phenylalanine.
4. What is galactosemia? What are the enzymes involved in it?
5. Give the list of foods to be included and excluded in galactosaemia.
6. Write short notes on fructosuria.
7. Explain Fructose-1, 6, biphosphatase deficiency.

TOPIC FOR DISCUSSION

- Collect information and discuss the food supplements available in the market for children affected by Inborn errors of metabolism.

23

Food Sensitivity

Food sensitivity denotes an adverse immunologic response to a specific substance with characteristic symptoms whenever food is ingested. It can also be defined as 'altered reaction of the tissue to foreign protein or antigen.' It is also called food hypersensitivity reaction.

TYPES OF REACTIONS

Sensitivity reaction arising due to food may be immediate or delayed.

Immediate Response

This is IgE mediated which results from an interaction between the allergen and target cells sensitised by IgE which is synthesised and secreted by plasma cells. As the interaction proceeds, there is release of mediators like histamine from mast cells and basophils. These mediators act on blood vessels, smooth muscles, mucous glands of skin, respiratory tract and digestive tract to produce symptoms which appear within minutes or few hours of exposure to small quantity of the allergen. They usually clear off within 24–48 hours. Food protein commonly cause this type of reactions. Individuals who are sensitive to egg and nuts experience immediate violent symptoms following ingestion of even minute quantities of food.

It is well known that milk and egg allergy commonly seen in younger children further peanut and tree nut allergies in late childhood also fish and shellfish allergies in older children and pollen-cross allergies in teenagers and adults.

Delayed Response

These are cellular in nature and do not involve circulating antibodies. Symptoms appear in 24–72 hours after ingestion of food and may last for several days. T cell mediated hypersensitivity is also involved in some chronic forms of immune mediated food intolerance, such as cow's milk protein sensitive enteropathy with malabsorption and in coeliac disease.

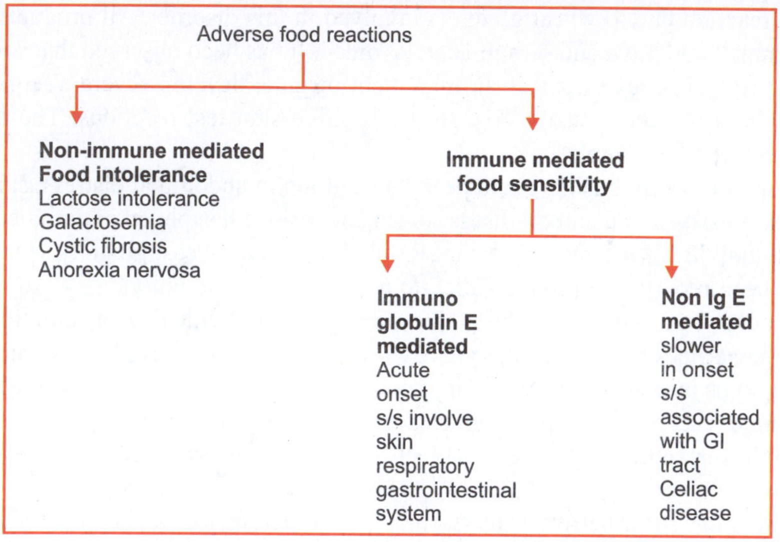

Fig. 23.1 Classification of adverse food reaction

FOODS INVOLVED IN SENSITIVITY

Animal Sources

In cow's milk, casein and β-lactoglobulin are known to be the major allergens. Cow's milk when consumed may cause allergic reactions like colic pain and passage of blood.

Milk intolerant children have positive weal and erythema reactions to one or more milk proteins. Egg is a common allergising agent among animal foods. Egg white is the allergising factor present in egg. Cutaneous manifestations occur more frequently than other symptoms.

Food labels should be checked carefully. Milk-sensitive patient should understand that the following terms indicate that milk may be present in the form of cheese, butter, casein, curds, lactalbumin, lactoglobulin, lactose and whey. Such foods also to be avoided. Baked foods may have glazed egg white. Egg white is also used to clarify coffee. Individuals sensitive to eggs must be aware of label ingredients including ovo globulin, livetin, albumin and of course powdered or dried egg.

Allergic symptoms due to consumption of fish is usually confined to a particular species. Any species of fish can, in principle, be responsible for allergic reactions. Crustacea (crab, lobster and shrimp) are the most common ones that cause allergy. As a rule, the allergic reactions appear very promptly as urticaria (skin eruptions, round smooth raised pinkish itchy weals) angioneurotic oedema of lips, dermatitis, gastrointestinal disorders and even asthma.

Meats of all kinds may give rise to allergic reactions in some individuals. It has been observed that in cases of hypersensitiveness to the meat of a certain animal, the liver, pancreas, kidney and brain of the same species can be eaten with impunity. Aged cheeses such as chedder are among the best known triggers.

Plant Sources

Wheat flour has been associated in precipitating symptoms of coeliac disease in some subjects. The findings that antibodies to wheat gluten appearing in the blood of these patients, indicate that allergic reaction due to wheat gluten is involved in this disorder. All products containing wheat like bran, bread, rava and semolina are avoided. It has been observed that some workers in glue factories using soya flour as an ingredient of glue, develop severe allergic asthmatic symptoms. These workers usually give strong positive skin test reactions. The allergen has been reported to be heat stable.

A few individuals may be allergic to peanuts resulting in abdominal distress, skin eruptions and asthmatic paroxysm. Peanut oil that has been cold-pressed, expelled or extruded may cause a reaction in individuals allergic to peanut. Refined oil is safe. Peas, gingelly seeds beans and lentils have been reported to produce allergic reactions in some individuals. Anything above 5 mg of peanuts can result in reaction for a high risk individual. Consumption of edible mushrooms sometimes may cause allergic reactions. Fats and oils have been found to produce allergic symptoms in a small number of individuals. The vegetables which have been found to produce allergic reactions in some individuals are carrot, spinach, cabbage, onion, garlic, sweet potato, cauliflower and pumpkin. The patient allergic to the raw need not be to the cooked vegetable and vice versa.

Among the fruits, straw berries, bananas, oranges, grapes, melons and apples are the principal offenders. Occasionally, allergic reactions can occur due to consumption of pears, cherries, plums, rasberries, gooseberries. Citrus fruits and tomatoes can cause atopic allergy.

Beverages

Alcoholic beverages may cause clinical manifestations of allergy, both specifically and non-specifically. Their specific allergic actions are due to traces of foreign substances derived from food materials employed in the preparations or clarifying the beverage, such as barley malt and yeast in beer; rye, corn, and wheat in whisky; fish; glue, egg white, or yeast in cheap white wine and champagne. The non-specific reactions are due to the effect of alcohol in increasing permeability of the membranes of gastrointestinal tract thus facilitating the absorption of incompletely digested food proteins which may cause allergic reactions. Allergic reactions to coffee and tea can occur occasionally. Chlorogenic acid, one of the active phenolic compounds found in coffee may be responsible for the allergic reaction.

Fermented Foods

Moulds can cause allergy. All fermented foods should be avoided as anything that has been fermented could harbour other strains of mould spores. Fermentation is involved in processing raisins, beer, wine, blue cheese, pickles and vinegar.

Food Contaminants

The contaminants of food for example preservatives, insecticides, and insect excreta or fragments may act as allergens and the food by itself may be harmless. Such contaminants may enter the plant food in the field or enter the food during storage, processing and shipping. The common additives include colour, flavouring materials, preservatives and insecticides. Additives most frequently cited as causing reactions are sulphites (preservative), tartrazine (colour), monosodium glutamate and aspartame (flavour and taste enhancers). MSG is associated with Chinese restaurant syndrome causing migraine with sensations of thoracic, cervical and facial tightness. For example, nordihydroguaiaretic acid (NDGTA) is an antioxidant used in food fats. It has been found to produce allergic reactions in some individuals. Workers in coffee industry (stripping the green coffee husk from the bean) develop occupational rhinitis and bronchial asthma. Commonly over looked contaminants are arthropod origin and their excreta may remain during the processing and preparation of stored food and may cause allergic reactions. Impurities in fermentation may also be responsible for allergic reactions.

Anaphylactic shock, the life-threatening food allergy reaction is most often caused by groundnuts, gingelly seeds, tree nuts, milk, eggs, wheat, soyabean, fish and shellfish. Children are more likely to outgrow allergies to eggs, milk and soya than allergies to peanuts. With an anaphylactic reaction, symptoms often develop quickly. The symptoms include extreme itching, swelling of the throat that makes breathing difficult, low blood pressure, cardiac arrest and shock.

SYMPTOMS

Manifestations of allergy can occur in any part of the body.

- Skin manifestations may include atopic dermatitis, oedema, fever, blisters and urticaria (rashes), eczema, erythema, edema and pruritus of the lips.
- Common gastrointestinal manifestations include occult fecal blood loss, cheilitis, stomatitis, colic in infants, malabsorption, abdominal pain and cramping, abdominal distention occult, constipation, diarrhoea, dyspepsia, flatulence, nausea and vomiting.
- Respiratory symptoms include sneezing, allergic rhinitis, asthma, bronchitis, shortness of breath, runny nose and nasal polyps.
- Neurologic symptoms such as migraine, neuralgias and tension fatigue syndrome (anxiety, fatigue, irritability, muscle and joints ache restlessness, stomach pain).
- Systemic symptoms include anaphylaxis, pallor, headache, cardiac arrhythmias and hypotension.

Table 23.1 Signs and symptoms in IgE- and non-IgE-mediated food allergy reactions

	IgE	*Non-IgE*	*Acute*	*Chronic*
Skin				
Urticaria (hives)	X		X	X
Angioedema (swelling of face, lips, and tongue)	X		X	
Atopic dermatitis	X	X	X	X
Respiratory				
Throat tightness	X		X	
Rhinitis (nasal congestion)	X		X	X
Gut				
Vomiting	X	X	X	X
Diarrhea	X	X	X	X
Pain	X	X	X	X
Anaphylaxis	X		X	

Source: American Dietetic Association

CHAPTER 23

DIAGNOSIS

Dietary History

A careful dietary history should be taken. In certain cases, if symptoms develop very rapidly and dramatically after immediate ingestion of the offending food, the patient can make his own diagnosis. But it is difficult to associate symptoms to any particular food especially when there is a delay of some hours and there may be an error sometimes. In cases of doubt, the patient is given a diary in which he should record all foods eaten and should also record any disturbances occurring due to food allergy.

Provocative Test

In this test, the patients are given a small quantity of the suspected food in a disguised form so the patient is unaware of the presence of particular food. Typical symptoms appear at the appropriate time after the meal. The test should be conducted for a minimum of 3 times before obtaining confirmative results. The provocative test should not be conducted in patients who develop severe allergic reactions as it may prove dangerous.

Elimination Diet

In this the patient omits one suspected food each day and keeps record of signs and symptoms. This can be adapted in infants and children because of the limited variety of foods they eat, for example, elimination of eggs, milk and wheat which are common allergens in children. This is difficult to follow in adults who live on a wide variety of foods to which sensitivity may develop. Various types of elimination diets have been devised with the object of finding out the offending food. These elimination diets are difficult and complicated and normally suited for investigation of patients in hospitals with a dietetic department and physician experienced in study of allergy.

Laboratory Testing

Skin test: The usefulness of this test in diagnosis of food allergy is limited. In intra dermal test, minute quantities of extracts containing suspected antigens are packed into the skin over the arm. In scratch test a small amount of the solution containing the antigen is placed into a series of scratches made into the skin. In patch test the antigen is applied to a piece of filter paper over the skin and covered with cellophane paper and kept for 24 hours. If a red inflammation or hive like wheal appears at the site of contact, the food is suspected to contain the allergen. Sometimes oedema or erythema due to vasodilation is seen.

Radio allergosorbent test: It is the skin prick test that aims to detect the presence of IgE antibodies. They aim to measure the binding of IgE to allergens such as milk, eggs or fish. An arbitrary score from 0–4 is given. Allergic patients usually have a score above 2. These tests are expensive and not very informative.

X-ray: An X-ray of the GI tract immediately after ingestion of suspected food, admixed with $BaSO_4$ will sometimes reveal changes associated with smooth muscle spasm. This only shows the abdominal distress after taking food.

Basophil histamine release assays: This measures histamine release from whole blood basophils which are exposed to various food antigens and can be used to test for IgE–mediated allergy. This method provides no additional information beyond standard in vitro and skin testing methods.

Food sensitivity in children

Food sensitivity in infants and children is common. Most children with food sensitivity and adverse reactions to food grow out of their sensitivities. The changed reactivity can be due to the decreased absorption of immunologic food proteins as the intestinal mucosa and secretory immune system nature.

Cow's milk is probably the most common single allergen in infants. It is reaction in infancy and usually appears in the first few months of life. Other common sensitivities seen in children are egg white and fish. The child may overcome egg white sensitivity but fish sensitivity often persists.

Milk sensitivity in infants can affect the gastrointestinal tract followed by respiratory system and skin. Most of the infants present with diarrhea and mucous. Vomiting, especially within an hour of feeding, is the second most common manifestation.

TREATMENT

Elimination Diets

Elimination diets have a proper place in the diagnosis and management of food intolerance. In elimination diets, the suspected food is excluded in the daily diet.

The common elimination diets are:

(*i*) *Simple Exclusion Diets:* When a single food like milk, egg or wheat is suspected, patients are advised how to consume a diet free of these. This is not simple in practice. Exclusion of foods like milk in children, require dietary expertise to ensure that nutritional requirements are met.

(*ii*) *Multi Exclusion Diet:* If it is not clear from dietary enquiry or simple exclusion diet which foods are responsible, a complex exclusion diet has to be tried on trial and error basis.

  (*a*) Initial exclusion diets: Initially a wide range of foods which may provoke intolerance is removed from diet and after a period of time, reintroduced singly into the diet so the offending item is identified.

  (*b*) Graduated exclusion diet: The number of foods excluded from a diet is gradually increased.

  One should read the labels carefully for 'under cover' allergens. While cooking, one should avoid any cross-contact between the food allergen and foods prepared without the allergenic ingredient. It is better to avoid all processed foods which contain many additives.

Figure 23.2 is a schematic diagram showing step-wise exclusion diet.

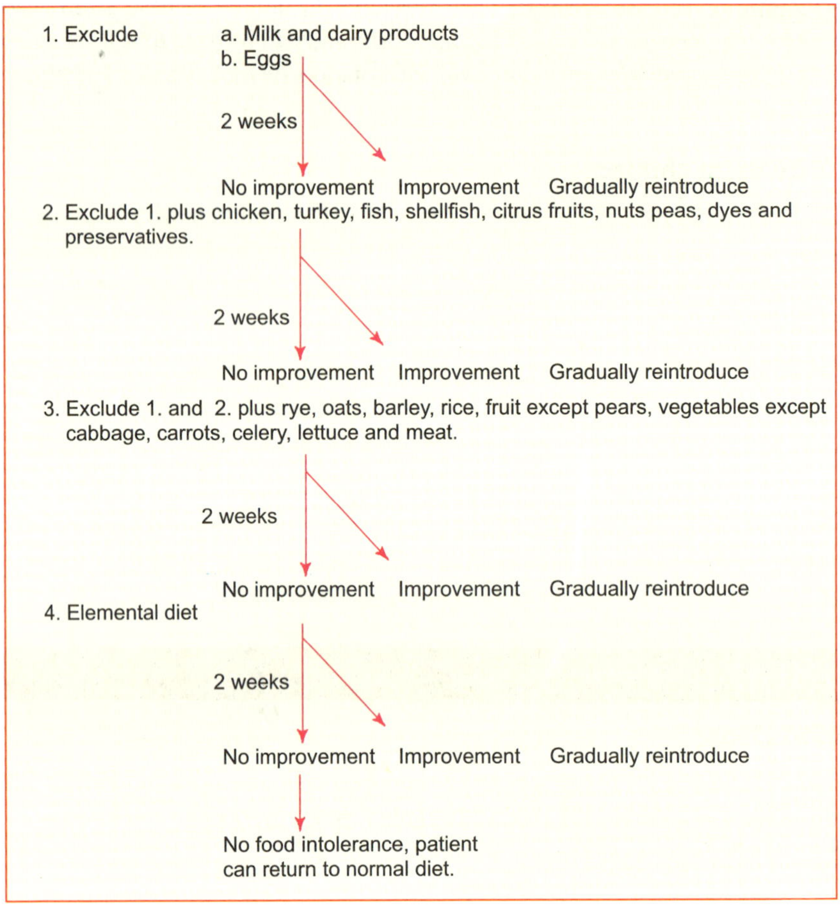

Fig. 23.2 Schematic diagram showing graduated exclusion diet

Source: Briony Thomas (The British Dietetic Association), 1988, Manual of Dietetic Practice, Blackwell Scientific Publications, Oxford, London.

Denaturation of Protein

Denaturation can help eliminate allergic activity of food, e.g., patient may be sensitive to raw milk but boiled may be suitable.

Hypersensitisation

Some physicians have been trying to help patients by giving repeatedly small doses of the allergen either by mouth or injection in the hope that their sensitivity may disappear.

Drugs

A number of drugs that mitigate the symptoms of allergy are available. Antihistamines are effective in controlling local forms of allergy like urticaria and angioedema. Although drugs causing somnolence are effective, these are likely to cause discomfort when taken regularly. Bronchodilator drugs are effective in treatment of bronchial spasms in attacks of asthma. Corticosteroids are highly effective in prevention of attacks. But they can cause adverse effects when used in long term especially in children. Sodium chromoglycate is a chemical substance in muciferous plants and is used as a herbal remedy. It acts by inhibiting the secretions of mast cells only if given before they are challenged by antigen.

Dietary Advice

Patients who are sensitive to eggs may be able to take egg yolk as egg white is the main allergen. Patient allergic to a particular food should avoid it for atleast a period of time. After six months, it can be tried but with great caution, if it is an important article in diet. The patient should be able to recognise the offending food and should inform the doctor before treatment and diagnosis.

Food allergies are often inherited and almost all are identified early in life. Infants are much more likely to have food allergies than adults and many allergies are outgrown. Milk allergy is usually outgrown by age three. The changed reactivity can be due to the decreased absorption of immunologic food proteins as the intestinal mucosa and the secretory immune system mature.

Compared with the complexity of diagnosis, the prevention is straightforward. Neither immunotherapy nor oral desensitisation has proved successful in preventing allergic reactions to food. Although many foods are easily avoided, some may be taken inadvertently in concealed form. Complications of avoidance may include growth retardation, vitamin deficiency disorders and impairment of musculature. These sequelae of long term nutritional deprivation are preventable. At all times patient should consume balanced diet avoiding the allergen.

Allergies can also be caused by inhaling pollen, cosmetics or perfumes.

Allergic reactions can adversely affect a child's nutritional status and health. The solutions may not be easy but can be found by identifying the allergen.

FOOD INTOLERANCE

Not all adverse reactions to food are food allergies. Monosodium glutamate and lactose intolerance may produce adverse reactions. As there is no antibody production they are not allergies but called food intolerances.

Food intolerance is different from food sensitivity. It is an abnormal, nonimmunologic response to an ingested food that may be pharmacological metabolic or toxic.

Pharmacologic reactions to food are the result of natural or added chemicals that produce an effect resembling that of a drug. Examples of natural constituents are alkaloids, such as those found in mushrooms; goitrogens, such as those found in cabbage; or pressor amines found in bananas. Metabolic reactions from the effect of the food on the metabolism of the recipient for example, lactase deficiency. Food toxicity is caused by toxins contained in the food or released by microorganisms that contaminate the product. Aflatoxin and pesticides are examples of contaminants.

Sixty percent of south Indians and 30–50 per cent of north Indians are lactose intolerant.

FODMAP Diet

Certain people have trouble in digesting all or some FODMAPs.

FODMAP stands for fermentable oligo, di, monosaccharides and polyols. FODMAPs are found in wide range of foods in varying amounts.

The main dietary sources of the four groups are

Oligosaccharides

– fructans in wheat, barley, legumes, garlic, onion, cauliflower.

Disaccharides

– Lactose in milk, yogurt and soft cheese.

Monosaccharides

– excess fructose in apples, figs, mangoes, pears, high fructose corn syrup, honey.

Polyols

– sorbitol, mannitol in mushrooms, cauliflower and low calorie sweeteners.

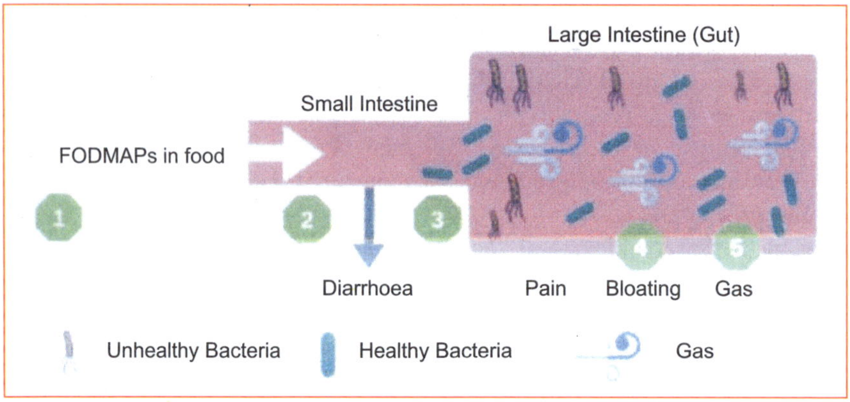

Fig. 23.3 In some individuals FODMAPs cause diarrhoea, abdominal pain, bloating and flatulance.
Source: Diet vs disease

Those saccharides and polyols are short chain carbohydrates that if poorly digested ferment in the lower part of large intestine. This fermentation process draws water and produces carbon dioxide, hydrogen and/or methane gas that causes the intestine to stretch and expand. The result is strong pain, bloating, visible abdominal distension and other related symptoms.

Table 23.2 Some effects of food intolerance

Symptoms	*Precipitating foods*
Skin disorders	
Urticaria and rashes	Almost any
Eczema	Dairy foods, fish, eggs, chocolate, citrus fruits, yeasts, nuts, food colours and preservatives, beef, chicken
Respiratory disorders	
Rhinitis and nasal polyps	Wheat, eggs, salicylates, azo-dyes, sodium benzoate,
Asthma	Milk, azo-dyes, sodium benzoate, monosodium glutamate, sulphur dioxide, sodium meta bisulphite
Nervous system	
Central nervous system	Food additives
Behavioural disturbances (hyperactivity)	Food additives
Migraine	Foods rich in vasoactive amines *e.g.* tyramine in cheese, caffeine in coffee and chocolate, yeasts, citrus fruits
Gastrointestinal disorders	
Vomiting, abdominal pain, diarrhoea	Almost any
Malabsorption	Lactose, sucrose, fructose, fat
Infantile colic	Cow's milk
Coeliac disease	Wheat, rye, oats, barley
Crohn's disease	Wheat, dairy products, yeasts, brassicas
Irritable bowel syndrome	Wheat, corn, dairy products
Inflammatory disorders	
Arthritis	Cereals, milk, cheese, fruit with skins.

A low FODMAP diet is designed to temporarily restrict the amount of FODMAPs consumed and is useful for treating conditions like IBS. A low FODMAP diet is not designed to be permanent. It is highly restrictive for several weeks, before foods are slowly reintroduced to determine the substance that causes symptoms.

FODMAPs exist mainly in dairy, legumes and many fruits and vegetables while gluten is not technically a FODMAP. Before giving up gluten one should consider whether FODMAP might be real problem. To treat troubled abdomen, a low FODMAP diet may be better especially when gluten free diet is not effective. FODMAP diet alters gut bacteria.

The signs and symptoms of food intolerance sometimes can be mistaken as food allergic reaction.

SUGGESTED READINGS

- American Academy of Allergy, Asthma and Immunology. www.aaaai.org.
- The Food Allergy and Anaphylaxis Network www.foodallergy.org.

QUESTIONS

1. Define food sensitivity and describe the two responses.
2. Explain food contaminants as allergens.
3. Write the types of allergic reactions.
4. List the common food allergens that have been identified. Describe treatment for food allergy.
5. Give symptoms of food sensitivity.
6. Explain food sensitivity in foods of animal origin.
7. Explain the diagnosis of food allergy.
8. Discuss different kinds of elimination diets used for detecting allergy.
9. What is the difference between food allergy and food intolerance?
10. If a child is sensitive to milk protein, list ten foods that he needs to avoid.
11. Explain FODMAPs diet.

24

An Overview of Diet and Mental Illness

Mental illness includes depression, anxiety and bipolar disorder, Parkinson's disease, Alzheimer's disease, migraine headaches, multiple sclerosis, epilepsy and so on. Presently they are all treated with medicines and given psychotherapy. However, treatment is not successful in many cases. Studies suggest that they may also require lifestyle modifications particularly improvement in diet quality.

Chronic, low grade inflammation characterized by an elevation in pro-inflammatory cytokines and acute phase proteins is implicated in the development *de novo* depression, schizophrenia and bipolar disorder. Studies have shown that lifestyle modification require particularly in diet. Observational studies show that healthy dietary patterns like Mediterranian diet with high PUFAs, fibre, fruits and vegetables are associated with lower levels of inflammatory markers.

In schizophrenic patients, oxidative and nitrosative stress are implicated with higher levels of oxidative stress markers observed, low levels of antioxidants such as vitamin E, vitamin C, Coenzyme Q_{10} and glutathione when compared with healthy controls. Consumption of fruits and vegetables rich in antioxidants may be beneficial.

Neurogenesis, particularly within the hippocampus is associated with learning, memory, and mood relation, while altered neurogenesis implicated in mental illness. In addition, to possessing nutrients such as ω-3-fatty acids, polyphenols, L-theanine and vitamin E can stimulate neurogenesis while energy dense diets high in fat and sugar impair this process.

The gastrointestinal microbiota has been implicated in several neurobiological pathways related to mental illness. Diet plays an important role in maintaining healthy gastrointestinal microbiota. Studies have shown that high fiber diets and Mediterranean diets, promote a diverse gut microbiota, and are associated with a reduced likelihood of depression. In addition, fermented foods may also have potential to modify the gut microbiota and to alter gut physiology and mental health. Thus, it is clear that gut health influences mental health.

Studies in adults have shown that there is inverse relationship between dietary patterns having high intake of fruit, vegetable, whole grain, fish, olive oil, fat, dairy products and increased risk of depression with high consumption of red processed meat, refined grains, sweets and high fat dairy products have been observed. Diet is likely related to mental health at all stages of life.

Gene-Diet interactions in Brain ageing and neurodegenerative disorders

Dietary factors may interact with disease-causing or predisposing genes in molecular cascades that either promote or prevent the degeneration of neurons. Epidemilogic findings suggest that high-calorie diets and folic acid deficiency increase the risk for Alzheimer's disease and Parkinson's disease.

Studies of animal models of these disorders have shown that dietary restriction (reduced calorie intake or intermittent fasting) and dietary supplementation with folic acid can reduce neuronal damage and improve behavirouʼal outcome. By keeping homocysteine levels low, folic acid can protect cerebral vessels and prevent the accumulation of DNA damage in neurons caused by oxidative stress.

The emerging data suggest that high calorie diets and elevated homocysteine levels may render the brain vulnerable to age-related neurodegenerative disorders, particularly in persons with a genetic predisposition to such disorders.

Alzheimer's disease involves the progressive degeneration and death of neurons in brain regions such as the hippocampus and basal forebrain, that are involved in learning, memory and emotional behaviours. Parkinson's disease involves the progressive degeneration of neurons in the substantia nigra, resulting in the patient's inability to control body movements.

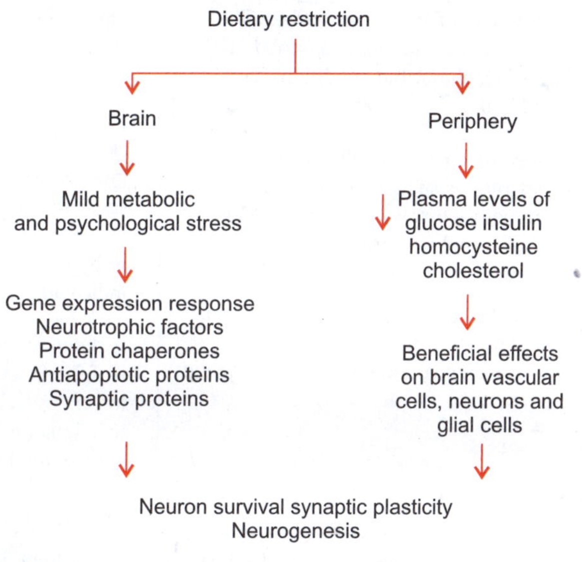

Fig. 24.1 Working model for the mechanism by which dietary restriction can increase brain health

Source: Mark P. Mattson, Gene-diet interactions in brain ageing and neurodegenerative disorders, Ann Intern Med., 2003; **139**.

Nutritional deficiencies

Deficiencies in vitamins can affect mental health. B_{12} deficiency causes mania, psychosis, poor memory, lethargy and fatigue. Thiamine deficiency leads beri beri, CNS symptoms and Wermicke's encephalopathy. Folic acid deficiency results in detrimental effects on neurodevelopment *in utero* and in infancy; greater risk of depression during adulthood.

These findings highlight the important role of a balanced diet in providing an adequate nutrient supply to support brain development for later cognitive function and the relevance of early life development in the vulnerability for (later) psychiatric disease, which may explain, at least in part, the observed heterogeneity in treatment.

Nutritional psychiatry is a rapidly growing field of research that has the potential to provide clinically meaningful interventions to both prevent and manage mental illness. Observational research has demonstrated a consistent relationship between diet quality and common mental illness, while biological pathways including inflammation, oxidative stress, gastrointestinal microbiota and neurotrophic factors provide viable mechanisms of action for this observed effect. Preliminary clinical evidence provides support for the feasibility and efficacy of dietary and some nutraceutical interventions.

DIET IN PARKINSON'S DISEASE

Parkinson's disease is a chronic progressive age related neurodegenerative disorder. The disease is characterised by bradykinesia, rest tremor, muscle stiffness, shuffling gait and flexed posture.

Table 24.1 Role of Dietary Macronutrients in Parkinson's Disease (PD)

Macronutrient	*Status*	*Dietary of Other Adjustments*
Fat	Animal fat, including diary, appears to increase risk of PD. High intakes of arachidonic acid are to be avoided. Otherwise, comoribid conditions should be considered.	Substitution of polyunsaturated fat, especially long-chain ω-3 fat, appears prudent.
Carbohydrates	No specific data are available. Theoretical considerations suggest minimizing inflammatory cytokine formation and metabolic consequences that may result from excessive simple sugar intake.	Maintain usual dietary range of carbohydrate with modifications: low glycemic index, reduced simple sugar intake, as little trans fat as possible through dietary means or by other appropriate agents as indicated.
Protein	Protein meals close to the time of levodopa ingestion reduce the therapeutic response.	Although partially effective, timing is difficult and frequently lowers overall protein intake. Taking levodopa on an empty stomach may suffice. Inadequate protein consumption may promote sarcopenia and loss of bone mass.

Source: Kones Richard Parkinson's disease; Mitochondrial Molecular pathology, inflammation stakins and the therapeutic neuroprotective nutrition, Nutrition in clinical practice, 2010; 25.

Inflammation, oxidative and nitrosative stress, accumulation of abnormal proteins and defects in the ubiquitin proteasome system are central events in the pathogenesis of Parkinson's disease. The CoQ10, creatine, ω-3-fatty acids may be beneficial in this condition.

DIET IN ALZHERIMER'S DISEASE

Alzhemier's disease is a degenerative brain disorder that manifests as a progressive deterioration of memory and mental function. The most common form of dementia - Alzheimer's disease imparis memory, thought and speech. The disease's final stage renders an affected individual totally helpless and unable to control bodily functions.

The disease is characterized by the formation of neurofibrillary tangles and amyloid plaques in the brain. These tangles and plaques are composed of various protein deposits and cellular debris. The result is the shrinkage and loss of nerve cells, including ones that produce neurotransmitters. As the nerve cells continue to die, the brain itself shrinks and the wrinkles along its surface start to smoothen.

Alzheimer's disease is the most common type of dementia and accounts for 60–80 per cent of dementia cases. Vasular dementia is the second most common and usually is the result of a stroke Dementia can have negative impact on self feeding abilities, swallow function and appetite.

Physiological changes associated with ageing in general such decreased thirst and hunger perception complicate nutrition, and hydration status in dementia patients.

The most notable approaches for Alzherimer's disease are the Mediterranean diet, MeDi Mediterranean, DASH Dietary Approaches to Stop Hypertension, intervention for neurodegenerative delay diet or more commonly the Mind diet which combines DASH and MeDi have been shown to improve cognition.

Table 24.2 DASH, Mediterranean, and MIND diets

	Encouraged components	*Limited components*	*Additional components*
DASH diet	– High in vegetables, fruits, fat-free and low-fat dairy products, whole grains, poultry, fish, and nuts	– Limit sodium to 1500–2300 mg/day – Limit saturated fat, *trans fat* – Limit sweets, sugar-sweetened beverages, and red meats	Maintain a healthy body weight or lose weight
Mediterranean diet	– High intake of olive oil, fruits, vegetables, whole grains, and cereals, legumes, fish, and nuts – Primary protein sources are seafood, legumes, and nuts – Moderate intake of red wine	– Limit intake of red meat, dairy products, and sweets	– Increase physical activity – Consume meals with family and friends
MIND diet	– Encourage green leafy vegetable (6 servings/week) – Other vegetables (1 serving/day) – Nuts (5 servings/week) – Berries (2 servings/week) – Beans (3 servings/week) – Whole grain (3 servings/day) – Fish (1 serving/week) – Poultry (2 servings/week) – Olive oil – Wine (1 glass/day)	– Limit red meats, butter and stick margarine, cheese, pastries and sweets, fried or fast foods	

Source: Ramirez-Salazar A. Sergio et al, Dietary insights in neurological diseases Current neurology and Neuroscience reports, 2021; 21.

The role that certain dietary supplements may play in preventing and managing the disorder is under experimentation.

Ginko Biloba and Hypnzine A which is an extract from moss and turmeric have been tried in the prevention of Alzheimer's disease.

Fatty acids, especially DHA, docosahexaenoic acid, may have a profound impact on the prevention and treatment of Alzheimer's disease. Because DHA supplementation is considered relatively safe, many patients with Alzheimer's disease or those at risk for Alzheimer's disease may decide to supplement with DHA. Those who decide to take a DHA, ω-3 fatty acid supplement should choose a reputable company whose products are free of heavy metals (e.g., mercury, lead, cadmium). In addition consumption of antioxidants and non steroidal anti-inflammatory drugs are associated with reduced risk for Alzeimer's disease.

In many pschiatric disorders particularly schizophrenia and MDD, major depressive disorders, have shown positive results when supplementation is given as adjunct to standard pharmacotherapy. Supplementation of ω-3-fatty acids have no deleterious side effects.

Healthy dietary interventions are crucial to decrease the progression and reduce disability in many neurological conditions, including multiple sclerosis, neurodegenerative diseases, stroke, and migraines. The dietary patterns shoule be plant based, limit meat intake, low fat, high fibre and rich in antioxidants. However, a healthy diet is a part of a continuum of an adequate lifestyle, including exercise, adequate sleep patterns, and appropriate stress management. The ketogenic diet is an essential component for the management of refractory epilepsy; its main limitation is adherence.

In general, nutrients and their metabolites act upon multiple targets in multiple organs. While many studies have examined the effects of individual nutritional components or foods on brain and behaviour, nutritional research is shifting from a focus on single nutrients or supplements to dietary pattern analysis. This is important because nutrients may act together to affect specific functions and interactions between specific nutrients may affect their bioavailability thus complicating the identification of specific substrates.

SUGGESTED READINGS

- Adau A.H. Roger *et al.* Nutritional psychiatry. Towards improving mental health by what you eat. European Neuropsychopharmacology 2019; **29**.
- Lee Song *et al.* Current Clinical applications of ω-6 and ω-3 fatty acids. Nutrition in clinical practice 2006; **21**.
- Joseph A James Grape juice, berries and walnuts affect brain aging and behaviour J Nutr 2009; **139**.

QUESTIONS

1. Explain diseases related to mental illness and diet.
2. Define Alzheimer's disease. Explain dietary modifications required in this condition.
3. Discuss diet in Parkinson's disease.
4. Explain nutritional deficiencies that cause mental illness.

25

Some Special Diets

PURINE-RESTRICTED DIET

This diet is suggested to patients with hyperuricemia, gouty arthritis or urinary uric acid lithiasis.

Purine occurs primarily in foods of animal origin with the exception of dairy products and eggs. Foods that contain 150 mg or more purines per 100g serving should be avoided.

Modification of diet

- Protein intake should be normal- 10–15 percent total calories or 0.8 g per kg. body weight for well nourished individuals.
- Patients who are poorly nourished or in the inflammatory phase of the disease should consume 1.5–2.0 g/kg. body weight.
- Carbohydrate intake should be normal.
- Fat intake should also be normal.
- Cholesterol intake should be less than 300 mg/day.
- Healthy body weight is maintained. If weight loss is indicated, it should be gradual. Rapid weight loss through fasting or use of low carbohydrate diets can cause the body to produce ketones which may increase hyperuricemia.
- Alcohol, especially beer should be avoided. Along with providing a source of purines, alcohol inhibits renal excretion of purines.
- Adequate fluid intake helps dilute urinary uric acid, which helps prevent formation of renal calculi. It is advised to drink 2–3*l* of fluid daily.

Hyperuricemia is caused by an overproduction or underexcretion of uric acid. The state of hyperuricemia is present in many people with gout. Hyperuricemia also increases the risk of developing urolithiasis.

Eating a high purine diet, regular alcohol consumption, obesity and hypertriglyceridemnia play a role in increased urate production. Other aspects of nutrition therapy such as controlling diabetes mellitus, hypertension and alterosclerosis are also recommended. Lifestyle changes along with medication are often needed to control hyperuricemia.

Although dietary purines contribute only 1.0 mg/dl to the serum urate concentration a diet moderate in purines is still recommended. Diet is generally considered an adjunct therapy to medication but may be used as an alternative treatment if medications are not tolerated.

In patients with gout weight reduction and abstinence from alcohol reverse hypertriglyceridemia, hyperuricemia urate over production and urate underexcretion. Obesity is associated with gout and may contribute to the onset of the disease. There is strong positive correlation between body weight and serum urate concentration. Weight loss should be gradual to prevent ketone production which inhibits uric acid excretion.

Uric acid nephrolithiasis occurs as a result of long-standing hyperuricemia and is seen 10–25 per cent of patients with gout. It is most common in those who excrete more than 700 mg uric acid per day.

Precipitation of the uric acid crystals in the urine is further encouraged by the acid urine formed by these patients. A high intake of protein increases the urinary excretion of calcium, oxalate and uric acid and reduces urinary pH and citrate. These changes markedly increase the risk of forming uric and/or calcium oxalate stones. Treatment is moderate intake of protein and an increase in the volume and alkalinity of the urine.

Food group	*Foods allowed*	*Foods restricted*
Beverages	Low fat milk, carbonated beverages, cocoa, coffee, tea	Alcohol
Breads	All refined breads and cereals	Whole grain breads and cereals oat meal, wheat germ and wheat bran.
Fats	All fats and oils	Meat gravies
Fruits	All fruits	–
Meat and Related foods	Low fat cheese, eggs	Fish, lamb, beef, pork, poultry, shellfish, dried beans and peas nuts, peanut butter
Vegetables	All	Mushrooms, green peas, spinach, cauli-flower
Miscellaneous	Iodized salt, herbs, spices	Baker's and brewer's yeast

Source: American Dietetic Association

KETOGENIC DIET

Ketogenic diet therapy is an established form of treatment for both paediatric and adult patients with intractable epilepsy. Ketogenic diet is a term that refers to any diet therapy in which dietary composition would result in ketogenic state of human metabolism.

Epilepsy has been defined as having two or more unprovoked seizures at least 24 hours apart.

The mechanism by which ketogenic diet impacts seizure control are not completely understood. Hypotheses are alterations in energy metabolism, including a decrease in glucose concentration with an increase in fatty acid oxidation and ketone production and alterations in neurotransmitter production, release and uptake.

The goal of the ketogenic diet is to reduce or eliminate seizures. The primary component of the diet is fat. At a 4:1 ratio, fat comprises approximately 90 percent of the child's total calorie intake. Protein is limited to 100 percent of RDA. Carbohydrate is severely restricted and excessive fluid intake is avoided.

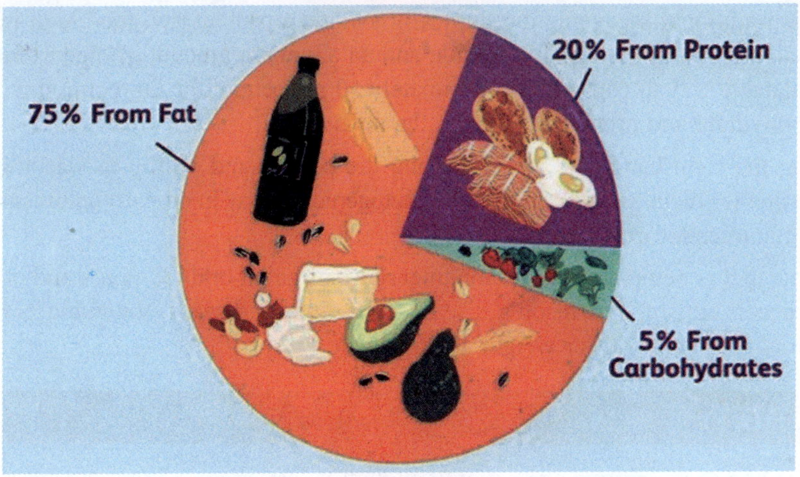

Fig. 25.1 Calorie distribution on a ketogenic diet

The purpose of the diet is to produce an acidosis by curtailing very severely the amount of available glucose and increasing markedly the intake of fat so that complete combustion of fats cannot take place.

Mechanism: In the absence of significant carbohydrate, mitochondrial β-oxygenation of fat in the liver generates large quantities of the ketone bodies acetoacetate and β-hydroxybutyrate, which unlike fatty acids, the brain can readily use as an energy source. Ketone bodies may also contribute to certain cerebral metabolic pathways, including those of the neurotransmitters glutamate and gamma-amino butyric acid GABA and increase brain adenosine triphosphate ATP concentration, cerebral energy reserves and GABA receptor sites, all of which are thought to contribute to the diet's inhibitory effect on seizures.

Nutritional side effects include stunted growth, hypoproteinemia and micronutrient deficiencies; these effects can be prevented or corrected, by providing adequate protein and calories and by supplementing the diet with vitamins and minerals.

Ketogenic diet lasts for a minimum period of two years. Eventually most children can gradually return to a normal diet with lasting seizure control.

The child is admitted to the hospital for 3–5 days to initiate the ketogenic diet. If needed a dextrose-free saline-based intravenous drip can be initiated without adverse effects on ketone levels. The initiation of the ketogenic diet can be tailored to the child. The child can be discharged once education of the caregiver has been completed, the child has tolerated solid food, blood glucose levels are stable and the child has urine ketone between 80 and 160 mg/dl.

After 1 to 2 years the child is weaned from ketogenic diet. During weaning the diet ratio is gradually reduced thereby reducing the amount of fat and increasing the amount of carbohydrate. If seizures return after weaning the diet may be restarted.

Ketogenic diet can be divided into 3 or 4 meals. Each meal must contain the correct ketogenic ratio of fat to protein and carbohydrate. Small, frequent meals throughout the day may be more appealing to children with appetite problems.

Meals on traditional ketogenic diet typically include a protein rich food high in biological value a small amount of fruit and vegetable and an abundant amount of dietary fat. Whipped cream is palatable way to consume approximately 50 per cent of the fat required without using all the carbohydrate and protein allowed in the meal.

Choosing the right candidate and involving the patient and family in selecting the most appropriate diet is crucial when implementing ketogenic therapy in order to optimise compliance and prevent unintended complications.

Ketogenic diet is being tried in the treatment of malignant brain tumours and other various forms of cancer, autism, Parkinson's disease, Alzheimer's disease, traumatic brain injuries, mitochondrial disorders and for weight management.

PALEO DIET

Paleo diet is one in which one can eat any amount of lean meat, poultry, seafood, fresh fruit and vegetables. Foods that are not part of the modern day Paleolithic diet include cereal grains, dairy products, high glycaemic fruits and vegetables, legumes, alcohol, salty foods, fatty meats, refined sugars and processed foods.

Some believe paleo diet is suitable as ergogenic diet for athletes.

There are basic reasons the paleo diet enhances athletic performance.

1. **Branched-chain amino acids:** This diet is high in animal protein which is the richest source of the branched chain amino acids—valine, leucine and isolecuine. BCAAS are potent stimulants for building and repairing muscle. These amino acids work best when consumed immediately after exercise. By consuming high amounts of lean protein and hence BCAA athletes can rapidly reverse the natural break down of muscle that occurs following a work out and thereby reduce recovery time and train at a greater intensity at the next session.
2. **Blood acidity versus alkalinity:** In addition to stimulating muscle growth via BCAA, the Paleo diet for athletes simultaneously prevents muscle protein break down because it produces a net metabolic alkalosis.

   All foods upon digestion produces net acid or alkali.

   A diet having grains, cheeses and salty processed foods produce acid. The athlete's body is even more prone to blood acidosis due to the by products of exercise. One way the body neutralises a net acid-producing diet is by breaking down muscle tissue. Paleo diet is rich in fruits and vegetables it reverses the metabolic acidosis produced by typical grain and starch laden diet for athletes, thereby preventing muscle loss.
3. **Trace elements:** Fruits and vegetables are also rich sources of antioxidant vitamins, minerals and phytochemicals.

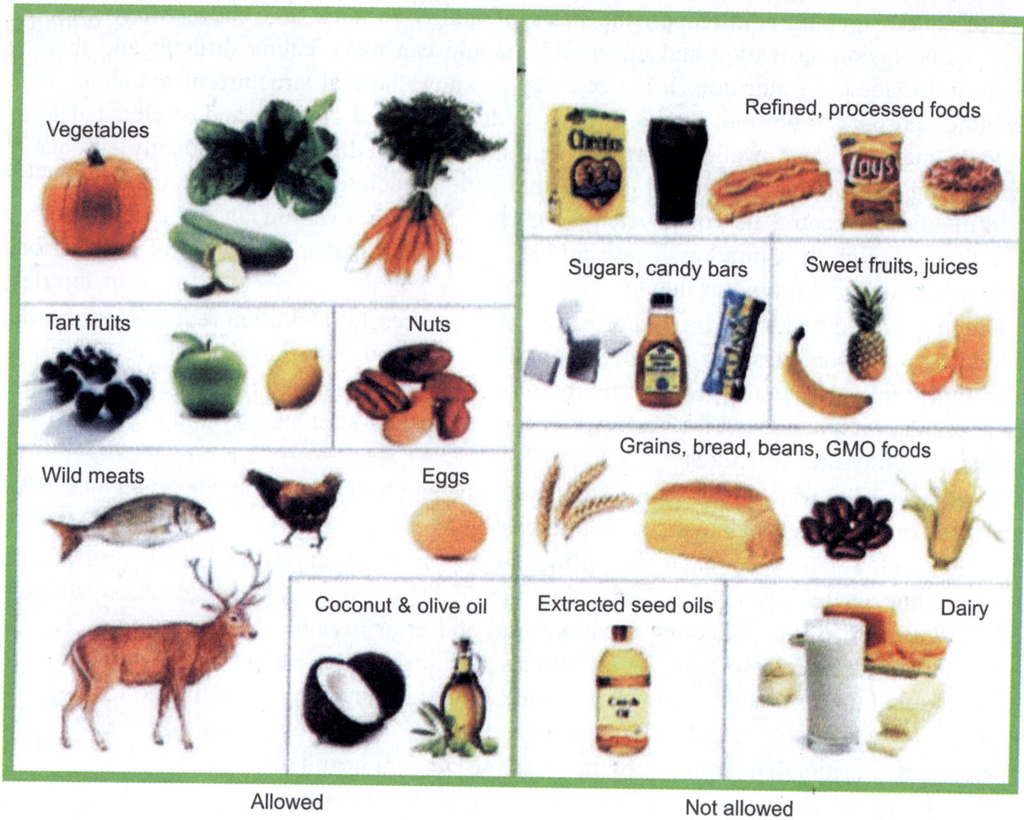

Fig. 25.2 Foods allowed and not allowed in paleo diet.

Paleo diet is low carbohydrate and high protein diet. It is also high in fibre, high in minerals and vitamins. It lacks in dairy foods hence poor in calcium and vitamin D. This diet causes stress on kidneys and not practical to use long term. Some find this diet also promotes weight loss.

Paleo diet is stone age diet of ancient ancestors. Microbiome – a billions of organisms that reside in the guts is vastly different now than paleo times and is not suitable now.

DIET IN CLEFT LIP AND /OR PALATE

The diet for a child with cleft lip and/or palate should be adequate for all nutrients based on the RDA. Oral supplements can be used to meet energy and nutrient needs if necessary.

A cleft is diagnosed in the neonate and may be a unilateral or bilateral cleft of the lip without palate involvement or it may be a unilateral or bilateral cleft of the soft and/or hard palate with or without a cleft lip defect or a submucous cleft palate. A submucous cleft involves the muscles of the soft palate and part of the hard palate. Feeding is usually not a major problem although an infant with milk coming through the nose may indicate a submucous cleft palate and therefore should be evaluated appropriately.

Children with a cleft lip and/or palate also have other associated medical conditions such as chronic otitis, hearing loss and dental and orthodontic problems.

The child's diet be adjusted on the basis of ability to suck and chew. Many children have malocclusion, crowding and bite problems and can make eating difficult and thereby compromise adequate nutrition. It is necessary to know the oral structure of the child when planning appropriate nutrient intake. Infants with an isolated cleft lip and/or cleft palate as the only medical issue swallow normally but suck abnormally. More frequently associated swallowing difficulties are found in infants with associated pharyngeal or esophageal abnormalities or central nervous system problems. Signs of swallowing difficulties include coughing, gagging or aspiration. These infants require nasogastric feeds and/or gastrostomy feeds with extensive oromotor therapy.

Feeding a child with cleft lip and/or palate may be stressful and often requires extra time, individualized techniques and patience. In addition to promoting growth and development, good nutrition is essential to enable the infant to build up resistance to infection, to acquire the necessary weight needed for surgery, to promote healing after surgery and to develop and maintain healthy oral structures.

Modifications of usual breast feeding and bottle feeding techniques help the infant to achieve goals. Infants with cleft palate are seldom breast fed.

Infants with a cleft palate find it more difficult to create a suction and are usually unsuccessful in maintaining a latch-on. Special attention should be given to achieve adequate latch-on. Infants with cleft of the palate require more trial and error in bottle feeding to be successful than infant, with a cleft lip only. As with breast feeding, bottle feeding should be limited to 30 mn to minimize excessive energy expenditure. Bottle feeding may be facilitated with special bottles.

Adequate nutrition is monitored by maintaining optimal health.

Cleft lip repair is often performed before the infant is old enough to begin solids. The lip repair allows the child to eat more easily from a spoon without food losses through the cleft.

After repair of the cleft, less food modification is necessary.

DIET FOR CHILDREN WITH AUTISM SPECTRUM DISORDERS

Feeding problems are common in children with autism spectrum disorder. Family meal time as stressful, chaotic and energy depleting. Food selectivity (eating a narrow variety of foods or rejecting one or more food groups) is the most widely documented feeding problems in ASD. Common dietary patterns in children with ASD include strong preference for processed foods, snacks and starches coinciding with a bias against fruits and vegetables.

Problematic meal time behaviour may occur when the child refuses to eat foods based on the secondary characteristics e.g. texture, taste or smell. Demands high intake of single food item e.g. eating the same food multiple times per day, insists on eating in a specific location or require certain utensils. There rigid meal requirements are often accompanied by crying, throwing objects and aggression toward caregivers when presented with just the sight or smell of non-preferred foods.

LOW CARBOHYDRATE HIGH FAT DIETS

Three tire definition of low carbohydrate diet

- Moderate carbohydrate diet (26-45% of daily kcal).
- LCHF diet (< 26% of total energy intake or < 130 g CHO /day).
- Very LCHF (ketogenic) diet (20-50g CHO/day or < 10% of daily kcal of 2000 kcal/day diet)

Ketosis occurs in people who restrict their carbohydrate intake below 20-50 g/day with some degree of protein restriction.

Since the carbohydrate content of the diet is significantly reduced, the relative proportion of energy derived from protein and fat will increase.

LCHF diets typically produce a reduction in hunger, with the result that the individual's total calorie consumption will usually decrease on the LCHF diet sometimes significantly. Therefore, even though the relative contribution of fat to dietary energy intake may increase the absolute fat intake may not. As a result, the term high fat diet may be misleading. Hence, the term low carbohydrates healthy fat is probably more appropriate.

Atkins, Banting, Paleo and South Beach diets are LCHF diets. All these diets focus on eating unprocessed food consisting primarily of cruciferous and green leafy vegetables, raw nuts and seeds eggs, fish, unprocessed meats, dairy products and natural plant oils and fats from avocado, coconuts and olives.

Banting diet

Banting diet–Foods recommended

Animal Protein	*Dairy*	*Fats*	*Nuts and seeds*	*Vegetables*
Eggs Meats Poultry Game Sea food	Cottage cheese Cream Full cream Greek Yogurt Cheese	Olive oil Avocado oil Coconut oil Macadamia Nut oil	Almonds Flax seeds Macadamia nuts Pecans Pine Nuts	All green leafy Vegetables Cruciferous Vegetables or above Ground Vegetables

Diabetic ketoacidosis is life-threatening and nutritional ketosis is a normal physiological response to dietary carbohydrate restriction, in which the body alters its primary fuel utilisation from carbohydrates to fat. This change spares blood glucose for use particularly by the brain which has an obligatory glucose requirement of about 25 g/day when using alternate fuels including ketones or lactate in fat-adapted persons.

In adults consuming a 'normal' diet blood ketone body concentrations vary between 0.1 and 0.3 m mol/L. In nutritional ketosis, the levels way rise to over 1 m mol/L and maximally upto 7-8 m mol/L, but without an acidosis. In contrast, the diabetic ketoacidosis, blood ketone body concentration usually exceed 25 mmol/L and blood pH decreases below.

Nutritional and ketosin is safe but also beneficial to many patients. Nutritional ketosis is beneficial in the management of cancer, acne, polycystic ovarian syndrome and neurological diseases including Alzheimer's disease. It increases athletic performance.

In any diet, optimal nutrition should emphasise high nutrient density while properly managing energy balance. LCHF controls energy balance through increased satiety and reduced *adlibitum* energy intake whole encouraging the ingestion of a nutrient-dense diet by replacing refined, nutrient-poor processed foods with nutrient-dense, natural foods.

The diet encourages weight loss and unique metabolic changes including marked improvements in glycaemic control and plasma triglyceride HDL-C, ApoB and saturated fat concentrations with reductions in the number of small dense LDL particles.

The unique effect is in part due to the reversal of (NAFLD) Nonalcoholic Fatty Liver Disease by carbohydrate restriction.

LCHF diets are proven to be a safe and efficacious strategy for weight loss and improved health outcomes for many patients, specially for those with insulin resistance, the metabolic syndrome, Alzheimer's disease and NAFLD.

Effects of LCHF diet

Low-carbohydrate high-fat (LCHF) diets are at least as effective as other dietary strategies for reducing body weight, with the additional advantage of increased satiety and spontaneous reduction in energy intake.

LCHF diets are an effective dietary strategy to improve glycaemic control and reduce hyperinsulinaemia in type 2 diabetes mellitus and in otherwise healthy patients with insulin resistance.

LCHF diets have unique effects on blood lipid concentrations and cardiovascular risk factors, characterised by decreased blood TG, ApoB and saturated fat concentrations, reduced small LDL particle numbers and increased HDL-C concentrations. The effect on LDL-C concentrations is variable.

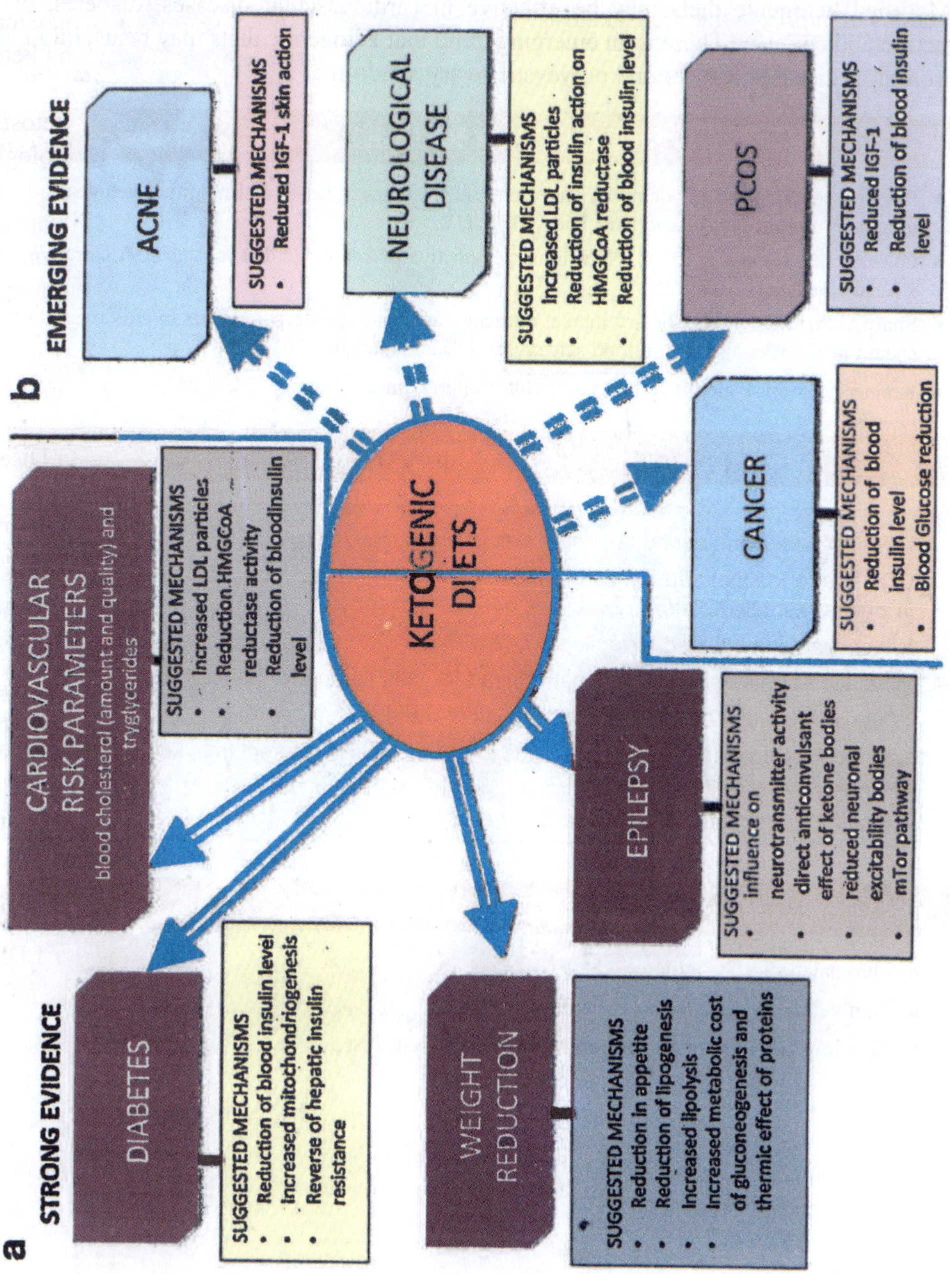

Fig. 25.3 **Effect of ketogenic diets in different conditions.**

Source: Noakes David Timothy and Johnn Windt, Evidence that supports the prescription of low-carbohydrate high-fat diets: a narative review, B.J Sports. Medicine 2016; 51.

Modified ketogenic diets may be effective in cardiovascular diseases, diabetes, weight reduction and epilepsy. There is an emerging trend that ketogemic diets may be useful in acne, neurological diseases, cancer and polycystic ovary syndrome.

SUGGESTED REFERENCES

- Practice paper of the Academy of Nutrition and Dietetics: Classic and modified ketogenic diets for treatment of epilepsy. J Acad Nutr Diet. 2017; **117.**
- Oliveira L.P. Camila *et al.*, A. Nutritional perspective of ketogenic diet in cancer: A narrative review J Acad Nutr Diet. 2018: **118**.
- Sharp G. William et al., Dietary intake, nutrient status and growth parameters in children with antism spectrum disorder and severe food selectivity. J Acad Nutr Diet. 2018; **118**.
- Konner Meltion, P aleolithic Nutrition, Nutrition in Clinical Practice, 2010; **25**.

QUESTIONS

1. In which conditions purine restricted diet is suggested? Why?
2. Give five foods that can be taken in foods allowed and five foods that should be avoided in purine restricted diets.
3. Which diet is suggested for epilepsy? Why?
4. What kind of dietary modifications required for cleft lip and for palate?
5. What is Paleo diet? Explain the limitations of the diet.
6. Low carbohydrate and high fat diet leads to ketoris. This is different from ketoris complication of diabetes. Explain.
7. Explain the problems in feeding autistic children.

TOPICS FOR ACTIVITY

- Plan paleo diet for athletes.
- Plan ketogenic diet for an epileptic patient.
- Plan low carbohydrate and high fat diet for weight loss.

26

The Dietitian

A dietitian is defined as a professional who applies the science of food and nutrition to promote health, prevent and treat disease and to optimise the health of individuals, groups, communities and populations.

CLASSIFICATION

International Labour office in Geneva, Switzerland, classified dietitians as Professional Medical Workers. In 1969, they were further classified by the labour office as follows:

Dietitian (General)

One who plans and supervises the preparation of therapeutic or other diets for individuals or groups in hospitals, institutions, other establishments and for workers in particular sectors, gives instructions in selection and proper preparation of food according to dietetic principles, performs duties related to nutrition programmes and may be responsible for food purchasing on behalf of an organization or establishment.

Public Health Nutritionist

One who appraises various factors related to nutrition and food problems in the community, plans and executes nutrition elements of health programmes; participates in programmes of nutrition activities for particular groups or the community.

Other Dietitians

Not elsewhere classified e.g., those acting as consultants to food processing and distributing firms or manufacturers of food processing equipment.

A modified definition given below has been suggested at the International Congress held in July, 1988 in Paris.

A dietitian is a person with legally recognized qualification in nutrition and/or dietetics who applies the science of nutrition to the feeding and education of groups of people and individuals in health and disease.

According to American Dietetic Associations Dietetics is the integration and application of principles derived from the science of nutrition, biochemistry, physiology, food management and behavioral and social sciences to achieve and maintain people's health.

ETHICS AND RESPONSIBILITIES

Dietetic practitioners have voluntarily developed a code of ethics to reflect the ethical principles guiding the dietetic profession and to outline commitments and obligations of the dietetic practitioner to self, client, society and the profession.

Ethical principles suggested by American Dietetic Association (2009) are given below:

Fundamental Principles

- The dietetics practitioner conducts himself/herself with honesty, integrity and fairness.
- The dietetics practitioner supports and promotes high standards of professional practice.

Responsibilities to the Public

- The dietetics practitioner considers the health, safety and welfare of the public at all times.
- The dietetics practitioner complies with all laws and regulations applicable or related to the profession.
- The dietetics practitioner provides professional services with objectivity and with respect for the unique needs and values of individuals.
- The dietetics practitioner does not engage in false or misleading practices or communication.
- The dietetics practitioner withdraws from professional practice when unable to fulfill his or her professional duties and responsibilities to clients and others.

Responsibilities to Clients

- The dietetics practitioner recognizes and exercises professional judgment within the limits of his or her qualifications and collaborates others, seeks counsel or makes referrals as appropriate.
- The dietetics practitioner treats clients and patients with respect and consideration.
- The dietetics practitioner protects confidential information and makes full disclosure about any limitations on his or her ability to guarantee full confidentiality.

Responsibilities to the Profession

- The dietetics practitioner practices dietetics based on evidence-based principles and current information.
- The dietetics practitioner presents reliable and substantiated information and interprets controversial information without personal bias, recognizing that legitimate differences of opinion exist.
- The dietetics practitioner assumes a life long responsibility and accountability for personal competence in practice consistent with accepted professional standards, continually striving to increase professional knowledge and skills and to apply them in practice.

- The dietetics practitioner is alert to the occurrence of a real or potential conflict of interest and takes appropriate action whenever a conflict arises.
- The dietetics practitioner permits the use of his or her name for the purpose of certifying that dietetics services have been rendered only if he or she has provided or supervised the provision of those services.
- The dietetics practitioner accurately presents professional qualifications and credentials.
- The dietetics practitioner does not invite, accept or offer gifts, monetary incentives or other considerations that affect or reasonably give an appearance of affecting his/her professional judgement.

Responsibilities to Colleagues and other Professionals

- The dietetics practitioner demonstrates respect for the values, rights, knowledge and skills of colleagues and other professionals.

DUTIES OF A DIETITIAN

NUTRITIONAL ASSESSMENT

Assessment of nutrition is done by the dietitian and may be required after any change in condition such as surgery or oral food and liquid intake status. Mini nutritional assessment or subjective global assessment (given in appendix) scoring can be done on admission of the patient.

To determine the nutritional inadequacy malnutrition screening tool is used.

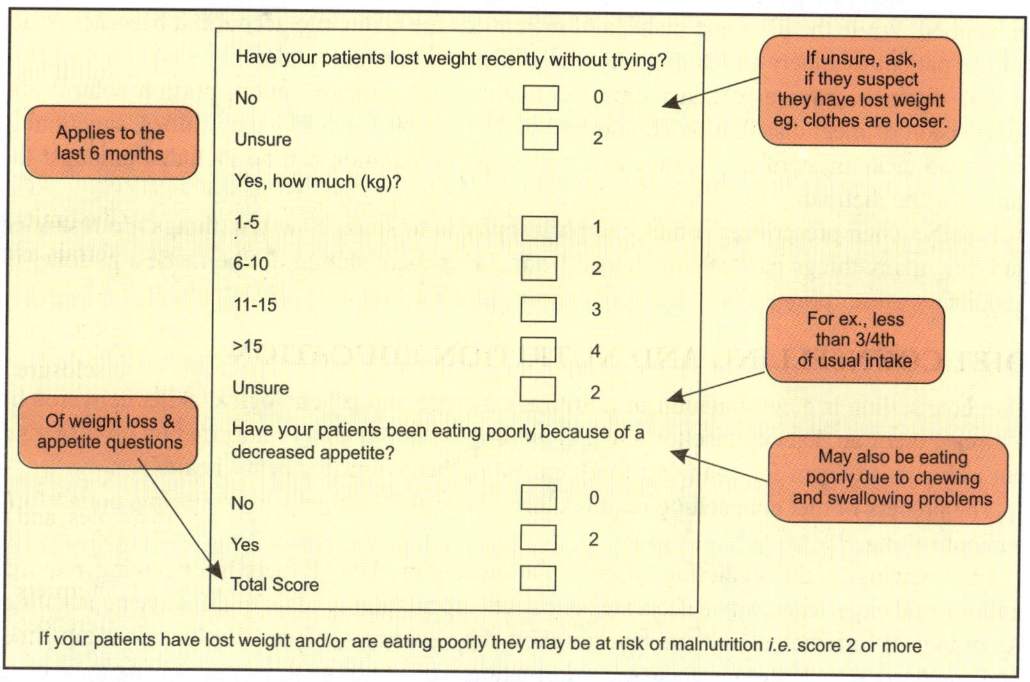

Fig. 26.1 Malnutrition screening tool

Source: Ferguson et al Nutrition 1999; 15.

To formulate the most appropriate nutritional therapy for each patient, individual requirements must be considered with initial metabolic, bio-chemical and anthropometric data obtained by nutritional assessment of the patient.

Mini nutritional assessment and subjective global assessment scoring and alternate measurements used for non-ambulatory patients are given in appendix.

DIET PLANNING

Since the dietary habits vary widely in Indian population, prescribing appropriate diet for an individual patient for a particular disease becomes challenging. The dietary prescriptions are made on the basis of the patient's age, sex, activity, body weight, and the type of treatment he is undergoing. Income, education level, ethnicity and marital status should also be considered for diet prescription.

A daily record of the intake of calories and other nutrients is very important. The convenient way is to administer a detailed questionnaire regarding the type of food item and the quantities consumed, throughout the day, in terms of cooked volumes. That is converted to raw ingredients and nutritive value is calculated using the standard food tables. Diet prescription should meet all the nutrient requirements of the patient. Further it is recommended to prescribe the therapeutic diet in terms of raw uncooked foods since the caloric and other nutrient values of the prepared foods differ in different households. However, it is very difficult for the patient to adhere to his diet prescription strictly in terms of raw ingredients, when food is cooked in bulk for the whole family. Therefore, counselling in terms of raw ingredients may not be feasible. Advice should be given in terms of cooked foods and volumetric measures in order to achieve better compliance.

To introduce variety and flexibility in diet prescriptions, provisions of exchange lists proves to be good. While the likes and dislikes of the patient are taken into account, it becomes easier for the patient to adhere to his recommended food and nutrient intake.

The dietitians have a role in recipe formulation and standardisation, portion control and supervision of meal distribution should be within their purview. Planning duties, sanctioning leave and cleanliness of staff concerned with meal preparation can be included amongst the duties of the dietitian.

Finally, when prescribing a diet, the philosophy is to stress how few things are restricted and how many things patient can choose from. The patient should not be made a prisoner of his dietary prescription.

DIET COUNSELLING AND NUTRITION EDUCATION

Diet counselling is a combination of nutrition expertise and psychological skills delivered by a trained dietitian. Diet counsellor's role is no longer seen as a mere information on dispenser but rather as an agent for changing food and eating behaviour for better health.

The process of diet counselling requires three basic skills namely, interviewing, counselling and consulting.

Interviewing is the gathering of information and/or data. Expert interviewing requires training and experience, since accurate, selective information is basic to effective counselling. A competent interviewer will be able to elicit the necessary information in minimum time. The emphasis is on gathering focussed information. The major goal in interviewing must be to participate with the person in such a way as to provide maximum help in resolving mutually recognized problems.

Counselling is listening, accepting, clarifying and helping the client to form his/her own conclusions, identify problems and develop his/her own plan of action. The focus is on the client. An effective diet counsellor must be able to guide the client's thinking, focus on objectives and interpret and evaluate information accurately and effectively.

Consulting involves developing plans or proposals for and with the client based on observations and evaluations, adding and enhancing knowledge and understanding of the individual seeking help.

The next millennium requires dietitians who will focus on disease prevention in addition to traditional responsibilities. The change in the role of dietitians will be driven by the shift in disease pattern from communicable to non-communicable diseases in the population. Epidemiological studies have implicated life style factors such as diet, lack of exercise and cigarette smoking in the growth of chronic diseases. The solution lies in educating people to change their behaviour e.g., eating healthy diets, exercising more and quitting smoking. Dietitians have access to patients and their relatives and they must exploit the opportunity to give them health and nutritional advice.

Dietitians can dispel myths and misconceptions about foods especially fads fed by media reports and advertisements.

Hospital dietitians could address large groups of patients attending clinics, such as the paediatrics and gynaecology, OPDs on the importance of nutrition. Dietitians could prepare easy-to-understand leaflets on nutrition for distribution to patients.

The major objective of dietary counselling should be to educate the patients regarding the nature of disease, its hazards, and how it can be recognized and prevented; advice on personal hygiene, individual instructions on diet and any specific therapy are essential. For effective dietary counselling, a team approach (physician-dietitian-nurse-patient) should be encouraged for success in diet therapy. A good rapport should be established with the patient. He should be made aware of the fact that diet plays an important role in the prognosis of disease and that he should strictly follow the guidelines of diet therapy; also he should be encouraged for a regular follow up programme in order to remain in sound health.

Apart from the food service, the diet clinic, an out-patient service helps in wider use of dietary counselling and serves to extend and clarify diet instruction, and have follow-ups. Whenever possible, home visits may also help in ensuring the adjustment of the patient to home environment. Programmed instruction through booklets, food models, charts and other audiovisual aids merit attention due to their great impact and flexibility of use for many kinds of people. In a food clinic or health centre, group therapy may also be used with advantage for such groups as pregnant and lactating women, women with preschool children, diabetic patients, weight-control groups and so on.

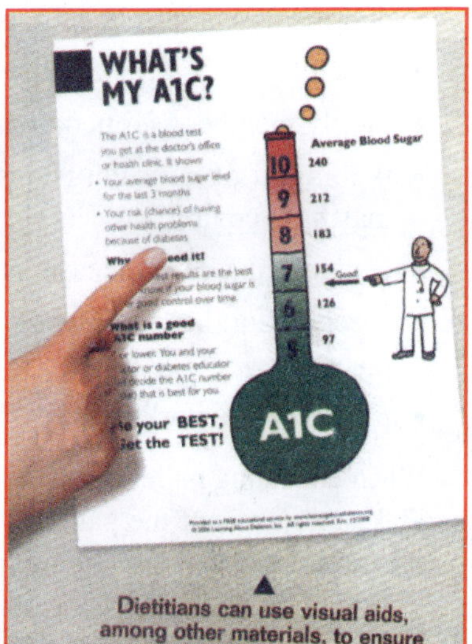

Fig. 26.2 **Visual aid to explain A1c**

Source: **Today's Dietitian, May 2010**

The advances in technology permeated in the health care industry dietitians have to use technology in diet counselling.

The dietitian can set up electronic food dairy, which the client would fill out over several days and submit with the click of the mouse. Dietitian analyses and discusses with the patient on his next visit.

General population who are well can seek diet information from the dietitian through e-mail or website. In this approach, computers are used and there is no verbal communication.

Counselling can also be done by the dietitian by combination of telephone and internet facilities. Specialised dietitians like those who have expertise in gluten free diets can counsel clients all over the world. Telephone consultation can be followed by face to face meeting. By using internet facilities, dietitian has the freedom and resources to serve people all over the world. A dietitian has a flexibility to work part-time and to work from home.

Offering on-line counselling gives dietitians a unique competitive edge as it offers clients something new, different and valuable.

Non-compliance to Dietary Advice: Large proportion of patients fail to adhere to advice on diet, exercise and blood glucose monitoring leading to risk of complications. Some of the possible reasons for non-compliance are:

- primary care providers (doctors) do not consistently provide counselling to their patients.
- patients are not referred for nutritional counselling.
- resistance to changing a diet.
- competing time and energy demands.
- genetic characteristics may have greater effects.
- lack of relevant educational material.
- diet therapy is infrequently prescribed.
- the changes required are life long, so life-style needs to be changed.
- family members cooperation is required.
- the impact of nutrition counselling is not dramatic and those who do not have patience may stop complying.
- festivals and party occasions may disturb the schedule.
- special effort has to be taken when patient eats outside home in the restaurant or relative's place.
- patients who work for long hours may not comply with dietary advice.

When educating patients about the disease, dietitians must first treat any existing depression and take into account the patient's education level and cognitive ability. Usually the older the patient and the longer the duration of disease and treatment the better is the compliance with dietary guidelines. Primary health care personnel need to give due importance to diet and exercise. Dietitians should focus on providing dietary alternatives for the married and working patients. They can suggest ways of modifying the family diet according to patient's needs.

Dietetics professionals should be aware that a short intervention, such as a one hour dietary counselling session or reading a brochure, will not achieve substantial reductions in a person's dietary intake. Repeated exposure to positive nutrition messages over a prolonged period of time brings out desired dietary goals.

RESPONSIBILITIES OF SPECIFIC DIETITIANS

Role of Gastroenterology Dietitian

A Gastroenterology (GE) dietitian has major responsibilities in both the branches of GE-Surgical GE and Medical GE. Surgical GE involves treating surgical patients after abdominal surgeries. Medical GE involves treating patients with GI disorders that may not require a surgical intervention, such as Crohn's disease, celiac disease, GERD (Gastroesophageal reflux disease) etc. The duties and responsibilities of a GE dietitian include the following:

- Nutritional assessment should be done to assess the nutritional status and a nutrition diagnosis has to be made.
- All symptoms related to GI disturbances that lead to poor oral intake should be clearly noted and understood. Dietary recommendations such as soft, bland diet, etc. and small frequent meal patterns can be suggested.
- Clinically appropriate diet regimens should be planned, executed and monitored by the GE dietitian. Counseling should be done to the patient and family.
- For surgical patients, the nutritional status prior to the surgery must be evaluated. Post-operative initiation of oral/enteral/parenteral nutrition must be done on time and monitored on a regular basis for tolerance and progress.
- Oral Nutrition Supplements, appropriate to the clinical condition of the patient, should be suggested whenever required. A classic example would be the advice of pre-digested formulas for patients with malabsorption.

Role of Diabetes Mellitus Dietitian

Medical Nutrition Therapy for Diabetes (MNT) is integral to overall diabetes care and management. Nutrition care should be research based and outcome focused.

"Registered Dietitian" who is knowledgeable and skilled in implementing current nutrition therapy recommendations into the medical management of diabetes is a core member of the multi-disciplinary diabetic care team.

The primary role of the dietitian in the team is to provide effective nutrition care, nutrition self-management education, counseling, and support both in prevention and management of diabetes. This can be achieved through individualized sessions or group based settings with patients, tailoring patient programs considering their anthropometric, biochemical, clinical, dietary and family medical history, food intolerances, personal and cultural beliefs, preferences, lifestyle and the willingness and ability of the person to change to motivate them to meet their specific needs.

Nutrition care process needs to be extended to type 1 diabetes, prediabetic, type 2 diabetes, secondary and gestational diabetes and also to those with euglycemic status post-partum, towards the prevention of type 2 diabetes mellitus in the near future.

The role of a dietitian goes beyond the identification of an appropriate meal plan including working individually with the patients to design meal algorithms, highlighting appropriate and realistic nutrition goals, negotiating dietary strategies, providing ongoing patient support.

Dietitians must regularly participate in comprehensive diabetes and nutrition education programs for patients, community, medical, nursing and allied health professionals.

In short, the role of a dietitian attached to diabetology department revolves around nutrition screening, assessment, counseling, training, education and glycaemic control related research activities.

To perform the duties and responsibilities effectively she needs to be well versed with food exchanges, carbohydrate counting, glycaemic index, glycaemic load, insulin to carbohydrate ratio related recent researches. She needs to update herself with the recent nutrition recommendations, newer anti diabetic medications and their nutrient interactions.

Role of a Bariatric Dietitian

- The dietitian plays a very important role in all three stages of a bariatric surgery. Pre, peri and post operatively.
- She has to assess, monitor and counsel the patient at all three stages for strict adherence to the diet and to ensure effective weight loss and attain optimal nutrition.
- She helps the patient to relearn the pattern of eating and lifestyle that is practiced for many years.
- Screening for any nutritional deficiency in the patients profile before surgery is done by the bariatric dietitian and ensure corrective measures are taken and prepare the patient before surgery.
- During and after the period of achieving the ideal body weight careful monitoring has to be done in the nutritional status so that the patient does not slip into any deficiencies or malnutrition.
- Healthy weight loss is when the patient loses the fat and not the muscle mass. Bariatric nutritionist has a very important role to ensure that the weight loss is a healthy one.
- Since the portion size reduces eventually, care has to be taken to ensure that little portion contains the necessary macro and micronutrients to help the patient maintain a healthy body and state of mind.
- She helps in problem solving, modification of current behaviour pattern and helps the patient with new skill and knowledge to establish and maintain new eating habits and food choices.
- Frequent monitoring and adjustments in the diet and supplements are monitored by the dietitian during post surgical weight loss and weight maintenance periods.
- Patient need to be in bariatric support groups. In a comprehensive surgical weight management program the role of a bariatric dietitian has evolved beyond the traditional role of a dietitian.

Role of Renal Dietitian

The renal dietitian plays a key role in managing various stages of renal disease. Poor oral intake is often observed in these patients due to the stringent diet restrictions advised and also due to poor appetite or lack of interest in food. Duties and responsibilities of a renal dietitian include the following:

- A thorough nutritional assessment should be done to assess the nutritional status and a nutrition diagnosis has to be made.
- An extensive diet counseling and explanation is required with respect to salt and fluid restrictions, protein intake, phosphorous and potassium restrictions Salt and fluid distribution throughout the day must be clearly explained as these restrictions are common in renal patients. Consistency of the diets can be altered to suit better intakes.
- After counselling the patient and family, a daily monitoring of intake has to be done. If intake is poor, appropriate ONS (Oral Nutrition Supplements) can be suggested by the dietitian.
- The biochemical parameters should be checked on a regular basis. These parameters include urea, creatinine, sodium, potassium, BUN (Blood Urea Nitrogen), phosphorous, etc. in order to monitor the renal function of the patients.

For patients undergoing dialysis, the renal dietitian needs to pay special attention to ensure that their nutrition needs are met and malnutrition is prevented.

Challenges of a dietitian

The main role of a dietitian is to provide the patients with the necessary information regarding diet lifestyle. In the present age patients have filled their mind with popular ideas and then approach the dietitian with preconcieved ideas whereas the dietitians responsibility is to erase the misleading beliefs and guide the patient in the right path.

INDIAN DIETETIC ASSOCIATION

Indian Dietetic Association was registered under Societies Registration Act, 1961.

Milestones of Indian Dietitic Association (J Acad Nutr Diet 2022; 122)

- **1962:** Dietetics profession organized. IDA Life Membership category created based on academic degree or for medical doctors interested in nutrition.
- **1981:** Honorary Registered Dietitian (RD; Unless specified as US RDN, the term RD will be used to refer to the credential issues by the Indian Dietetic Association and RD Board of the Indian Dietetic Association) credential introduced based on academic food and nutrition degrees and experience (in multispecialty hospital or teaching clinical nutrition).
- **1995:** RD credential created based on examination in addition to academic and experience requirements list of hospitals approved for internships published. Academic syllabus created.
- **2009:** Train-the-trainer workshops conducted for educators on a newly developed competency package.
- **2012:** Academic requirements changed to any graduate with degree in Food Nutrition and Dietetics with 1 or 2 years of postgraduate degree. Requirements introduced for dietetic trainers (preceptors) for internships. Alternate non-internship experience route added (2 years of experience in multispeciality hospitals).
- **2016:** Six-month continuous internship requirement added. Revised competency package to add research: 50 case studies required.
- **2018:** Non-internship multispecialty experience route increased to 5 years.

- **2020:** In response to COVID, a virtual program offered for students (orientation, case studies, and refresher course) and train-the-trainer workshops. Increased the number of examination centers to seven.

Since the inception of the association, one of the major activities of the IDA is to organize seminars and lectures in which eminent scientists from India and abroad participate.

Objectives

- To present and discuss important advances and problems in dietetics, nutrition and other relevant sciences and to adopt measures for the advancement and popularisation of dietetics, nutrition and other relevant science.
- To promote the cause of science, particularly the branch of dietetics, nutrition and related disciplines of the social science and to encourage the spirit of active pursuit of knowledge and original scientific research.
- To support and project the status and interests of the members of the Association and work for their general welfare.
- To encourage the study of dietetics, nutrition and other sciences relating to human health and raise funds to institute for this purpose scholarships, prizes, awards and travel grants.

Fig. 26.3 Logo of Indian Dietetic Association

- To generate scientific and cultural fellowship and cultivation of goodwill among its members and to safeguard the professional interests of its members.
- To promote knowledge of dietetics and nutrition by lectures, discussions, publication of books, correspondence with government officials, public bodies and individuals.
- To publish journals, monographs, souvenirs, commemoration volumes and other matter.
- To promote close contact and exchanges among persons following different branches of pure and applied science and to facilitate the evolution of a wider outlook and integration of available scientific knowledge.
- To accept, receive, purchase, take on lease on hire or otherwise acquire any movable or immovable property or any rights or privileges necessary or convenient for the purposes of the Association on terms and conditions as considered appropriate.
- To secure, accept, receive and to manage gifts, funds, endowments, donations from governments, public bodies, persons or other agencies for the promotion of dietetics, nutrition and other sciences.
- The income and property of the Association, whensoever derived, shall be applied solely towards the promotion of aims and objectives of the Association.
- To enable the institution of foundations by donations received from persons or agencies interested in the furtherance of the cause of Association.
- To invite scientists of eminence in India or abroad to deliver lectures and to participate in the scientific deliberations of Association.

- To create public opinion in favour of the aims and objects of the Association through its publications, holding seminars, conferences and press campaigns.
- To perform any other acts that may assist in, conducive to or be necessary for the fulfillment of the aims and objectives of the Association.

The Journal of Indian Dietetic Association is published by the Indian Dietetic Association.

Membership

Any person having a minimum qualification of the first degree in college with interest in the field of dietetics can become a life member or ordinary member. Student studying for a degree in science or medicine in the field of nutrition, dietetics or allied fields can become a student member.

Chapters

The chapters work closely with institutions training students for a degree in dietetics as well as dietetic department of hospitals and nursing homes. They run dietetic counselling centres, annual exhibition of therapeutic diets, symposia on dietary management of different diseases and conduct research projects in the field of dietetics sponsored by different funding agencies. The chapters have been able to increase the awareness of dietetic management of the diseases among the administrators of government and private hospitals. The chapters are in touch with their respective State Governments to establish Dietetic Department in every hospital and improve the condition of dietitians.

Registration Board

To maintain high standard of quality of dietitians who will be employed by hospitals and public health institutions, IDA has instituted a registration board to conduct Registration Examination for dietitians who would like to get registration as dietitians. Those who pass the examination will be registered as dietitians and given Registration number.

Pattern of Examination

There are two test papers:

Paper-1: Physiology, Microbiology, Biochemistry

Paper-2: Nutrition, Dietetics, Food Service Management.

Each paper will consist of three sections–Section A and B: Objective questions (50 marks) and Multiple choice questions (20 marks) and Section C: Clinical oriented questions (30 marks).

Detailed syllabus and references are usually given in the handbook supplied to candidates along with the examination application form.

The candidate is required to obtain at least 50 per cent marks for "qualifying" with a minimum of 45 per cent for each paper.

Usually the eligibility examination is conducted on the first/second Saturday of November every year.

Eligibility Requirements for R.D. Examinations

- Life membership of IDA.
- Graduate in Nutrition and Dietetics/P.G. Diploma or Master's degree in Nutrition and Dietetics.

- Six months Internship after completion of qualifying exam in a multispeciality hospital recognised by IDA for internship and supervised by an R.D. who is a full time employee of that hospital. The internship should be done continuously or in two installments of 2–4 months each, with a break of not more than 6 weeks.

or

Two years of experience as a full time dietitian in a multispeciality hospital of minimum 150 beds.

Centres to write Registration Exam

- Dietary Department, Christian Medical College Hospital, Vellore.
- S.V.T. College of Home Science, S.N.D.T. University, Juhu Road, Mumbai.
- Dietary Dept. All India Institute of Medical Sciences, Delhi.

Application forms are available in April every year. RD eligibility examination is usually conducted every year on first/second Saturday in the month of November.

The website of Indian Dietetic Association is www.idaindia.org

Registered Dietitian Day is on 10th March.

SUGGESTED READINGS

- Social media and the dietetics practitioner: Opportunities, challenges and best practices. Practice paper of the Academy of Nutrition and Dietetics, J Acad Nutr Diet. 2016: **116**.
- Tremelling Kaylee *et al.*, Orthorexia Nervosa and eating disorder symptoms in Registered Dietitian nutritionists in the United States, J Acad Nutr Diet. 2017: **117**.
- Mitchell J. Lana *et al.*, Effectiveness of Dietetic consultations in primary health care: A Systemic review of randomised controlled trials, J Acad. Nutr Diet. 2017: **117**.
- Shanthi Dhandapami *et al.*, Clinical Dietetics Practice Audit in India. A collateral collaboration of dietitians from India and the limited states J Acad Nutr Diet 2022; **122**.

QUESTIONS

1. Define dietitian. What are the responsibilities of a dietitian?
2. What are the pre-requisites to become a registered dietitian?
3. What are the challenges faced by dietitian in an Indian hospital?
4. Suggest ways of using technology in diet counselling.

TOPIC FOR DISCUSSION

- Should Indian Registered Dietitian be called 'Registered Dietitian Nutritionist' in line with other countries? Discuss.

Appendices

Appendix 1

CONVERSION FACTORS

1. Conversion of kcal to kJ: 1 kcal = 4.18 kJ
2. Conversion of Interactional Units of vitamin A to Retinol Equivalents of vitamin A:

   From an animal source divide by 3.33; From a vegetable or fruit divide by 10
3. Milligrams to milliequivalents

   Divided milligrams by the atomic weight of the ion and multiply by the valence number.

$$\frac{\text{Milligrams of an ion}}{\text{atomic weight of ion}} \times \text{valence}$$

Element	*Atomic weight*	*Valence*
Sodium, Na	23	1
Potassium, K	39	1
Calcium, Ca	40.08	2

- To convert m mol/L triglyceride to mg/dL multiply m mol/L by 88.6.
- To convert mg/dL triglyceride to mmol/L, multiply mg/dL by 0.013 triglycerides of 80 m mol/L = 159 mg/dL,
- To convert mmol cholesterol to mg/dL multiply m mol/L by 38.7.
- To convert mg/dL cholesterol to m mol/L, multiply mg/dL by 0.026. Cholesterol of 5.00 m mol/L = 193 mg/dL.

Appendix 2

AVERAGE NUTRITIVE VALUE OF FOODS

per 100 grams of edible portion

Food Name	*Energy kcal*	*Protein g*
Ragi, rice and rice products	343	7.4
Bajra, jowar, wheat	334	10.4
Dals	328	22.4
Milk, cow's	72	3.2
Meat	135	20.3
Nuts and oil seeds	570	20.2
Green leafy vegetables	27	2.6
Roots and herbs	70	1.2
Other vegetables	27	1.8
Fruits	58	0.6
Oils and fats	900	–

Source: Longvah T., R. Ananthan, K. Bhaskarachary and K. Venkaiah 2017. Indian Food Composition Tables. National Institute of Nutrition, Hyderabad.

Appendix 3

NUTRITIONAL ASSESSMENT FOR NON-AMBULATORY PATIENTS

Height

The knee height measurement (KH) is used to calculate the value for deriving body height equivalent.

$$\text{Height (women)} = [(1.83 \times \text{KH}) - (0.24 \times \text{age})] + 84.88$$

$$\text{Height (men)} = [(2.02 \times \text{KH}) - (0.04 \times \text{age})] + 64.19$$

Weight

Calf circumference (CC) is used with three other measurements-knee height (KH), and mid arm circumference (MAC) and subscapular skin fold (SSF) to derive body weight.

$$\text{Weight (women)} = (1.27 \times \text{CC}) + (0.87 \times \text{KH}) + (0.98 \times \text{MAC}) + (0.4 \times \text{SSF}) - 62.35$$

$$\text{Weight (men)} = (0.98 \times \text{CC}) + (1.16 \times \text{KH}) + (1.73 \times \text{MAC}) + (0.37 \times \text{SSF}) - 81$$

Appendix 4

SUBJECTIVE NUTRITIONAL GLOBAL ASSESSMENT

Patient Name: ________		**Anthopometric**	
Age:	Sex: Male/Female	Height: cm	Weight: Kg
Consultant:		Ideal Body Weight:________Kg	
IP No.:	Room No.:	BMI: (18.5–25)	
		☐ Under Weight ☐ Normal	☐ Over Weight ☐ Obesity
Diet Recommended by Consultant:			

A. History:

1. **Weight Changes:** ☐ Yes ☐ No $\%\text{Wt. change} = \frac{\text{Wt. 6 months ago} - \text{current wt.}}{\text{Wt. 6 months ago}} \times 100$

   Overall loss in past 6 months ☐ Kg Percent Loss ☐ %

   Change in past 2 weeks ☐ Increase ☐ No Change ☐ Decrease

2. **Dietary Intake change (relative to normal)**

   No change ☐

   Change: Duration ☐ Weeks ☐ Months

   Type: Sub-optimal Solid Diet ☐ Full liquid diet ☐ Hypo calorie liquid diet ☐ Starvation ☐

3. **Gastro intestinal symptoms (persisting more than 2 weeks)**

   None ☐ Nausea ☐ Vomiting ☐ Diarrhea ☐ Anorexia ☐ Loss of Appetitis ☐

4. **Functional Capacity**

   No dysfunction ☐

   Dysfunction: Duration ☐ Weeks ☐ Months

   Type: Working sub-optimally ☐ Ambulatory ☐ Bed ridden ☐

5. **Disease and its relationship to nutritional requirements**

   Primary diagnosis________________________

   Metabolic demand/Stress: None ☐ Low ☐ Moderate ☐ High ☐

B. Physical Examination

(For each specify: 0 = Normal, 1+ = Mild, 2+ = Moderate, 3+ = Severe)

Loss of subcutaneous fat (triceps, chest) ☐

Muscle wasting (quadriceps, deltoids) ☐

Ankle edema ☐ Sacral edema ☐ Ascites ☐

C. Subjective Global Assessment Rating:

Well Nourished A ☐

Moderately (or suspected of being) malnourished B ☐

Severely Malnourished B ☐

Diet Plan: Energy________Kcals, CHO:________gm, Protein____________gm,
Fat________gm, Salt____________gm, Fluid______________ml

Date: Signature of the Dietitian

Appendix 5

MINI NUTRITIONAL ASSESSMENT

Name

Age *Weight in kg*

Complete the screen by filling the boxes with the approximate numbers. Add the numbers for the screen. If score is 11 or less, continue with assessment to gain a Malnutrition Indicator score.

Screening

A. Has the food intake declined over the past 3 months due to loss of appetite, digestive problems, chewing or swallowing difficulties
0 = severe loss of appetite
1 = moderate loss of appetite
2 = no loss of appetite ☐

B. Weight loss during last 3 months
0 = weight loss more than 3 kg (6.6 lbs)
1 = does not know
2 = weight loss between 1 & 3 kg (2.2 & 6.6 lbs)
3 = no weight loss ☐

C. Mobility
0 = bed or chair bound
1 = able to get out of bed/chair but does not go out
2 = goes out ☐

D. Has suffered psychological stress or acute disease in the past 3 months
0 = yes
2 = no ☐

E. Neuropsychological Problems
0 = severe dementia or depression
1 = mild dementia
2 = no psychological problems ☐

F. Body Mass Index (BMI) (weight in kg)/(height in m^2)
0 = BMI less than 19
1 = BMI 19 to less than 21
2 = BMI 21+ to less than 23
3 = BMI 23 or greater ☐

Screening score (subtotal max 14 points) ☐☐

12 points or greater	Normal-not at risk no need to complete assessment
11 points or below	Possible malnutrition-continue assessment

Assessment

G. Lives independently (not in a nursing home or hospital) ☐
0 = no
1 = yes

(Contd...)

H. Takes more than 3 prescription drugs per day 0 = yes 1 = no	☐
I. Pressure sores or skin ulcers 0 = yes 1 = no	☐
J. How many full meals does the patient eat daily? 0 = 1 meal 1 = 2 meal 2 = 3 meal	☐
K. Selected consumption markers for protein intake * Atleast one serving of dairy products (milk, cheese, yoghurt) per day? yes ❍ no ❍ * Two or more serving of legumes or eggs per week? yes ❍ no ❍ * meat, fish or poultry every day yes ❍ no ❍ 0.0 = if 0 or 1 yes 0.5 = if 2 yes 0.1 = if 3 yes	☐
L. Consumes two or more servings of fruits or vegetables per day? 0 = no 1 = yes	☐
M. How much fluid (water, juice, coffee, tea, milk . .) is consumed per day? 0.0 = less than 3 cups 0.5 = 3 to 5 cups 1.0 = more than 5 cups	☐
N. Mode of feeding 0 = unable to eat without assistance 1 = self-fed with some difficulty 2 = self-fed without any problem	☐
O. Self view of nutritional status 0 = view self as being malnourished 1 = is uncertain of nutritional state 2 = view self as having no nutritional problem	☐
P. In comparison with other people of the same age, how do they consider their health status? 0.0 = not as good 0.5 = does not know 1.0 = as good 2.0 = better Q. Mid arm circumference (MAC) in cm 0.0 = MAC less than 21 0.5 = MAC 21+ to < 22 1.0 = MAC 22 or greater	☐ ☐
R. Triceps Skinfold thickness (TSF) 0 = >20% 1 = up to 10-19% 2 = up to 10% 3 = Normal	☐

(Contd...)

APPENDICES

Assessment (max. 18 points)	☐	☐
Screening score	☐	☐
Total Assessment (max. 32 points)		
Malnutrition Indicator score	☐	☐
17 to 25.5 points — at risk of malnutrition		☐
less than 17 points — malnourished		

Appendix 6

DIALYSIS MALNUTRITION SCORE

A. PATIENTS RELATED MEDICAL HISTORY:

1. Weight change (overall change in past 6 months)

1	2	3	4	5
No weight change or gain	minor wt loss (< 5%)	Wt loss 5 to 10%	Wt loss 10 to 15%	Wt loss > 15%
2. Dietary Intake:				
1	**2**	**3**	**4**	**5**
No change	Sub - optimal Solid diet	full liquid or decrease	hypo-caloric liquid	starvation
3. Gastrointestinal symptoms:				
1	**2**	**3**	**4**	**5**
No symptoms	nausea	vomiting or Mod GI symptoms	diarrhea	severe anorexia
4. Functional capacity:				
1	**2**	**3**	**4**	**5**
None (improved)	difficulty with amputation	difficulty with normal activity	light activity	bed/chair ridden
5. Co-morbidity:				
1	**2**	**3**	**4**	**5**
Dialysis <12mths and healthy	dialysis 1-2 yr or mild comorbidity	dialysis 2-4 yr or moderate comorbidity	dialysis>4yr or severe comorbidity	very severe or multiple comorbidity
B. PHYSICAL EXAM:				
6. Decreased fat stores or loss of subcutaneous fat:				
1	**2**	**3**	**4**	**5**
None		moderate		severe
7. Signs of muscle wasting				
1	**2**	**3**	**4**	**5**
None		moderate		severe

Appendix 7

APPROXIMATE CALORIFIC VALUE OF SOME COOKED PREPARATIONS

Recipe	*Measure*	*Calories*
1. Cereal		
Rice	1 cup	170
Phulka	1 No.	80
Paratha	1 No.	150
Puri	1 No.	80
Bread	2 Slices	170
Poha	1 cup	270
Upma	1 cup	270
Idli	2 Nos.	150
Dosa	1 No.	125
Kichidi	1 cup	200
Wheat porridge	1 cup	220
Semolina porridge	1 cup	220
Cereal flakes with milk (corn/wheat/rice)	1 cup	220
2. Pulse		
Plain dal	1/2 cup	100
Sambhar	1 cup	110
3. Vegetable		
With gravy	1 cup	170
Dry	1 cup	150
4. Non-Vegetarian		
Boiled egg	1 No.	90
Ommelette	1 No.	160
Fried egg	1 No.	160
Mutton curry	3/4 cup	260
Chicken curry	3/4 cup	240
Fish fried	2 big pieces	190
Fish cutlet	2 Nos.	190
Prawn curry	3/4 cup	220
Keema kofa curry	3/4 cup (6 small koftas)	240
5. Savoury snacks		
Bajji or pakora	8 Nos.	280
Besan ka pura	1 No.	220

(Contd...)

Recipe	Measure	Calories
Chat (Dahi-pakori)	5 pieces	220
Cheese balls	2 Nos.	250
Dahi vada	2 Nos.	180
Vada	2 Nos.	140
Masala vada	2 Nos.	150
Masala dosa	1 No.	200
Peak-kachori	2 Nos.	380
Potato bonda	2 Nos.	200
Sago vada	2 Nos.	210
Samosa	1 No.	200
Sandwiches (butter-2 tbsp)	2 Nos.	200
Vegetable puff	1 No.	200
Pizza (Cheese and tomato)	1 slice	200
6. Chutneys		
Coconut/groundnuts/til	2 tbsp	120
Tomato	1 tbsp	10
Tamrind (with iaggery)	1 tbsp	60
7. Sweets and Desserts		
Besan barfi	2 small pieces	400
Chikki	2 pieces	290
Fruit cake	1 piece	270
Rice puttu	1/2 cup	280
Sandesh	2 Nos.	140
Double ka meetha	1/2 cup	280
Halwa (kesari)	1/2 cup	320
Jelly/Jam	1 tbsp	20
Custard (caramel)	1/2 cup	160
Srikhand	1/2 cup	380
Milk chocolate	25 g	140
Ice-cream	1/2 cup	200
8. Beverages		
Tea (2 tbsp sugar + 50 ml toned milk)	1 cup	75
Coffee (2 tbsp sugar + 100 ml)	1 cup	110
Cow's milk (2 tbsp sugar)	1 cup	180
Buffalo's milk (2 tbsp sugar)	1 cup	320

(Contd...)

Recipe	*Measure*	*Calories*
Lassi (2 tbsp sugar)	1 cup/glass (200 ml)	110
Squash	1 cup/glass	75
Syrups (Sharabats)	1 cup/glass	200
Cold drinks	1 bottle (200 ml)	150
Fresh lime juice	1 glass	60

Source: Dietary Guidelines for Indians. A Manual, 2011, National Institute of Nutrition, Hyderabad.

Appendix 8

NOMOGRAM FOR DETERMINING BODY MASS INDEX (BMI)

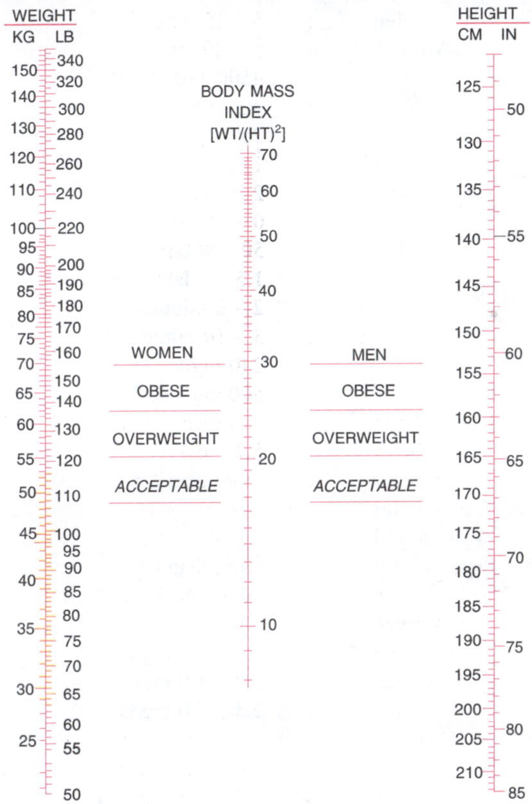

To use this nomogram, place a ruler or other straight edge between the column for height and the column for weight connecting an individual's numbers for those two variables. Read the BMI in kg/m^2 where the straight line crosses the middle lines when the height and weight are connected. Height and weights are without shoes or clothes.

Overweight: BMI of 25-30 kg/m^2; Obesity: BMI above 30 kg/m^2.

Cited from Wyngarden., B.J., *et al.*, 1992. Textbook of Medicine W.B. Saunders Company Philadelphia, London, Toronto, Montreal, Sydney, Tokyo.

Appendix 9

NORMAL BLOOD COUNT AND BIOCHEMICAL TESTS

RBC count	Men	:	4.5 – 5.5 million/cu mm
	Women	:	3.8 – 4.8 million/cu mm
Haemoglobin	Men	:	13.0 – 17.0 g |d|
	Women	:	12.0 – 15.0 g |d|
Packed cell volume	Men	:	40 – 50%
	Women	:	36 – 46%
Mean corpuscular volume		:	80 – 101 cub µ
Mean corpuscular Hgb		:	27 – 32 pg (Picogram = One trillionth of a gram = 10^{-12} gram)
Mean corpuscular concentration		:	31.5 – 34.5 g |dl
Mean corpuscular Diameter MCD		:	6.7 – 8.0 micron
Reticulocyte count		:	0.5 – 1.5%
ESR 1st hour	Men	:	5 – 15 mm
	Women	:	5 – 20 mm
Total WBC count		:	4500-11000/cells/cmm
Polymorphs		:	40 – 65%
Lymphocytes		:	20 – 45%
Eosinophils		:	1 – 6%
Monocytes		:	2 – 10%
Basophils		:	0 – 1%
Eosinophil count		:	50 – 400/µl
Platelet count		:	1.5 – 4 lakh cells/µl
Bleeding time		:	2 – 6 minutes
Clotting time		:	3 – 10 minutes
Plasma vit. A. (Retinol)		:	240 mg/l
Carotenoids		:	500 mg/l
HbA1c	Non diabetic	:	less than 5.6 %
	Risk of developing diabetes	:	5.7 – 6.4%
	Diabetes	:	more than 6.5 %
	In known diabetics Good control	:	6 – 7%
	Fair control	:	7 – 8%
	Poor Control	:	more than 8%
B. Urea	Men	:	16.6 – 48.5 mg/dl
	Women	:	10 – 30 mg/dl
S Creatinine	Men	:	0.6 – 1.2 mg/dl
	Women	:	0.4 – 1.0 mg/dl
S Uric acid	Men	:	2.5 – 7.0 mg/dl
	Women	:	1.5 – 6.0 mg/dl
S calcium		:	9.0 – 110 mg/dl
S In. phosphorus		:	3.0 – 4.8 g/dl
S Total proteins		:	6.0 – 8.0 g/dl
S Albumin		:	3.8 – 5.0 g/dl
S Total bilirubin		:	0.3 – 1.2 mg/dl
S Direct Bilirubin		:	0.0 – 0.3 mg/dl
SGOT (Serum glutamic oxaloacetic trans aminase)			
	Male	:	upto 40 U/L
	Female	:	upto 32 U/L
SGPT (Serum glutamic pyruvic transaminase		:	5–40 IU/l

S Alkaline phosphatase			
	Adults	:	100 – 250 IU/L
	Children	:	200 – 770 IU/L
S Gamma GT		:	6 – 28 IU/L
S Acid phosphatase total		:	1.0 – 4.0 KA units
	Prostatic #	:	0.0 – 0.8 KA units
S Amylase		:	5 – 30 IU/L
S Total CPK (CK) Creatinine	Men	:	0.7 – 1.2 mg/dl
	Women	:	0.5 – 0.9 mg/dl
SCPK-MB SLDH (Lactate dehydrogenase)		:	170 – 365 IU/L

Electrolytes

S Sodium	:	136 – 145 mEq/L
S Potassium	:	3.8 – 5.0 mEq/L
S Bicarbonate	:	20 – 28 mMol/L
S Chloride	:	99 – 111 mEq/L

The values can vary depending on methods and instruments used.

Appendix 10

LIPID PROFILE: NATIONAL CHOLESTEROL EDUCATION PROGRAM GUIDELINES

Total cholesterol	Child – upro 19 years		
	< 170 mg |d|	:	desirable
	170 – 199 mg |d|	:	borderline high
	> = 200 mg |d|	:	high
	Adult above 19 years		
	< 200 mg |d|	:	desirable
	200 – 239 mg |d|	:	borderline high
	> = 240 mg |d|	:	high
HDL cholesterol	coronary heart disease risk		
	< 40 mg |d|	:	high risk
	40 – 60 mg |d|	:	normal risk
	> = 60 mg |d|	:	low risk
Triglycerides	< 150 mg |d|	:	desirable
	150 – 199 mg |d|	:	normal risk
	200 – 499 mg |d|	:	high risk
	> = 500 mg |d|	:	very high risk
LDL cholesterol	< 100 mg |d|	:	optimal
	100 – 129 mg |d|	:	near optimal
	130 – 159 mg |d|	:	borderline high
	160 – 189 mg |d|	:	high
	> = 190 mg |d|	:	very high
Total cholesterol : HDL ratio			
	Less than 3.5	:	low risk
	3.5 – 5.0	:	normal risk
	> 5.0	:	high risk

Appendix 11

GLOSSARY OF DIETS

Bland diet: This diet is mechanically, chemically and thermally non irritating. Diet suggested for peptic ulcer patient and other gastro intestinal disorders.

Karell diet: This is a regimen of undernutrition allows 800 ml of milk daily in four feedings of 200 ml each administered at four-hour intervals. After 3 or 4 days this routine is liberalised to include toast, eggs, cream soup and fruit. This diet is given in acute type of heart disease.

Portfolio diet: This diet combines in one diet the plant foods that lower cholesterol. Their effect may better than lipid lowering drug therapy. This diet is for atherosclerosis patient.

Atkins diet: This diet is low in carbohydrate and calories and high in protein.

The four stages include: The fortnight induction diet, The ongoing weight loss diet, Premaintenance and Maintenance diet.

The induction diet limits carbohydrate to 20 g/day (1 cup permitted vegetables and 1 cup salad vegetables). Unlimited amounts of beef, turkey, chicken and eggs as well as fats are allowed. This phase of the diet allows no fruit, bread, grains, starchy vegetables or dairy products other than cheese, cream or butter. Carbohydrate restriction in lessened during the other stages until individuals determine the level of carbohydrate they can consume while maintaining their weight loss.

Calories are not specified, diet nutritionally inadequate providing lower than recommended intakes of vitamin E, vitamin A, thiamin, vitamin B_6, folate, calcium, magnesium, iron, zinc, potassium and dietary fibre. No calcium or potassium supplements are prescribed. Diet is high in saturated fat, cholesterol and animal protein.

Atkins diet is extremely low in carbohydrates which helps to regulate insulin production and decreases circulating insulin. Less insulin may result in less fat storage and fewer food carvings.

Ornish diet: Ornish's multifaceted approach focuses on reversal of heart disease but is also recommended for weight loss. His programme incorporates aspects of nutrition, exercise, stress management and love and intimacy. Moderate exercise like walking is recommended. Stress management techniques include one hour per day of stretching, breathing, meditation or prayer, progressive relaxation and group support. Love and intimacy is accomplished through group support facilitating their adherence to the programme.

Very low fat (10% fat) plant-based diet based on adlibitum intake of fruits, vegetables, whole grains, beans and soya products. It incorporates moderate quantities of egg whites and nonfat dairy or soya products and small amounts of sugar and white flour. Fish is permitted; 3 g of ω-3 fats should be taken daily.

The following daily supplements are recommended:

Vitamin C-2 to 3 g; vitamin E-100-400 IU; Folate-400-2000 µg;

Women: flax seed oil-2 g and fish oil-2 g; Men: fish oil-2 g

Slenium-100-200 µg; Multivitamin

Diet is low in vitamin E, B_{12} and zinc; problems in adherence and palatability

Willett diet: This diet consist of abundant fruits, vegetables, whole grains and vegetable oils as well as optimal portions of fish and chicken. Risk of heart disease is reduced by replacing saturated fat with unsaturated fat like Mediterranean diet (2004).

All three Atkin, Willet and Ornish share an emphasis on reducing blood sugar spikes by reducing glycaemic load. All three condemn trans fats, white flour and sugar.

Summer bell *et al.*, diet: This diet consists of milk and one other food each day. Low calorie diet for reducing.

The South Beach Diet: It is developed by Arthur Agatson.

Phase 1: According to the South Beach Diet right carbohydrates and fats should be taken. Normal size helpings of meat, chicken, turkey, fish and shell fish should be taken. Plenty of vegetables, eggs, cheese and nuts can be taken. Salads with olive oil can be included. Three balanced meals can be taken till hunger is satisfied. Midmorning and midafternoon snack and dessert can be taken after dinner. Water, coffee and tea can be taken. For fourteen days no bread, rice, potatoes, pasta or baked goods. No fruit. No candy, cake, cookies, ice cream or sugar for two weeks. No beer or alcohol.

Phase 2: After 14-day period, source of those avoided foods can be taken. Bread, pasta, rice or potatoes can be reintroduced but sparingly. Fruit and chocolate also is back on the diet. Should stay in phase 2 until target weight is reached.

Phase 3: This stage that lasts the rest of life.

Normal foods in normal size portions. There will always be times when one overindulges a little even after years on the diet. Those are the times to switch back to phase 1 for a week or two.

On South Beach Diet one loses 8 to 13 pounds in the first two weeks without feeling hungry. There is no mandatory exercise and never left craving more food.

The Zone diet: It was created by Dr. Barry Sears. At the heart of the zone diet is its nutrient ratios. The zone diet follows a formula of 40 per cent carbohydrate, 30 per cent protein and 30 per cent fats (sometimes called as 40 : 30 : 30). This must be followed at every meal. It's biggest criticism is that the diet is simply too complex to follow. It can be considered 'low carb', due to the fact that the average person consumes about 50-60 per cent carbohydrates in their diet. The good thing about the zone diet is that it encourages a combination of all the nutrients in each meal and it stresses the risks of processed carbohydrates (white pastas and breads).

The grape fruit diet: This diet claims that grape fruit contains a special fat-burning enzyme. Half a grape fruit for each meal should be taken.

Dr. Fed on Lindberg diet: Eating often is better than going for long periods without food as this risks overindulging later.

Eat mainly foods with a low GI. Sugary high GI foods should be strictly limited and eaten as small snacks only after a low GI meal.

Cut down on starchy high-carbohydrate foods such as white bread, baked potatoes and rice.

Encourages plenty of protein and fats.

Unprocessed vegetable fats found in nuts, seeds, avocado and olives, cold pressed vegetable oils such as canola and olive oils and fatty fish are all favourite on his menu.

Cheese, gram and butter should be eaten moderately. Alcohol and caffeine should be limited because they kick off a desire for sweet foods.

General Motors Weight loss Programme: The following health programme was developed for the employees and dependents of General Motors Inc. USA and designed a target weight loss for 5-6 kg/week. During the first seven days, one must drink 10 glasses of water each day.

Day one—All fruits (except bananas)

Day two—All vegetables—cooked or raw without oils or coconut

Day three—Any mixture of fruits and vegetables. No banana. No potatoes

Day four—Bananas and milk, vegetable soup

Day five—One cup of rice; 6 whole tomatoes; 12 glasses of water

Day six—One cup of rice; vegetables cooked and raw

Day seven—One cup of rice, fruit juice and vegetables

Macrobiotic diet: This diet is similar to a strict vegetarian diet; all meat and dairy products are excluded and replaced with many soya based products. Supplemental foods such as white meat fish, seasonal fruits, nuts and seeds may be included 2 to 3 times a week. Vitamin and mineral supplementation is discouraged.

The standard macrobiotic diet ranges 50-60 per cent whole grains, 25-30 per cent vegetables, 5-10 per cent soups, 5-10 per cent beans and sea vegetables.

Nutrition concerns: Protein, vitamin B_{12} and calcium deficiency investigated for its potential cancer preventive effects.

Planetary health diet: It improves both human and planets health and is suggested by "The Eat-lancet commission". This gives 2500 kcals per day and the target is global population.

The details of the diet are as follows:

Food	*Intake g/day*	*Caloric intake (kcal/day)*
Whole grains	232	811
Tubers	50	39
All vegetables	300	78
Fruits	200	126
Dairy foods	250	153
Beef, lamb, pork	14	30
Chicken	29	62
Eggs	13	19
Fish	28	40
Legumes	75	284
All sugars	31	120

This diet is expensive as it includes foods of animal origin and fruits and vegetables. More than the minimum requirement for nutrition adequacy and much higher quantities are prescribed.

Even if many poor consumers were to aspire to consume healthier and more environmentally sustainable foods, income and price constraints frequently renders this diet unaffordable.

Appendix 12

HEALTH CARE ON NET

- All India Institute of Medical Sciences—www.pugmarks. cons/aims.
- American Institute of Child Nutrition—www.faseb. org.
- American Society for Nutritional Sciences—www.faseb. org/as ns.
- American Public Health Association Food and Nutrition Division—www.apha.org.
- American Dietetic Association—www.eatright.org/.
- American Diabetes Association—www.diabetes.org.
- American College of Sports Medicine—www.acsm.org.
- American Heart Association—www.americanheart.org.
- American Cancer Society—www.cancer.org.
- American Institute for Cancer Research—www.aicr.org.
- Gatorade Sports Science Institute—www.gssiweb.com.
- Healthy Recipes and Nutritional Facts—www.nutrition.about.com health/Nutritions.
- Health and Nutrition Guide—www.healthrecipes.com.
- Health Information Library—www.allindia.com/helplib.
- Health Canada Nutrition—www.hc-sc.gc.ca/hppb/nutrition/.
- Institute of Cardiovascular Disease—www.pppindia.com/mmm.
- Jaslok Hospital—www.madein India. com/industry/medical/jaslok. Health and Nutrition store—www.the nutrition connection.com.
- Journal of American Dietetic Association—www.eatright.org.
- Lifelines Nutrition and Fitness Links—www.lifelines.com/ntnlnk.html.
- Medline—www.nebi n/m.nili. gov/pub med.
- Medical Computer Society of India—www.hostindia. com/mcsi.
- National Center for Education in Maternal and Child Health—www.neemch.org.
- National Institute of Health—www.nih.gov/od/oar.
- NIH Osteoporosis & Related Bone disorders National Resource Center —www.osteo. org
- UN World Food Programme—www.wfp.org.
- Nutrition foundation of India—www.nutrition foundation in org.
- Nutrition Software—www.nutrigenie.biz/products.html.
- Nutrition and Weight Maintenance—www.niddk.nih.gov/health/nutrit/nutrit.htm.
- Peerless Hospital and Medical Research Centre—www.123 india.
- President's Council on Fitness and Sports—www.whitehouse.gov/WH/PCPFS/html/fitnet. html.

- Surgeon General's Report on Physical Activity—www.cdc.gov/nccdphp/sgr/sgr.htm.
- Tata Consultancy Service—www.web health centre.com.
- Vegetarian Resource Group—www.vrg.org.
- Vegetarian Pager—www.veg.org/veg/.
- World Health Organization—www.who.org/nut.
- 5a Day For Better Health—www.5aday.com.

Appendix 13

CAREER OPPORTUNITIES FOR DIETETICS PROFESSIONALS

Dietitians are experts in food and nutrition. Their purpose is to optimise the health and nutrition of the population. The job opportunities are many. Some are listed here. Registered dietitians can work in a hospital or can become specialised dietitians like

- renal dietitians
- ICU dietitians
- bariatric dietitians
- diabetes dietitians
- sports dietitians
- gastroenterology dietitians
- transplant dietitians
- cardiology dietitician
- can become free lance dietitians
- or diabetes care and educationist
- work at health clubs
- join in hotel industry
- join in gym and sports clubs
- join in noon meal centres at the planning levels
- join large food store chains
- work in food and pharmaceutical industry
- join in product development of food industry
- plan healthy meals for corporate bodies
- join as consultant to super markets and speciality food store
- do research on the effect of foods on the health status
- take up teaching at collegiate level after completing post graduation and passing National Eligibility Test conducted by UGC
- join as nutrition experts in international organisations such as UNICEF, WHO and FAO
- take up hospital management as career
- join school nutrition services
- take charge of fast food centres

- become food and culinary professionals
- become free lance writers on dietetics and nutrition
- can work with NGO
- can do private practice

Appendix 14(A)

Balanced diet for sedentary man with nutrient content values ICMR-2020

Food Composition	Amount (g/day)	Nutrient	Vegetarian diet	Non-vegetarian diet	EAR	RDA
Cereals and Millets	275	Energy kcal	2130	2650	2710	–
		Protein g	67.2	81.7	43	54
Pulses (Legumes)/ flesh foods[1]	80	Visible fat g	25	35	30	30
Green leafy Vegetables	100	Calcium mg	968	1054	800	1000
Other Vegetables	200	Iron mg	27.4	31.1	11	19.0
Roots and Tubers (excluding potatoes)	100	Zinc mg	13.5	15.9	14.1	17
Fruits	150	Magnesium mg	798	891	370	440
Milk	300	Vitamin A μg*	1768	1796	460	1000
Fats and oils	25	β-carotene μg	9638	9779	2760	6000
Oil seeds and Nuts (gingely seeds and Pea nuts)	30	Thiamine mg	1.7	1.6	1.2	1.4
Spices	10	Riboflavin mg	1.6	1.6	1.6	2.0
		Niacin mg	15.6	16.0	12	14
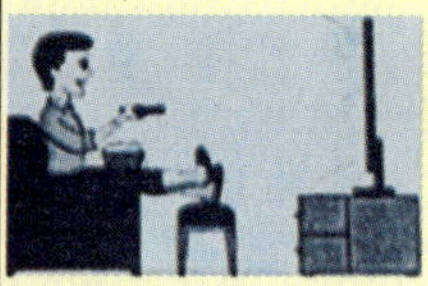		Vitamin B_6 mg	2.0	2.0	1.6	1.9
		Vitamin C mg			65	80
		Total Folates μg	483	450	250	300
		Vitamin B_{12} μg	1.5	2.0	2.0	2.2

Note: Total protein from the above diet = 71 g, Digestible protein = 58 g, PDCAAS = 85%

[1]Pulses can be replaced with animal foods (egg, meat, fish, and chicken) for non-vegetarians.

*Retinol derived from β-carotene from diet was also added to the total Vitamin A.

For cereals and millets, it is recommended to consume 50% as whole grains.

Appendix 14(B)

Balanced diet for sedentary woman with nutrient content values ICMR-2020

Food Composition	*Amount (g/day)*	*Nutrient*	*Vegetarian diet*	*Non-vegetarian diet*	*EAR*	*RDA*
Cereals and Millets	200	Energy kcal	1690	1650	1660	–
		Protein g	58.2	57.4	36.0	46.0
Pulses (Legumes)/ flesh foods[1]	60	Visible fat g	15	15	20	20
Green leafy Vegetables	100	Calcium mg	905	895	800	1000
Other Vegetables	200	Iron mg	23.8	22.8	15.0	29.0
Roots and Tubers (excluding potatoes)	100	Zinc mg	11.0	10.5	11.0	13.2
Fruits	150	Magnesium mg	684	649	310	370
Milk	300	Vitamin A μg*	1730	1727	390	840
Fats and oils	15	β-carotene μg	9412	9380	–	–
Oil seeds and Nuts (gingely seeds and Pea nuts)	30	Thiamine mg	1.36	1.30	1.1	1.4
Spices	10	Riboflavin mg	1.5	1.48	1.6	1.9
		Niacin mg	13.0	13.5	9.0	11
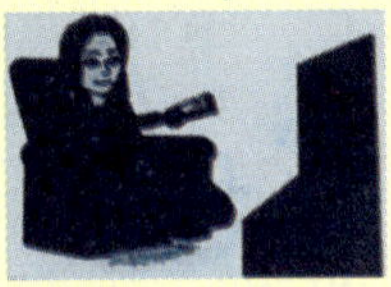		Vitamin B_6 mg	1.7	1.7	1.6	1.9
		Vitamin C mg	187	187	55	65
		Total Folates μg	426	395	180	220
		Vitamin B_{12} μg	1.5	2.0	2	2.2

Note: Total protein from the above diet = 60 g, Digestible protein = 50 g, PDCAAS = 87%

[1]Pulses can be replaced with animal foods (egg, meat, fish, and chicken) for non-vegetarians.

*Retinol derived from β-carotene from diet was also added to the total Vitamin A.

For cereals and millets, it is recommended to consume 50% as whole grains.

Appendix 15

Body weights (kg) of children and adolescents (5-18y) reported from IAP and WHO growth standards

Age (y)	*Boys*		*Girls*	
	IAP 2015	*WHO 2007*	*IAP 2015*	*WHO 2007*
5	17.1	18.5	16.4	18.3
6	19.3	20.5	18.7	20.2
7	21.9	22.9	21.2	22.4
8	24.8	25.4	24.0	25.0
9	27.9	28.1	27.2	28.2
10	31.1	31.2	31.0	31.9
11	34.7	34.6	35.4	36.2
12	39.0	38.9	39.8	41.1
13	43.3	44.3	4.6	46.0
14	48.2	50.6	46.4	50.1
15	53.1	56.5	48.4	52.8
16	56.8	61.3	49.7	54.7
17	59.5	64.8	50.9	55.7
18	61.6	67.3	52.0	56.7

Height (cm) of children and adolescents (5-18y) reported from IAP and WHO datasets

Age (y)	*Boy*		*Girls*	
	IAP 2015	*WHO 2007*	*IAP 2015*	*WHO 2007*
5	108.9	110	107.5	110
6	114.8	116	113.5	115
7	120.7	122	119.4	121
8	126.4	127	125.4	127
9	131.8	133	131.4	133
10	137.2	138	137.4	139
11	142.7	143	143.3	145
12	148.4	149	148.4	151
13	154.3	156	152.2	156
14	159.9	163	154.7	160
15	164.5	169	155.5	162
16	168.1	173	156.9	163
17	171.0	175	157.4	163
18	173.6	176	157.8	163

The 3rd, 50th and 97th percentiles values for body weights were plotted against age which showed a considerable overlap between the IAP and WHO data, suggesting that either of these datasets could be used as reference for the Indian population.

Source: Nutrient requirements for Indians Report of the expert group, 2020. National Institute of Nutrition. ICMR Hyderabad.

Appendix 16

TOLERABLE UPPER LIMIT (TUL) FOR NUTRIENT-ICMR-NIN, 2020

Age Group	Category of work	Protein (PE ratio)	Calcium (mg/d)	Magnesium* (mg/d)	Iron (mg/d)	Zinc (µg/day)	Iodine (mg/d) (day)	Niacin (mg/d)	Vit. B6 (mg/d)	Folate (µg/d)	Vit. C (mg/d)	Vit. A (µg/d)	Vit. D (IU/d)
Men	Sedentary Moderate Heavy	< 40%	2500	350	45	40	1100	35	100	1000	2000	3000	4000
Woman	Sedentary Moderate Heavy	< 40%	2500	350	45	40	1100			1000	2000	3000	
	Pregnant woman	< 30%	2500	350	45	40	1100	–	–	1000	2000	3000	4000
	Lactation 0-6 m 0-6 m 7-12 m	< 40%	2500	350	45	40	1100	–	–	1000	2000	3000	4000
Infants	0-6 m	< 15%	–	–	40	4	–	–	–	–	–	600	1000
	6-12 m	< 15%	–	–	40	5	–	–	–	–	–	600	1500
Children	1-3 y	< 15%	1500	65	40	7	200				350	600	2500
	4-6 y	< 15%	2500	110	40	12	300	–	–	–	550	900	3000
	7-9 y	< 15%	2500	110	40	12	400			300	800	900	3000
Boys	10-12 y	< 15%	3000	350	40	23	600	–	–	600–800	1050	1700	4000
Girls	10-12 y	< 15%	3000	350	40	23	600	–	–	600-800	1300	1700	4000
Boys	13-15 y	< 15%	3000	350	45	34	900	–	–	600-800	1550	2800	4000
Girls	13-15 y	< 15%	3000	350	45	34	900	–	–	600-800	1800	2800	4000
Boys	16-18 y	< 15%	3000	350	45	34	1100	–	–	600-800	1950	2800	4000
Girls	16-18 y	<15%	3000	350	45	34	1100	–	–	600-800	2000	2800	4000

The TUL is the maximum level of habitual intake from all sources of a nutrient or related substance judged to be unlikely to lead to adverse health effects in humans.

***Note:** For magnesium the TUL values are only for non-dietary pharmacological doses.

Appendix 17

Key micronutrients in different food groups

(All values are for 100 g edible portion) ICMR 2020

Micro-nutrients	Cereals[a]	Pulses[b]	Leafy Vege-tables[c]	Other Vege-tables[c]	Roots and Tubers[d]	Fruits[e]	Milk (Buffalo)[f]	Milk (Cow)[f]	Egg	Chic-ken	Mutton	Beef	Fish	Liver (Sheep, Goat, Lamb)
Iron (mg)	3.00	5	8.5	2.12	0.6	0.56	0.2	0.2	1.82	1.5	1.3	2.2	0.6	6.3
Zinc (mg)	2.16	2.1	0.2	0.3	0.3	0.11	0.4	0.3	1.2	1.7	3	4.6	0.6	3.6
Vitamin A (μg)	2.43	8.6	259.1	22.4	70.0	32.36	49.8	58.3	198	21.4	9	15.5	5.6	6690
Riboflavin (mg)	0.15	0.14	0.1	0.07	0.0	0.01	0.13	0.11	0.2	0.09	0.16	0.12	0.03	0.36
Dietary Folate (μg)	24.03	127.7	16.7	24.4	31.3	17.61	8.6	7	49.3	9.3	6.4	8.1	15.4	92
Vitamin B_{12} (μg)	Nil	Nil	Nil	Nil	Nil	Nil	1.5	1.5	1.8	NA	2.8	1.7	1.4	91.9

a Mean values of nutrients from commonly consumed cereals (67% weightage) such as rice and wheat were taken and 33% weightage was also given to millets such as Bajra, Jowar, Maiz and Ragi.

b Mean values of nutrients from Lentils, Tur dal, Bengal gram, Black gram, Cowpea, Green gram, Peas, Rajmah, Red gram and Soyabean were considered.

c Carotenoid conversion to retinol equivalents.

d Mean values of nutrients from Beetroot, Carrot, Colocasia, Onion, Radish, Tapioca and Yam were considered.

e Mean values of nutrients from Amla, Apple, Banana, Cherries, Grapes, Guava, Jack fruit, Lemon, Lichi, Mango, Melon, Orange, Papaya, Pine apple, Pomegranate, Sapota, Custard apple, Strawberry were considered.

f Good source of bioavailable calcium.

NA = Not available; NR = Not reported

- Low absorption of non-heme iron can be improved by consuming more vitamin C rich foods (Amla, Lemon, Oranges, Guava, etc.) in raw form as much as possible.
- Meat, poultry and liver contains high bio-available heme iron and also increases absorption (meat factor) of non-heme iron (including fish).

Appendix 18

Different dietary fiber fractions in selected Indian foods

Food Group	Food Name	Dietary fiber (g/100g)		
		Total	Insoluble	Soluble
Cereals and millets	Bajra (*Pennisetum typhoideum*)	11.49	9.14	2.34
	Jowar (*Sorghum vulgare*)	10.22	8.49	1.73
	Ragi (*Eleusine coracana*)	11.18	9.51	1.67
	Rice, raw, milled (*Oryza sativa*)	2.81	1.99	0.82
	Wheat, whole (*Triticumaestivum*)	11.23	9.63	1.60
Grain legumes	Bengal gram, whole (*Cicer arietinum*)	25.22	22.70	2.52
	Green gram, whole (*Vigna radiata*)	17.04	14.59	2.44
	Rajmah, red (*Phaseolus vulgaris*)	16.57	13.86	2.70
	Soya bean, brown (*Glycine max*)	21.55	16.56	5.00
Green leafy vegetables	Amaranth leaves, green (*Amaranthus gangeticus*)	4.41	3.21	1.20
	Colocasia leaves, green (*Colocasia anti-quorum*)	5.60	4.32	1.29
	Drumstick leaves (*Moringa oleifera*)	8.21	6.12	2.10
	Tamarind leaves, tender (*Tamarindus indica*)	10.70	9.34	1.36
Other vegetables	Brinjal (*Solanum melongena*)	3.98	2.84	1.14
	Drumstick (*Moringa oleifera*)	6.83	5.60	1.23
	Ladies finger (*Abelmoschus esculentus*)	4.08	2.80	1.28
Fruits	Apple, big (*Malus sylvestris*)	2.59	1.43	1.16
	Pineapple (*Ananas comosus*)	3.46	2.88	0.59
	Sapota (*Achras sapota*)	9.60	8.46	1.14
Roots and tubers	Carrot, orange (*Dacus carota*)	4.18	2.81	1.37
	Potato, brown skin (*Solanum tuberosum*)	1.71	1.13	0.58
	Tapioca (*Manihot esculenta*)	4.61	3.85	0.76
Condiments and spices	Chillies, red (*Capsicum annum*)	31.15	26.55	4.60
	Fenugreek seeds (*Trigonella foenumgraecum*)	47.55	27.63	19.92
	Pepper, black (*Piper nigrum*)	33.16	30.61	2.54
Nuts and oil seeds	Almond (*Prunus amygdalus*)	13.06	10.55	2.52
	Gingelly seeds, black (*Sesamum indicum*)	17.16	13.57	3.59
	Mustard seeds (*Brassica nigra*)	14.10	10.63	3.47
Mushrooms	Buttom mushroom, fresh (*Agaricus* sp.)	3.11	2.76	0.35
	Shiitake mushroom, fresh (*Lentinula* sp.)	3.02	2.03	0.99
	Oyster mushroom, dried (*Pleurotus* sp.)	39.12	35.64	3.48

Source: Indian Food Composition Tables (www.ifct2017.com)

Index

A

D

E

F

G

H

I

J

K

L

M

N

O

P

Q

R

S

T

U

V

W

X

Y